COMPREHENSIVE FACIAL REJUVENATION

A PRACTICAL AND SYSTEMATIC GUIDE TO SURGICAL MANAGEMENT OF THE AGING FACE

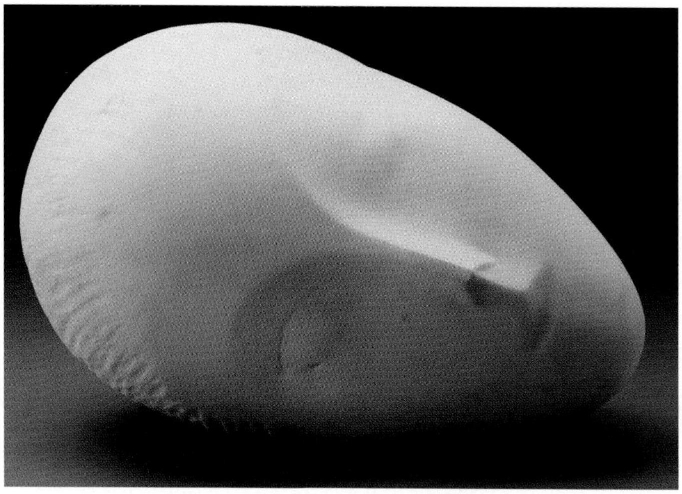

per aspera ad astra

COMPREHENSIVE FACIAL REJUVENATION

A PRACTICAL AND SYSTEMATIC GUIDE TO SURGICAL MANAGEMENT OF THE AGING FACE

EDWIN F. WILLIAMS III, M.D.

Associate Clinical Professor
Albany Medical College
Albany, New York
Medical Director
Williams Center for Facial Plastic Surgery
Latham, New York

SAMUEL M. LAM, M.D.

Medical Director
Lam Facial Plastic Surgery Center
Director
Willow Bend Wellness Institute
Plano, Texas

Illustrations by Samuel M. Lam, M.D.

LIPPINCOTT WILLIAMS & WILKINS
A **Wolters Kluwer** Company
Philadelphia • Baltimore • New York • London
Buenos Aires • Hong Kong • Sydney • Tokyo

Acquisitions Editor: Jim Merritt
Developmental Editor: Alyson Forbes
Production Editor: Karina Mikhli
Manufacturing Manager: Benjamin Rivera
Cover Designer: Vina Lam
Compositor: Maryland Composition
Printer: Walsworth

530 Walnut Street
Philadelphia, PA 19106 USA
LWW.com

Printed in the USA

Library of Congress Cataloging-in-Publication Data
Williams, Edwin F.
Comprehensive facial rejuvenation : a practical and systematic guide to surgical management of the aging face / Edwin F. Williams, Samuel M. Lam ; all illustrations by Samuel M. Lam.
p. ; cm.
Includes bibliographical references and index.
ISBN 0-7817-5093-8
1. Facelift. 2. Face—Surgery. 3. Surgery, Plastic. I. Lam, Samuel M. II. Title.
[DNLM: 1. Face—surgery. 2. Reconstructive Surgical Procedures—methods. 3. Practice Management, Medical. 4. Surgery, Plastic—organization & administration. WE 705 W722c 2003]
RD119.5.F33W556 2003
617.5′20592—dc22

2003058812

---

10 9 8 7 6 5 4 3 2 1

To my father who has inspired everything I do; and
to my mother who has nurtured and supported me throughout.
SML

To my professors who have taught me so much;
to my residents and fellows who continue to teach me;
to my dear wife Cherie who remains my constant support; and
to my children, Katie, Riley, Lydia, and Evan who fill my days with joy.
EFW

CONTENTS

DVD VIDEOS

Disc One

Chapter 4. Upper and Midfacial Rejuvenation

- Transconjunctival Lower-Lid Blepharoplasty
- Skin-Muscle Flap Lower-Lid Blepharoplasty with Midface Extension
- Upper-Lid Blepharoplasty
- Minimal Incision Brow and Midface Lift

Chapter 5. Lower Facial Rejuvenation

- Chin Augmentation with Gore-Tex Alloplast
- Primary Facelift
- Secondary Facelift with Gore-Tex Sling

Chapter 6. Hair Restoration

- Follicular Transfer Hair Transplantation Session
- Scalp Reduction Sessions

Disc Two

Chapter 7. Rejuvenation of the Aging Nose

- Rhinophyma

Chapter 8. Adjunctive Procedures for Rejuvenation

- Alloderm Lip Augmentation
- Collagen Injection Sequence (Lips and Nasolabial Folds)
- Botox Reconstitution and Injection Sequence (Zones I, II, IIIA, B, C)

Chapter 9. Cutaneous Rejuvenation

- Full-Face Jessner's/35% Trichloroacetic Acid Peel
- Carbon Dioxide Laser Resurfacing
- Combined Resurfacing Technique for Acne Scarring (Wire-Brush Dermabrasion/Chemical Peel/Carbon-Dioxide Laser Resurfacing)
- Postoperative Care of the Chemical Peel Patient (Including Cosmetic Camouflage Session)

FOREWORD

Comprehensive Facial Rejuvenation: A Practical and Systematic Guide to Surgical Management of the Aging Face encompasses not only surgical procedures but also practice management procedures including business plans, staff leadership, marketing, aesthetic skin care, and more. This information, which is so important to the novice surgeon, is presented in a practical and balanced manner. The authors discuss effective strategies for patient care, such as recommendations on patient communication, preoperative imaging, and office forms. These initial chapters succinctly present key issues facing the young surgeon beginning a practice, and also provide useful insights for more experienced practitioners; they are highly recommended for all surgeons interested in improving their facial plastic surgery practice. The section on surgical procedures presents current techniques of facial rejuvenation in a clear, practical, and organized manner. Surgeons unfamiliar with any of the procedures will find essential information on preoperative evaluation, operative management, and postoperative care. In addition to upper and lower facial rejuvenation, the authors discuss rhinoplasty of the aging nose and hair restoration.

The authors recognize that most patients seeking facial rejuvenation prefer nonsurgical options when possible. Adjunctive procedures such as soft tissue fillers or botox, and cutaneous rejuvenation with both ablative and nonablative resurfacing techniques are thoroughly discussed. Although technology in this area changes rapidly, the comprehensive approach recommended remains useful.

Facial plastic surgery is both an art and a craft: procedures and techniques are visual and difficult to translate into words. The two supplemental DVD videos complement the text and demonstrate key procedures well. The primary authors and their contributors are to be congratulated for developing this unique, high-quality, multimedia resource. *Comprehensive Facial Rejuvenation* will be a welcome addition to the bookshelves of all facial plastic surgeons.

Wayne F. Larrabee, M.D.
Director
The Larrabee Center for Facial Plastic Surgery
Seattle, Washington

ACKNOWLEDGMENTS

The authors would like to thank the numerous individuals whose invaluable assistance has made this project a reality. Dr. Edward Buckingham provided immeasurable help in manuscript preparation for Chapters 2 and 3, as well as contributing significantly to principal photography and videography. Cassie Audette has worked tirelessly behind the scenes to ensure that every minor and major task related to this project was completed successfully. Brian Hempstead offered his insight and resources to complete the medical management for hair-loss section of this book; his advice helped to ensure that only up-to-date, unbiased, scientifically-based information was presented. Sandy Lasher and Kathy Bergeron helped compile all the requisite patient-care forms, instrument and suture lists, and other related documents. Lori Daggett and Myong Chong offered their extensive experience and knowledge about basic skin care that has been incorporated into Chapter 9. Susan Sullivan provided her expertise with management of the postresurfacing patient and kindly allowed herself to be filmed for the daily encounters she had with the patient in the postoperative setting. Vina Lam, Carol Lam, and Isabell Rossignol reviewed Chapter 2 and provided their unique insight and criticism to website design, business strategy, and marketing strategy, respectively. Dr. Thomas Takoudes was instrumental in the initial phases of project development by interceding on my behalf with the current publisher and convincing them that this project would have a broad readership. Dr. Steven Dayan gave a very helpful perspective on the marketing strategies that have worked well in his clinical practice. All of Dr. Williams' staff was diligent in their help to complete this project, and the authors would like to apologize if they have overlooked anyone that contributed in any way.

COMPREHENSIVE FACIAL REJUVENATION

A PRACTICAL AND SYSTEMATIC GUIDE TO SURGICAL MANAGEMENT OF THE AGING FACE

1

INTRODUCTION

SAMUEL M. LAM
EDWIN F. WILLIAMS III

The past decade has witnessed a revolution in facial plastic surgery, particularly in the management of the aging face. In the past, the facelift represented the principal method of facial rejuvenation, which could only serve to restore the lower third of the face. The traditional browlift that addresses the upper third of the face involved a wide coronal incision that left patients with protracted or permanent scalp anesthesia, lingering edema, potential alopecia, and occasionally unsightly scarring. The midface was uncharted terrain until recently. Techniques now have evolved to provide global rejuvenation of the face without an extended healing period. This book outlines the latest surgical strategies that exist to rejuvenate the face. Although many advances in surgical techniques have proven their efficacy over time, other novel approaches that have failed to withstand the test of time have been abandoned. The surgical techniques that are covered in this book are not untested methods but reflect the extensive clinical experience that has validated the procedures described herein.

Incisional-based surgery only constitutes one strategy for facial rejuvenation today. The surgeon need not brandish the scalpel as the only weapon in the fight against aging. Cutaneous resurfacing is integral to facial restoration for those patients who require this form of intervention either in combination or apart from incisional surgery. Chemical exfoliation represents the oldest method of skin resurfacing and has regained popularity; the luster of laser therapy has been tarnished somewhat by the accompanying lengthy erythema and recovery time. Nevertheless, carbon dioxide (CO_2) laser resurfacing still has its role in the treatment of more recalcitrant rhytids, particularly in the perioral region. Mechanical dermabrasion also exhibits unique properties that make it effective in certain circumstances, such as deep acne scarring or post–scar revision management. This book covers the different treatment modalities separately—laser, chemical, and mechanical—and then addresses how to combine these techniques effectively in the apposite setting. Recently, the new technology of nonablative resurfacing has arisen as an alternative method to efface mild to moderate rhytidosis; and the results of research that the authors have conducted reveal remarkable histologic improvement. The chapter endeavors to guide the reader in the selection of a suitable candidate who will benefit from nonablative laser or light therapy. The topic of basic skin care is reviewed at the conclusion of this chapter; every cosmetic surgeon should have at least a rudimentary knowledge of this subject so that he or she can reasonably respond to patients' queries. Also, safe and effective skin care is a fundamental concern in the postresurfacing period, and the physician should be able to navigate the patient through this often-trying time.

Myriad adjunctive procedures, including paralytic agents and soft-tissue fillers, have been introduced over the past decade that offer a wider range of options for facial rejuvenation. The savvy consumer, bombarded on all fronts by the Internet and other media propaganda, must determine the best rejuvenative option in a smorgasbord of choices. The fast-paced life of workaday America has placed an ever-increasing premium on minimal downtime and less invasive surgery. Quick fixes are the norm, and prolonged recovery is not tolerated. Patients are seeking incremental treatments to ward off ineluctable aging at an earlier age. Botulinum toxin and collagen offer the younger and older patient effective treatment without any notable downtime. In addition, permanent soft-tissue fillers, such as acellular dermis and expanded polytetrafluoroethylene, have entered the market to provide more enduring soft-tissue augmentation. This book details not only how to execute every step of these procedures, but also how to select the right patient for a particular modality.

True to its title, the covered topics are comprehensive in scope, including hair restoration surgery and rhinoplasty of the aging nose. The hair-restoration chapter not only discusses the technique of follicular grafting in detail, but also elaborates on scalp rotation (the twice-delayed temporoparieto-occipital, or Juri, flap) and reduction (with extender) procedures in the context of when these techniques are appropriate. A thorough review of medical hair management is undertaken as well, with mention of both traditional techniques (e.g., finasteride and minoxidil) and newer, more experimental therapies. The chapter on rejuvenation of the aging nose addresses both functional and aesthetic flaws that typify the aging nose. For instance, a reliable and straightforward method for correction of rhinophyma is presented. The chapter on upper facial rejuvenation also covers another functional disorder, blepharoptosis, which affects the cosmesis of the aging face. Although this book is primarily directed at aesthetic facial surgery, corrective functional surgery is included when appropriate, as enumerated.

Besides in-depth review of surgical techniques for the aging face, this book also covers practice management that may be instructive to both the junior and more seasoned surgeon. Chapter 2 addresses how to develop an effective business strategy and media presence as well as how to select and retain the physician's most valuable asset, the staff. Another chapter is dedicated to the development of an effective strategy for patient care, including how to enlist the services of a patient-care coordinator, use digital imaging effectively, and conduct a rewarding preoperative consultation. The surgeon should always make a concerted effort to develop his or her practice by diligent review of current tactics and creative thinking for future strategies. This book serves as a framework within which the surgeon and office team can build an effective business and marketing plan.

The entire book is structured in a format that the surgeon can readily appreciate: Each chapter is partitioned into preoperative, operative, and postoperative sections. The reader is guided through the pearls and pitfalls of each stage and is trained to think in a logical, systematic fashion: how to decide when a particular surgical procedure is appropriate (preoperative), how to perform the procedure (operative), how to manage the patient after surgery, and how to avoid and handle any complications that might arise (postoperative). This book is not intended as an academic dissertation on arcane matters of facial plastic surgery but as a strictly practical manual that will benefit both the novice and more experienced surgeon who is unfamiliar with any of the many procedures enumerated in the text. In accordance with the objective for relaying as much useful information as possible, the principal chapters also contain a detailed list of all surgical instrumentation and equipment necessary to perform a procedure; a review of all the salient technical points that are described within the body of the text; and full copies of all patient instructions, both preoperative and postoperative.

Besides step-by-step photography; informative, computer-rendered illustrations; and lucid text, the authors realize that the amount of practical knowledge that can be conveyed in a book format is limited. Therefore, this project is as much a video manual as it is a printed textbook. Two high-quality double-density DVDs have been included that illuminate each procedure in detail. Being surgeons, the authors realize that text and photographs alone cannot present the amount of information that even a short video can. The video sequences inform the reader about every conceivable aspect of surgery: how to reconstitute and use botulinum toxin properly, what instrumentation is required for hair transplantation, how to inject collagen correctly, how to perform a scalp reduction, how to perform a trichloroacetic acid (TCA) peel, and how to manage that patient during the intensive 10-day postoperative period, and numerous other videos. The total video length included totals 6 hours and covers all the major aspects in this book.

The authors sincerely hope that this book and video project will serve as a foundation within which the reader will be comfortable in undertaking the procedures delineated herein. The reader who has sought a career in aesthetic facial surgery should be rewarded with a lifetime of fulfillment in making people look and feel better about themselves.

2

DEVELOPMENT OF AN EFFECTIVE PRACTICE

EDWARD D. BUCKINGHAM
SAMUEL M. LAM
EDWIN F. WILLIAMS III

True to the aim of this book, this chapter strives to offer the reader a practical and informative guide that reflects the 10-year experience of a busy facial plastic surgical practice. Often medical texts neglect the very important aspect of practice management, partly because of the limitations of scope and ambition, and partly because of the lack of authoritative information on the subject. After completion of years of professional training, many physicians find themselves ill equipped to handle the exigencies of daily business affairs that are integral to a medical or surgical practice, and thereby fail to succeed. Constant and ongoing ambition to achieve excellence in business and marketing should be a fundamental part of every plastic surgical practice. Unlike other sectors of medical care, plastic surgery caters exclusively to an elective patient base that can easily go elsewhere for their care if every nuance of the practice has not been properly managed. In this endeavor, the surgeon should also not overstep his or her budgetary limitations in the short-sighted effort to attract patients without the long-term foresight for continued financial viability. Although certain sections of this chapter are targeted at the junior surgeon, the practical advice contained herein should benefit even the seasoned veteran. A flourishing plastic surgical practice demands constant nurturing through resourceful and informed business and marketing tactics. This chapter addresses the following topics: starting a practice, developing and maintaining an effective business strategy, hiring and retaining a first-rate office staff, designing a successful marketing plan, and integrating profitable aesthetic skin care services into the practice.

DEVELOPING AND MAINTAINING AN EFFECTIVE BUSINESS STRATEGY

Starting a Practice

The old real estate adage "location, location, location" should be well heeded by the plastic surgeon embarking on a new career, because it applies to both the physical address of the practice as well as to the greater metropolitan or suburban landscape that surrounds that site. The first task is selection of a city or town that can support the practice of a new plastic surgeon. Research should endeavor to determine two key factors: the characteristics of the population and the present market penetration. No substantive documentation exists to answer the question of how large a population is required to support the practice of a plastic surgeon who is interested in building an aesthetic practice, but an estimate falls in the order of 200,000 to 250,000. Other features of the population that should carry weight are the relative age of the population, affluence, and local acceptance of cosmetic surgery. The age of the population serves as a more important factor for a plastic surgeon who endeavors to only practice facial cosmetic surgery, because a large part of the practice often may be dedicated to rejuvenative procedures for the more mature individual (unless the practice is geared more toward rhinoplasty, which has a broader age appeal). Likewise, if the facial plastic surgeon pursues reconstructive aspects of the face (excluding trauma) for both skin and soft-tissue tumors of the head-and-neck region, then an older patient profile is more likely to receive these services. The plastic surgeon who performs body surgery may have a younger patient base, particularly because of the demand for augmentation mammoplasty that is currently in vogue. The existing market penetration of plastic surgeons may be more difficult to assess. Often the number of plastic surgeons in an area may not be the single most important factor to dissuade a prospective surgeon from entering that market. If the surgeon should elect to perform facial surgery alone, then he or she should ascertain how many other plastic surgeons in the area have really dedicated themselves to promotion of facial cosmetic surgery. In addition, a well-established group of plastic surgeons with a sizable, collective budget may pose a more tangible threat to the junior plastic surgeon, who may be restricted in financial and marketing options.

After the city has been selected, the surgeon must decide on the particular part of town that will best suit his or her new practice. The location of the office need not be in the most upscale area, in which real estate prices may come at an unreachable premium; instead, a compromise should be struck between an expensive site and a more affordable location so that some finances can be reserved to outfit a capacious and well-decorated interior space. If a partnership is arranged with a sponsoring hospital or physician group, the office location may be partially or wholly dictated by that organization. They may require rental of office space within their building as part of the financial arrangement. Selecting an office location nearby the surgical suite affords an easier commute between the two locales when shuttling between office visits and operative cases. Although the office need not be in a high traffic area, visibility from passing commuters provides increased recognition and recall of the practice as well as the surgeon's name. Another key feature of a good office location is accessibility: a convenient location (short travel time), easy parking, and a relatively straightforward path from the outside lot to the interior office space. Any of these physical encumbrances could unfavorably detract from return patient visits or future physician referrals.

Acquiring Capital

As part of a location search, the new surgeon should seek local health care institutions regarding their willingness to aid in the acquisition of capital. Specifically, marketing or medical directors may be in a position to assist in the capital outlay for a new office with the understanding that the new physician will generate revenue for that institution through operative cases and hospital admissions. Open dialog with a hospital director about his or her interest in this type of reciprocity also may reveal insight into the need for a plastic surgeon in that area, and thereby guide the decision about a suitable practice location. Having another institution carry some of the financial burden of initial setup costs distributes part of the substantial risk to which a starting physician is subjected. In general, financial institutions as sources of capital should be avoided if possible. Bank loans require personal guarantees and immediate monthly repayment, which can add to an already negative cash flow. Even if immediate payments are not required, interest begins to accrue, being capitalized, and thereby adds to the principle balance of the loan as well as the overall debt and eventual cash outflow.

The federal government outlines very specific rules and regulations regarding the appropriate relationship between hospitals, communities, or health care delivery organizations and physicians. These rules prohibit the use of certain types of loans, income guarantees, and other financial incentive agreements between the institution and physician unless certain criteria are met; these usually are related to an underserved population by a particular specialty. Contracts can be written to fulfill these criteria, and hospitals should be familiar with what is deemed acceptable. As mentioned, hospitals or similar health care institutions enter into an arrangement with a physician only if that physician's presence will serve the financial interest of that institution. Therefore, special favors are not to be expected: Only a mutual financial benefit for the institution and physician alike determines the likelihood that a workable contract can be attained. The physician should be ready to draft a business plan that projects the budgeted income and expenses for anywhere from a 3- to 12-month period. Accordingly, the physician should approach the institution with the amount of financial assistance he or she requires. The projected figure is often a challenging proposition, because it depends on the estimated payer mix of Medicaid, Medicare, private insurance, and cosmetic fee-for-service. The starting surgeon should expect that the majority of his or her practice will be derived from insurance-based income until a cosmetic referral basis arises. Insurance referral patterns can also be quite entrenched and established ties, difficult to break. Three to six months of operating capital is required before any significant receivables begin to be collected, and this time allotment needs to be built into the budget. Even if income generated from insurance payments begin to accrue from the first day of practice, a delay of 3 to 4 months should be expected from the time of billing to actual receipt of payment.

Once a potential source of capital has been identified—preferably a hospital or physician group rather than a financial institution—the newly established physician should try to rely on that institution's accounting services. Hiring an accountant may be an expensive option; also, that individual may not have the extensive medical experience of his or her counterpart in the hospital's employ. Besides a detailed pro forma that estimates the long-term income and expenses, the physician and institution should arrange a method of repayment, including an interest-free loan period (18 months is a reasonable time frame), graduated repayment, and periods of free rent. These concessions should be recouped easily by the interest that the institutions are levying as well as the income that the new physician will generate in terms of hospital admissions and operative cases.

Initial Office Space

The tendency to acquire too little space is a common mistake but must be balanced against the cost of the space. In most communities, around 2,500 sq ft is sufficient as long as that space is properly allocated. In general, storage and closet space usually are underestimated and should be accounted for when proportioning space. The physician's private office should not assume an unreasonable size because it is a non–revenue-generating room. Instead, office space should be outfitted to impress the patient who is seeking services for the first time: Space and resources should be allocated primarily to the reception area and consultation rooms. Generally speaking, the office requires a reception area, a front desk, consultation rooms, examination rooms, physician-and-nursing charting areas, and a procedure room. A discrete rear entrance should be designed to permit inconspicuous entry and exits for the physician and staff as well as for bandaged and swollen postoperative patients, who may alarm prospective patients and deserve added privacy. The entrance should be designed to fit a standard-size stretcher if an emergency should arise. Two-to-three examination rooms should be adequate in number, and each room should measure approximately 8 × 10 feet as a guideline. A medical (or dental) chair should be situated in each room with the capacity for electrically controlled elevation but without an external light source, automated recline, or other advanced features that can add to the cost unnecessarily. An attractive cost-saving option is the use of a vinyl-covered recliner for one postoperative examination room rather than a formal medical-grade chair. Frugality in all aspects of office design is imperative for the starting physician but should be tempered with judicious taste to maintain the proper image befitting a plastic surgical practice. "Perception is reality" should be the modus operandi. A patient often judges the potential quality of surgical services based on the overall appearance of the office suite.

Each examination room should be equipped with ample cabinet space to house all necessary patient care items. The physician and staff can then manage all postoperative care without having to leave the room. A countertop with a sink should be installed in each examination room and ideally should accommodate a hidden trash receptacle that can be concealed from view and minimize use of valuable floor space. One examination room can be designed slightly larger, at 10 × 12 feet, to permit a photography lane, thereby eliminating a dedicated photography room when space is at a premium. A minimum of one consultation room that is styled with decorum adds considerably to the ambiance and should provide a nonmedical, intimate feel. Accordingly, the size requirement for this room can be less than a standard examination room: approximately 8 × 8 feet or 8 × 10 feet generally is sufficient to foster a more personal but still maneuverable environment.

A larger procedure room measuring a minimum of 14 × 18 feet is a necessity. Many procedures can be undertaken in an office setting with local anesthesia, intravenous medication, or conscious sedation at a substantial cost savings to the practice and patient. The limits of office surgery are determined by the willingness of the surgeon to perform the procedure and the patient to tolerate it. Keep the patient's comfort ultimately in mind, because most referrals are derived from prior patients who have been satisfied with both the surgical result and the treatment they received before and after surgery. The procedure room should be fitted with an adjustable chair, overhead operative lighting, and a countertop and cabinet storage space for all necessary equipment, including a small autoclave. At this time, office-based surgery does not require any accreditation by a governing agency, but future legal restrictions on office surgery are an imminent prospect. Several legitimate agencies offer accreditation, including the Joint Commission on Accreditation of Healthcare Organizations (JCAHO) and the Accreditation Association for Ambulatory Health Care (AAAHC)*. Medicare approval for the surgical facility is both cost prohibitive and unnecessary unless the surgeon desires to obtain a facility fee for operative cases and is often only profitable if the individual is considering running a multisurgeon, dedicated, outpatient surgical facility. The surgeon is advised to consider the benefits of accreditation (e.g., prestige, safety, and future compliance) and at least review the guidelines so that basic compliance can be assured to avoid expensive retrofitting if accreditation is sought at a later date.

When leasing office space, the cost often includes only the amount for basic "fit-up" or "white-box finish out." Therefore, the physician has to expend an additional amount to complete the interior space to his or her desired specifications. Because all of these leasehold improvements are fixed entities (ceiling-mounted lighting, window blinds, carpeting, etc.), it is imperative that the contract outlines whether the added value that the physician inputs ultimately belongs to the building owner or tenant. In addition to these fixed properties, capital should be outlaid for movable furniture and equipment. Often additional costs for leasehold improvements can be included in the lease, for example, by increasing the payment from $18/sq ft to $22/sq ft. This arrangement avoids payment for additional improvements at the outset. Most contracts request a 5-year lease. When negotiating this contract, one should consider the option for an additional 5- to 10-year term following execution of the original lease. Often, the cost for this additional time may be less than the original if cost of leasehold improvements were already included. However, if they were not, then costs may be higher depending on the market value of the property. The option does not bind the lessee to remain in the space after the expiration of the original lease period but gives him or her the first right of refusal. If the option to extend cannot be arranged with the original lease, then the physician should proceed with lease renewal at least 1 year in advance to allow sufficient time to relocate if the new terms are deemed unfavorable.

Staff and Salaries

Physicians often place an undue emphasis on the importance of the office manager in the success of a fledgling practice. The physician may function effectively as the manager until this duty encroaches on his or her time and effort. The first employee for hire should be an individual who is flexi-

*JCAHO can be reached at *www.jcaho.org* or 630-792-5259 (Ambulatory Care Program), One Renaissance Boulevard, Oakbrook Terrace, IL 60181. AAAHC can be reached at *www.aaahc.org* or 847-853-6060, 3201 Old Glenview Road, Suite 300, Wilmette, IL 60091-2992.

ble in his or her capacity in that he or she is willing to play many roles, including answering phones, removing sutures, and disposing of waste. That individual should express sincere interest in the success of the practice and be motivated to support its growth rather than assume merely a mechanical role of carrying out assigned responsibilities. Incidentally, the physician also must be willing to assist in even the most menial tasks, because a full complement of office personnel may be lacking at first. Operating-room technicians are an excellent source of potential hires. The specifics of how to find and retain employees is discussed in a later section.

The second person to hire is a front-desk receptionist: This staff member should be present only on a part-time basis when the physician or assistant is occupied with other affairs, for example, during an operative case or with a busy office visit schedule. Part-time assistance eliminates the need to offer health benefits, vacation time, and so on. Nevertheless, the quality of every staff member cannot be overemphasized. The individual who answers the phone may have the most significant impact on whether a patient ultimately decides to book a consultation visit based on that staff member's knowledge, attitude, and salesmanship. Training the staff is a fundamental responsibility of the principal physician if success is to be achieved. Personnel who have been accustomed to working in a non–elective care environment may not be service-oriented and should be reeducated on the value of patient rapport (e.g., answering phone calls promptly, not permitting long hold times, etc.). Ideally, the physician should instruct by example and serve as the model of proper etiquette with patients. With regard to employee salaries and benefits, the county medical society is an excellent resource for this information and the new physician is encouraged to become a member. The local medical society is able to provide details about normative values for salaries, expected benefits, and allotted vacation time. Additionally, often employee health insurance can be obtained for a reasonable rate through the county or state medical society.

Practice Organization

The options for legal organization of a practice vary from state to state. A business attorney should be consulted to learn about the rules in a particular area. Additionally, the state medical society is a valuable resource. In general, the types of business organizations include sole proprietorship, partnerships, and corporations. The advantage of a corporation is that it offers some protection for the shareholders; that is, the physician, from personal general liability. Unfortunately, it does not shield one from financial liability because any source of capital requires the physician's personal guarantee. However, it protects the physician from personal financial crisis if an unforeseen catastrophe should occur in which the physician has not played a direct role in the adverse event; for example, if a patient elects to commit suicide on the premises by leaping out of a window. If one is a sole practitioner, it may be unnecessary to form a more elaborate business organization than simple registration with the county. However, if one takes a partner into the practice, then a formal partnership or limited liability corporation may help establish guidelines for this arrangement. Again, consultation with an attorney can ensure that the correct avenue is pursued. Alternatively, an accountant can offer valuable advice and provide a different perspective than an attorney.

Hospital Privileges and Office-Based Surgery

If a physician is targeting his or her practice toward cosmetic surgery, then most of the surgical procedures may be performed in an ambulatory surgical facility. Developing an office with a self-contained fully accredited surgical facility is a lofty but attainable goal. However, initially this ambition may prove to be a taxing emotional and financial liability. This objective is better set aside as a long-term goal after a busy practice has been established. Many procedures can be performed in the office setting at a reduced cost to the practice and patient. Smaller procedures (e.g., eyelid surgery) can be undertaken without an exorbitant setup cost; however, lengthier procedures (e.g., facelift and browlift) mandate a higher expense to outfit the office properly for safety and sedation. Accordingly, shorter procedures can be undertaken in the office setting, and longer surgeries may be reserved for an ambulatory surgery center until it becomes financially affordable to build one's own facility. However, facility fees extracted from an ambulatory surgery center can prove to constitute a significant portion of the total cost to the patient and thereby motivate a physician to construct his or her own surgical facility when the volume of cases justifies this action.

Hospital privileges should be obtained for multiple facilities and surgery performed in those facilities for reasons that are explained in the following. Albeit not currently legally mandated, laws eventually may require a physician to maintain hospital privileges for procedures in order to be authorized to perform those procedures in an office-based setting. Once hospital privileges have been acquired in one facility, gaining privileges elsewhere is facilitated. Occasionally, a patient may require an overnight hospital stay, and maintaining privileges at a nearby facility with an overnight capacity is vital. A comorbid patient may be better serviced regarding anesthesia in a hospital setting, where emergency care is readily available. Also, patients may request that surgery be performed in a certain facility for personal preference.

Once hospital privileges are secured, the physician should approach the emergency room, which can serve as a valuable base for patient referrals, to offer his or her services for any trauma that might enter. Assuming trauma call at the hospital can be an important way to build a practice. Each laceration that is repaired may provide several patients for referral. Name recognition stands as the most important reason to acquire privileges at multiple facilities and frequent those facilities on a regular basis. Being on the operating-room schedule, the surgeon can be afforded one opportunity to disseminate his or her name to the medical community. Proper attire and behavior should always be observed in the hospital setting, as the medical staff can serve as an invaluable referral basis.

Office Purchases

The decision whether to purchase or lease office equipment must be based on the particular article and the budgetary constraints of the practice. An accountant can offer sound advice as to which avenue is most suited to a physician's needs. Different accounting rules apply to leasing expense versus depreciation expense and vary based on the anticipated life of the equipment. Therefore, not only does the initial cost of the equipment and its potential revenue play into the decision but also how the accounting will affect the bottom line of the income statement and taxable income. A general rule of thumb to consider is that any piece of durable equipment with a serviceable life greater than 5 years should be purchased, whereas equipment with a shorter life span should be leased. Of course this rule is not universally applicable, and other factors should be taken into consideration.

Some specific items will be discussed to clarify the preceding recommendations. Desktop computer hardware and software should be purchased. Although the computer industry continues to evolve rapidly, computers have become very reasonably priced and usually survive in excess of 5 years with proper maintenance and software upgrades. In addition, some manufacturers offer hardware upgrade options to keep a computer system current. Lasers for the practice are very expensive acquisitions and need to be justified before purchase. A laser device is never as productive per unit time financially as a scalpel in a surgeon's hand, unless the staff has been trained to operate the laser. However, this latter option may expose a surgeon to excessive liability, especially if the staff is inexperienced with laser use. Therefore, do not consider a laser as a substitute for surgery. If a laser is purchased, it is advisable to calculate the number of procedures that need to be performed to pay it off, preferably within 2 to 3 years. If this goal cannot be accomplished, then the transaction is a questionable profit-making endeavor. Laser technology is rapidly evolving; therefore, one should beware of the life span of a particular laser and its projected future utility. Additionally, many lasers require frequent maintenance that can add considerably to their cost and that should be budgeted. It takes a creative surgeon to make a laser profitable; a portion of the practice needs to be structured and marketed to support its use. Regarding software purchases, combined software for office management, including scheduling, billing, accounting, marketing analysis, and so on is very expensive and is not required initially, if ever. Billing is discussed later, but other cash outlays are more important at the outset. For example, imaging software is a recommended early purchase. Patients often need to be convinced that a particular surgical endeavor is a worthwhile venture, and digital morphing software affords the surgeon a more precise method of communication.** As the practice develops, preoperative and postoperative images of former patients become available to inform prospective patients of envisioned surgical results, but initially this option may not be available.

Leadership and Effective Staff Management

A trip to the local bookstore to inquire about resources for managing a business will yield scores of results but only few that are fruitful or cogent. Every decade new ideas and concepts emerge describing the recent trends for successful management strategies. Although the practice of tyrannical management has thankfully passed, the latest quick-fix methodologies may not offer the best solution to effective managerial supervision. In fact, the dynamics of a medical practice differ markedly from the typical business or corporate model. In very few business settings is the Chief Executive Officer or President of the Board the sole revenue generator, as the physician is in a medical practice. Although an omnipotent mantle may be easily assumed, the physician should exhibit restraint in this regard because of the devastating consequences on employee morale and motivation. It has been wisely stated that one joins a *company* but leaves a *manager.* At the helm of the ship, the physician must exercise judicious leadership skills to help shape the work of his or her employees through example and instructive remarks. The hallmark of good leadership is "emotional intelligence," in which the captain senses the emotional disposition of the team at a given moment and responds to that situation accordingly. Some concrete examples of this leadership skill are elaborated to illustrate this concept more fully.

In an ideal practice, the surgeon should be busy operating on surgical cases with delegation of other duties to his or her staff. Because operative cases are the prime source of income, all staff efforts should be channeled to this ultimate goal. Proper physician–staff rapport facilitates the attainment of this objective, and the following recommendations can help ensure that a physician achieves this aim. It is imperative that the physician treats his or her staff in a manner that encourages them to desire excellence and to contribute in a material way to the practice rather than mechanically

**The next chapter discusses in detail exactly how and when digital-imaging technology should be effectively employed, including how to discuss its limitations and how to minimize potential liablility.

biding their time as hourly employees. An employee must share in the excitement for growth potential and be rewarded accordingly. Financial incentives may be the most direct method to stimulate employee motivation, but the caliber of the staff should be such that they seek opportunities to build the practice through desire derived from within rather than from a *quid pro quo* monetary exchange. One can *inspire* another person to excel, but rarely can one *motivate* another to act. If someone is work adverse, then no amount of training will change that inert character. Choosing the right person (then treating that person well) may be the most fundamental aspect to success.

Employee turnover is a good measure of an employer's managerial success. High turnover suggests that a managerial flaw may be undermining staff satisfaction. Rather than discount one's own managerial failure, one should instead dwell on those leadership attributes that may be interfering with proper staff contentment. Employees must be regarded as the most valuable assets and should be treated accordingly. Loss of an employee translates into an incalculable injury to the practice in terms of time to locate another qualified individual and time to retrain that person from scratch. The erosion of staff morale and loss of patient-care continuity are other factors affected by an employee's departure. Although the physician must remain the leader of the team, he or she should not micromanage the daily affairs of the practice. Micromanaging is construed as distrust for the staff's capabilities and prohibits an individual's talent to flourish; it can also prove to be an immense burden on a physician's valuable time and energy. Permitting a staff member to fail, on a small scale, encourages that individual to learn from that mistake and mature from the misadventure. The physician's character should stand above repute. He or she should exercise a certain sangfroid in adverse situations and be equitable in the treatment of all employees. Quick and irrational temper is a sign of poor leadership that ruins employee morale and decimates the staff. Negative comments about other staff members should not be tolerated, because gossip can fester like a cancer on the unanimity of the work team. Respecting an employee's feelings and opinions is a prerequisite to a healthy working relationship. Understanding a person's needs outside of the office and accommodating those needs indicate a fundamental respect for that individual as a whole person rather than just as a functioning employee. If an employee needs to transport his or her children from school early, then the physician should permit earlier arrival to compensate for that lost time. If the employee has trouble arriving punctually in the morning, then the physician should not assign duties that require an early presence, but instead ask that the staff member be available to perform services later in the day when others may need to leave. Rather than dwell on the weaknesses of an individual, the leader should strive to identify personal strengths and capitalize on those attributes. Respect of an employee's time should be a top priority: The physician should complete daily office affairs and operative cases on a timely basis and employees should be permitted to leave at a regularly scheduled time. The physician always should be mindful that an employee has a personal life after work and should honor that time with dependable, predetermined closing times. Respect of employee time also entails appointed rest breaks during the workday. Rotating a schedule of breaks and lunches permits a continuous circle of care while affording a much-needed respite in a hectic day. The physician always should support a staff member despite a patient's protestations to the contrary. Manipulative patients attempt to drive a wedge between the physician and staff member by commenting on the inadequacies of physical skill or personality of the staff. The physician should not be tempted to side with the patient. The physician should remain supportive of the staff member while attempting to address the patient's needs. In summary, loyalty to one's staff will be repaid in a commensurate fashion, and respect for their valuable presence at every level will likewise be returned in contentment and dedication.

Billing Services

Billing services should include everything involved in the generation of fees and collection of receivables. The process encompasses negotiating contracts with insurance companies, coding, assigning fees, billing, collecting, and tracking all of the data. Three approaches may be used to address billing: (a) hiring an employee and purchasing billing software; (b) hiring an employee or assigning the task to an existing employee to enter the data into the system and then recruit an outside billing agency to process the claim; or (c) contracting an outside billing service to perform all of the services.

Many offices consider internal billing the preferred route because of cost effectiveness and better control over when services are billed and how account receivables are collected. From experience, internal billing may be justifiable if several physicians work in a practice to maintain a capable billing staff. Clearly, filing insurance-based claims is the type of payment that is discussed herein, as it requires the level of sophistication absent in the more straightforward task of cash collection for elective services. For a smaller outfit (for example, a single physician office), a dedicated, full-time individual or staff may not be warranted for several reasons. In most market environments, numerous insurance carriers compete; and each year and each time a new carrier enters the market a new or renewed contract must be negotiated. An outside billing service has ongoing relationships with these insurance carriers so that they will be in a better position to negotiate contracts on behalf of their physician clients and maintain current knowledge about companies' contracts and negotiating practices. In a small office, billing duties that are assigned to one individual also may be detrimental, as it creates a situation in which one employee becomes indispensable who can then demand salary or benefit increases with undue leverage. Additionally, this person needs to be monitored and audited either internally or externally to assure that all services are being billed, collected, and, if not collected, followed up. The rationale that internal billing is more cost effective may be offset by the cost of additional office space, the maintenance and cleaning of that space, and the taxes and benefits accrued by the added employee.

The advantages of an outside billing service are manifold. The billing service is experienced with bill payments on a large scale and therefore tends to be more up to date on all of the new coding rules and contract variations with insurance carriers. The billing company, because they do the task regularly, should be experts in contract negotiations and should accomplish this task as well as insuring that the practice is contracted with all the necessary regional payers including filing the necessary paperwork. A good billing company should track what all the carriers will pay and bill out 20% or so above the highest payer: If the billing service asks for less than the amount that the insurance company is willing to pay, the difference will never be recouped.

Research is paramount when selecting a reputable and reliable service. The billing service should be experienced with handling similar specialties that use the same coding and bill payments. After contacting the prospective billing services, one should ask for the physicians who are contracted with them in order to determine their level of satisfaction with the respective billing companies. The fee for a billing service depends on and should be negotiated based on the type of payment mix: The more heavily weighted the practice is on office visits and smaller insurance procedures, the higher the percentage required by the service since a proportionate effort is needed to make collections. An approximate estimate of this charge falls between 3.5% and 7% of collections. As mentioned, cosmetic services do not require an external biller, because obviously these payments do not involve negotiation with a third-party payer. Once a service has been contracted, the physician or trusted office staff should meet with the billing service on a routine basis, at least monthly, to discuss how account receivables are progressing and to ensure that a minimum of outstanding accounts receivables are carried over.

Management of Payables

As the practice becomes busier, it becomes increasingly difficult for the physician to keep track of cash outflow. Accordingly, the physician is tempted to assign the task of check signing over to a member of the office staff. Although the volume of outgoing checks may become unmanageable, the physician should retain responsibility for check signing. By doing so, the physician can keep track of expenditures without burdensome micromanagement of this task. The bookkeeper can attach a copy of the bill to each outgoing check so that the physician can confirm the nature and necessity of each payment. If it becomes necessary to hire or assign payables to an employee, it is imperative to ensure that a check-and-balance system be maintained to prevent large checks from being written without dual signatures, one of which should bear the physician's imprint. Further, cross-verification of smaller payments must be periodically undertaken by an independent person to prevent the temptation of embezzlement.

A system should be established to manage purchases, and records should be maintained for all aspects of purchasing. When an order is placed, that record should be cross-referenced with the actual delivery to ensure completion of the transaction. If items remain outstanding, then the cause of the discrepancy should be pursued until the matter is properly resolved. Ideally, a copy of the original order should be placed with the shipper's inventory, which have been confirmed to be complete, and then placed with a copy of the check or other method of payment and filed as a purchase unit for later reference. This accounting method minimizes any payable errors and maximizes efficiency of financial audits and statement preparation.

Basic Business and Personal Finance

Physicians are notorious for spending whatever income they generate. These bad spending habits are rooted in the delayed gratification that follows a poorly compensated, protracted, and demanding medical education process. By the time the physician finally embarks into practice, a feeling of entitlement arises to justify frivolous purchases: "I've been in school for 12 years. I've earned the right to spend money." In most medical practices, new physicians are hired and offered a guaranteed salary. The potential that future earnings will exceed the present salary is high and the risk is low; therefore, spending comes easily. A similar guarantee does not exist for a plastic surgical practice, because the business takes time to mature and the risk of failure is ever-present and real. Financial institutions contribute to the ease of spending because they often lend money generously to physicians based on earning potential. It is quite easy to become over-leveraged because of this false security. The physician should exercise restraint in personal spending habits as well as professional expenditures. When the business turns profitable, a portion of the gain should be reserved for savings and retirement, with financial reserves available for economic downturns or to cover other unforeseen necessities.

Early on in the practice, a budget must be formulated to determine whether income will exceed expenses, thereby allowing continuation of the practice without further capital infusion. A budget can be developed with the assistance of an accountant or a more experienced colleague. As the practice grows, a budget remains an efficient method for keeping fixed spending on target and assessing how variable expenses are fluctuating with income generation.

HIRING AND MAINTAINING EFFECTIVE OFFICE STAFF

The single greatest investment a physician will ever make is his or her staff who should be treated with appropriate respect if they are to be retained. Some of the key points of staff interaction have been addressed in a previous section but are reiterated and elaborated herein. A successful practice must be able to hire productive personnel, train them effectively, and retain them as employees. Hiring an employee is a significant investment in time and money at every phase, including recruiting, hiring, and training. It is estimated that the loss of one trained employee may be valued at 30% to 100% of that person's salary. The following section details how to find good employees, what positions are needed, and how to maintain their employment.

Hiring Office Staff

When seeking employees, the personality and work ethic of the individual are much more important than the level of training. Although certain services (e.g., medication dispensing) require certification, many positions demand little if any prior training. An employee who exhibits a good work ethic, strives to be an active participant in the operation of the practice, understands its goals, and works hard to achieve them is much more valuable than a highly trained individual who only cares about how little he or she can accomplish in order to obtain a paycheck. Much of this work ethic is internally derived and cannot be taught. However, it remains crucial to foster a healthy work ethic at the office and to rally everyone around this constructive behavior. If a person is a hard worker but appears ill suited to a particular position, the physician should try to identify that individual's strengths and relocate him or her to a more conducive workstation that will allow that talent to flourish rather than dismissing that staff member. A solid work ethic is a rare character trait that should be sought and retained at almost any cost.

When a position becomes available, one should identify what traits are required to fill that post. If that position carries more responsibility, compensation, or prestige, the physician should find an employee in the practice with the talent to move into that position rather that hiring a new person to fill that role. This arrangement communicates that hard work will be rewarded with advancement in the practice rather than that lower positions are stagnant without room for promotion. If no qualified person is available within the keep of the practice or if the position is entry level, then the physician must seek a new employee to fill the post. Classified advertisements are a less trustworthy source of new personnel than networking or word of mouth. The physician is encouraged to retain a list of key individuals who work in larger institutions who may know of qualified individuals seeking employment. A good work ethic, bright smile, pleasant demeanor, and intelligence often supersede level of training.

Several other positions need to be added once a practice begins to grow. The position of dedicated patient care coordinator should be filled near the beginning. This individual needs to possess a mature personality in order to relate to facial cosmetic patients. Because a large percentage of today's facial aesthetic procedures are dedicated to facial rejuvenation (hence, the need for this book) and are aimed primarily at women, a more mature woman is able to convey more empathy and rapport with patients of a similar age than a recent college graduate. At a minimum, the patient care coordinator should be in her late thirties and needs to exude an elegant conservatism in her demeanor and attire. She should be the one who receives all prospective cosmetic phone calls and dedicates time to answer all questions posed and to secure the consultation. The complete role of the patient-care coordinator is discussed in the following chapter.

Once the practice is highly developed and profitable, it may be wise to hire a practice manager, who can serve as the office–staff supervisor as well as marketing director. This individual can also function as a business manager, but the physician is encouraged to retain some if not all responsibility in this sphere in an oversight capacity. The practice manager's responsibilities should include developing a marketing plan and overseeing its execution, as discussed in the forthcoming section. Additionally, this individual should be responsible for the day-to-day management of the staff including hiring new staff. It is also important for this person to remain involved in patient care in order to judge the ongoing needs of the practice and to determine how decisions are affecting its present operation. In the senior author's practice, this individual is also primarily responsible for the preconsultation process, as discussed further in the following chapter. In addition to the positions already discussed, individuals who can work on a per diem basis are helpful to cover vacations or unexpected absences. Often, these part-time employees seek this limited role because of family obligations or regular professional duties elsewhere. Although an accountant should not be a full-time employee of the practice, he or she should be available as a consultant to manage the preparation of financial statements and tax documents as well as for other personal or professional financial consultations. Ideally, the accountant is willing to assist in the training of a new hire that is managing the bookkeeping records.

Maintaining Staff

The best way to maintain staff is to ensure that their job is challenging and financially as well as personally rewarding and that they are respected and appreciated. Motivation is important with staff, and the physician needs to set the pace as well as the mood of the practice. If the physician is distracted or disturbed, then this perturbed temperament will be transferred to the staff. Additionally, the staff mimics the tone and social interaction that the physician takes with patients. They will act by following that example. Financial motivation needs to be clear in that benefits, including vacation time, pension plans, sick time, and health insurance are provided. Additionally, raises should be based on the financial performance of the practice from the preceding fiscal year. Scheduled bonuses are not recommended because the staff will come to expect and depend on them and will be disappointed if they do not receive the allotted income at the predetermined time. Instead, bonuses should be offered on a less rigorously defined timetable that parallels the financial success of the practice.

Although the physician needs to assume the leadership of the practice, that role should not be as a totalitarian dictator or overzealous micromanager. A tyrannical management style only fosters resentment and stifles talent, ultimately leading to employee resignation. A forum should be established to air grievances and to ensure that all staff problems are properly attended and a viable solution reached. If an unfavorable event should occur, preventative measures need to be evaluated to preclude this situation from recurring. No accusatory tone ever should be taken toward an employee; rather, nurturing words should be offered to improve and redirect that employee's performance. The physician should be prepared to complete any task that is assigned to a staff member so that every undertaking is perceived as a team effort. Cross training employees in other areas promotes an appreciation of another's duties and help minimize resentment that one's responsibility exceeds that of another's. Additionally, cross training ensures that when one employee is unavailable for any reason that all tasks remain covered. Above all, equitable treatment of all employees and a zero tolerance policy of internal gossip foster a healthy work environment and help to retain valuable staff.

Weekly staff meetings permit a suitable forum in which all practice issues may be discussed in a team setting, thereby facilitating the aforementioned goals. These meetings should be maintained at a set time, and an agenda should be outlined. These sessions should provide an opportunity to cover patient issues, instruct about cosmetic surgery, discuss practice development, and staff assignments to carry out the overall plan. It should also be a time when both practice issues and individual concerns can be broached. However, each staff member should be reminded that a problem should be presented with a possible solution in mind and that other resolutions should be solicited from the group. Presenting problems without possible solutions creates a negative environment in which the meetings devolve into mere complaint sessions with very little if any productive outcome.

In summary, hiring and maintaining staff is a costly enterprise that deserves careful attention and constant nurturing. Those who possess a quality work ethic should be retained and trained in positions that fit their skills. Employee satisfaction should be frequently evaluated and addressed: Scheduled meetings provide for a forum for this assessment. Talent should be allowed to thrive, and a good work ethic, rewarded. By hiring and maintaining effective office personnel the practice has unlimited potential for growth and requires decreasing personal management time from the physician.

DEVELOPING AND MAINTAINING AN EFFECTIVE MARKETING STRATEGY

Marketing of a medical practice is a recent invention that has paralleled the growth of the elective-care sector. Unlike traditional medicine that addresses the treatment of physical ailments, cosmetic surgery caters to nonobligatory care. Accordingly, marketing is a primary method to generate interest and knowledge about the services and products that are available to increase one's quality of life. Marketing may assume many different incarnations and permutations, all of which are discussed in detail in the following text. First of all, the concept of "branding" is explained as well as how to position oneself in a competitive market. The external-marketing section explains how to develop a marketing plan as it relates to efforts outside the practice such as yellow page advertisements and other media sources. Internal marketing discusses the daily activities within the practice used for self-promotion, and a public-relations strategy—which essentially constitutes external marketing via means that do not require expenditure—are elaborated.

Branding

The most fundamental aspect of successful marketing is so-called "branding." Successful corporations (e.g., Nike, Sony, McDonald's, etc.) have developed a well-formulated corporate identity through unified marketing strategies that rely on stunning logos, memorable tag lines, and a repeated market presence. For instance, when one thinks of Nike, the automatic mental image conjured up is the indelible "swoosh" logo that bears all the hallmarks of classic design: simplicity, elegance, and recall. The practice should try to develop a striking graphic logo that can be imprinted on all practice-related paraphernalia, including stationery, business cards, advertisements, and so on. Often, the artistry of an aesthetic surgeon becomes manifest in the choice and design of a logo. If the physician cannot devise a workable logo by his or her own effort, it may be excessive to hire a firm to complete this task during the initial phases of practice development, because precious funds should be allocated toward other more profit-oriented endeavors. In the creation of a logo, one is advised to meditate on the form that the logo will assume more than the color scheme. Although color can help define the image of a practice, it should not be the primary focus of logo design for several reasons. First, one cannot brand a color; that is, one cannot own a color per se. Again to use Nike as a good example, the "swoosh" design can assume any color and still retain its complete identity. Moreover, some advertisements are only in black-and-white format, so color is not an option. Alternatively, a two-color printing setup may incur too high a cost and is unnecessary in most cases. Nevertheless, color identification can serve as an added brand recognition tool for the consumer and should be exploited when possible. If the logo is an abstract entity, the full or contracted name of the practice can be integrated with the logo to increase the link between the non–concrete design element and the more concrete typeface. For instance, "Lam Facial Plastics," which appears under one author's every logo, describes in three simple words that the practice is centered on the surgeon who specializes in facial plastic surgery (Fig. 2-1). The choice of font also should reflect an artistic sensibility and be used consistently as another tool to aid in consumer recall. Nevertheless, a logo does not make a practice. Despite the inherent value of marketing, the reader is reminded that the core of a successful practice is centered on patient satisfaction. Marketing cannot replace quality patient care and excellent surgery. A plastic surgical practice is built one patient at a time.

As part of "branding," every advertisement should focus on what makes a physician's services, training, perspective, and so on unique in the marketplace; that is, why a prospective patient should seek services with that particular physician. As a fruitful exercise, one is encouraged to write down a list of 10 items that set forth the defining characteristics of a particular practice and then organize that list in a hierarchical fashion. Selecting two or three of the most salient items from the list may assist the physician in determining the unique characteristics that define his or her practice. For instance, if a surgeon is of a certain ethnic or racial background, marketing strategies can be focused on capturing that demographic without exclusion of the principal White market by advertising differentially in the local papers targeting particular ethnic or racial readerships (Fig. 2-2). A memorable tag line also can be used to reinforce the unique qualities of a given practice. For instance, if the physician is female, then "plastic surgery from a woman's perspective" may be a selling point to a largely female-based patient pop-

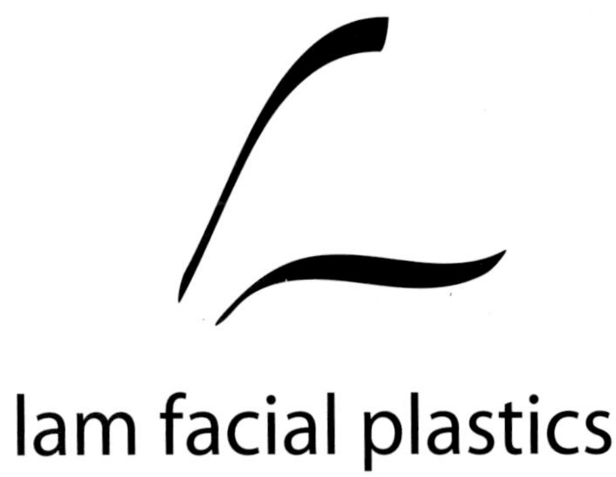

FIGURE 2-1. The logo design should exemplify simplicity and elegance. These qualities serve to embody the ideals of the practice and reinforce public recall through brand identity. The logo should be open to interpretation because it is an abstract entity. The logo shown here has been viewed as an arching eyebrow, an aquiline nose, or (the designer's original intent) an open configuration of the letter "L." The words below the logo work to make the abstract shape more concrete and memorable and essentially have become incorporated into the logo design. The choice of font (in this case, myriad roman) and the use of all lowercase letters are meant to connote an impression of modernity. In order to ensure that the caption "lam facial plastics" is kept as part of the logo design rather than lost in a larger body of neighboring text, no other accompanying text is ever written in this particular font.

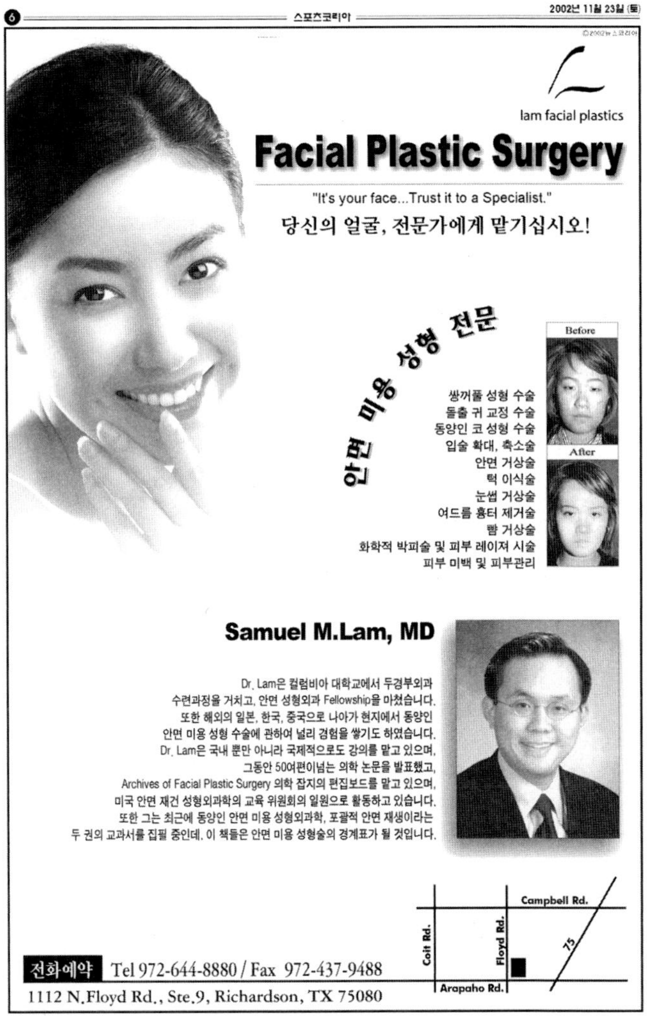

FIGURE 2-2. This advertisement is focused on the Korean market and contains some key elements that try to brand the identity of the practice. The use of a Korean model (as opposed to a White or even another Asian model of a different ethnicity) shows cultural sensitivity, draws the attention of the reader, and visually anchors the advertisement. The logo design and tag line are exhibited on every advertisement for brand recognition. A convincing before-and-after photograph is an invaluable tool to convince the reader that the surgeon is skilled in his or her art; and it is changed on weekly basis so that different aspects of the practice can be highlighted.

ulation. If the physician has been in practice for many years, then the phrase, "with over 25 years of experience" may be a marketable line. Many of these concepts have been gleaned from contemporary thinking, and some ideas have been derived from the senior author's experience.

To reiterate, every advertisement should bear the logo and tag line to create recognition and recall in the public's mind. In addition, the advertisement should focus on the services that can be offered to the patient–consumer. For instance, advertising "over 10 lasers on the premises" fails to convey the advantages those laser devices will offer to the prospective patient. Instead, "no-downtime laser rejuvenation" or "lasers to remove spider veins" communicates how that technology will benefit the recipient. According to some state medical laws and the American Medical Association ethical guidelines, the physician should be cautioned not to boast unsubstantiated claims, for example, "the most experienced plastic surgeon" or "the best . . . ." State law may also prohibit patient testimonials in advertising. One other important tenet that should be remembered in any marketing campaign is the necessity for ongoing, repeated exposure. Even in a downturn economy, the physician must continue to sustain a market presence in order to retain the public's recall and recognition of a particular practice and physician. The advertising budget need not be as heavy during certain periods of the year but should represent a sustained effort and commitment. The physician's "mugshot" photograph should be included in every advertisement, which can increase "brand" familiarity as much as a logo, and establish an intimacy with the potential patient. Because a picture is worth a thousand words, a good "before-and-after" photograph can convince a reader or viewer of the quality of the surgical services offered. Conversely, poor photographs (inconsistent positioning, bad lighting, mediocre surgical result) should not be included, because these images will most likely dissuade the prospective patient from calling. Finally, if the surgeon perceives that a discount or free giveaway will not tarnish his or her image (and if done tastefully, it should not), then these promotional measures can entice a prospective patient to make the initial phone contact.

External Marketing

The purpose of external marketing is to make the phone ring. Once the patient has placed the call, it is up to the internal workings of the office to keep that patient engaged and assure that an in-house consultation is arranged. Accordingly, the staff should be well trained on how to answer phone calls; they should be knowledgeable and courteous, consummate salespeople. The most common mistake made in development of a marketing strategy is failure to plan. Before making any marketing expenditures, a plan with an overall strategy for the upcoming year should be in place. Part of planning entails how to brand a practice and create an advertising strategy, as outlined in the preceding. Marketing is an expensive endeavor, and many different media sources attempt to convince the physician that their particular offering is the best. The physician should ensure that an overall plan is in place before making this significant financial commitment. Once the decision has been made to proceed with the plan, it is imperative that a tracking system be in place to confirm the effectiveness of the media or its relative ineffectiveness. It must be stressed that omission of an effective tracking system constitutes the single, biggest error in any marketing strategy. This task can be accomplished by simply inquiring how the practice's phone number was obtained when the patient initially calls. This information then can be recorded in a database to determine which media strategies are effective and which are ineffective, thereby tailoring future efforts toward productive sources. Although tracking is a relatively straightforward affair, determination of marketing effectiveness may be hampered by a long delay between the time that a prospective patient sees a media source and the time that he or she actually follows through with a phone call. Although marketing appears on the financial statements as an expense and is perceived as negative cash flow, it should be viewed more like an investment and measured by its return. Not only does the source of the patient's call need to bc tracked but also the surgery that is ultimately undertaken and the related revenue generated from the procedure. A general rule of thumb favors a four-to-one return on marketing investment.

When first embarking on a media strategy, a conservative policy should be followed. As the practice grows and develops, marketing power will increase because of name recognition. Yellow page advertisements are a necessity and are a costly expenditure for a young practice (Fig. 2-3). External marketing beyond this may prove cost prohibitive at the outset. Instead, public relations strategies that require more effort and less money may be a preferred avenue to pursue for the fledgling practice. Estimates for a marketing budget should fall between 2% and 15% of gross revenue. In actuality, 2% is probably too low, and 15% represents quite high a figure. Regardless, it is wise to decide on a marketing budget and be faithful to it. Just as spending too much on marketing too early can be detrimental so can spending too little—once again emphasizing the importance of tracking. At some point it will hopefully become impossible to see any more consultations or book any more surgeries owing to time constraints. If the practice matures to this level, then marketing efforts can be tapered to see if practice volume can be sustained with a smaller expenditure.

After patient and physician referrals, yellow page advertisements are the third most common source of patient calls. The advertisement should be as large or one size larger than the competition and display contrasting colors to draw attention. Most cities have several different providers for yellow pages and each one should be approached. When a patient calls, the office staff should inquire which yellow page

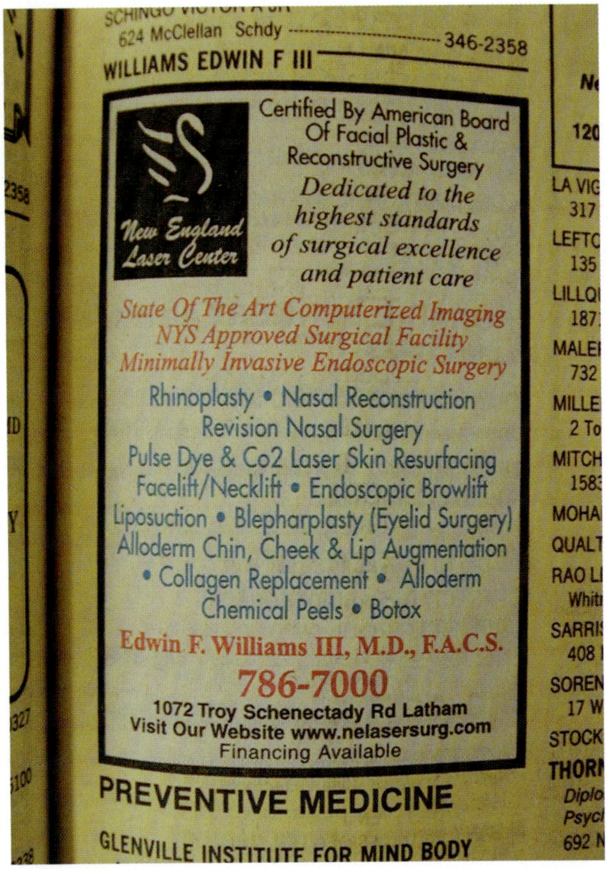

FIGURE 2-3. This yellow page advertisement does not occupy a full page but stands out from the surrounding advertisers because of its color scheme and relative size. The use of color attracts the eye and helps to delineate the different elements of the text. Choice of a white background for a yellow page advertisement renders it more visually striking without being overbearing or distasteful.

advertisement the patient glimpsed for tracking purposes. Yellow page advertisements have declined in their popularity by virtue of the Internet (see below). Often, yellow page advertisements may capture a mature demographic that is more accustomed to this format. Another confusing and costly attribute of yellow page advertising today concerns the many sections in which a physician may need to put his or her advertisement (e.g., under plastic surgery, physicians, skin care, hair loss, etc.). Obviously, a judicious policy should be followed depending on the target consumer the physician is trying to pursue.

Print advertising can be a good venue for an aesthetic surgeon dedicated primarily, if not exclusively, to the face. Television and radio advertising appear not to be as effective media choices for promoting a facial plastic practice. Conversely, body liposuction and breast augmentation services tend to reap more benefit from these electronic media sources. However, television and radio public relations efforts can be remarkably effective, not to mention cost effective, in an overall marketing strategy. As part of an advertisement, the physician may elect to promote an upcoming seminar with a phone call listed to make reservations for the event. Seminars held every other month should be viewed as an integral part of a successful practice and should be tracked accordingly to determine revenue generated from these events (Fig. 2-4). Topics that focus on "minimally invasive, no downtime" aspects of surgical and nonsurgical interventions can attract patients and serve as an introduction to other procedures that require longer convalescence. We know from experience that individuals who may not book surgery immediately after a seminar may do so months to years later.

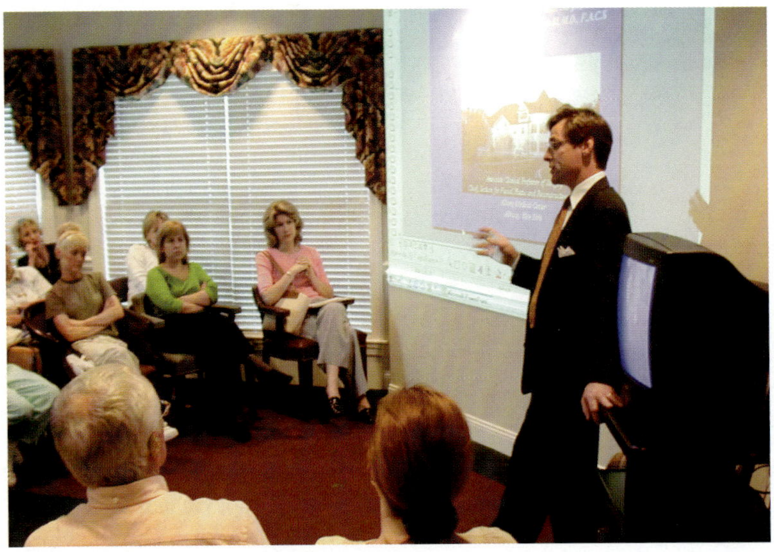

FIGURE 2-4. Seminars held every other month should be an integral part of a successful practice in order to maintain and continue to grow the practice. On-site seminars are advisable for several reasons: (a) cost; (b) convenience; and (c) increasing the patient's familiarity and comfort with the office environment.

Developing a Web presence is almost mandatory today (Fig. 2-5A,B). The Internet may provide a national and international patient base for the more seasoned practitioner. However, even for the junior surgeon, a Web presence can afford a 24-hour, 7-day-a-week advertisement that is relatively inexpensive to maintain after initial setup costs. In fact, reviewing click times (i.e, when patients seek the Web for information) reveals that late evening and nighttime hours are the primary window when Web browsers go online for medical (and nonmedical) information. Therefore, a website can effectively extend one's business hours into the night, so that information and interest about the practice can still be generated after the office has closed. Developing a website requires an ongoing commitment and should not be viewed as

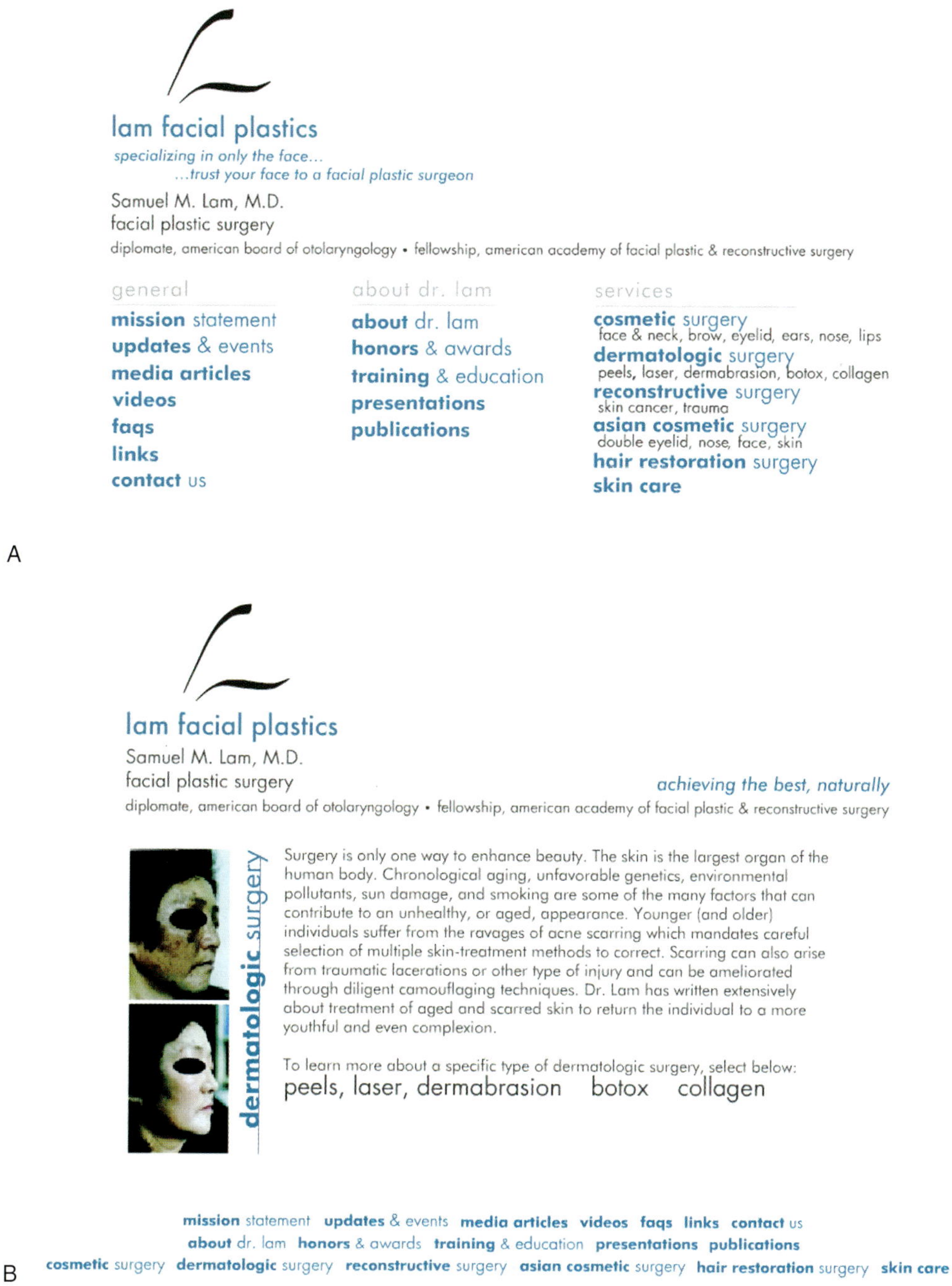

FIGURE 2-5. A: The home page should be clearly laid out for the potential patient. The displayed page is divided into three groupings: general information **(left column),** information about the surgeon **(middle column),** and information about services **(right column). B:** The subpages should be easily navigable as well. Note that the bottom and side directories permit the individual the freedom to enter any other subpage directly without returning to the home page.

a static, one-time outing. Instead, the Website should have a section dedicated to "what's new" or "events & updates," encouraging patients to return to the Website to see what seminars will be offered, what discounts are available, and in which recent media coverage the physician has been featured. In addition, the physician is encouraged to review periodically his or her recent and not-so-recent before-and-after photographs to determine whether any likely candidates are suitable for the Website.

Meeting with a qualified Web developer is a first step. However, the physician should be savvy about some key elements of good Web layout that will facilitate dialog with the developer. The single most frustrating event for a prospective patient is a long delay in opening a Web page because of burdensome graphics or a lengthy introduction. Fortunately, broadband connections are making these problems less frequent. Heavy animation also can prove to be a distracting element for the returning customer who has already been dazzled by the glitzy introduction. Instead, a static home page or a very brief introduction is encouraged. Fortunately, animation programmed in Macromedia's Flash permits fluid, elegant movements and transitions without any significant load time, because it requires very little memory capacity. However, not every household has Flash preinstalled, and older computers and more mature individuals may be too frustrated to load the requisite, albeit free, software to run Flash. Also, different versions of Flash exist, and an individual may have an older version that is incompatible with the later edition. Recent data claim that 97.8% of Internet users have Flash already installed, because it comes preinstalled on Windows 98, XP, Netscape Navigator, America Online, and the Macintosh operating system. Flash animation can be done with subtlety and be well integrated into the Website to enhance transitions between screens when an icon is clicked (known as a "rollover"). In order to maximize the widest possible audience and still retain the elegant feel of Flash animation, twin Websites can be built, one in Flash and one in standard HTML (hypertext mark-up language). The introductory sequence can bear the line, "If you do not see this page animated, please click here to download a free version of Flash software, or click here to enter the HTML site." Of course, this option adds some expense and may not be the preferred route to take for starting physicians but may be a good option for the established practice that possesses greater financial resources. Languages and formats are constantly evolving, and this information may be outdated by the time this book is published. Therefore, the reader is advised to consult his or her Web developer for the most current information.

A basic element of good Web design is easy and straightforward navigation: The individual should be able to enter the subdirectories or subpages, travel between subdirectories, and return to the main home page simply and seamlessly. Part of good navigation requires that no "dead links" exist (i.e., one does not encounter a dead end when clicking on an icon). Of course, good writing and excellent photography are prerequisites for an outstanding Website. Having all of the text, photography, and artwork prepared and labeled for the Web developer will eliminate confusion and facilitate an expeditious and accurate completion of the Website. A virtual office tour is a wonderful feature that can offer the patient a walking tour of the office to minimize fear of what the consultation, surgery, and postoperative care entail. The least expensive way to build this feature into the site is simply to photograph each room in the office and have accompanying text share what each room is designed for. A printable or electronic datasheet that the patient can fill out before coming to the office also may help reduce the labor of the office staff and decrease wait times for the patient when he or she arrives at the office. However, electronic correspondence is fraught with liability in terms of privacy, dispensing medical advice (especially if the communication is interstate), and so on, and should be weighed carefully against the potential benefits of drawing new patients with this feature. If the physician would like to add updates to a particular section (e.g., "what's new" or "events & updates"), he or she may ask the Web developer to build a *database* into which the physician or office staff can directly add information without assistance from the Web developer. On the other hand, the physician may decide to pay the Web developer a small retainer fee for a periodic update of the Website, for example, on a monthly basis.

Tracking return on a Website can be done the old-fashioned way, by asking the patient where he or she found information about the practice or by assessing click rates. The latter method is informative in terms of overall traffic to the Website but does not reveal how many visitors to the Website became actual patients or who decided on additional procedures based on a visit to the Website. Information about the number of clicks, the time that the Website was visited, error messages, and so on, typically can be obtained from one's Web-hosting site. "Metatags" are HTML codes that are embedded within a Website for certain keywords (e.g., rhinoplasty, otoplasty, etc.) that may be used as searchable terms in a search engine when the Website has been formally registered with that search engine. However, external (nonembedded) keywords can be registered directly with search engines for a fee charged to the physician based on the number of clicks per given time period and the popularity of that term. For instance, if the searchable term "plastic surgery" is determined to cost $3 per click, and 300 consumers clicked on the physician's Website based on a search for that keyword, the charge for the month is $900. The cost for keyword listings is constantly changing based on demand and the particular search engine, and keywords have come to supersede the relevance of free "metatags" in the current Web landscape. Determining which search engine(s) is the most popular can be obtained from *www.searchenginewatch.com.* As mentioned, these rules are not fixed but are incessantly evolving: A Web developer's current advice should be heeded over any suggestions made in this book.

Internal Marketing

Everything that occurs in the office may be considered internal marketing. The moment the patient walks through the door he or she begins to form an impression of the practice; therefore, it is vital that an investment is made in the upfront section of the office. The receptionist should be properly attired in a conservative style and convey a sense of warmth and congeniality. The reception area should be tasteful and tidy, representing the aesthetic ideals that the physician exemplifies. Fresh flowers, classical music, and soft illumination are aspects that are inviting and generate a positive impression in the prospective patient. Every patient encounter can be classified in the following manner: positive, neutral, and negative, with the latter two categories representing equally bad outcomes. If the patient does not walk away raving about the staff, physician, and care, then that "neutral" encounter should be interpreted as negative because of the lost opportunity to impress the patient in a favorable way.

The reception area represents the single most important room where internal marketing can be exploited. Instead of a room filled with outdated magazines and other clutter, the physician should truly concentrate on how that room can serve to educate the patient about services and products that the physician offers. For instance, a Web terminal can be installed that has the physician's home page prominently displayed. The patient can find out more about available services than he or she may have otherwise known. Brochures can be purchased in a generic format, but the physician is strongly advised to create his or her own brochure that is tailored to the particular services offered in that practice with before-and-after photographs included. A cabinet can be installed that prominently presents all of the aesthetic skin care products available, so patients can browse while they wait. A binder that holds all of the physician's publications, awards, thankful patient letters, and curriculum vitae also can be placed on the coffee table; lamination of all the inclusive papers adds a polish to the look and preserves the integrity of the documents. The same brochures and displays can be exhibited in each of the examination rooms so that the patient can reach for one before the physician enters the room. However, the consultation room probably should not have all these marketing paraphernalia so that the patient will remain focused on the dialog rather than be distracted by the surrounding material. Diplomas and awards should be prominently displayed in the consultation room or another heavy traffic location rather than tucked away in the physician's office, because these framed documents substantiate the physician's credentials to the patient.

Although different policies exist concerning discounted cosmetic services for employees, the physician is encouraged to offer unlimited free cosmetic surgery to any employee for several reasons. First and foremost, a beautiful cosmetic result is the most tangible evidence to the patient that the physician is credible in his or her surgical skills. The employee who has undergone surgery is the most active spokesperson for the practice and can share empathy with a patient who is considering surgery. That employee also is able to answer questions about what is involved in surgery and postoperative care better than anyone else. Employees with beautiful cosmetic results constitute the best internal marketing strategy for a physician.

Public Relations

Public relations may be defined as making a concerted effort to extend one's time, energy, or skills to improve the perception of one's image in the public's eye. Although advertising simply requires monetary expenditure to accomplish this feat, public relations necessitate no financial obligation other than time commitment. For the junior and senior plastic surgeon alike, the dividends reaped from good public relations may far outweigh those derived from straightforward advertising. Public relations begin in the office where the definition becomes blurred with internal marketing. An example includes a patient-concern book: Disgruntled patients' names are recorded in a directory, and the entire office staff is made aware of that patient and his or her concern. If that patient should call, extra time and care should be dedicated to alleviate his or her concern, rebuild the lost trust, and convert that person into a potential return customer and referral source. Patients should be routinely called after surgery, preferably the night of surgery and the day after (at a minimum), to check on how the recovery process is going and answer any outstanding questions. Patients appreciate the call and expression of concern, and the time commitment is minimal. Additionally, when a patient calls the office or answering service, the physician or office staff should ensure to return calls promptly and patiently. The patient's call to the office should never be the last phone contact: A follow-up call should be made, preferably by the physician, at the end of the day, once again to confirm proactively the patient's recovery status. These simple courtesies impress on patients that one truly cares about his or her progress and expeditious recovery.

Outside the office, many things can be done to improve the image of the physician and practice. The junior surgeon, who has very modest financial resources, is strongly advised to take full advantage of all public relations opportunities and to seek those prospects in a creative way. For instance, forwarding a press release to the local newspaper about one's upcoming speaking engagement or one's reflections regarding a new surgical technique is an economical but effective method to elevate one's prestige and exposure. An article written about a physician is much more convincing to readers than a simple advertisement. If three competing advertisements surround an article devoted to a physician, clearly the latter is much more authoritative and costs nothing. The same technique can be used to work with radio and television stations. Often, the press is looking for a good story, and a press release can offer them what they want without their doing the work to find it. If a good relationship is established, a physician becomes the media expert—a much-coveted position that elevates a physician above his or her colleagues in a community, at least in the public's estimation.

Attendance at charitable functions and other high-society gatherings increases a physician's exposure in the desired, influential circles. When participating in these kinds of events, a quantifiable return of investment may not always be rigorously calculable. Nevertheless, because no expenditure has been laid out, tracking may not be as critical as when real money is committed. Involvement with the local medical school can be a very enriching experience for the physician interested in teaching since he also benefits from the increased exposure in this academic setting. Affiliation with a prestigious institution, even as a clinical instructor or lecturer, can be construed favorably by the public seeking a physician with a professorial reputation. Charitable work is a very personally rewarding experience as well. Medical mission work to underdeveloped countries or gratuitous treatment of domestic violence patients can be gratifying activities that in turn also benefit one's prestige in the community. Although a physician may believe that declaration of his or her charitable endeavors may be a boastful gesture, making the public aware of one's sincere contributions is important. In reality, every public appearance may be deemed a public relations outing, and the physician should act commensurately. Conservative attire, sobriety, and proper conduct should be exhibited whenever a physician leaves the confines of his or her domicile.

DEVELOPING AND MAINTAINING AN EFFECTIVE AESTHETIC SKIN CARE STRATEGY

The Role of the Aesthetician

Whether or not a plastic surgeon engages in dermatologic resurfacing, the role of an aesthetician can enhance the value and prestige of a cosmetic surgical practice (Fig. 2-6). Product sales can add considerable revenue to a physician's practice, and unlike surgery, entail very little effort and potential headache. An aesthetician can offer the patient elective services, such as microdermabrasion, massage, makeup, and facial treatments other than retailing skin care products. With extensive products and services offered, patient visits to the office will increase several-fold and may translate into potential surgical revenue. Obviously, patients who seek elective aesthetic care by an aesthetician may be considered "positive" traffic flow in that these individuals are also likely to spend money on cosmetic surgery. Furthermore, a trained medical aesthetician can provide invaluable advice and care during the postoperative setting when patient handholding is necessary. Lymphatic massage and vitamin regimens may be added to hasten recovery in those individuals who so desire these services. Tedious and prolonged care is mandatory for the postresurfacing patient (Chapter 9), and can be partly alleviated by the assistance of the aesthetician. Nonirritating products and proper camouflaging makeup can help the patient return to normal activity efficiently and expeditiously.

Business Arrangement with an Aesthetician

The primary responsibility that faces the plastic surgeon that elects to partner with an aesthetician is defining the precise nature of that professional relationship. Should the aesthetician manage a completely independent business or function as an employee of the physician? The answer to this question must be made on an individual basis, and the following text describes the benefits and drawbacks of each scenario.

If an aesthetician functions as a solo business apart from the plastic surgical practice, then the physician need not be concerned about the revenue generated; the aesthetician's liability per se (see the following); the salary, commission, and related benefits; and product inventory. Instead, the aesthetician's area can be turned into a rentable space subleased to the aesthetician, who then assumes all of the risk for the

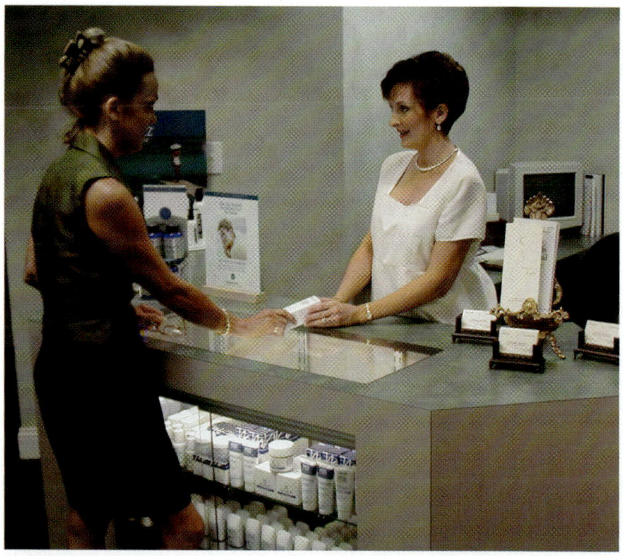

FIGURE 2-6. An aesthetician can enhance the value and prestige of a cosmetic surgical practice. Skin care products should be prominently displayed in an area of heavy traffic flow. The aesthetician can either function as an employee or as an independent contractor (see text for more details).

undertaking. Clearly, with this independent association, the physician still should show significant interest in the aesthetician's success, because the business relationship is symbiotic in nature. The aesthetician also benefits from this arrangement in that the aesthetician earns all the profits on products and services rather than handing them over to the physician. However, with greater reward comes greater risk, which the aesthetician rightfully incurs. With this risk, the aesthetician also is more likely to promote his or her practice diligently and seek avenues for growth and new strategies for marketing. If the aesthetician is functioning independently from the physician, then the aesthetician must obtain his or her own liability coverage. Also, in this circumstance patient records cannot be shared and patient charts must be kept confidential and separate. The licensing of an aesthetician varies from state to state. If a separate license is required for the aesthetician, no financial arrangements can be made that involve profit sharing for mutually shared patients. This policy violates kickback laws imposed on physicians. The exception to this restriction involves the sale of products—if the products do not require a prescription—because many states permit only pharmacies to sell prescription products.

If the physician chooses to have the aesthetician as an employee, then all the contrary arguments are valid. The aesthetician must then be compensated for his or her time based on an hourly wage, commission, or both. If a full-time position is involved, then health insurance, vacation time, and other benefits must be extended. The area dedicated to aesthetic care is no longer a space from which a physician can extract rent, but instead from which he or she can earn revenue from products and services. Another consideration is that the aesthetician working under the employ of the plastic surgeon may in turn subject the physician to increased liability caused by negligence or error on the aesthetician's part. For instance, if a patient suffers a corneal abrasion from a microdermabrasion session, then the physician may be liable if the aesthetician is an employee. Nevertheless, by law, some states mandate that certain services—including microdermabrasion in several states—be under physician supervision. In these circumstances, the physician is not exempt from legal responsibility regardless of the working relationship with the aesthetician. Similarly, hair laser removal and aesthetician-strength chemical peels also have been the target of shifting state regulations; and the physician is strongly advised to research current state laws when deciding on what relationship and services ultimately will be provided in a particular setting. If the aesthetician serves as an employee, the physician should consult his or her medical malpractice coverage to determine whether an "extension" needs to be granted to cover the aesthetician's liability under that policy.

Although the advice rendered herein is in no way meant to be infallible, the recommendations are derived from substantive experience rather than mere conjecture or arcane reasoning. The chapter has been dedicated in large part to the starting physician but scattered throughout the text are many helpful hints that may serve to advance the practice of even the veteran practitioner. A successful plastic surgical practice mandates constant nurturing, and the reader is encouraged to review parts of this chapter on occasion to ensure that business and marketing strategies have been effectively exploited.

3

AN EFFECTIVE STRATEGY FOR PATIENT CARE

EDWARD D. BUCKINGHAM
SAMUEL M. LAM
EDWIN F. WILLIAMS III

The previous chapter focused on business and marketing strategies that could help build and sustain a plastic surgical practice. This chapter continues that discussion but focuses on specific concerns related to patient care. Like each successive chapter, this chapter is structured according to preoperative, intraoperative, and postoperative considerations. The preoperative process is addressed first with particular attention paid to the role of the patient-care coordinator. Also as part of the preoperative evaluation, the dynamics of the consultation process are elaborated, from the preconsultation and consultation to the postconsultation period. Although some physicians staunchly defend the merits of 35-mm film, this chapter endeavors to convince the reader that digital imaging is a less costly, less labor intensive, more flexible, and more effective medium for every phase of patient care. Intraoperative discussion attempts to delineate the appropriate operating-room environment conducive to optimal patient care and to delve into other nuances that favorably affect delivery of care. Postoperative concerns include developing and maintaining patient rapport and managing the difficult patient. At the conclusion of this chapter, sample copies of all preoperative and postoperative instructions for the patient are provided as a ready reference for the reader.

PREOPERATIVE CONSIDERATIONS: EVALUATION, CONSULTATION, AND IMAGING

Role of the Patient-Care Coordinator

Often patients consider cosmetic surgery for quite some time before placing the initial call for consultation. Once this call has been made, it becomes imperative to ensure that the patient will schedule a consultation by establishing immediate rapport, by answering all queries fully but succinctly, and by engaging the patient's interest and motivation. A well-trained patient-care coordinator can fulfill this role in a dedicated fashion. In a busy practice, the phone may be answered by a receptionist, the patient-care coordinator, or another staff member. The physician should ensure that every staff member is fully trained to answer the initial phone consultation in a professional and knowledgeable manner. Mock telephone conversations can be used to assess the level of competency of the staff in this regard: The physician or senior staff can role play as a prospective patient to ask each staff member in turn how he or she would respond in a given scenario. These sessions should be nonjudgmental in nature and be emphasized to be simply a didactic tool. Any deficiencies in telephone aptitude should be identified and critiqued for betterment of the staff. Besides the skill of salesmanship, the physician should also ensure that basic fund of knowledge concerning all products and services is upheld through formal, scheduled didactic sessions. This fundamental skill in patient dialog that all staff members should possess underscores the importance of cross training (Chapter 2); that is, the entire staff should feel comfortable with multiple office roles. A related section has been included that offers sample questions that can be used in training the staff and to stimulate discussion. Although every staff member should be well versed in answering the phone, the patient-care coordinator should make every effort to be the primary person in charge of this responsibility to provide needed continuity of care and breed a sense of familiarity when the patient arrives for the consultation. Perhaps the most effective way for this arrangement to be executed is for the receptionist to answer the majority of incoming calls and to direct potential consultations or other patient-related questions to the patient-care coordinator. Any overflow of calls should be then handled by the patient-care coordinator or other staff member in that order of priority.

The responsibility of the patient-care coordinator begins with the initial patient call. When a cosmetic call is received, the patient should be referred by name to the coordinator. It is important to reinforce the coordinator's name to the patient in order to encourage a more durable relationship between the two parties. Once the patient has become comfortable with the coordinator, it is more likely that meaningful dialog will ensue. After the coordinator has been relayed the telephone call, it is then his or her responsibility to transform the discussion into a consultation with the physician. Although many of the patient's questions can and should be answered during the initial call, the goal should not be to conduct a formal telephone consultation but to exchange enough information to secure an office appointment. Additionally, the coordinator should be selling the primary product of the practice—the physician—to the patient. The coordinator should endeavor to enlighten the patient of the physician's impeccable credentials and why the physician is best qualified to address the patient's cosmetic concerns. Additionally, designation of one individual in the office as the primary contact for patient care opens the door for convenient, comfortable reestablishment of that contact at any time. It allows the patient who has never visited the office before to step into that environment and feel an intimate rapport through the established contact with the patient-care coordinator, a relationship that can be nurtured during every return visit. Women tend to value this relationship greatly, which can manifest as a greater likelihood to schedule surgery, return in the future, and refer friends for consultation.

When a prospective cosmetic patient arrives for the appointment, the patient-care coordinator should greet them, explain how the visit will proceed, and assist with any preliminary paperwork. The coordinator should then escort the patient to the consultation room and begin the preconsultation process or turn that responsibility over to another designated staff member (the details of which are discussed in a following section). After the patient's consultation with the physician, the coordinator assumes responsibility again for the patient. Initially, the physician needs to be comfortable and responsible for determining and discussing fees with the patient. However, as the coordinator gains experience and confidence, he or she is able to engage in the explanation of fee schedules and payment options (Fig. 3-1). These fees should be individualized and totaled for the patient on a personal price sheet that should be placed in the chart with a copy given to the patient. It may be a wise policy to have the patient sign and date the price sheet to acknowledge agreement to the price, payment schedule, and expiration of the quoted price after a particular date. If the patient decides to proceed with surgery, the patient-care coordinator should then schedule a date for the procedure. If the patient defers decision for surgery, the coordinator should offer both the physician and coordinator's business cards to the patient and welcome the patient to call any time to inquire further or to return for another consultation. Within a few days the coordinator should then compose a follow-up letter thanking the patient for the visit and thereby reinforce the relationship and open communication. The authors feel that telephone calls to the patient after a consultation may be too intrusive or improperly construed as an overly assertive gesture.

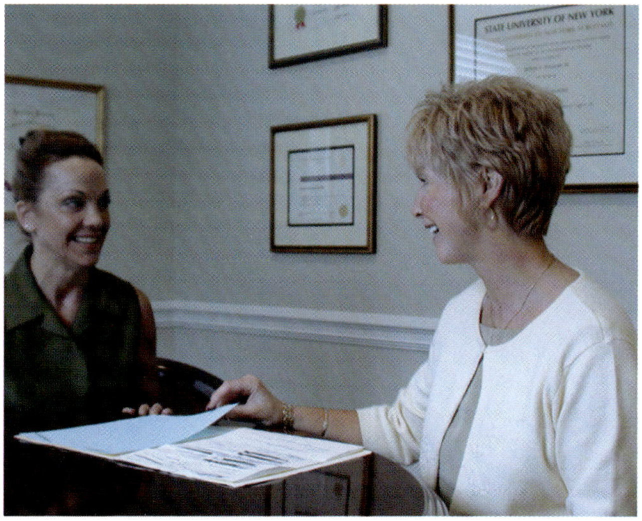

FIGURE 3-1. The patient-care coordinator *(right)* discusses the surgical fees and payment options with a prospective patient. The conversation is conducted in a dedicated "booking" room that provides seclusion away from office traffic and that is uniquely designed. The diplomas mounted on the wall can be most effectively displayed in this room when the patient is contemplating whether to proceed with surgery. The circular desk also permits a nonconfrontational encounter between the patient-care coordinator and the patient.

Although the staff should be knowledgeable about procedures and the surgeon's particular background and credentials, the staff should not dispense medical advice. As mentioned in the text, the objective of the telephone conversation with the patient is to answer any preliminary questions or concerns about the physician and related services and, more important, to secure a formal consultation with the physician. The person answering the phone must promote the surgeon and the practice and encourage the prospective patient that a consultation with the surgeon will be worthwhile.

The "Preconsultation"

The preconsultation provides the forum for a member of the staff with intimate knowledge of cosmetic procedures to make preliminary contact with the patient and build on the relationship initiated by the patient-care coordinator. Obviously, the most thorough knowledge that a staff member can possess of a particular procedure would be gained if that individual has already undertaken that procedure himself or herself. The best example of the success that a procedure can afford is living proof. Accordingly, the authors encourage all staff members who would like to undergo cosmetic surgery to do so at cost.

The purpose of the preconsultation session is manifold. The staff can answer some questions about the surgical process, recovery time, expectations, aesthetic objectives, or other concerns before entering the consultation room. This interaction saves valuable time for the physician and also alleviates some fear that the patient may have in addressing

Training Questions for the Staff

1. What is the cost of the procedure/procedures?
 The cost of surgery is solely dependent upon the procedure/procedures being performed which is based on a realistic goal to be achieved and is determined after a consultation between Dr. X and the patient. The patient can phone the office for a convenient time to schedule a consultation.
2. What is the recovery period?
 Usually, the recovery period is 7 to 14 days, depending on the patient and the procedure/procedures performed.
3. Will there be discomfort?
 The level of discomfort varies depending on the patient and the procedure/procedures involved. With today's modern anesthesia techniques, most patients experience minimal if any discomfort. Because it is our goal to achieve the maximum level of comfort for all of our patients, a prescription to relieve discomfort will be provided if necessary.
4. When can I exercise?
 You may exercise approximately 2 days to 3 weeks afterward, depending on the procedure/procedures.
5. Will there by a significant difference in the way I look after surgery and will people notice?
 There should be a significant improvement in your appearance, including a more youthful rested look, bearing in mind that it is our goal to provide you with an improved look based on your natural assets.
6. How long does the procedure/procedures last before I need surgery again?
 The surgery results in an improvement ranging from approximately a few to 10+ years, depending on the procedure/procedures chosen. However, the surgery does not arrest the aging process.
7. How long before I can wear makeup?
 You can start wearing makeup approximately 7 to 14 days after the procedure/procedures.
8. How much bruising and swelling will occur?
 The amount of bruising and swelling depends on the patient and the procedures chosen. However, both preoperative and postoperative recommendations are given to the patient, including care performed by the nursing staff and our clinical aestheticians, that can substantially diminish the bruising and swelling.
9. Is the physician board certified?
 Every staff member should know the surgeon's board certification status, including when it was obtained, what the proper name of the board is, and what distinguishes that board from other related specialty board certifications. The staff also should know where the surgeon trained and in what field, any honors that the surgeon has accumulated, and other biographic details about which the patient may inquire.
10. Why does Dr. X perform a certain procedure?
 The staff should know what kind of facelift (deep-plane, SMAS [superficial musculoaponeurotic system], etc.) the surgeon practices, and why that technique is the most beneficial for the patient. The staff member should always remember not to denigrate another surgeon's technique, but simply sell the practice's surgical philosophy and techniques.
11. What is Botox?
 Botulinum toxin (Botox, Allergan, Inc., Irvine, CA) is a purified toxin that paralyzes the targeted muscles in order to prevent wrinkles in that area. It is only temporary in nature, lasting anywhere from 3 to 8 months, but typically endures for a 6-month period. There are no untoward long-term side effects; however, the procedure should be performed only by qualified physicians who are trained and experienced in its use in order to avoid short-term complications (e.g., brow or eyelid drop and asymmetry). The staff member should know all of the clinical indications for which the surgeon uses Botox (e.g., migraines, axillary hyperhidrosis, etc) and the surgeon should try to enlighten the staff about Botox pricing as well: The Botox preparation is not overly dilute, which may account for lower pricing elsewhere.
12. What is collagen?
 Collagen is a soft-tissue filler that can enhance the fullness of one's lips, fill in depressions such as acne scarring, and soften deep smile or marionette lines. The patient should know that a test patch is required and that he or she must wait 30 days for a negative result before augmentation can be undertaken. The staff members should know if a test patch is offered free of charge. The benefit of the collagen should be stressed as temporary in nature, lasting between 3 to 8 months, depending on the body's resorption of the material. Also, if the patient inquires, it should be stated that collagen is derived from a bovine source; for this reason a test patch for hypersensitivity must be conducted first in the antecubital region. A formal didactic session should be carried out by the surgeon to instruct the staff members about the differences between Zyderm I, Zyderm II, and Zyplast; why the physician selects one type of collagen over another; and other related properties and clinical uses for collagen.
13. What kind of payment options are available?
 The staff member should know what credit cards are accepted, whether cash is acceptable, how far in advance a personal check must be written before a procedure, and whether any financing is offered. Current discount or other promotional pricing should be known and extended to the patient if the surgeon has endorsed the policy. Deposits, return of deposits, and cancellation policies must be clearly understood and

communicated to the patient if asked. Consultation fees, if charged, should be disclosed; also, it should be understood by every staff member whether these fees are deducted from surgery. The surgeon and office manager must ensure that current pricing is communicated to every staff member.

14. I am quite unhappy with the surgical result.
Any concern or dissatisfaction a patient expresses regarding a surgical outcome must be communicated to the surgeon immediately. Rather than try to handle the situation over the telephone, it is usually wise to have the patient come to the office for direct inspection by the surgeon. This tends to build rapport and ensures that any problems can be addressed promptly and accurately. In addition, as advocated elsewhere in this book, the patient's name, nature of the complaint, and date all should be recorded in a notebook so that the surgeon can follow the patient's progress and ensure that ongoing rapport is not lost.
15. I decided to cancel my consultation.
Rather than simply allow this to happen, the diligent staff member should gently seek the reason that the patient is canceling the appointment. In addition, the staff member should try to establish whether the patient could select an appropriate alternative date for consultation.
16. Where does Dr. X perform his or her surgery? What kind of anesthesia is offered?
The staff member should know basically where the surgeon elects to perform a procedure, whether in the office or a surgery center, but not be dogmatic in telling the patient where the surgeon is likely to do so unless obviously clear. For instance, if the surgeon typically performs lower-eyelid surgery in the office, he or she may decide to do so in an ambulatory surgery facility because of the patient's health status or comfort level. The location and general directions to the surgical facility also should be given, and the phone number of the facility should be readily available. The type of anesthesia that is possible in the office or surgery center should be known as well (e.g., local anesthesia, intravenous sedation, monitored anesthesia care, or general anesthesia).
17. What can I do before or after surgery? What restrictions will there be on activity and so on before or after surgery?
Every staff member should be well acquainted with the routine preoperative and postoperative care and restrictions that are outlined in the appended forms at the end of the chapter. For instance, use of aspirin-related products, herbal medications, certain vitamins, alcohol, tobacco, and so on should be abstained from. During the preoperative phone confirmation call, the patient should be reminded to wear a button-down shirt that does not have to be pulled over the bandaged head, not to wear fingernail polish that can interfere with the pulse-oximetry reading, not to engage in heavy cardiovascular exercise the morning of surgery, and not to eat food that morning. In summary, every staff member should be well versed with the stated policies for routine preoperative and postoperative care. Any questions or concerns that cannot be readily answered should be directed to the physician. No matter what the level of medical training, the staff must understand fully that they are not medical physicians and should never offer formal, medical advice without the physician's assent or knowledge.

these concerns with the physician. Often, the patient may feel more at ease with an individual of the same gender and age group than with the physician, who may be of a different age or sex. During the preconsultation, the patient may confess dissatisfaction with another surgeon or disdain about a type of rejuvenative procedure that can ultimately help steer the physician away from these pitfalls if he or she knows about them in advance. The staff member then may glean what is principally bothering the patient about his or her aesthetic appearance so that any pertinent information can be relayed to the physician. The preconsultation also can enlighten the patient about various surgical options over which he or she can ruminate before seeing the physician. The preconsultation session can be used to reinforce the physician's reputation and credentials before the actual consultation. While this process is taking place, information also can be garnered regarding the patient's expectations both financially and surgically. Invaluable information can be obtained about the patient's financial standing that may help the physician decide what procedures would be within the patient's budgetary constraints. The preconsultation also affords the opportunity to determine what digital "morphing" images need to be obtained and rendered before the physician speaks with the patient. Although this saves precious time during the actual consultation, the patient is informed that the physician may or may not decide to use these images based on his or her professional judgment. The preconsultation must remain relatively concise, because the consultation itself may be involved and taxing to the patient.

The Dynamics of an Effective Consultation

Just as the goal of the initial phone contact is to book a consultation, the goal of the consultation process is to convert a visit into a surgical case. Ideally, every consultation produces a surgical case. However, this goal is neither feasible nor realistic. Although the ambitious goal of a surgeon is to convert every consultation, the surgeon comes to realize over time that certain patients are simply not good surgical candidates, either physically or mentally. Like traditional medicine, the surgeon must establish a diagnosis and recommend appropriate surgery based on the clinical findings. However, unlike traditional medicine, the surgeon must endeavor to follow the patient's concerns carefully without prematurely interjecting his or her own opinions. If the patient asks for the surgeon's professional opinion, the surgeon should refrain from commentary until the patient professes an initial aesthetic complaint. For instance, if the surgeon should state that the patient's neckline requires rejuvenation, the patient may express resentment or confusion over this advice if he or she was principally interested in rhinoplasty or brow surgery alone. Another clinical scenario may prove illustrative: If the patient asks what should be done to improve her skin, the surgeon may immediately respond that carbon dioxide laser treatment is the best option. The patient may then reply that she has already undergone laser therapy without much benefit. Instead, the surgeon should inquire a bit more about the patient's past experiences and projected expectations before a quick reply.

The primary goal of the consultation is to gather and exchange information. However, this task must be undertaken in a caring manner with the utmost caution not to offend the patient. The possibility of offending the patient and therefore losing him or her as a customer may arise because of recommending surgery too liberally or conservatively. Thoughtful attention to the patient's desires and constant feedback are required to adjust the conversation accordingly. Once the patient's preliminary concern is solicited (e.g., "my eyes look tired"), the surgeon should delve into the motivation and expectation that the patient has regarding this aesthetic complaint. After the patient has been permitted to articulate some basic concerns about his or her aesthetic interests, the surgeon can offer a tentative recommendation based on an expeditious and targeted examination. Feedback about the patient's understanding and agreement should be elicited before moving forward with the discussion. If the patient assents to the general line of thinking, then the surgeon may continue to elaborate more fully. Constant interaction and adjustment of the discussion must take place to ensure that the conversation is progressing in accordance with the patient's expectations. Nevertheless, the surgeon must direct the conversation at times, even redirecting it if need be. For example, if the patient exhibits only minimal jowling along the jaw line but notable brow ptosis, the surgeon can introduce the idea of a browlift judiciously if the patient appears receptive to this idea. Although the surgeon must remain sensitive to the patient at all times, he or she should not hesitate to offer the patient an educated opinion that may step somewhat outside of the patient's initial concerns so long as the patient appears to demonstrate the right temperament to accept these suggestions. The patient may achieve the maximal rejuvenation possible and see a more dramatic benefit by undergoing the procedure the surgeon advises. With experience, the physician will know when and how to direct the conversation. In certain circumstances, the physician should exercise caution when introducing other aesthetic flaws about which the patient has not yet remarked. For instance, drawing attention to a prominent nasal hump of an aging face is rarely indicated when unsolicited, even if the nose is suffering from the effects of aging; suggesting the removal of an unsightly mole may prove disastrous. These kinds of concerns may be safely addressed once the patient introduces them. As a general guide, the surgeon should remain within the sphere of the patient's general complaint; that is, only speak about the aging face if that is the principal concern of the patient (with the aging nose as an exception for inclusion).

It is important to focus the patient during the consultation. A great deal of information must be exchanged, and patient fatigue may become an issue. As mentioned, the preconsultation aids in focusing the consultation. Once the patient's principal concern is recognized, the physician must manage to accomplish a brief, targeted physical examination, recommend appropriate procedure(s), and describe the precise nature of the surgical endeavor. However, details about the risk involved with surgery may be better deferred to a separate session. (See the following section on Preoperative Counseling.) Selection of an appropriate candidate for surgery is a critical skill that must be developed. Refusal to operate on unsuitable individuals, especially those with unrealistic expectations, will prove to be a prudent decision in the end. If the surgeon once undertakes elective surgery on an unreasonable or (worse yet) litigious patient, then he or she will hesitate to repeat this costly error in the future. A good admonition is only to agree to proceed on one's own terms rather than acquiesce to the patient's every caprice. Often, patients are not ready to book surgery at the time of consultation because of deficient financial or mental preparedness. Therefore, the surgeon should try to convert patients to surgery who have reasonable expectations, psychological readiness, and the financial resources for elective surgery. A practical estimate for this figure is approximately 50% to 60% of all consultations. In a maturing practice (5 to 10 years of clinical practice), the objective should be to schedule enough consultations in a given week with an estimated conversion rate to fill the operating schedule for 2 to 4 weeks in advance. A schedule that falls below this quota will permit valuable operating time to be left idle. In a mature practice (10 to 15 years of clinical experience), booking beyond this period, approximately 1 to 2 months in advance, avoids fluctuations in monthly revenue. With this objective in mind, patients will not turn away because of a prolonged waiting period but perceive that the surgeon is in demand because of the need for advanced booking. Nevertheless, bountiful surgical volume is a welcome problem.

Preoperative Counseling

Preoperative counseling initially takes place during the consultation. Risks, benefits, and alternatives are briefly explained to the patient, but the focus throughout remains on the aesthetic objectives of surgery. If the patient is interested in scheduling surgery at the conclusion of the session, then a date should be chosen for the procedure, and either a partial (deposit) payment should be collected or the entire amount to reserve the scheduled surgical date. Also at the time of the initial consultation, a separate session should be scheduled during which formal, preoperative counseling may be undertaken. Because the consultation process may be quite taxing to the patient, this separate appointment can permit the patient some time to regain composure and concentration to digest the extensive amount of information that must be conveyed during the preoperative counseling meeting. In addition, the surgeon need not be present throughout the entire preoperative counseling session and thereby be alleviated the burden of the added time commitment.

During the preoperative counseling session, one must explain in detail the exact risks the surgery entails in more graphic terms than were expressed at the time of consultation. The two negative aspects of the surgical endeavor that must be truthfully and carefully explained to the patient are the material risks and surgical limitations. Material risks include all major complications that can, but only infrequently, occur (e.g., facial nerve paralysis), or minor complications that more commonly occur (e.g., milia after resurfacing or prolonged ecchymosis and edema). The surgeon should relay all of this information systematically, sincerely, and clearly but without labored commentary that might otherwise engender undue trepidation on the part of the patient. In addition, surgical limitations must be forthrightly stated, which include the unattainable goal of symmetry, specific anatomic constraints, and reasonable cosmetic/functional improvement. After all of these details have been elaborated, the patient must be granted the opportunity to ask any pertinent questions about the stated limitations, risks, benefits, and alternatives before a formal, informed consent is obtained. The patient then is given the informed consent and left undistracted during careful review of the written document and then signature. The authors have relied on a standardized, detailed dictation "macro" that elaborates all of the material risks and limitations for each procedure and that is incorporated into a typewritten preoperative evaluation note. Although many legitimate alternatives exist for medico-legal documentation, the surgeon always should ensure that some form of written documentation exists that outlines all of the potential negative consequences that may follow surgery.

After the consent is properly obtained, the surgeon should conduct a more formal history and physical examination that covers all aspects of the patient's health and family history in order to determine how extensive a preoperative medical evaluation is required to ensure patient safety during the operation. Guidelines for requisite laboratory studies, related radiographic imaging, cardiac evaluation, and preoperative medical clearance lie beyond the scope of this textbook and should be determined on an individual basis.

After this portion of the preoperative counseling session is completed, the surgeon may delegate the rest of the work to a reliable staff member who can dutifully complete the remaining tasks. The entire surgical process, from arrival at the surgery center through the postoperative recovery period, is explained to the patient as part of preoperative counseling. Details of postoperative care may be overwhelming for the patient at this point, particularly for the individual who will undergo resurfacing, and is best left to the postoperative period. However, the patient should understand clearly the appointed time of arrival, location of surgery, and other related information. For instance, the patient should know that no fingernail polish should be worn on one finger to accommodate the pulse-oximetry meter or that a button-down shirt is preferred in order to avoid the difficulty of a pullover shirt after facial surgery. All of these details are printed in the preoperative instruction sheet (included at the end of this chapter), which should be explained to the patient line by line. Other salient concerns include perioperative use of aspirin, aspirin-related products, herbal medications, or vitamins that can adversely affect hemostasis or exacerbate photosensitivity. Again, the reader is referred to the specific documents that cover these details (appended at the end of this chapter). After everything has been explained to the patient, prescriptions handed over, and postoperative appointments scheduled, the patient should sign a preoperative checklist sheet that states that he or she has been thoroughly counseled, given the opportunity to ask any questions, and has understood all of the presented material. All standardized photographs also should be taken at this session.

The Role of Digital Imaging

Digital imaging has become an indispensable and sole means for photographic documentation, retrieval, and presentation in the authors' practices. This section expounds on how digital imaging can be effectively incorporated into a plastic surgical practice at every level so that 35-mm film may be entirely abandoned. Although technology continues to evolve rapidly, certain basic tenets that relate to setup and execution remain steadfast and are included herein. Some of the material presented will become obsolete, and the reader is referred to the latest periodicals, the Internet, or other reliable sources for updated advice on these matters. Forthcoming sections discuss the effective use of digital morphing and photography separately.

Although 35-mm film has become the standard of professional plastic surgical communication and documentation, digital imaging has quickly made incursions into this exclusive domain. The initial set-up costs for digital imaging clearly exceed that of 35-mm photography, but that margin is diminishing daily. In addition, the savings that accrue over time in terms of expended cost, labor, and time over conventional film will manifest clearly in a relatively short time frame. Paper and ink consumables for ink jet printing remain relatively expensive but fall short of 35-mm transparency film purchases. More important, the time needed to catalog 35-mm film when it returns from the photography laboratory translates into excessive staff labor that could be redirected more profitably elsewhere. Retrieving and reviewing standard transparency film can also be a labor-intensive effort. The added sorting and storage space for film-based photography can also prove burdensome. Over time, film in whatever format fades, scratches, or (even worse) gets lost; whereas digital imaging remains in pristine condition and can be infinitely backed up even in remote locations in order to prevent against theft, loss, or force majeure. The unmatched flexibility of the digital medium should be considered in that electronic communication between physicians can be facilitated and the capacity for digital morphing is possible. Also, because images can be immediately reviewed on the digital viewfinder or computer monitor, the chance of a poor outcome is reduced and the ability to use that information immediately for patient communication is enhanced. Hopefully, the reader has been persuaded that digital imaging offers a viable, photographic medium for a plastic surgical practice.

Two principal input devices exist to capture an image digitally: digital cameras and scanners. Digital cameras have become increasingly affordable, and advanced features can be found even on budget-conscious models. A thorough discussion of the requisite features and options of a digital camera that would be necessary for a plastic surgical practice cannot be persuasively undertaken given the risk of obsolescence of the material presented. Nevertheless, certain fundamental considerations are addressed. The pixel war continues to wage, and resolution quality always has been a preeminent concern. The poor image resolution that accompanies the digital format is the major drawback of digital imaging that diehards of the film medium cite. Although ISO 50 speed film may provide exceptional quality, the grain-versus-pixel debate carries little meaningful value in the world of plastic surgery. Most images obtained on a routine basis never become enlarged beyond an 8-×-10 inch printed format. Even so, no consensus exists as to the equivalent conversion of a film grain to a digital pixel, and estimates have fallen anywhere from 2 to 80 million pixels to achieve parity with a high-quality 35-mm print. The true bottom line is that digital cameras provide superb image quality and ultimately conserve time, labor, and expense.

The key to consistent photography is use of the same camera for all preoperative and postoperative photographs owing to the nuances in the way a digital camera captures an image. Each camera possesses a different dynamic range; that is, the ability to capture the darkest blacks to the lightest whites and all of the intervening colors as well. Color accuracy (discussed under scanners) also can vary significantly among digital cameras. The exact methods by which the reader can achieve consistent, reproducible photographs digitally are discussed in a following section.

Scanners provide a method by which 35-mm film (transparencies, negatives, and prints) can be converted over to the digital medium. For film transparencies or negative exposures, dedicated film scanners so far have provided the optimal conversion quality to digital in terms of accurate translation of color, resolution, and restoration of imperfections in the source image (scratches, color fade, or other noise). In lieu of a film scanner, a flatbed scanner provides versatility and affordability: besides transparencies and negatives, printed images and text also can be transformed into the digital medium. Generally, four parameters exist that define a scanner's optical reproduction quality: optical resolution, bit depth, color accuracy, and optical density. Optical resolution simply refers to the number of pixels per inch (ppi). Pixels per inch is a linear measurement and is different from dots per inch (dpi; also linear), which a printer outputs. Bit depth or color bit depth refers to the maximum number of colors that each pixel of an image can display. For convenience, color depth is defined in terms of power of 2. A black-and-white image, for instance, has two colors or 2 to the first power; therefore, it is termed a one-bit image. At the other end of the spectrum, an RGB True Color image may display 16.7 million colors, which is equivalent to 2 to the 24th power, or 24 bits. Most consumer output devices, printers, and monitors are limited to 24 bits. However, scanners can be 30, 36, or even 42 bits. These scanners actually create a better image. Color accuracy refers to the overall ability of a scanner to reproduce faithfully the original colors of the scanned image. The standard developed by the International Color Consortium (ICC) has allowed testers to measure precisely the "Delta E," or variance of the scanned from the original color. A Delta E of one correlates to the barely perceptible difference between colors seen in a controlled lighting situation by an experienced viewer. Good Delta Es fall below 10, and poorer values may exceed 30. The fourth major specification for a scanner is optical density (OD), and generally is not a descriptor of lower-end models. Optical density refers to the brightness that a scanner is able to capture. Optical density is measured in a logarithmic fashion. Therefore, a scanner with a 3.6 OD has 10 times the brightness of one with a mere 2.8 OD. Generally, OD is not as critical when scanning text or prints but greatly influences the quality of a scanned negative or slide. If a scanner does not boast an OD rating, then one should consider the OD to fall between 2.8 and 3.0. It is recommended that a minimum of 3.2 OD be present for transparencies and 3.4 OD for negatives.

The image must be stored appropriately to permit rapid and easy retrieval once it has been captured. Archiving programs abound, each with touted claims of superiority. More advanced software programs permit attachment of "metatags" to an image (e.g., "crooked nose," "Susan Smith") that facilitate the search for these titles during routine image retrieval or academic research. A simple, reliable method that dispenses with dedicated archiving software is placement of patient images into a folder labeled by the date that the image was taken (e.g., 03-11-6) with the year as the leading value to maintain chronologic integrity, which in turn is placed into a folder with the patient's name (Smith, Susan). All of these images should be backed up on a routine basis to avoid any potential loss owing to a host of unforeseen factors.

After the image has been captured and stored, it can then be outputted via two main techniques, a printer, or a digital projector. Three main types of printers exist on the market today: the laser printer, ink jet printer, and dye-sublimation printer. The ink jet printer remains the mainstay of printing affordable, photographic-quality images but still can extort a high toll for the price of consumables (ink and paper). Nevertheless, the cost of these consumables can be markedly reduced by printing only select photographs for the patient. Generally, the authors print a set of photographs for the patient at 1 week or 1 month in order to show the patient the difference between before-and-after surgery. Of note, these images can be an excellent marketing tool, because enthusiastic patients often show their colleagues and friends the remarkable transformation that has occurred in their appearance. Color laser printers have decreased in price and can provide a cost savings if a heavy volume of printing is projected. The quality of a color laser print typically falls short of the photographic potential of a color ink jet print produced on specially treated paper. However, the cost per page of a laser color print is markedly less than for an ink jet print because of the less expensive consumables used for laser printing (ink and paper). Finally, dye-sublimation printers provide unparalleled quality in even-tone transition that can mimic film photography but may not truly be necessary. Their versatility is also limited, because only photographs of a certain prescribed size may be output and text-based copy cannot be effectively reproduced. Nevertheless, prices for these printers have continued to fall to consumer-friendly levels, and their widespread distribution may be imminent.

As film transparencies have been replaced with digital equivalents, old slide projectors have given way to the advent of digital projectors. Digital presentations are more elegant than film-based presentations in that subtle animation and edited video clips can be embedded into the lecture. In addition, any aspect of the talk can be updated or altered easily at any time without added expense or labor. Portable projectors are a handy way of presenting seminars on-site or off-site. There are many types of projectors available on the market today, all of which can provide excellent image reproduction, including cathode ray tube (CRT) projectors, liquid crystal display (LCD) projectors, digital light projectors (DLP), and plasma display panel (PDP) projectors. Another factor to consider is "native," or uncompressed and unexpanded, resolution level of one of the following grades: VGA (640 × 480), SVGA (800 × 600), XGA (1,024 × 768), SXGA (1,280 × 1,024), and UXGA (1,600 × 1,200). Cathode ray tubes that use an analog-based technology, do not have a native resolution level, but are considered resolution independent, which means that they can handle most computer monitor resolutions without needing to be matched to the monitor's exact resolution. Digital projectors, on the other hand, must be matched to the monitor's resolution. Ideally, they should match the monitor resolution exactly. However, if several computers with different monitor resolutions are to be used with one projector, then the projector should be matched with the highest resolution screen. A minimum of SVGA for simple graphic presentations is recommended, but an SXGA is preferred for improved resolution and display of more detailed images. The other major parameter that defines a projector's quality is the brightness, defined in ANSI lumens. A *minimum* of 300 to 500 ANSI is recommended for dimly lit rooms; a 1,000-ANSI minimum is recommended for well-lit rooms; and larger venues such as auditoriums demand a minimum of 1,500 ANSI. The contrast ratio—which refers to the range of brightest whites to darkest blacks that a projector can display—also affects image quality and can range from a low value of 100:1 to a high value of 2,000:1. Zoom lenses can aid in changing the projected image size without the cumbersome need for physically repositioning the unit. Digital keystone correction refers to the ability of the projector to correct any distortions that may be displayed when the projector is aimed at a wall from an angle.

Digital Morphing Software

Digital morphing software allows a surgeon to alter a patient's image digitally to provide an envisioned surgical outcome. Although this medium can be used effectively for patient communication, it must be properly harnessed to maximize its benefit but minimize confusion and limit liability. Digital morphing is only appropriate in select facial cosmetic surgery. Because any kind of photographic imaging is only a two-dimensional medium, conveyance of three-dimensional information using digital imaging may be poor or inaccurate. For example, digital translocation of tissue may not be readily apparent on the frontal view, because flesh color is moved on top of each other from one part of the face to another. Instead, profile views can be particularly informative when the tissue is moved against the uniform blue background. For instance, the nasal profile can be augmented, rotated, or refined using the digital imager quite effectively (Fig. 3-2A,B). Similarly, a hypoplastic chin, submental fullness, or platysmal diastasis may be very easily depicted with the digital imager (Figs. 3-3A,B; 3-4 A–C; and 3-5 A,B). More important, the patient often fails to appreciate his or her own profile view; therefore, the digital imager provides valuable information that can convince the patient of a cosmetic benefit that would otherwise be incommunicable. The frontal view, on the other hand, still can be used for select purposes in digital morphing. A browlift result can be approximated using digital subtraction techniques between two digital photographs, one showing the native ptotic brow position, and the other the manually lifted brow position (Fig. 3-5 C, D). The brow must be overcorrected somewhat to eliminate the redundant upper-eyelid skin by pulling upward on the brow manually until all of the excess soft tissue and skin have been effaced—a process that typically imparts a startled expression. In order to correct this unnatural appearance, the brow then should be readjusted downward somewhat. Despite the benefit that digital imaging may afford for the patient entertaining brow rejuvenation, simple use of a hand-held mirror and manual elevation of the brow may be a more direct, natural-appearing, and effective technique (Fig. 3-6). Effacement of wrinkles similarly can be very difficult to undertake given the stated limitation with flesh-on-flesh alterations; or worse, digital resurfacing may promise the patient too much (especially the acne-scarred patient), or look bizarrely artificial with a smeared, textureless appearance. Although nasal changes can be appreciated best on lateral view, the width and attitude of a nasal tip, alae, or dorsum can be adjusted or straightened on frontal view using digital imaging with meaningful results. In summary, digital morphing software must be used only in the select cases (e.g., the profile view), in which it would prove beneficial to convince the patient of a cosmetic benefit to surgical intervention.

Despite its benefits, digital morphing software can be a two-edged sword. Liability remains a key reason why many surgeons have not adopted this technology. Fear that an envisioned result may be misinterpreted as a promise of guarantee has hindered even the brave. However, care can be taken to educate the patient that morphing only provides a method of communication and does not represent any claims that the surgical results will approximate the digitally conceived image. Patients are asked to sign a waiver that states their acknowledgment of this fact, which becomes incorporated into the medical record. Further, no altered image is ever given to the patient to take home or saved in the hard drive; therefore, no record is retained of the retouched image. As an important side note, if the patient has already decided on surgery, the surgeon should not endeavor to

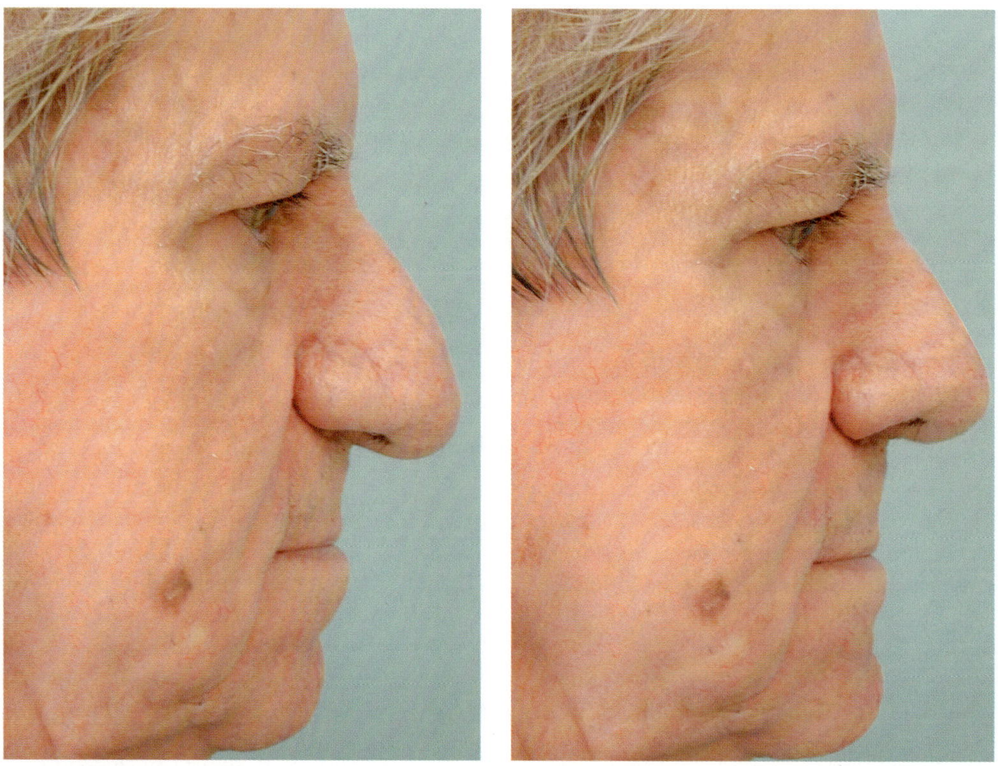

A B

FIGURE 3-2. A,B: These photographs show the projected surgical result of a rhinoplasty and chin implant for the aging nose using a digital imager, which can help enhance patient communication, especially when discussing the profile view.

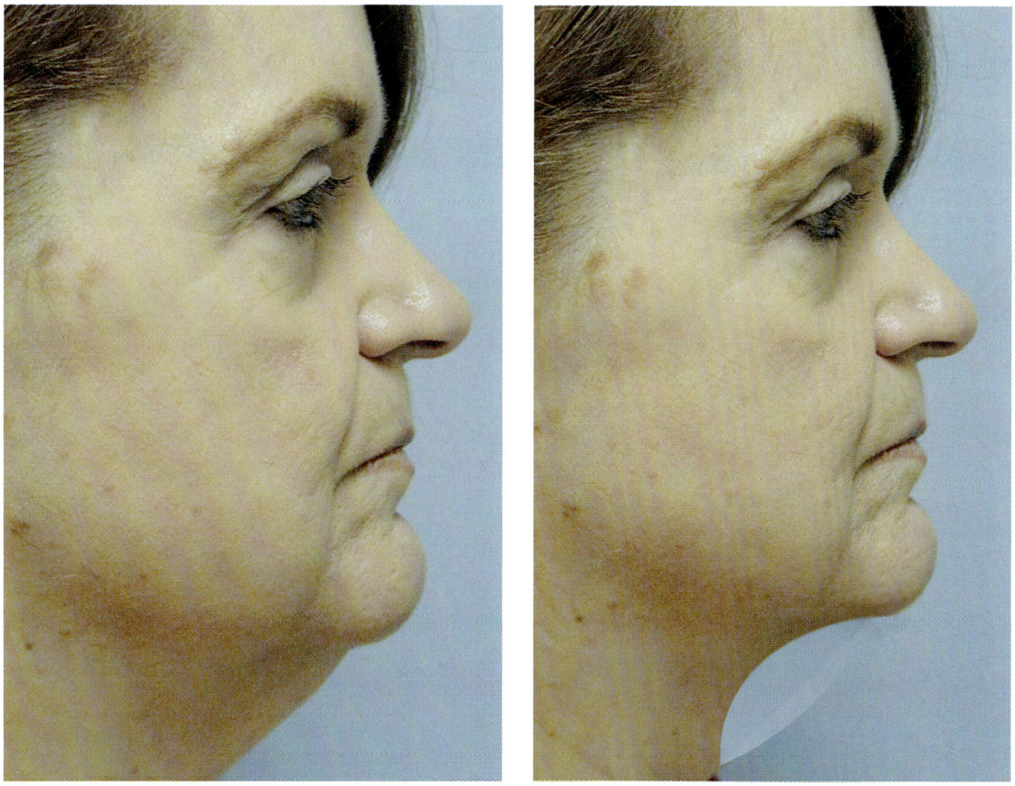

FIGURE 3-3. A,B: The digital imager is used to convince the patient that a facelift and submentoplasty would improve the patient's profile view dramatically. Of note, jowling is a more difficult entity to correct naturally on digital imaging software because the flesh-tone tissue is moved over similarly contrasted tissue.

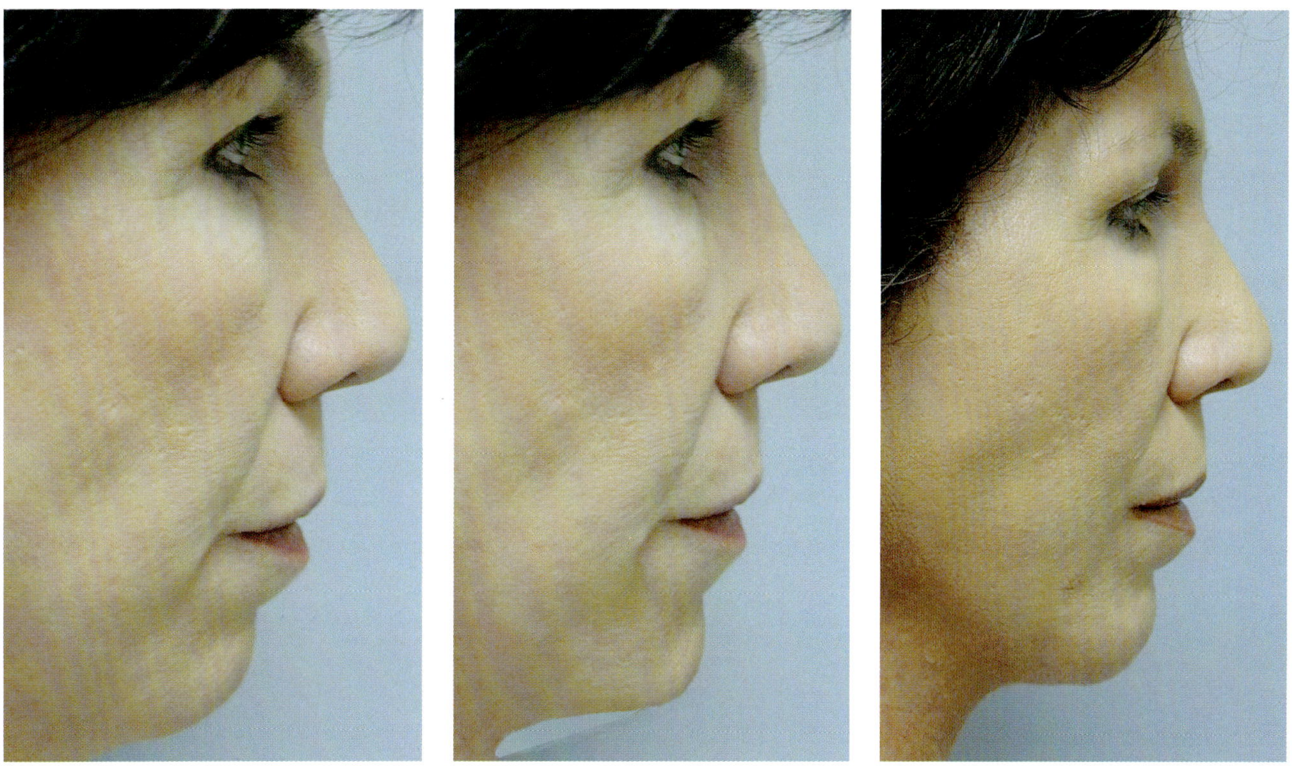

FIGURE 3-4. A–C: The patient is shown with the projected benefit of a chin augmentation, submentoplasty, and facelift on the digital imager **(B)** and 2 months after surgery **(C)**.

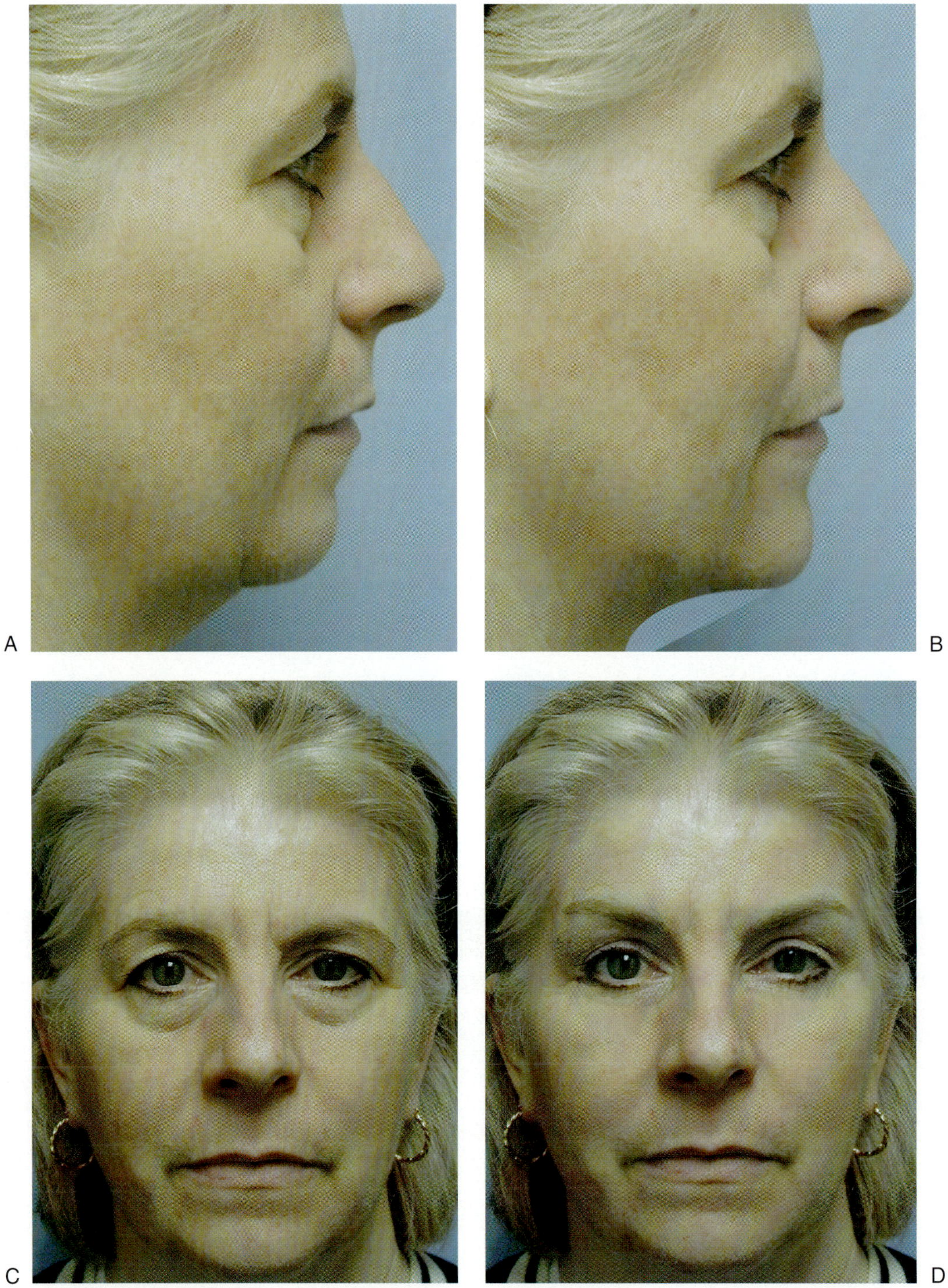

FIGURE 3-5. A,B: The lateral view of the patient shows the projected benefit that a submentoplasty and facelift will give the patient using the digital imaging software **(B)**. Of note, the patient's brow ptosis is not digitally corrected on the lateral view because of difficulty in accomplishing this objective. **C,D:** On frontal view, the patient is shown before and after digital modification of her brow ptosis. Of note, the jowling and neck region are left unretouched because of the difficulty in conveying this information on frontal view. If the patient would like to see a simulation of how a facelift/submentoplasty would appear on frontal view, the surgeon should simply lift the tissues manually and show the benefit to the patient in a hand-held mirror.

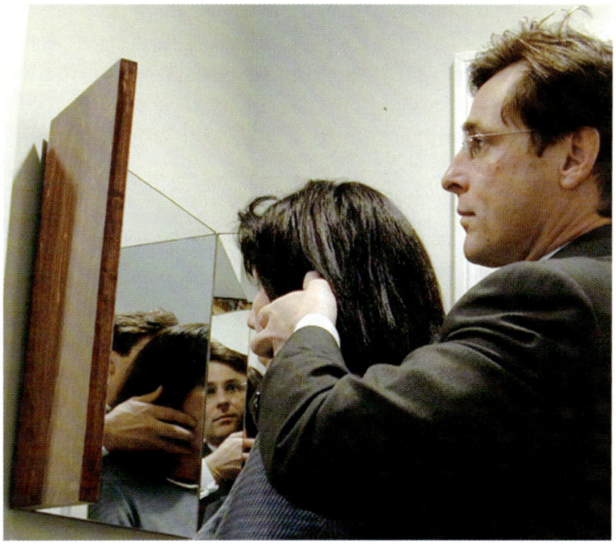

FIGURE 3-6. A mirror and manual elevation of the brow or neckline can be sufficient to convince the patient that surgery would be beneficial. Digital imaging software is not always required or even desirable.

show the patient the digitally morphed image at that point. Doing so may convince the patient that surgery is not indicated and thereby jeopardize the transaction.

Achieving Standardized Photography

Standardized photography is the basis for accurate documentation and dialog. Many physicians are already knowledgeable about how to achieve desired consistency with 35-mm film but may be fearful that digital photography may not provide the same degree of reproducibility. Fortunately, a digital camera can provide excellent, standardized results with the right technique. Primarily, the same camera must be used for all preoperative and postoperative photographs. The differences between images created by two digital cameras even from the same manufacturer will be immediately apparent. In addition, all of the same settings should be maintained (i.e., the exposure value, compression method [JPEG, TIFF, etc.], white balance, and f-stop). Because every camera is different, the physician must experiment with the ideal combination of settings that will provide an optimal image given the setting in which the photograph is taken. Accordingly, a room must be dedicated to take all preoperative and postoperative photographs in order to ensure that the same ambient lighting conditions are maintained. Although flash photography can provide the most even illumination if done properly with balanced lighting, the authors have relied on fluorescent or photoflood lamps and then adjusted the camera's exposure value (usually to the plus side) in order to compensate for any slight deficiency in lighting.

Preferably, the same photographer should be used to take every preoperative and postoperative photograph, but this task may be impractical. To minimize camera shake, the camera can be mounted onto a tripod, which in turn may be poised on a moving dolly, to permit easy positioning. A tripod head that can quickly shift between vertical and horizontal compositions also is helpful. A remote shutter release eliminates any chance of camera blur owing to unsteady hands (Fig. 3-7). Maintenance of camera-to-subject distance is also a critical feature. A line should be drawn across the floor to mark certain prescribed distances where the photographer should be situated vis-à-vis the subject in order to maintain a reproducible distance. If a zoom lens is affixed to a digital camera, the exact same zoom distance must be set to ensure that the image will be kept at the same camera-to-subject distance. For SLR-based digital cameras, a higher image quality may be obtained and greater flexibility is possible. In order to achieve a true 1-to-1 aspect ratio, the size of the CCD (which is analogous to the 35-mm film

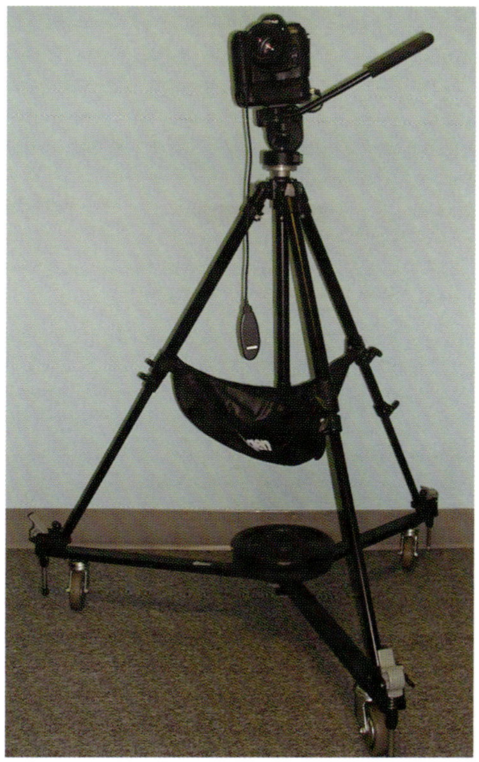

FIGURE 3-7. A Nikon D100 digital camera is outfitted with a 105-mm Nikkor Micro Lens that permits 1-to-1 distortion-free reproduction. The camera is mounted on a tripod, which in turn is poised on a moving dolly that can permit flexibility in camera movement while minimizing camera shake. A quick-release tripod head allows easy removal of the camera from the tripod, and the design of the tripod head permits rapid change of the camera position from a vertical to a horizontal orientation and vice versa. A remote shutter release button also alleviates the risk of any camera shake owing to unsteady shutter release. This camera has an on-demand grid in the viewfinder that facilitates proper alignment of the subject according to the Frankfort Horizontal Plane.

plate) must be known. The manufacturer should be consulted to determine exactly what type of lens offers a 1-to-1, distortion-free image with that particular camera model. Advanced, SLR, digital cameras may also permit an on-demand grid that facilitates accurate composition of the image along the Frankfort horizontal plane. Finally, use of the same compression algorithm is important. The two principal types of compression used today are JPEG and TIFF. Although the latter provides a lossless (no appreciable loss of resolution) compression, JPEG may be the preferable format to capture digital images for speed of retrieval (i.e., opening and closing images) and to minimize storage space. The amount of JPEG compression should be kept low to moderate in order to maintain high quality if a print is desired.

Unlike preoperative and postoperative photography, the authors use slightly different tactics for intraoperative photography to achieve the optimal image (Fig. 3-8). Two overhead operating room lights are positioned at 45-degree angles to the subject, and all of the ambient room lights are turned off. Instead of matrix-style metering, the image is spot metered on the area of interest. This combination of lighting techniques permits the subject to be composed against a uniform black background rather than needing to hold up a blue background or, worse yet, see the wrinkled texture of a blue surgical gown in the background. Again, experimentation with the camera's particular settings ensures that the best image is taken.

Effective Use of Photography

Actual preoperative and postoperative photographs of patients and projected digital morphing images are both effective tools in communicating surgical goals to the patient. Perhaps the most effective method to demonstrate reasonable surgical outcomes is to provide actual preoperative and postoperative photographs of the surgeon's patients. Unfortunately, this option is not possible initially. As patients are accrued, those individuals with desirable outcomes should be approached for consent to use their images in an album that can be shown in turn to the prospective patient. The photographs should be of high quality; that is, standardized poses, proper illumination, and sharply in focus, and, more important, show a convincing improvement. Poor photographs should never be used because they ultimately dissuade the patient about the quality of surgical services. Superior images are absolutely de rigeur for medicolegal documentation, patient communication, and scientific dialog. The photographs selected for display should be bound lavishly in a leather "wedding-album" style binder in which only one set of preoperative and postoperative photographs is displayed on an open page. By maintaining only one set of images per page, the surgeon can control what the patient sees more effectively. An alternative to this style of presentation is to keep all the display images on a PowerPoint presentation on the computer's hard drive. The physician can then access this information easily from any room through a central server without having to maintain several albums or to request that album for every patient visit. Images can be added easily and deleted according to acquisition of better examples of a particular technique. Several PowerPoint presentations should be made, each with a distinct theme (e.g., Rhinoplasty, Skin, Aging Face, Hair Transplantation, etc). The physician exercises ultimate control over patient viewing; he or she can click forward or backward and select only those images he or she wants to present to the patient. If images are captured digitally to begin with, no consumables (paper and ink) are expended; therefore, cost and labor are reduced. To add even greater control over the image, the surgeon should have a monitor that he or she can easily swivel away from the patient when the surgeon does not want the patient to view an image or to maintain the privacy of other patient images. Alternatively, the surgeon can assign a "hot corner" of the screen so that when the mouse is positioned to that corner the monitor fades to black or a screen saver is displayed. However, a swiveling monitor affords the optimal image control for the surgeon. The surgeon should be the only person to show the collective preoperative and postoperative photographs to the patient, because an office staff member may misconstrue or misrepresent the surgical endeavor or perceived outcome. Effective use of preoperative and postoperative photographs along with the use of a hand-held mirror to show the patient the proposed lifting procedure often obviates the need for a digital imaging, or morphing, system.

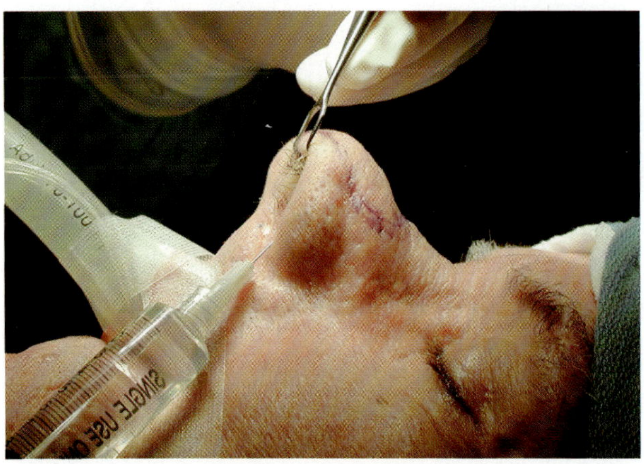

FIGURE 3-8. An intraoperative photograph that shows the preferred technique for proper illumination. Two overhead lights are focused on the subject at 45-degree angles, room lights are turned off, and the camera is set to spot meter off the central aspect of the image. This technique permits a uniform, black background that accentuates the subject without the visual clutter of a wrinkled blue surgical gown or other distracting background elements.

Although ideally the surgeon has an image that matches the prospective patient's precise ethnicity, age, sex, and aesthetic pathology, this objective is not always feasible. Often, a dramatic before-and-after photo may be preferable to an exact age and sex match in every case. For instance, if a 40-year-old patient would like some improvement in the jaw line, an image of a more mature lady who has a very convincing preoperative and postoperative photographic difference may prove more beneficial than a patient of a similar age group who shows only a mild improvement. The key, as always, is to show photographs that will impress the patient. The "wow factor" should underscore selection of every photograph used for display.

INTRAOPERATIVE CONSIDERATIONS: THE OPERATING ROOM EXPERIENCE

The Operating Room Environment

Undergoing surgery for any reason is an anxiety-provoking experience. Every aspect of the presurgical and surgical experience should be tailored to reduce surgical anxiety and achieve as relaxed an environment as possible. The patient should be asked to arrive shortly before the anticipated surgery in order to allow adequate time to prepare, but not excessively early to limit the anxiety engendered by a protracted wait. Once the patient arrives to the surgical facility and has been properly greeted, the necessary paperwork should be completed expeditiously so that an intravenous line can be started and anxiolytic medications delivered as needed.

As the patient is brought into the operating room, the environment should exude tranquility and order. On entry, warm blankets should be offered to the patient to limit the shivering that manifests because of anxiety and cool, ambient temperature. All personnel should remain focused on the patient, and irrelevant conversations kept to an absolute minimum. Soothing music played at low volume can reinforce the appropriate mood and somewhat mitigate the sterile, medical character of the operating room experience. Classical music remains an unobtrusive and innocuous choice that can encourage the right temperament in the patient. Preparation of electrocardiogram (ECG) leads, oxygen-saturation monitors, and other equipment should proceed in an efficient and orderly manner, allowing the induction of anesthesia to begin as soon as possible. Another option that may further enhance patient relaxation is use of medical massage before entry into the operating room suite. A licensed masseuse can alleviate stress and create a favorable mood for the patient, which should be maintained until the patient has received induction of anesthesia. Although all of these points may seem rather intuitive, they are worthy of reiteration herein and to the staff who assist the surgeon, especially if the procedure is performed in an off-site facility where cosmetic patients are a rarity and the staff is less mindful of these attributes.

Patient positioning is very important for facial cosmetic procedures. The patient's head should be far enough away from the anesthesiologist/anesthetist to permit a comfortable, working space. For the aging face, the surgeon often needs to be above and on either side of the patient at various times. Accordingly, turning the table 90 degrees away from the anesthesiologist facilitates easy maneuverability around the patient's head without interfering with the anesthesiologist's work. If the patient does not require any direct airway support (e.g., endotracheal intubation or laryngeal mask airway), the operating room table should be positioned at a 90-degree angle to the anesthesiologist when the patient enters the room. In addition, a bed whose head can be easily raised or lowered also may be beneficial, especially for brow surgery or a chemical peel in which the patient should be in a semierect posture for part of the time (Fig. 3-9). A comfortable head rest that extends beyond the principal stretcher is also a welcome feature. A headrest is more comfortable for the patient and keeps the head in the desired position during the procedure. In addition, the surgeon can approach the patient more closely than if the head were resting on the main table itself, and the surgeon can rest his or her feet more easily under the table to ease back strain if the surgeon is seated. A stretcher that can double as an operating table has provided the optimal solution in the senior author's practice: The patient can be brought into and out of the operating room without significant labor and with utmost efficiency.

Another notable attribute that should be installed in every operating room is a computer monitor that can display the patient's preoperative images in all standardized views (Fig. 3-10). Accessing the images from a central server permits easy retrieval and display of the digitally acquired images. Display of preoperative images can guide surgery by reminding the surgeon of the precise anatomic deficits when the patient was in an upright, undisturbed pose. When the patient is supine on the operating room table, has received local infiltration, and exhibited edema from prolonged surgery, the exact preoperative pathology may be forgotten easily. For off-site surgery, a laptop computer loaded with the patient's images or a printed hard copy of all the preoperative views should be prominently displayed in the operating room.

Anesthesia Considerations

For most cosmetic procedures, anesthesia can be administered using inhalational agents with the use of an endotracheal tube or laryngeal airway mask (general anesthesia) or alternatively with monitored intravenous anesthesia (monitored anesthesia care, MAC). Both techniques are combined with local injectable anesthesia with a vasoconstrictive agent in order to provide regional analgesia and vasoconstriction, thereby allowing a lighter plane of overall anesthesia. Occasionally a patient is encountered, usually a young male rhinoplasty patient, who will not tolerate MAC, but in most instances anesthesia is a choice made by the patient, surgeon, and anesthesiologist. The patient who also tends to

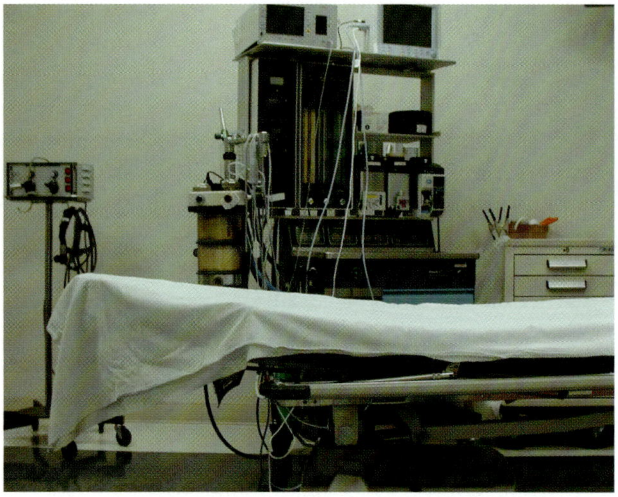

A

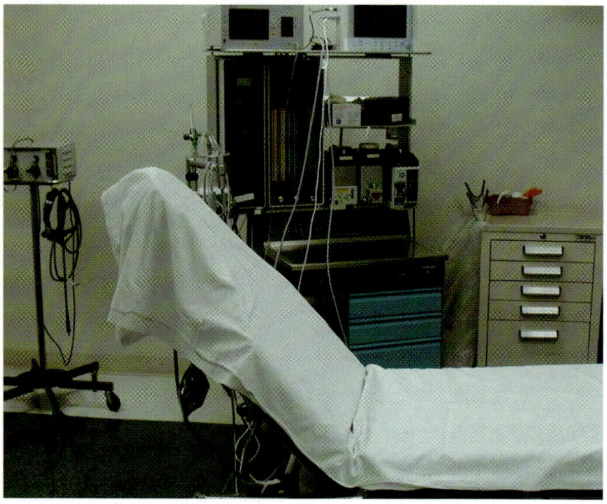

B

FIGURE 3-9. A,B: The ideal operating table for elective, ambulatory facial cosmetic procedures should have the following attributes: (a) a headrest that allows comfortable surgeon positioning around the patient's head; (b) the ability to incline and decline the upper torso; and (c) the table can double as a stretcher so that the patient can be transported out of the room without having to transfer him or her onto a separate, recovery bed. The position of the operating table should also be situated 90 degrees to the anesthesiologist to provide maximal working space.

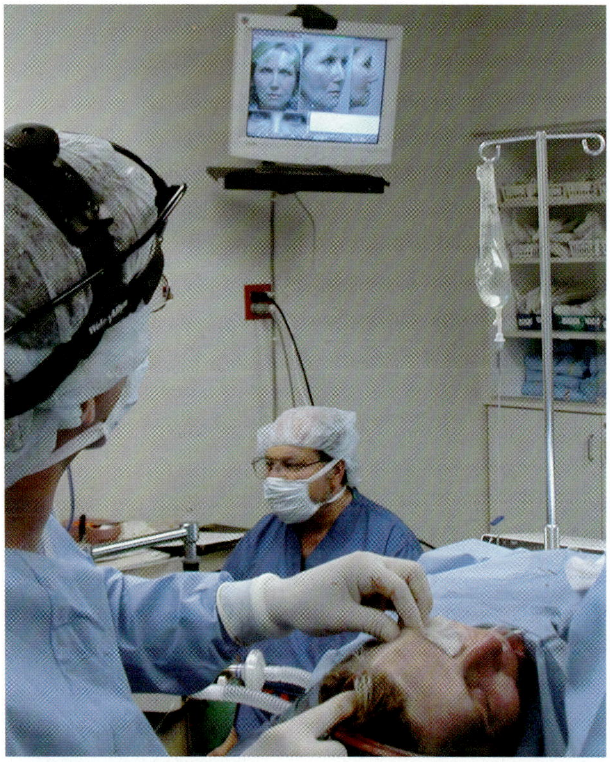

FIGURE 3-10. Intraoperative display of all standardized views of the patient permits review of the patient's salient aesthetic deficits in his or her undisturbed, upright state during the procedure. When the patient is supine, local anesthesia has been infiltrated, and the edema has set in, the surgeon may fail to grasp the precise surgical objectives without the aid of these photographic references.

consume alcohol on a routine basis may have a very high anesthetic requirement owing to faster hepatic metabolism. Accordingly, if the proclivity for this social habit is gleaned from the patient's history, a general anesthetic may be preferable to reduce overall anesthetic burden and increase patient compliance during the procedure. The advantages of general anesthesia for facial cosmetic procedures are few: convenience of the anesthesiologist and surgeon or occasionally the required deeper level of anesthesia in the difficult patient. The disadvantages are many, including longer recovery with greater risk of postoperative nausea, throat discomfort from the endotracheal tube, inconvenience of the tube obstructing the operative field (especially for lower facial surgery), greater fluctuations in blood pressure on emergence, and the rare possibility of dental injury or failure to obtain an airway. The major advantages of MAC are that the patient awakens promptly after the cessation of anesthesia, is able to tolerate fluids shortly thereafter, and may be discharged to the comfort of home usually after a relatively brief observation period. Other advantages mirror the disadvantages of general anesthesia, including lack of laryngeal manipulation and related throat discomfort, absence of the endotracheal tube in the operative field, less nausea and vomiting, and more stable blood pressure readings. With regard to cost, general anesthesia is probably less expensive to deliver. However, the overall cost savings may be lost when considering staff time to recover the patient and the cost of oxygen during that time. Monitored anesthesia care has the distinct disadvantage that it requires a skilled anesthesiologist comfortable with this type of delivery, who is willing to deal with the variable level of anesthesia and occasional apneic spells that the patient may experience. If the anesthesiologist expresses unease about MAC anesthesia, it may be best to avoid this option for patient safety and compliance during the procedure. Additionally, the surgeon occasionally must tolerate patient responsiveness and the associated movement. However, with skilled delivery and communication between the surgeon and anesthesiologist, MAC is greatly preferred.

Regardless of whether MAC or general anesthesia is elected, thoughtful use of local anesthesia with a vasoconstrictive additive (e.g., epinephrine) is encouraged. Adjunctive local anesthesia provides the advantage of allowing a lighter level of anesthesia because of increased local-pain threshold as well as the benefit that vasoconstriction affords in terms of overall hemostasis. The precise sites for anesthetic injection are discussed in the following chapters that cover specific surgical procedures; they will not be reiterated here. However, general principles are emphasized. Infiltration of local anesthetic should begin shortly after the onset of general or MAC anesthesia in order to take advantage of the initial deep state of anesthesia associated with this phase and to allow adequate time for the onset of vasoconstriction and anesthetic effect. Generally, 10 minutes of delay are necessary to meet these objectives. Only the surgical area to be addressed first should be infiltrated, and those facial regions that will be violated after 45 minutes should be injected in a staged fashion. For instance, when the surgeon is 10 minutes away from concluding one side of a facelift, the contralateral side should be infiltrated to permit uninterrupted surgical progress. The surgeon should announce to the anesthesiologist that additional local anesthesia is about to be delivered for two reasons: (a) the anesthesiologist can adjust the level of sedation to minimize patient discomfort during the injection process; and (b) the anesthesiologist will be attuned to any vital sign changes caused by the vasoconstrictive agent. In addition, areas that have just been completed should receive immediate application of ice packs to limit postoperative edema. An ice pack may be held in place by repositioning the towel that circumscribes the hair to accommodate the ice pack as well. However, no amount of ice substitutes for a gentle surgical hand and expeditious surgery.

The patient should receive adequate oxygen delivery (2 to 3 L/min via nasal cannula or greater with humidified face tent) in the immediate postoperative setting, which may limit postoperative nausea. In addition, adequate hydration and continued warming with air-inflated devices or warming blankets continue patient comfort and possibly minimize postoperative nausea. A prophylactic dose of an intravenous antiemetic agent also may preclude against unwanted nausea. The patient should remain in a semiinclined position with liberal use of ice packs to the operated facial regions to counteract undesirable edema throughout the immediate recovery period and be reminded to do so on return home. Visual contact with the surgeon at every phase of the operation also provides comfort and reassurance that the surgeon is at the helm of the team and is up to date with the patient's progress.

POSTOPERATIVE CONSIDERATIONS: CARE, FOLLOW-UP AND COMPLICATIONS

Maintaining Patient Rapport

Patient rapport should be maintained from the initial encounter through the postoperative period. The surgeon only constitutes one individual in the chain who must maintain excellent patient rapport. The patient-care coordinator serves as the common link between the patient and the practice for any concerns and acts as the spokesperson of the practice. However, the presence of the patient-care coordinator should never be used as a convenient crutch for the surgeon to dodge patient contact. No substitute exists for an outstanding, sustained relationship between the surgeon and patient, no matter how strained this bond may become postoperatively. If a poor surgical outcome arises or the patient perceives the outcome to be such, then the surgeon should devote extra effort to nurture this relationship. The single most important factor for patient dissatisfaction and eventual legal action is poor physician–patient rapport, *not* a bad surgical outcome. When the patient appears disgruntled or dissatisfied with any part of patient care or the actual surgery, then the physician must attend to these concerns immediately and on a continued basis until a resolution can be attained. All staff members should be aware of the dissatisfied patient and the exact nature of the concern so that a uniform front can be established to help assuage the patient and address the problem at hand. A logbook also should be retained that lists all dissatisfied patients and their concerns in order to minimize phone contact; if not, ask for frequent return visits to improve their disposition. Ignoring the patient is the absolutely worse course of action and only exacerbates the condition.

The question then becomes: How does one develop rapport? The answer may be more elusive than can be easily addressed here, but certain mannerisms and behavior during patient interaction can assist in developing good rapport. First, on entering the room the physician should greet the patient with a warm smile and good eye contact, and then sit down alongside the patient. Even in the maelstrom of a busy clinic, sitting while interacting with a patient affords the illusion of patience even if the elapsed time remains relatively brief. When a patient expresses a concern, the physician should recognize that it bothers the patient and therefore acknowledge that concern even if the problem is imperceptible to the physician. Patients may peer into the mirror for a long time, lamenting over the most negligible imperfection that may be transformed into a glaring emblem of poor surgery in their fixated mind. At times, patients may focus on minor flaws only because they are uncertain whether what they see represents normal healing or an aberrant departure from that norm. Gentle reassurance often is all that is needed. No two patients are identical in their need for physician or staff encouragement, or hand holding, in the postoperative setting. In addition, the resurfaced patient requires more guidance and dedication on the part of the staff to ensure that the postoperative instructions are carefully adhered to and that the patient remains at ease with his or her appearance. Maintaining good patient rapport not only reduces the risk of litigation, but also prevents the patient from expressing dissatisfaction vocally to friends, neighbors, and acquaintances. Gaining a new patient is much more difficult than maintaining an established patient, and every effort should be undertaken to preserve that trust.

Managing the Difficult Patient

Managing the difficult patient is a natural extension of the concepts elaborated in the previous section on maintaining patient rapport. However, several, specific issues related to patient management also should be addressed individually. In many ways difficult patients who behave badly may be viewed as toddlers who act out to gain attention or for other secondary gain. The physician must assiduously delineate justified from unjustified behavior and not encourage the latter. A very fine distinction exists between providing good care and promoting bad behavior. Several clinical examples may prove illustrative. A patient who has been receiving regular collagen injections now for several years calls to request that the injection be performed that day without a scheduled appointment because of an important, upcoming social engagement. The physician should try his or her best to accommodate this request, if possible, because the patient has an established relationship with the practice that the physician desires to maintain. This scenario differs from the new patient who calls and says that he or she cannot make the appointment tomorrow and must be seen today. This is an unreasonable request and should be declined unless the schedule conveniently permits. To do otherwise supports a behavior pattern destined to disrupt the practice in the future. Another example is a patient who presents for evaluation of a nevus and demands its excision during that visit despite the fact that the appointment time does not allow for it. This patient should be informed that if the excision were undertaken at that time, it would delay the remainder of the clinic and be unfair to the remaining patients. Additionally, the surgeon can reinforce that the patient would not like to be similarly delayed because of another patient's need for personal gratification. As discussed in the section regarding developing employee trust, a patient must not be allowed to interfere with the physician–staff relationship. Even if the staff has committed an obvious mistake, the patient must be expected to treat the staff with respect. Discussion with the staff about the error should take place in private. The staff should be supported. The physician should never undermine a valued staff relationship in order to appease a patient. Office policy should dictate that every staff member who has been treated inappropriately by a patient should notify the physician of the transgression.

The unhappy patient may be categorized into two broad groups: those unhappy with a good result and those unhappy with a bad result (as interpreted by the physician). In either case, the physician must acknowledge the patient's dissatisfaction and suggest a resolution, even if that simply entails further observation. In the case of the unhappy patient with a reasonably good result, the source of the displeasure may lie in the divergent expectations that the patient and physician hold. Preoperative and postoperative photographs often help to instruct the patient in a concrete way as to the notable, aesthetic improvement. The photographs should reveal a degree of improvement even if they fail to measure up to the patient's expectations. If the patient continues to express discontent, then the surgeon should try to delineate more precisely the cause and offer to correct the problem if deemed possible. If it is a minor surgical endeavor, the surgeon can readily absorb the cost. Greater differences in perceived outcome may require that the patient accept some responsibility until a reasonable course of action is determined. In the event that the surgeon and patient are unsatisfied with the result, corrective surgery can be offered at no charge. If surgery is performed at an ambulatory surgical facility, the patient may need to incur a facility fee. Alternatively, the physician may offer to cover this expense as well. As an example of an easily correctable problem, the rhinoplasty patient with a dorsal contour irregularity can be rasped in the office setting to satisfy both the patient and physician. Patients who suggest that a refund should be given must be firmly declined. Payment for medical services compensates for the physician's training and best surgical effort but never implies a guaranteed result. Additionally, return of funds is an admission of wrongdoing that has potentially adverse medico-legal ramifications.

Patients who have visited another surgeon and been unsatisfied with the result may be categorized in the same fashion: those with a legitimate complaint and those who bear unrealistic expectations of the surgical result. Above all, the surgeon should never denounce a colleague, because it speaks poorly of his or her own professional demeanor, may engender medico-legal action, and would not be well received if a colleague did likewise. For the patient without a legitimate complaint, the surgeon should reinforce that the other surgeon performed an adequate surgery. For a patient with a reasonable complaint, the surgeon should encourage the patient to return to the erstwhile surgeon to seek further advice. If the patient refuses and the surgeon believes that the result can be improved, then the patient should be asked to return for another consultation. In these circumstances, an additional consultation session with the patient may help establish trust, delineate expectations clearly, and expose any of the patient's irrationalities. If a staff member expresses reservation about a potential patient, the surgeon should seriously listen to the comment and contemplate whether any kind of surgery is advisable. Using every measure of information that can be collected about a prospective patient allows the surgeon the best effort to avoid a potential problem. Some manipulative patients berate the staff but hold the surgeon with respect. These patients prove to be genuine problems after surgery. If the surgeon feels that the patient may be litigious, it is always better to refuse surgery than to embark on surgery that will be fraught with long-term regret.

SUMMARY

Although surgical excellence should form the underpinning of every successful plastic surgical practice, uncompromising and superb perioperative care is equally important to sustain growth of the practice. The patient-care coordinator ensures that a friendly, personal face is stamped on each patient encounter and facilitates a smooth transition between every phase of patient care. Excellent photography optimizes medico-legal documentation, patient dialog, and scientific communication; and the digital medium may provide the most effective method to accomplish these objectives. The operating room should provide the patient an embracing and comforting environment during a trying, anxiety provoking time and further reinforce positive patient rapport. The postoperative period must continue excellent patient care and maintain rapport, especially in those patients who may exhibit signs of discontent, whether justifiable or not. Despite the exceptional marketing strategies enumerated in the previous chapter, a successful plastic surgical practice is built one patient at a time. This chapter has endeavored to provide a blueprint for a jubilant, return patient.

AUTHORIZATION AND INFORMED CONSENT

Patient's Name: ____

I request and authorize ____________________________, M.D. (the physician) to perform an operation on me or my ____________________________ entitled (description of procedure):

____

____

____

The nature and effects of the operation, the risks, ramifications, complications involved, as well as alternative methods of treatment, have been fully explained to me by the Doctor and I understand them.

I authorize the Doctor to perform any other procedure that he or she may deem desirable in attempting to improve the condition stated in paragraph one (1) or any unhealthy or unforeseen condition that may be encountered during the operation.

I consent to the administration of anesthetics by the Doctor or by the Anesthesiologist or Nurse Anesthetist responsible for the service.

I have been thoroughly and completely advised regarding the objectives of the operation. Because I understand that the practice of medicine and surgery is not an exact science and therefore that no reputable surgeon can guarantee results, I acknowledge that imperfections might ensue and that the operative result may not live up to my expectations. I certify that no guarantees have been made by anyone regarding the operation(s) I have requested and authorized. I understand that in the unlikely case where an imperfection results that the patient and the doctor determine the necessity of a secondary procedure, such revisions are not included in the initial surgical facility or anesthesia fee, but they will be billed at a lesser rate.

I understand that the two sides of the human body are not the same and can never be made the same. If during the consultation(s) Dr. ____________________________ used computerized imaging he or she emphasized to me that this was used for communication purposes and in an attempt to determine if my expectations for surgery were realistic. He or she emphasized to me that the image created is an ideal goal. However, because of the unpredictability of wound healing and biology, the desired goal was in no way promised as an outcome of surgery. I give permission to Dr. ____________________________ or a staff member to take still or motion clinical photographs with the understanding that such remain the property of the doctor.

If, in the judgment of the Doctor, medical research, education, or science will benefit from their use, such photographs and related information may be published and republished in professional journals or medical books, or used for such publication or use, including as presentation material. I shall not be identified by name.

I understand that if Dr. ____________________________ judges at any time that my surgery should be postponed or canceled for any reason, he or she may do so.

I hereby authorize that the information furnished to Dr. ____________________________ by me during my diagnostic evaluation is correct.

I have received complete instructions given to me by Dr. ____________________________ and his or her staff and I have agreed to follow the instructions to the best of my ability before, during, and after my surgical procedure.

The risk of complications despite proper treatment exists in all cases but can be reduced by carefully following my aftercare instructions and by notifying the office at ____________________________ if a problem develops. I agree that a full set of instructions and prescriptions were given to me and again reviewed by the staff, including ____________________________

I certify that I have read the above authorization, that the explanations referred to therein were made to my satisfaction, and that I fully understand such explanations and the above authorization.

Signed ____

(Patient or person authorized to consent for the patient.)

Witness ______________________________ Date ____________

PHOTOGRAPHIC RELEASE FORM

Record of Authorization for Taking and Publication of Photographs

In connection with the medical services, which I am receiving from my physician, Dr. __________, I consent that photographs may be taken of me or parts of my body under the following conditions:

A. The photographs may be taken only with the consent of my physician and under such conditions and at such time as may be approved by him or her.

B. The photographs shall be taken by my physician or by a photographer approved by my physician.

C. The photographs shall be used for medical records and media purposes, and if in the judgment of Dr. __________, medical research, education, or science will benefit from their use, such photographs and information relating to my case may be published and republished, either separately or in connection with each other, in professional journals, books, pamphlets, or the Internet, or used for any other purpose that he or she may deem proper in the interest of medical education, knowledge, or research; provided, however, that it is specifically understood that in any such publication or use I shall not be identified by name.

Patient's Name (PRINT) ______________________________

Patient's Signature ______________________ **Witness** ______________________

Date ______/______/______ **Phone No.** (____)______-________

Type(s) of Surgery ______________________________

If a minor or patient is unstable to affix signature:

Proxy/Guardian's Name (PRINT) ______________________________

Proxy/Guardian's Signature ______________________ **Relationship** ______________________

HISTORY AND PHYSICAL FORM

Patient's Name ______________________________ Date of Birth _____/_____/_____

Procedure Planned ______________________________

____

Present Problem/Indication for Procedure ______________________________

____

Significant Past Medical History ______________________________

Diabetes	Y N		Heart Disease	Y N	
Lung Disease	Y N		MI	Y N	
Asthma	Y N		MVP	Y N	
Hepatitis	Y N		Hypertension	Y N	
Neuro/Stroke	Y N		Abx	Y N	

Significant Surgical History

____

____

Significant Family History of Cardiovascular Disease

____

____

Tobacco Use	Y N	Amount _________
Alcohol	Y N	Amount _________
Drug Use	Y N	Amount _________

History of Anesthesia Problems/Reactions: Self Y N Family Y N

Explain ______________________________

____

Medications

____

____

Allergies (Including Reactions)

____

____

Latex Allergy Y N

Physical Examination (Pertinent to Procedure)

V/s HR _________ BP _________ Temp _________

Normal Abnormal (Explain)

Head & Neck ______________________________

CV/Lungs ______________________________

Body ______________________________

Examiner ______________________________ Date _______/_______/_______

PERSONAL PRICE SHEET

for

(Place Name Here)

	PROCEDURE(S)	*PRICE*
1.		
2.		
3.		
4.		
FACILITY FEE		
ANESTHESIA FEE		
TOTAL		

As a reminder, you must have someone pick you up and stay with you overnight if you have had anything more than local anesthesia.

In addition to the surgeon's fee, other charges may include blood work, ECG, pathology, x-ray, and prescription medications (if necessary). The preceding quotation is valid provided any surgery is schedule within 1 year of the date signed below, for surgeons fees only, unless a discounted price is offered in which case, the surgical fee is valid for 90 days only. If more surgery is performed other than originally estimated (i.e., moles, skin lesions, or medically indicated functional surgery), there will be an additional charge.

A deposit of $500 is required in order to insure your scheduled date of surgery. Full payment is due 2 weeks prior to your surgery; at that time your consult fee will be deducted if the procedure is over $1,000. If the surgical date is canceled less than 7 days before surgery, 20% of the surgical fee will be deducted. If the surgery is canceled on the date of surgery, no refund will be offered.

____ _______/_______/_______

Please sign here Date

CONSENT FOR OFF-SITE COMPANION SERVICES

I ______________________________ understand that ______________________________ will be staying with me, not to perform nursing care, but as a companion. I understand that I will employ ____________________ from the time I leave the office/hospital after my procedure until I return to the office the following day for my postoperative visit. The service is in no way associated with Dr. __________________'s practice.

Signature: ______________________________

Witness: ______________________________

Date: ________________

PREOPERATIVE CHECKLIST

Patient's Name ____

Procedure(s)____

Date of Surgery ____________________ Date of Consult #2 ______________________

Phone Number Where Patient Can Be Reached the Night of Surgery ____________________

- ☐ Photographs taken
- ☐ Preoperative Instruction Sheet reviewed with patient
- ☐ Surgical Consent Forms signed by patient
- ☐ Prescriptions given: (Please circle)
  Keflex 250 mg po q.i.d. (or if allergy to PCN, then Emycin 250 mg po q.i.d.), one refill
  Clindamycin 150 mg po q.i.d., disp. three pills (if mitral valve prolapse), no refill
  Sig.: two tabs 1 hour prior to surgery, take one tab 6 hours after surgery
  Darvocet N-100 one tab po q 4 prn, disp. 15 pills, one refill OR
  Lortab 5/500 one tab po q 4 to 6 prn, disp. 15 pills, one refill OR
  Tylenol #3 1 to 2 tabs po q 4 to 6 prn, disp. 15 pills, one refill (for smaller office-based procedures)
  Valtrex 500 mg po b.i.d., #14 pills (for perioral resurfacing), one refill
  Phenergan 25 mg pr q6 prn, disp. four pills, no refill (after general or MAC anesthesia)
  For browlift and facelift surgery, Decadron 4 mg two tabs q8 after surgery, two tabs 8 hours after first dose (patient cannot have diabetes, peptic ulcer disease, immunosuppression; for example, HIV, malignancy), no refill

- ☐ List medications the patient is taking
- ☐ Make sure patient is not taking aspirin-related products, herbal or vitamin supplements
- ☐ List allergies to medication:
- ☐ Anesthesia: Review type of anesthesia (local, oral sedation, MAC, general)
- ☐ EKG if (a) + family history and/or symptoms; (b) female over 50 years old; or (c) male over 45
- ☐ Transportation arrangements:
- ☐ NPO 8 hours prior to surgery. Patient may take sip of water for BP meds.
- ☐ Make appointment for postoperative visits (if not already done):

  Rhinoplasty, Blepharoplasty: suture excision at 1 week Date: _________ Time: _________

  Facelift (Tuesday): next day, Friday, Monday, Wednesday Date: _________ Time: _________

  Browlift (Tuesday): next day, Friday, MondayDate: _________ Time: _________

  TCA Peel: next day, day #2, day #3, day #7, day #9, day #14 Date: _________ Time: _________

- ☐ Make sure someone is staying with the patient after surgery.
- ☐ Payment is due 2 weeks prior to surgery. Make checks payable to: ____________________
- ☐ Make sure that Gore-Tex is ordered or already in office for patient. AlloDerm (LifeCell Corporation, Branchburg, New Jersey) should be made on Friday prior to surgery for delivery Monday, if surgery is to be performed on Tuesday.
- ☐ Does the patient have a health care proxy? If so, he or she needs to bring the paperwork with him or her the day of surgery so OR can make a copy for their chart.
- ☐ The patient should not drive or operate heavy machinery during the first postoperative week or when the patient is taking narcotic painkillers and should only resume these activities after explicit approval by the physician.

I have carefully read the foregoing information regarding my preoperative procedures and have had any and all questions answered to my fullest understanding.

______________________________ ______________________
Patient Signature Date

______________________________ ______________________
Physician/Nurse/Office Staff Signature Date

GENERAL PREOPERATIVE INSTRUCTION SHEET

Aspirin and Aspirin-Related Products

Aspirin and aspirin-related products (see following list) should not be taken 2 weeks before or after surgery because they increase the tendency of bleeding. For this reason, it is very important that contents of any over-the-counter preparations be checked carefully prior to their use. Many headache preparations, cold remedies, and "hangover cures" contain aspirin. The chemical name of aspirin is acetylsalicylic acid.

Examples of drugs containing salicylates (aspirin) follow:

Acetidine	Bufferin	Liquiprin
Alka-Seltzer	Coricidin	Midol
Anacin	Darvon Compound	Pepto-Bismol
Anahist	Dristan	Persistin
APC	Ecotrin	Sal-Sayne
Aspirin	Empirin Compound	Stanback
BC	Excedrin	Theracin
Bromo-Quinine	4-Way Cold Tablets	Trigesic
Bromo-Seltzer	Inhiston	

Examples of aspirin-related products follow:

Advil	Ibuprofen	Orudis
Anaprox	Indocin	Oruvail
Ansaid	Indomethacin	Piroxicam
Arthrotect	Ketoprofen	Ponstel
Cataflem	Ketorolac	Relafen
Celebrex	Lodine	Sulindac
Celecoxib	Mefenamic Acid	Tolectin
Clinoril	Mobic	Tolmetin
Daypro	Motrin	Toradol
Diclofenac	Naprelan	Vioxx
Dolobid	Naprosyn	Voltaren
Etodolac	Naproxen	
Feldene	Nuprin	

You can substitute **TYLENOL** (acetaminophen) for these products if you require pain medication before surgery. Check with your pharmacist if you are uncertain whether a medicine contains aspirin.

Herbal Medications and Nutritional Supplements

Some herbal medications and nutritional supplements may also increase bleeding or photosensitivity (i.e., sun sensitivity). Please discontinue all herbal medications and nutritional supplements 2 weeks before and after surgery. In particular, discontinue use of the following medications and supplements 2 weeks before and after surgery. Some of the following plant foods (e.g., celery, dill, fennel) may be used in moderation in your diet.

Some herbal medications that may make you bleed:

Bilberry	Hawthorne	Sweet vernal grass leaves
Black cohosh rhizome	Horse chestnut bark	Sweet-scented bedstraw plant
Bromelain	Kava kava	Tonka bean seeds
Cayenne	Licorice root	Valerian
Dong quai	Ma huang (ephedra)	Vanilla leaf leaves
Echinacea	Meadow sweet flower	Willow bark
Feverfew	Melatonin	Wintergreen leaves
Fish oil caps	Poplar bark or buds	Woodruff plant
Garlic	St. John's wort	Yohimbe
Ginseng	Sweet birch bark	
Ginkgo biloba	Sweet clover plant	

Some herbal medications that may make you sensitive to the sun:

Angelica root and fruit	Cow parsnip	Fig
Celery	Parsley	Goosefoot
Dill	Queen Anne's lace	Lemon peel
Fennel	Agrimony	Psoralea seeds
Khella fruit	Bergamot peel	Rue leaves
Lomatium root	Bitter orange peel	St. John's wort
Lovage root	Buttercup plant	Yarrow plant

Vitamins

If you are taking a routine multivitamin, you may continue doing so. However, if you are taking *any vitamin E pills*, please stop 2 weeks before and after surgery, because this may increase your chance of bleeding.

Prescribed Medications

If you are taking prescription medications (e.g., for high blood pressure), please continue to do so even the morning of surgery, except:

1. If you are diabetic, please refrain from taking your diabetic pills or insulin injection the morning of surgery because you will not eat or drink anything that morning. Please also check your blood sugar level that morning prior to coming to the hospital or clinic. If your blood sugar is excessively low (below 80), you may take a few sips of orange juice.
2. If you are taking prescription pain medications (e.g., for arthritis), please ask us if you can safely continue these medications. Some medications contain aspirin or aspirinlike products that may cause you to bleed. (See the previous page for list of aspirin-related products.)

If you are asthmatic, please take your inhaler(s) the morning of surgery as well as per your routine schedule.

Diet

Do not eat or drink anything (including gum, mints, etc.) after midnight the night before surgery. On the morning of surgery, you may have a few sips of water when you take your prescription medications. Otherwise, do not eat or drink anything that morning.

Tobacco

Nicotine in any form, including cigarettes, cigars, chewing tobacco, and even transdermal patches and gum can adversely affect your wound healing. If possible, you are advised to stop all forms of tobacco 2 weeks before and after surgery, especially if Dr. ________ is performing a flap reconstruction (e.g., facelift, cancer reconstruction, etc.). You may compromise the success of your surgery if you continue to take tobacco.

Alcohol

Try to abstain from any heavy drinking 2 weeks before and after surgery. If possible, curtail even moderate social drinking 1 week before and after surgery.

On the Day of Surgery . . .

1. Please wear a button-down shirt instead of a pullover shirt so that you may change clothes afterward without disturbing your wound or soiling your clothing.
2. Do not engage in any vigorous cardiovascular exercise the morning of surgery. Increasing your blood flow with exercise the morning of surgery may increase your chance of bleeding.
3. Please make sure that you have arranged to have someone transport you home after the surgery if you're scheduled to go home afterward. We believe it is mandatory in many cases to have a companion or family member stay with you for the first 24 hours after surgery.
4. If you wear fingernail polish, please ensure that at least one fingernail is free of polish so that the pulse oximeter (the device that reads your oxygen levels) may function properly.
5. Please wash your face the morning of your surgery, preferably with *PHisoDerm* soap.

Also . . .

Please read all your *postoperative* instructions very carefully now before your surgery. You will notice that you should clean your wounds with hydrogen peroxide and bacitracin using Q-tips or cotton balls. Also, applying vitamin E ointment to the wound edges is recommended. In addition, a package of frozen peas or corn should be purchased to decrease swelling after surgery. It would be convenient if you bought all these over-the-counter items prior to your surgery.

We greatly appreciate the confidence you have shown in us by allowing us to assist you in improving your appearance and/or health, and you may be assured of our best efforts to achieve the most satisfactory surgical result possible for your particular individual anatomy and condition.

GENERAL POSTOPERATIVE INSTRUCTION SHEET

Postoperative Anesthesia

(This section applies only if you have had some form of sedation or general anesthesia.)

After anesthesia, you may feel nauseated and may even experience vomiting for the first 24 hours. You may take the prescribed antinausea medication to alleviate your symptoms. Please contact us immediately if your vomiting persists despite medication. You should feel much better by the next day. Please let us know if you are still suffering nausea and vomiting after the first 2 days. If you were sedated or underwent general anesthesia, do not drive or operate any machinery because you may injure yourself or others. Sometimes, the narcotic pain medications you are taking may also cause some upset stomach and/or nausea. Try taking these medications with food, or abstain from taking them if they cause undue nausea and vomiting. It is also natural for you to feel a bit of fatigue for the first 2 to 3 days after surgery as your body recovers from the combined effects of surgery and anesthesia.

Showering and Water Exposure

Please do not get your wound area wet until all bandages have been removed. (If you are having nasal plastic surgery, please follow the bathing directions on that sheet.) If you do not have bandages, please do not shower or get your wound wet for the first 24 hours. After this period of time and after your bandages are off, you may shower and gently dry your wounds. After the first day, you may gently wash your face with mild soap and water. Try to avoid any vigorous cleaning of the suture line.

Wound Care

1. The suture line should be cleaned two to three times daily with a Q-tip or cotton ball soaked in hydrogen peroxide. (Be careful near the hairline if you have dark hair to avoid bleaching the hair.) Again, care should be taken because the sutures are delicate and can be broken if vigorously cleaned. Blot dry and apply an antibiotic ointment, such as Bacitracin, to the wound edges with a clean Q-tip so that a crust (scab) does not have a chance to form. Any over-the-counter antibiotic ointments will suffice (Bacitracin or Neosporin). If you develop a red, itchy, blistery area after you apply the antibiotic ointment, stop applying it because a small percentage of patients may develop an allergic reaction to it. Also, you may refrain from applying any ointment at night so as not to soil your bed sheets. Try to use a Q-tip or cotton ball instead of your fingers when applying ointment, because your fingers may be dirty and cause an infection in your suture line.
2. Apply ice packs over the wound for the first 24 to 48 hours because it will significantly reduce your postoperative swelling and cut down on your recovery time. You may do so every 20 minutes to 1 hour as convenient. After the first 2 days, ice packing will not lessen any swelling.
3. Sleeping at night with your head elevated with a couple of pillows will also help reduce the amount of swelling and reduce your recovery time. Sleep on your back or side only.
4. Avoid any hot packs to your face because you may unknowingly burn yourself. After your surgery, your wound area will be numb for several weeks, and you may burn yourself if you apply too hot an object (such as a curling iron to your hair, or even if you blow dry your hair) near or on your operated skin.
5. If you routinely wear makeup, please refrain from doing so for at least the first week after surgery. Makeup may cause significant irritation to the skin and also adversely affect your wound healing. Further, perfumes and colognes may irritate your wounds, so try to minimize or abstain from using these kinds of products near your wounds during the first week as well. If you had a brow lift or facelift, or any surgery near the hairline, please postpone any planned permanent waves or hair coloring for 4 weeks following surgery.
6. You may stop applying Bacitracin when your sutures have been removed. You may then start to apply vitamin E ointment to the suture line, which will also help with wound healing. Application of vitamin E prior to this time may cause undue irritation and should be avoided. You may continue to apply vitamin E for the next 2 weeks once or twice a day. If your skin becomes irritated please stop using vitamin E. (As advised in your Preoperative Instruction Sheet, taking vitamin E *pills,* however, is prohibited so as to minimize any chance of bleeding.)
7. Avoid any excessive rubbing or scratching of the wound area because this may disrupt the suture line or cause darkening of your skin. If you should have severe itchiness around the wound area, contact us immediately so that we may prescribe medication to alleviate your symptoms.

Antibiotics

If we prescribed antibiotics, please take them as directed. It is recommended that you take your antibiotics with food to minimize any chance of an upset stomach. If you are nauseated, please wait until the nausea has subsided before resuming your antibiotics. If you develop diarrhea, please stop taking your antibiotics. If your diarrhea should persist, please contact us regarding this matter. If you should develop a fever (>100.5°F) after the first 2 days, please let us know as well.

Pain Management

Please take the prescribed pain medication if you have significant discomfort after surgery. Please be sure not to take your pain medication more frequently than prescribed. Also, because this medication is a narcotic, you are advised against driving or operating any machinery while taking it. Further, you should not partake of any alcohol when using narcotic pain medications. If you have only mild pain, you may take plain Tylenol to alleviate your symptoms. However, if you take plain Tylenol, you should wait 4 hours before resuming your other pain medications because they frequently already have Tylenol in them, and you do not want to overdose on Tylenol. You should also avoid taking any other pain medications, especially aspirin or aspirin-related products (See the Preoperative Instruction Sheet for a partial list of aspirin and aspirin-related medications.) You should report any unexplained pain to us immediately.

Bruising and Swelling

It is normal that you have moderate or even significant bruising and swelling after surgery for the first 2 weeks. You will notice every day that the bruising and swelling are diminishing. However, if you develop any new-onset swelling, especially in the first 2 to 3 days, please let us know immediately.

Sun Exposure

Excessive exposure to sun in the first 3 weeks after surgery may result in prolonged facial swelling and injury to the skin. Also, excessive sun exposure to your wound area may cause your wound to darken (hyperpigment) in relation to the surrounding skin. If you must go into the sunlight, wear a wide-brimmed hat and apply one of the SPF 15 sun-block preparations, preferably with titanium dioxide or zinc oxide, available at your pharmacy or our clinic.

Exercise and Activity

For the first 2 weeks, please refrain from bending over or straining very hard. If you are constipated, please inform us so that we may prescribe a laxative. It is acceptable to begin light walking 24 hours after surgery. Jogging and light noncontact exercise should not be resumed until 2 weeks, whereas strenuous sports require 6 weeks of healing before being safely resumed. If you feel that you are too weak to perform a given activity, then you should listen to your body and rest appropriately. Remember your body is healing and some of your energy is expended in the healing process.

Other Things to Avoid

Please reread the Preoperative Instruction Sheet carefully and review all the medications, vitamins, and herbal supplements that you should avoid before and after surgery, including the advice about smoking and drinking. If you should have any questions about your surgery or any of the instructions written above, please do not hesitate to contact us.

BLEPHAROPLASTY (EYELID SURGERY) INSTRUCTION SHEET

Before Your Surgery

Please follow all the preoperative instructions outlined in the General Preoperative Instruction Sheet carefully. Avoid any aspirin-containing or aspirin-related products as well as herbal medications and nutritional supplements as outlined in the Preoperative Instruction Sheet.

After Your Surgery

1. Please follow the Postoperative Instruction Sheet carefully.
2. Blepharoplasty usually causes little if any postoperative discomfort. If you notice any significant sharp or dull pain that persists, notify the office immediately.
3. As recommended, use cold compresses (a bag of frozen peas or corn) over your eyes for 20 to 30 minutes six times per day as tolerated. This only helps for the first 2 days.
4. Apply only a **tiny** amount of ointment on the incision lines with a Q-tip. (If you had a transconjunctival [incision inside the eyelid and not on the skin] blepharoplasty, you may not have any incisions at all on which to apply ointment, so skip this step.)
5. You may use your eyes for reading or television viewing as frequently as you wish.
6. Do not use contact lenses for at least 2 weeks. Pulling on the eyelids while inserting or removing lenses may interfere with precise incision healing. Glasses may be used at any time.
7. Do not use mascara, eyeliner, or eye shadow until approved by us (usually 10 to 14 days). Minimal makeup applied to any bruising of the lower lid is acceptable at any time, but do not pull on the lids or incisions.
8. Any apparent redness of the whites of the eyes is only a form of bruising and will subside during the early healing process.
9. Do not engage in vigorous exercise or sports for at least 3 weeks or until approved by our office.
10. It is not abnormal to feel slight itching and tightness of the eyelids during the early healing period.
11. DON'T TAKE ANY CHANCES! Please do not hesitate to contact us if you are concerned about anything you consider significant.

AFTER BOTOX INSTRUCTION SHEET

After Your Botox Injection

1. You may have bruising, swelling, mild discomfort, and/or a headache following the injection. You may use an ice pack to the treated area and take Tylenol for the discomfort.
2. Do not massage the injected area. This may diffuse the Botox into surrounding muscles, causing unwanted effects.
3. Call our office with any rashes or persistent abnormal swelling (3 or more days).
4. Botox typically has its effect in 3 to 7 days following the injection. Effectiveness increases during the first week. The effect lasts approximately 3 to 6 months.
5. Call our office with any questions or concerns.

PREOPERATIVE AND POSTOPERATIVE INSTRUCTIONS FOR HAIR TRANSPLANTATION

Preoperative Instructions

1. It is very important that you do not drink any alcohol or take aspirin 2 weeks prior to surgery. Please let us know if you are on any type of medication.
2. Do not mix alcohol with any medication.
3. Hair should *not* be cut prior to surgery. I will trim a very small area on the back of the scalp, where the grafts will be removed. However, this should not be noticeable.
4. Most patients purchase a baseball or loose fitting cap or hat that can be worn after the procedure. Wearing a cap or hat makes it much less conspicuous that you have had a surgical procedure. **Do not wear pullover clothing, which would be difficult to put on over the postoperative bandage.**
5. ***IT IS ABSOLUTELY ESSENTIAL THAT YOU ARRANGE FOR TRANSPORTATION HOME.*** Under no circumstances should you attempt to drive home, because the sedation given at the beginning of your surgery can affect your ability to drive.

Postoperative Instructions

1. Most patients experience minimal or no discomfort. If you should have some mild discomfort, Tylenol is generally sufficient to ease it. You can be given a prescription for a small amount of stronger medication, but most patients find it unnecessary to take these. Significant pain or discomfort is very unusual and should be reported to our office.
2. When you return home and for approximately 72 hours afterward, use ice packs liberally on your surgical site(s) while you are awake. Twenty minutes on and then 20 minutes off usually works well.
3. The morning after your surgical procedure, it is permissible and recommended that you very gently shampoo your hair with a baby shampoo. It may take 1 to 2 weeks for scabs to fall off.
4. Infection is very rare. *Any significant swelling that is new and begins after the first 48 to 72 hours should be reported to our office.*
5. The donor site or area where the grafts were obtained from the back of the scalp will be relatively unnoticeable. For the first 2 weeks following surgery there will be sutures in this area; however, shampooing is necessary. Care should be taken to avoid catching the suture line while combing or brushing hair.
6. During the first week following your procedure, you may have some swelling of the forehead and occasionally the eyebrows or eyelids. The amount of swelling is extremely variable; most patients experience minimal or no swelling. You need not be alarmed because it should completely resolve over 2 to 3 days. It is helpful to eliminate salt from your diet at that time and sleep with your head elevated on one or two pillows.
7. It takes 3 months to 1 year to see the benefits of our hair transplant surgery. During this time, I strongly recommend the following regimen to maximize the benefit of your transplant:
   a. Maintain excellent scalp and hair hygiene with products that do not contain Sodium Lauryl Sulfate.
   b. Use Minoxidil and/or Finasteride for a minimum of 1 year following transplant surgery. Both Minoxidil and Finasteride have been shown to increase transplant viability in long-term studies. Minoxidil also contains a sulfur group that is necessary for hair growth.
8. Follow-up appointments are at 1 week, 2 weeks for suture removal, 3 months, 6 months, and 1 year.
9. Finally, it is *very* important to your well-being that you follow completely all instructions given to you by this office, and that we check your progress regularly following surgery. Failure to comply with instructions completely could lead to less than satisfactory results.

DO NOT TAKE ANY CHANCES! Please contact us immediately if you are concerned about anything you consider significant.

We greatly appreciate the confidence you have shown in us by allowing us to assist you in improving your appearance and health. You may be assured of our best efforts to achieve the most satisfactory surgical result possible for your particular individual anatomy and condition.

BEFORE PEEL/DERMABRASION/LASER INSTRUCTION SHEET

Two Days Prior

Valtrex (antiviral medication): **Only use this prescribed medication if the area around the mouth will be treated. This tablet should be started 2 days prior to the chemical peel and continued for a total of 7 days as instructed. This helps prevent a breakout of cold sores. If you experience breakouts that burn or tingle, or a cold sore, please notify Dr. ______________________________ and his or her staff.**

Items to be Purchased Prior to Your Procedure

Q-tips, cotton pads (or cotton balls), ice pack (a bag of frozen corn or peas works well), white vinegar, distilled water, Aquaphor ointment, Cetaphil Cleanser, Cetaphil Ointment (without SPF)

On the Day of Your Procedure

Thoroughly cleanse your face and neck with an antibacterial soap. We recommend you wear a shirt, blouse, or sweater that unbuttons in the front for easy removal postoperatively. Please bring a hair band for your hair if it is long.

AFTER TRICHLOROACETIC ACID PEEL INSTRUCTION SHEET

General Cleaning Instructions for the First 5 Days

1. Remove ointment with a damp, soft cloth. Ensure that all ointment is removed.
2. Wash gently in a circular motion with a damp cloth using a mixture of 1/2 tablespoon of white vinegar and 1 cup of distilled water.
3. Rinse off with distilled water by gently splashing the face over the sink or squeezing a soft, damp cloth over the area.
4. Dry area gently by patting off the water with a soft cloth.
5. Apply **Aquaphor** ointment evenly over entire peeled area using a Q-tip. We recommend applying ointment at least twice daily, or more frequently, to avoid drying out your skin. Be generous in your application. A thick coating ensures that all your skin is well moisturized.
8. Initially for the first day, cleansing should be done twice daily. You may then begin cleaning up to four times per day as tolerated. Wash your face less often if it causes too much discomfort.

General Cleaning Instructions for Days 6 Through 10

1. Remove ointment with a damp, soft cloth. Ensure that all ointment is removed.
2. Wash gently in a circular motion with a damp cloth using Cetaphil cleanser (instead of the vinegar and water). If the Cetaphil cleanser feels too astringent on your skin, then continue use of the vinegar and water until you are better able to tolerate the Cetaphil cleanser.
3. Rinse off with distilled water by gently splashing the face over the sink or squeezing a soft, damp cloth over the area.
4. Dry area gently by patting off the water with a soft cloth.
5. Apply **Aquaphor** ointment evenly over entire peeled area using a Q-tip. We recommend applying ointment at least twice daily, or more frequently, to avoid drying out your skin. Be generous in your application. A thick coating ensures that all your skin is well moisturized.

Showering

For the first 3 days, you may clean your hair in the sink and your body in the shower or bath, but try to keep water from the area of your face that has undergone a chemical peel. Your skin is usually too sensitive to tolerate direct exposure to water at this point. After the first 3 days, you may rinse your face in the shower by letting water gently hit your forehead and run down your face. You should avoid any extremely hot water because this may cause a significant burn. The goal is to have your skin peel off easily. Sometimes you may see yellowish build-up or crusting. Gently remove this build-up with a wet Q-tip. *It is strongly advised that you apply or remove ointment, crusting, etc. with Q-tips and not your fingers because you may contaminate your open wounds with bacteria.* Listen to your skin. You don't need to be aggressive.

After the First 8 to 10 Days

After the first 8 to 10 days, a new skin layer typically will have formed. At this point, you may stop applying Aquaphor to your face and start Cetaphil lotion. HOWEVER, DR. ______________________________ AND HIS OR HER STAFF WILL INFORM YOU WHEN IT IS SAFE TO TRANSITION FROM AQUAPHOR TO CETAPHIL LOTION AFTER CAREFUL EXAMINATION IN THE OFFICE. Avoid any direct and prolonged sun exposure.

What to Watch Out for

Your skin will remain a light-red to pink color for 1 to 3 weeks, but may return to your normal skin tone earlier. You may be experiencing dermatitis (i.e., an irritative reaction) if you notice that your skin turns significantly redder (or bright red), becomes irregular in contour (lumpy-bumpy), or you begin to feel a significant burning sensation. If you begin to notice these changes, stop applying whatever products to your skin might be irritating it, and contact us immediately. Little white bumps (known as milia) in the peeled area usually resolve; however, sometimes we need to unroof them with a sterile, surgical instrument if these cysts persist.

SUMMARY OF CARE INSTRUCTIONS AFTER A PEEL

Days After a Peel	Ointment	Cleaning	Makeup
1-5	Aquaphor	Vinegar and water* twice a day for the first day, then four times a day thereafter	None (avoid any perfumes or fragrances)
6-10	Aquaphor (until new skin is formed)	Cetaphil cleanser twice a day	None
11-30	Cetaphil lotion (without sunscreen)	Cetaphil cleanser twice a day	Natural, powder-based make-up with titanium dioxide or zinc oxide sunblock (only when new skin is complete)

* 1/2 tablespoon of vinegar is mixed with 1 cup of distilled water, then rinsed of with distilled water. You may begin showering on the third postoperative day.

RETIN-A/RENOVA INSTRUCTION SHEET

Retin-A/Renova

Initially, this cream/medication should be applied every other evening before going to bed for the first 2 to 3 weeks, slowly increasing to every evening. It is not unusual to experience some mild tingling and irritation during the first few weeks. If you are experiencing a burning sensation, or the skin appears to be cracking, discontinue Retin-A/Renova for two evenings and apply Vaseline to the irritated areas. You may resume using Retin-A/Renova when your skin is feeling and looking better. It is important to moisturize your skin in the morning as well as using a good SPF sunscreen. Please feel free to call us if irritation persists.

Directions for Applying Retin-A/Renova

1. Wash your face thoroughly with a mild soap or gentle alcohol-free cleanser and pat dry. (Do not rub.)
2. After washing, wait at least 10 minutes before applying Retin-A/Renova to be certain that the skin is totally dry. Skin that is wet, damp, or even moist tends to absorb cream quickly, which may cause unnecessary irritation.
3. After your face is totally dry, squeeze a pearl-sized amount (about a 1/4″ diameter) of Retin-A/Renova onto your fingertip. Using more than a pearl-sized amount will not increase your results and may cause irritation.
4. Dab it on your forehead, chin, and both cheeks but not immediately under your eyes.
5. Pat your skin so the small dabs begin to spread into a thin layer that covers your entire face. Smooth into skin until all white streaks have disappeared.
6. After applying Retin-A/Renova, you may apply a moisturizer. However, for best results, wait 1 hour in between if possible.

NOSE PLASTIC SURGERY (RHINOPLASTY) INSTRUCTION SHEET

Before Your Surgery

1. Please follow all the preoperative instructions outlined in the General Preoperative Instruction Sheet carefully. Avoid any aspirin-containing or -related products as well as herbal medications and nutritional supplements as outlined in the Preoperative Instruction Sheet.
2. Make sure that you wear clothing that fastens in the front or back and continue to do so for 1 week following the procedure. Avoid anything that slips over the head (e.g., sweaters, t-shirts, and turtlenecks).

After Your Surgery

1. Please read the General Postoperative Instruction Sheet carefully.
2. Do not blow your nose until instructed. Wipe or dab the nose gently with tissue if necessary. You may clean around the nostril area gently with a Q-tip and hydrogen peroxide.
3. Change the dressing under the nose (if present) as needed. It is no longer necessary to wear the dressing that has been placed under your nose once drainage has stopped.
4. A dressing also is placed in each nostril. Unless instructed otherwise, the dressing in each nostril should be removed the morning following surgery. Be sure you are in a sitting position and in front of a mirror. Remove the dressing by grasping it between your thumb and index finger. Repeat these instructions for the opposite side. You may clean the nostrils with a Q-tip and hydrogen peroxide.
5. Brush your teeth gently with a soft toothbrush only. Avoid manipulating the upper lip to keep the nose at rest.
6. You may wash your face carefully, avoiding the dressing. Take tub baths until the splint/nasal dressing is removed. Do not get the splint/nasal dressing wet.
7. The outer splint/dressing will be removed at your 1-week postoperative visit. It is advised to shower the morning of that visit to get the entire splint wet. This helps to slide the splint off easily with no discomfort.
8. Sleep with your head up, and sleep only in the supine position (i.e., keep your head facing the ceiling and not turned to either side for the first week). You can use sandbags or heavy pillows on either side of your head so that you do not turn your head to either side.
9. DO NOT TAKE ANY CHANCES! Please do not hesitate to contact us if you are concerned about anything you consider significant.

4

UPPER AND MIDFACIAL REJUVENATION

SAMUEL M. LAM
EDWIN F. WILLIAMS III

At first, a chapter devoted to both upper and midfacial rejuvenation rather than an individual chapter for each topic may seem illogical. However, after completing this chapter, the reader should appreciate how these two facial zones are intimately linked. Midfacial elevation may be achieved via a browlift incision, which is the authors' preferred approach. Alternatively, the midface may be lifted through an extended lower-blepharoplasty incision. This approach is less ideal for reasons that are enumerated herein; however, it is still a viable technique. The authors discourage midfacial rejuvenation via a rhytidectomy incision, because the favored vector of lift is vertical, which cannot be accomplished easily with a laterally based incision.

This chapter covers the pertinent details in brow elevation via a minimal-incision technique that can rejuvenate the upper and midface as a unit. Midfacial rejuvenation is described via a lower-blepharoplasty incision and alloplastic implantation. Eyelid rejuvenation is discussed in the many complex variations that exist to achieve the desired objective: ptosis repair, upper-lid blepharoplasty (with and without medial fat excision), transconjunctival lower-lid blepharoplasty (with and without skin pinch), and transcutaneous skin–muscle flap (with or without midfacial extension). The proper selection of technique is as critical as the execution, and the relevant preoperative considerations are also addressed. Finally, the reader is guided through the postoperative period to care for the patient during the normal postoperative course as well as to formulate the appropriate decision making required if complications arise.

PREOPERATIVE CONSIDERATIONS: PATIENT SELECTION AND RELEVANT ANATOMY

Upper Face (Brow and Eyelid) Rejuvenation

Interestingly, the authors have observed that many patients begin to exhibit brow ptosis about 10 years before any evidence of lower facial jowl formation. Obviously, this finding is not universally present. (On the other hand, submental fullness, as an independent phenomenon, can occur at any age because of heredity, obesity, or aging.) Surgeons in the past have been reluctant to undertake brow elevation because of apprehension over the potential morbidity associated with traditional coronal-type browlifts. Patients in turn have at times expressed some reticence to accept the added recovery time associated with this technique. Newer minimally invasive techniques have been able to restore the upper face with potentially less morbidity (smaller incisions, faster recovery, shorter and temporary scalp anesthesia, and less risk of scarring and alopecia) than the coronal lift while maintaining commensurate longevity and achieving equally favorable aesthetic results. Despite the fanfare that accompanied the midbrow lift, it still may be an arduous task to convince a patient, especially a younger patient, to agree to a brow lifting procedure that involves incisions in a highly visible location. Similarly, the direct browlift (at the eyebrow) has assumed a less prominent role in brow rejuvenation for a host of reasons, including poor scar camouflage, irregular alopecia, and technical difficulty. The authors rely on the "endoscopic" approach (five abbreviated incisions) to rejuvenate the brow, but have eliminated use of all endoscopic equipment and further can achieve midfacial rejuvenation via the same incision by carrying the dissection over the zygomatic arch. Although the endoscopic technique for brow rejuvenation is well known, a more accurate term, "minimally invasive" browlift, which reflects the technique advocated in the text, is substituted for the remainder of this volume.

Unlike the traditional facelift that solely addresses an aesthetic deficit along the lower face, brow and eyelid surgery may restore youth but also correct a functional visual impairment. Furthermore, the somewhat prosaic aphorism still captures the essence of upper facial rejuvenation: "The eyes are the window to the soul." When an individual engages in conversation or even casually gazes at another, he or she usually fixates on the others' eyes, which makes upper facial rejuvenation a critical aspect of restoring vibrancy and vitality to an individual that a facelift can less often accomplish. Patients who exhibit brow and eyelid aging often are accused of looking "angry," "sad," or "tired"—comments that belie that individual's true temperament and disposition. These unjustified remarks levied at the patient add another dimension of psychological burden for which the patient may desire a remedy other than correction for the stigma of aging alone.

Patients often present to the physician confused about what they actually want corrected. Often, the mass media has indoctrinated them into equating blepharoplasty with the cure for their woes. However, the surgeon must carefully select between upper-lid blepharoplasty (skin pinch with or without fat removal), lower-lid blepharoplasty (transconjunctival with or without skin removal versus transcutaneous), browplasty, and blepharoptosis repair, or a combination thereof to achieve the proper desired result. This section elucidates this thinking process so that the surgeon will possess a systematic appraisal of the aesthetic and functional deficits that require surgical intervention.

First, a simplified algorithm should be introduced that may facilitate easy analysis (but should be used with discretion and judgment). A vertical line can be drawn through the midpupil. Generally, any tissue ptosis medial to this line may be thought of as upper eyelid in origin and may be corrected with an upper-lid blepharoplasty. Conversely, any ptosis that presents lateral to this imaginary line may be assumed to be principally caused by brow ptosis rather than excessive upper-lid skin (or dermatochalasis) (Fig. 4-1). The fallacy that bedevils many junior surgeons is the same unsophisticated thinking that encumbers patients—that all upper-lid tissue ptosis is a byproduct of redundant eyelid skin rather than brow ptosis. Quite the contrary is true: The brow tends to age chronologically earlier than the onset of upper-eyelid skin redundancy. Furthermore, the absence of a developed lateral depressor brow complex (the orbicularis oculi provides weak counter pull to the brow laterally) as opposed to the well-developed medial depressor brow complex (corrugator and procerus) may contribute to the disproportionate lateral-brow descent. Anatomic studies also have highlighted the weaker development of the lateral-brow musculature that may serve as the principal cause for more significant lateral-brow ptosis, among other factors.[1–3] If an upper-lid blepharoplasty is performed in lieu of a recommended browplasty, the brow actually may be further depressed; and if excessive upper-lid skin is removed, a browlift may be precluded in the future because of risk of lagophthalmos. Also, an aggressive upper-lid blepharoplasty alone, especially if the adjacent, thicker brow skin is removed together with the thinner upper-lid skin, may result in an unnatural appearance.

The aesthetic position of the brow always should be recalled when considering a browlift. In the ideal female eyebrow, the eyebrow configuration assumes a tapered contour with a thicker, medial club of the eyebrow narrowing laterally to a fine point. The medial brow should rest at or slightly below the orbital rim with the peak of the eyebrow situated either at the lateral limbus (classical description, Fig. 4-2A) or at the lateral canthus (revised description, Fig. 4-2B) lying above the orbital rim. Laterally, the eyebrow descends somewhat to end at a point drawn through the imaginary line that joins the alar–facial groove through the lateral canthus. The descended brow often assumes a more flattened appearance that resembles the ideal male eyebrow; that is, a straight line that runs along the orbital rim (Fig. 4-3). Because the ideal female brow is arched laterally and the brow descends disproportionately laterally, the primary efforts to raise the brow position should be concentrated laterally. All fixation sutures are laterally based, and no medial suspension is undertaken. This surgical technique properly restores the ptotic brow without unnaturally producing the startled or frightened appearance that is a stigma of an improper browlift.

Another fallacy that has ensnared the neophyte surgeon is the thought that the eyebrow (the hairy portion of the brow) is the exclusive aspect of the brow that requires rejuvenation. Instead, the entire lateral brow complex should be viewed as a unit, which includes both the hair-bearing eyebrow and the adjoining soft tissue. As part of the physical assessment, the surgeon should place his or her thumb along the ptotic lateral brow and lift the tissue upward, carefully observing the improved position of the descended soft tissue and hair-bearing eyebrow. The patient also should be educated about this aesthetic deficit and confronted with the rejuvenated appearance using a mirror while the surgeon gently lifts the ptotic brow. Any excessive eyelid skin that remains after appropriate brow elevation may be pinched with a forceps or between the surgeon's fingers to illustrate how a concomitant blepharoplasty would further enhance the intended objective. However, if the patient desires only an upper-lid blepharoplasty despite a thoughtful education, the surgeon should plan for a conservative upper-lid skin excision that will not compromise a prospective future browlift or exacerbate the brow ptosis.

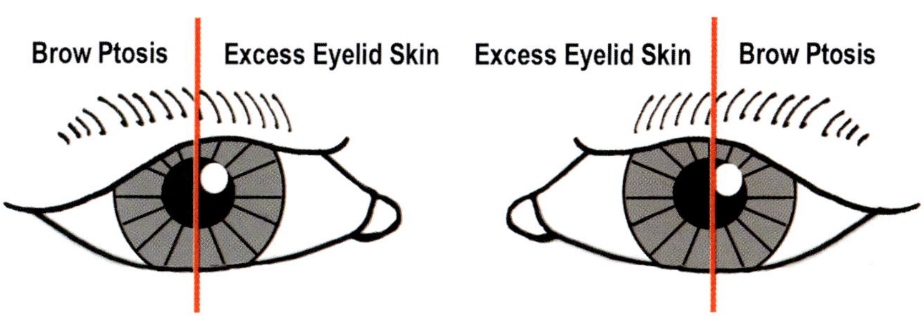

FIGURE 4-1. Illustration showing a simplified view of upper-facial aging. A vertical line drawn through the midpupil divides two distinct compartments of facial aging: lateral tissue excess is attributed in large part to brow ptosis, whereas medial, excess typically results from upper-lid skin redundancy. Clearly, this illustration is an oversimplification in that some tissue descent medially often may be attributed in part to brow ptosis and lateral tissue excess may be a result of upper-lid skin redundancy.

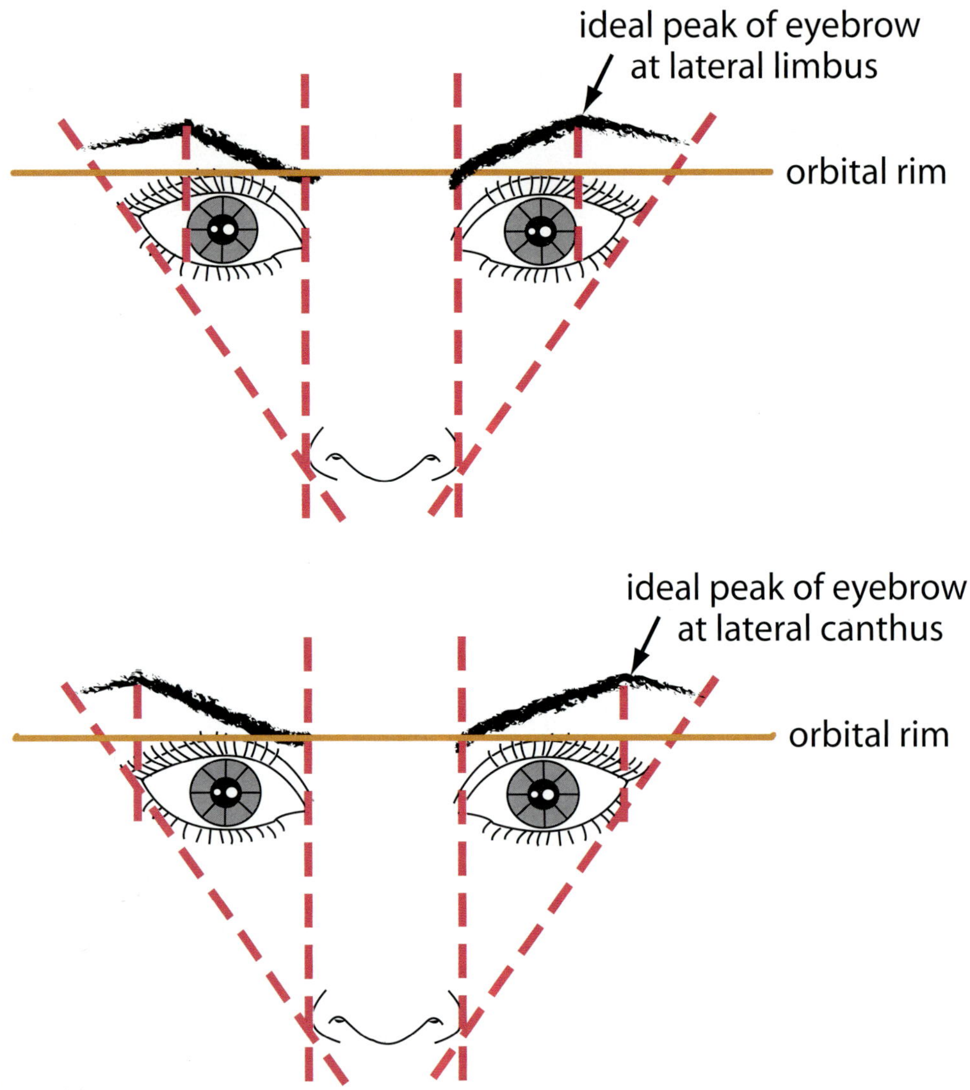

FIGURE 4-2. A: Classical description of the ideal female brow position. The medial brow head starts at or slightly below the level of the orbital rim, arching to a peak at the lateral limbus and tapering laterally to an imaginary point derived from the intersection of two points: the alar–facial groove and the lateral canthus. **B:** Revised description of the ideal female brow position. The description of the revised brow configuration matches that of the classical description, except the height (or peak) of the brow should lie above the lateral canthus rather than the lateral limbus. Both descriptions are acceptable alternatives, although some feel that the latter is more ideal given the less "startled" look that this shape imparts. Fashion and style change, so there are no absolutes to these guidelines.

After a careful inspection of the lateral brow for signs of ptosis, the surgeon then should pay meticulous attention to the upper lid that lies medial to the imaginary vertical midpupillary line. Again, this area represents principally upper-eyelid pathology—excessive upper-lid skin and/or pseudoherniation of fat (steatoblepharon). The redundant upper-eyelid skin should be pinched with a pair of fine forceps to determine the amount of skin that must be excised to achieve the optimal rejuvenation and demonstrate the intended surgical goal to the patient. Unlike the lower lid, which may have pseudoherniation of fat along the entire border, the upper lid suffers from fat protrusion chiefly medially. The central pocket is less likely to be herniated, and the lateral pocket is comprised entirely of the lacrimal gland, the repair of which lies beyond the scope of this textbook. This medial fat bulge should be noted and explained to the patient so that a proper preoperative plan for fat excision can be established.

The last consideration for upper brow and eyelid pathology that should be studied is evidence of blepharoptosis; that is, levator dysfunction and actual eyelid descent over the pupil. This condition should be differentiated from pseudoptosis that results from excessive upper-eyelid skin (dermatochalasis) that causes the lid to appear descended.

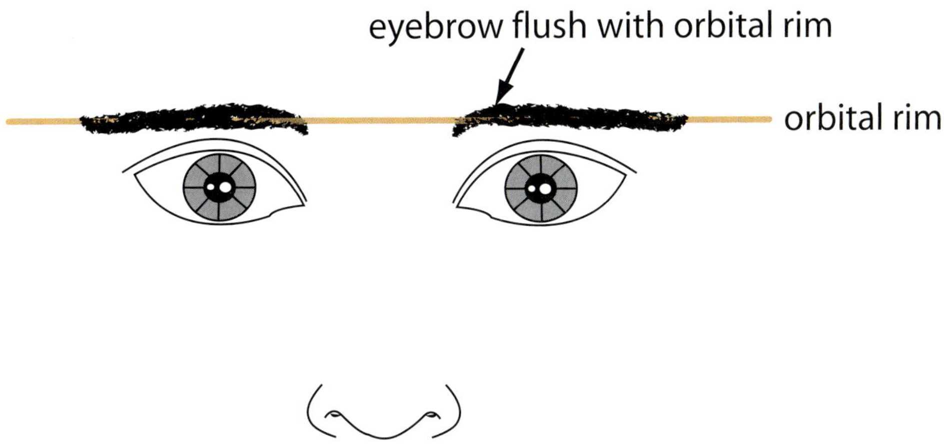

FIGURE 4-3. The ideal male brow is heavier than the female counterpart, in terms of the soft-tissue component, the hairy eyebrow itself, and the bony orbital rim. Classically, it should rest along the orbital rim in a flatter, straighter configuration as opposed to the arched shape of the ideal female eyebrow that extends superior to the bony rim.

Both true ptosis and pseudoptosis can obscure the visual axis and lead to visual field restriction. Most cases of eyelid ptosis are a result of senility and exhibit the following characteristic hallmarks:

1. Normal lid excursion (usually 8 to 12 mm), which can be tested by fixating the brow in position with a finger so that brow elevation is eliminated and true lid excursion can be assessed.
2. High or absent supratarsal lid crease because of disinsertion or weakening of the levator.
3. Thin, upper-eyelid skin that renders the underlying iris visible through the attenuated skin.

The palpebral fissure should be about 7.5 to 10 mm in distance. However, a more useful measurement is the margin reflex diameter-one (MRD-1), which is defined as the distance from the corneal light reflex (situated at the mid-pupil during primary gaze) to the upper-lid margin (Fig. 4-4). A normal MRD-1 should be 2.5 to 5 mm, and an abnormal value is considered less than 2 mm. If the lid overhangs the corneal light reflex, then every millimeter below the light reflex is considered a negative value. The MRD-2 is defined as the distance from the corneal light reflex to the lower-lid margin and is important in the evaluation of lower-lid malposition. A normal value of the MRD-2 is 4 to 5.5 mm. If the patient exhibits unilateral ptosis, then the ptotic lid should be elevated to the normal position, during which time the contralateral lid position is observed. Often the contralateral lid is seen to descend because of a central tonic mechanism that maintains lid position until the affected ptotic lid is digitally suspended. This phenomenon is known as Hering's Law. During assessment of lid ptosis, formal visual-field assessment should be obtained by an ophthalmologist or optometrist. If Hering's Law appears to be in effect, the ptotic lid should be taped in an elevated position while the contralateral visual field is measured.

Finally, the lower lid should be assessed for its aesthetic qualities. Pseudoherniation of fat, dermatochalasis, and hypertrophic roll of the orbicularis-oculi muscle typically are the targets for rejuvenation. Pseudoherniation of fat can be assessed effectively on the frontal and lateral views and accentuated on upward gaze. Patients with a significant amount of fat protrusion may even show well-demarcated fat pockets (medial, central, and lateral). Dermatochalasis, or excessive lid skin, may be assessed with a simple pinch using forceps to estimate the amount needed for removal. A hypertrophic orbicularis oculi muscle may be evident as a roll of tissue that is exaggerated during muscular contraction such as smiling.

Besides these aesthetic issues, the surgeon must be fully cognizant of the potential for postoperative lid malposition, which may arise even in the most qualified hands. Preoperative evaluation of lid tone and position must be an integral facet to every physical examination before embarking on a surgical undertaking. Lower-lid position should be assessed on primary gaze without digital distraction or other manipulation. If the patient already exhibits scleral show, lateral rounding, or frank ectropion, then a lid shortening procedure such as a tarsal strip, should be entertained. A lid distraction test should be performed in which the lower lid is pulled downward with one finger in order to assess lower-lid laxity. If the lid is in normal position before distraction and can be pulled downward with little resistance, then a lid-shortening procedure should be considered. However, if the lower lid is already malpositioned and moves very little with distraction, then vertical shortening of the lower lid may be present (e.g., an anterior, middle, or posterior lamellar deficiency). Usually, vertical shortening arises because of overzealous blepharoplasty in the past and requires replacement with the appropriate tissue. It is recommended that ophthalmologic guidance be sought if such a deficiency exists. A lid retraction test (or snap test) also should be performed to

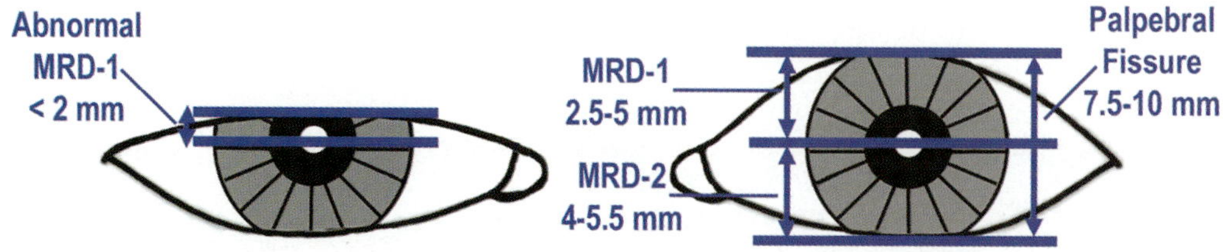

FIGURE 4-4. This illustration describes different measurements that are helpful in determining blepharoptosis, whether owing to excessive upper-lid skin (pseudoptosis) or levator dysfunction (senile ptosis), as well as measurements for lower-lid malposition. The palpebral fissure should measure 7.5 to 10 mm in distance. The margin reflex diameter-one (MRD-1) is defined as the distance from the corneal light reflex (situated at the midpupil during primary gaze) to the upper-lid margin. A normal MRD-1 should be 2.5 to 5 mm with an abnormal value measuring less than 2 mm. If the lid overhangs the corneal light reflex, then the MRD-1 value is read as a negative value for the distance from the corneal light reflex. The MRD-2 is defined as the distance from the corneal light reflex to the lower-lid margin and is important in the evaluation of lower-lid malposition. A normal value of the MRD-2 is 4 to 5.5 mm.

test the resilience of the lower lid. The lower lid is pinched between the index finger and thumb and pulled away from the globe. If the lid returns to contact the globe after 1 second or not at all, then poor lid elasticity is diagnosed and a lid-shortening procedure may be indicated. The patient also should be assessed in the lateral position to determine the relative globe to orbital-rim position. A prominent globe and recessed orbital rim predisposes the patient to the potential for postoperative lid malposition. This relationship is known as the negative vector in that the line drawn from the midpupil to the orbital rim on lateral view falls backward from superior to inferior (Fig. 4-5). If a lower lid is tightened in this situation, the lid may actually assume a worse, or lower, position, like an obese man's belt slipping further down his paunch when the belt is cinched tighter. The mnemonic "big eyes, big trouble" is a worthy phrase that the prudent facial aesthetic surgeon should always heed. A careful ophthalmologic history is also critical (e.g., history of dry eyes, ocular surgery, glaucoma, or prior blepharoplasty). These are all important clues to establish the patient's candidacy for elective eyelid surgery.

Besides evaluating the patient for possible eyelid surgery, the surgeon should recall the benefit that botulinum toxin alone may provide in the younger patient, who only exhibits rhytidosis during animation. Please refer to Chapter 8 for a detailed discussion of this treatment modality. Lower-lid resurfacing (CO_2 laser or trichloroacetic acid [TCA] peel) also may be frequently incorporated with lower-lid surgery to efface fine rhytidosis.

Midfacial Rejuvenation

One of the most challenging areas in facial rejuvenation surgery is the aging midface. Several approaches have been advocated to address the midface: laterally via a deep-plane rhytidectomy incision, superiorly via a lower-eyelid incision, and supero-laterally via a temporal-brow incision.[4–7] Despite these varied options, enthusiasm for these procedures has been tempered by the potential complications of each technique. The favored plane of dissection that unites these disparate approaches is subperiosteal, in which the malar fat pad and orbicularis-oculi muscle may be elevated as a unit. Since 1996, the senior author has performed a midface lift via the temporo-parietal browlift incision. However, reluctance has been noted in the literature to endorse this approach fully because of perceived concomitant morbidity. Protracted dissection time, risk to the frontal branch of the facial nerve, temporal wasting, and unnatural elevation of the lateral canthus all have been cited as drawbacks to this surgical approach to the midface.[9,10] Because of these touted shortcomings, the authors critically reviewed the technique, outcome, and complications in an objective scientific study that revealed little morbidity combined with dramatic improvement.[11]

The midface may be an elusive entity to some but may be simply defined as the facial zone that overlies the malar eminence. As one ages, two principal pathologies contribute to an unattractive midfacial appearance: draping of the orbicularis-oculi muscle (festooning) and malar-fat ptosis (malar bagging). These two entities may appear indistinguishable at first glance, because they both manifest as unsightly bulges in the cheek region. However, orbicularis redundancy and ptosis may be effaced when the patient squints and contracts the muscle: This finding may not always be evident. Malar fat descent usually does not respond to contraction of the orbicularis-oculi muscle. This distinction between festooning and malar bagging however may be a bit arcane, because the surgical treatment for both is essentially the same, a midface lift.

INTRAOPERATIVE CONSIDERATIONS: TECHNIQUE AND SALIENT TECHNICAL POINTS

Lower Blepharoplasty (Transconjunctival with Chemical Peel or CO_2 Laser)

A Jessner's/TCA peel serves as an effective adjunct for rejuvenation for fine rhytidosis of the lower lid without significant lower-lid redundancy (Figs. 4-6 and 4-7). The peel is performed first, because the patient should be under no or minimal sedation during this part of the procedure. In

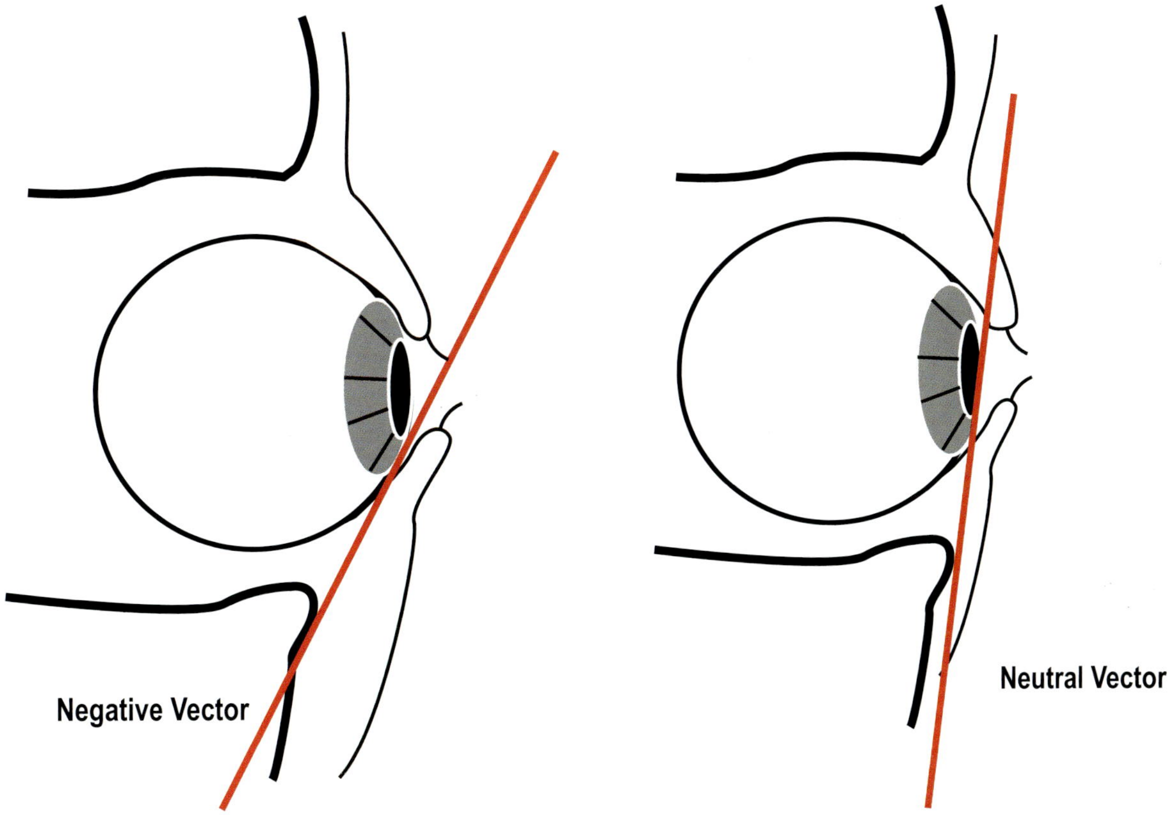

A B

FIGURE 4-5. A: The illustration describes the so-called "negative vector." A line from the globe to the inferior orbital rim is drawn on lateral view, and if the line falls from an antero-superior to a postero-inferior inclination, then a negative vector is present. This condition usually is attributed to prominent globes that rest anterior to the orbital rim shelf. The mnemonic "big eyes, big trouble" recalls the danger of operating on these patients who exhibit a "negative vector" in that lower-lid tightening may only exacerbate rather than improve lower-lid position. The analogy is likened to an obese man whose belt extends just under the widest diameter of his paunch, and any efforts to tighten the belt only move it further southward. The belly represents the globe; and the belt and pants, the lower lid. **B:** The illustration shows a more "neutral vector" that is a safer configuration for lower-eyelid surgery.

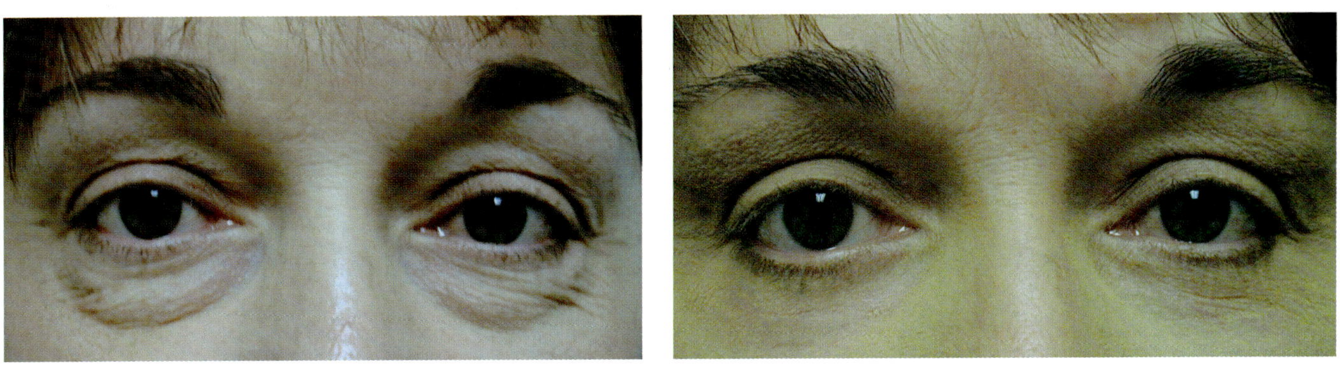

A B

FIGURE 4-6. A, B: This is a 39-year-old woman who appears older than her stated age principally because of her lower-eyelid appearance. She stated that her lower eyelids have always been somewhat "puffy" but that over the past 8 years a considerable worsening has occurred to the fullness in this area that has made her look chronically tired. On clinical examination, she exhibits fair skin and minimal rhytidosis except along her lower-eyelid region, which reveals numerous, fine rhytids and significant pseudoherniation of fat. The patient also had moderately good lid tone by a two-finger snap test. The patient wanted selective improvement in this area and did not entertain any further intervention other than lower-eyelid rejuvenation. She underwent a Jessner's/35% TCA peel to her lower eyelid region, transconjunctival blepharoplasty with a pinch excision of her redundant lower eyelid skin. She is shown 6 months after the procedure with notable improvement in skin appearance as well as reduction of the prolapsed fat.

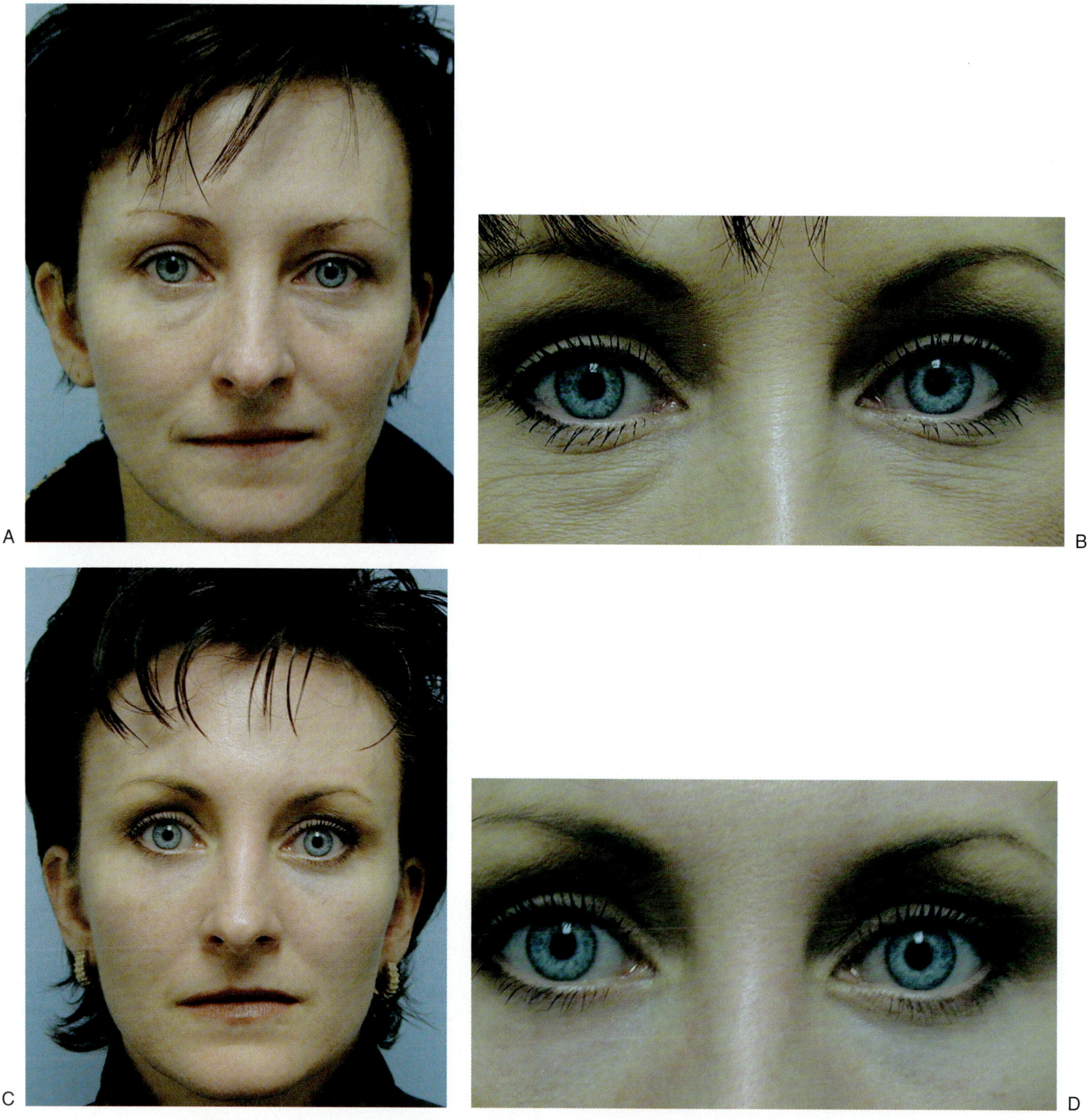

FIGURE 4-7. A–D: This is a 33-year-old aesthetician who presents with minimal pseudoherniation of fat along the lower eyelids but also fine rhytids of her lower-eyelid area that worsen on smiling. She is satisfied with the appearance of her remaining face but would like to have her lower eyelids addressed. She underwent a transconjunctival blepharoplasty with very conservative fat removal in the middle and medial fat pockets along with resurfacing of her lower eyelids using Jessner's and 35% TCA peel and of the remaining face using Jessner's and 20% TCA. She is shown 15 months after the procedure with notable aesthetic improvement. In this particular case, given the patient's minimal fat protrusion as well as relatively young age, it is very important to remain conservative with the amount of fat removal to prevent a hollow-eye appearance immediately after surgery or many years later when the patient matures.

Instrumentation and Equipment

Basic Soft-Tissue Instrument Set

Army–Navy retractors (2)
#3 knife handles (2)
Tonsil clamp
Medicine glass (1)
Suction, 10 French
Small double-pronged hook retractors (2)
Large double-pronged hook retractors (2)
Single hooks (2)
Bayonet forceps (for bipolar cautery)
Brown–Adson forceps (2)
Toothed Adson forceps
Bayonet toothed forceps
Bishop–Harmon toothed forceps
Castro–Viejo toothed forceps
Towel clip
Curved Mayo scissors
Medium Metzenbaum scissors
Serrated scissors
Tenotomy scissors
Iris scissors
Small curved sharp scissors
Needle holders (with scissors built-in) (2)
Needle holders (without scissors) (2)
Straight hemostats (2)
Curved Crile clamps (2)
Curved plane Crile clamps (2)
Converse retractor
Bowl
Freer elevator

(*Note:* These instruments constitute the basic instruments used on most major facial procedures. Other instrument lists that include a "Basic Soft-Tissue Instrument Set" refer to the preceding catalog of equipment.)

Instrumentation/Equipment for Brow/Midface Lift

Prep Stand:

Nonsterile gloves
10-cc syringe (2), 27-gauge (1¼ inch long) needle (2) with lidocaine 1% and 1:100,000 epinephrine
Hair comb
1/2" Micropore tape (to bind hair)
Surgical marking pen

Instruments:

Basic soft-tissue instrument set (see the preceding)
Hand-drill set (Drill bit, 1.5 × 6 mm)
Bovie handpiece and tip
Three curved, ebonized brow elevators:

1. Small, flat dissector
2. Large, flat dissector
3. Round dissector

Sutures:

CV-3 Gore-Tex,* Th-26 needle

Other Supplies:

Skin stapler
Laparotomy pads
10-cc syringe (2), 27-gauge (1¼ inch long) needle (2) with lidocaine 1% and 1:100,000 epinephrine

Dressing:

4 × 4 gauze
3" Conforming gauze bandage, or Kling (Johnson & Johnson, New Brunswick, NJ) (3)
Cotton padding
Bacitracin ointment in 5-cc syringe
1" clear tape
Scissors

Instrumentation/Equipment for Blepharoplasty/Ptosis Repair

Prep Stand:

Nonsterile gloves
1-cc tuberculin syringe (2), 27-gauge (1¼ inch long) needle (2) with lidocaine 1% and 1:50,000 epinephrine
Bowl with eye pads (2) soaked in iced saline
Surgical marking pen
4 × 4 gauze

Instruments:

Basic Soft-Tissue Instrument Set
Allis clamp
Castro–Viejo needle holder
Jaeger plate

*The trade name Gore-Tex is employed in the text to refer to the suture material for the sake of clarity, because the needle sizes used refer to those manufactured by W.L. Gore & Associates (Flagstaff, AZ). All other references to Gore-Tex material in the text are made to the generic name, expanded polytetrafluoroethylene, or ePTFE. The authors emphasize that they do not hold any financial arrangements or obtain any direct or indirect gain from the manufacturer.

Hand-held hot-tip wire-loop cautery
Bipolar cord and handpiece

Sutures:

6-0 silk, P-1(P-10, PRE-1) [C1] <EDR-1>[**] needle (traction suture)
7-0 nylon, P-1 (P-10, PRE-1) [C1] <EDR-1> needle (for wound closure)
5-0 polydioxanone P-3 (P-13, PRE-2) <RE-3>(for ptosis repair)
4-0 polydioxanone PS-3 (P-11, PRE-3) [PC-34] (for an extended skin–muscle dissection to tack the flap to the lateral–canthal periosteum)

Other Supplies:

Steri-Strips (3M, St. Paul, MN) (to hold medial end of lower blepharoplasty suture in place)

[**]The first needle size refers to the Ethicon code. The second parenthetical code refers to the equivalent needle size manufactured by US Surgical/Davis & Geck. Of note, the first code within the parentheses refers to the new US Surgical code and the second number within the parentheses refers to the older Davis & Geck code. The third bracketed code refers to the equivalent needle size made by Look. The fourth code in brackets refers to the Deknatel needle equivalent.

Cotton-tipped applicators
4 × 4 gauze

Dressing:

Bacitracin ointment
Aquaphor ointment (for lower-lid resurfacing)
N-terface occlusive dressing (for laser resurfacing)

Instrument/Equipment for Malar Augmentation

Prep Stand:

10-cc syringe (2), 27-gauge (1¼ inch long) needle (2) with lidocaine 1% and 1:100,000 epinephrine

Instruments:

Basic Soft-Tissue Instrument Set
Hand Drill with a drill bit sized 1.5 × 12 mm (the screw should measure 2 mm × 10 to 12 mm)

Other Supplies:

ePTFE (Gore-Tex) Malar Implant (small, medium, or large)

Dressing:

None

addition, the patient should be positioned upright during the peel (inclined about 60 degrees). A detailed review of technique may be found in Chapter 9. CO_2 laser resurfacing may be required if deeper etched lines are present, so long as the patient is amenable to the longer recovery period (upward of 3 months versus 2 weeks for the peel). Laser resurfacing may be undertaken before or after blepharoplasty; however, the authors routinely elect to perform laser ablation at the end of all surgical intervention. The surgeon should be extremely wary about performing additional skin excision after lower-lid resurfacing, because the risk of ectropion or vertical lid shortening is increased. After resurfacing, the lid continues to undergo some contraction and may pull away from the globe even without skin removal. The inexperienced surgeon is advised to wait several weeks if uncertain about the extent of additional skin excess and to undertake a pinch of skin as needed in the office setting at this later date.

A transconjunctival approach is preferred for the majority of lower-lid blepharoplasties, because the integrity of the orbicularis oculi is maintained, and an external incision is avoided if no skin redundancy exists. Both the skin and muscle sling act to retain the lower-lid position against the globe, and a skin–muscle flap predisposes to a higher likelihood of lid malposition. If a browlift is carried out concomitantly, a transconjunctival blepharoplasty should be performed first, because the brow suspension increases lower-lid tension and makes transconjunctival entry particularly arduous.

The first step in performing a lower-lid blepharoplasty involves proper local anesthetic placement, which is achieved with a mixture of 1% lidocaine to 50,000 epinephrine. The local anesthesia is injected into the conjunctiva in the medial, central, and lateral aspects in the preseptal plane while the conjunctiva is exposed with a Desmarres or wide, two-pronged retractor. Additional local anesthesia may be infiltrated into the lower-lid skin as well if skin excision is planned. The patient should be under sedation or general anesthesia for the infiltration of anesthesia as well as for the actual procedure because transconjunctival surgery may elicit patient discomfort. The anesthesiologist also should be advised that ocular lubrication should not be instilled before a transconjunctival blepharoplasty because the ophthalmic gel tends to obscure the surgical field.

After 10 minutes are allowed to transpire for maximal hemostasis, the Desmarres or wide, two-pronged retractor is properly positioned to retract the lower lid by the first assistant (who is stationed to the right of the surgeon and patient) while the surgeon (above the head of the patient) gently protects the globe and applies countertraction with a Jaeger plate. With a bipolar cautery, the surgeon seals the superficial conjunctival vessels before transconjunctival entry (Fig. 4-8). A hand-held, hot-tip, wire-loop cautery is used to incise the conjunctiva just past 5 mm from the lid margin (i.e., beyond the edge of the tarsal border) (Fig. 4-9).[†] The

[†]Monopolar cautery should be limited in use near the eye because of the known risk of electrical arc that can ignite and incinerate the eyelashes.

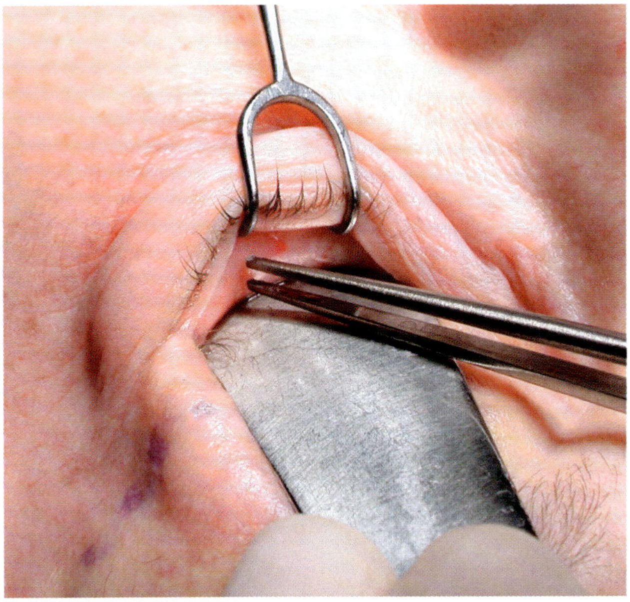

FIGURE 4-8. Lower Transconjunctival Blepharoplasty, Step 1. After infiltration with 1% lidocaine and 1:50,000 epinephrine, the first step in a lower-lid transconjunctival blepharoplasty entails cauterization of any superficial conjunctival vessels before conjunctival entry. A sharp, wide two-pronged retractor should be held upward to distract the lower lid by the assistant (seated to the right of the patient and surgeon); and a Jaeger plate used to protect and displace the globe.

Jaeger plate is removed; the inferior aspect of the transected conjunctival border (i.e., the side closest to the surgeon) is grasped with a Bishop forceps; and a 6-0 silk suture with a P-1 needle is passed through the conjunctiva so that the conjunctival flap can be retracted upward over the globe for protection and retraction (Fig. 4-10). The silk loop is secured with a hemostat and placed on the patient's forehead resting on a moist 4 × 4 gauze to provide adequate tension on the conjunctival flap.

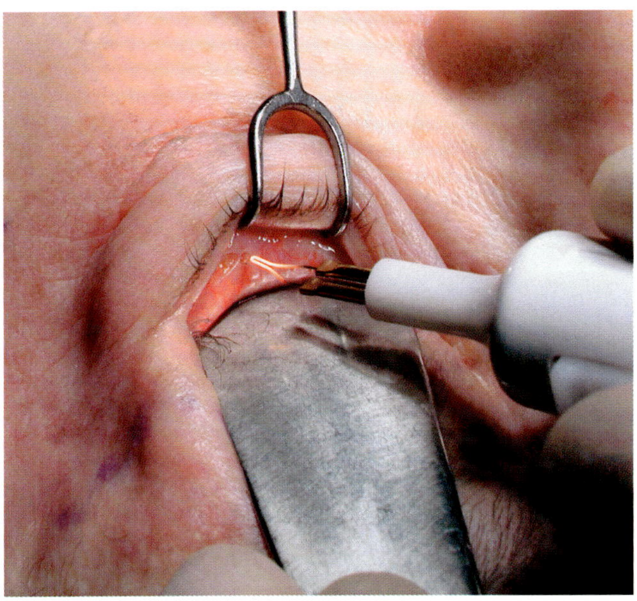

FIGURE 4-9. Lower Transconjunctival Blepharoplasty, Step 2. A hand-held, hot-tip, wire-loop cautery is used to incise the conjunctiva just past 5 mm from the lid margin (i.e., below the edge of the tarsal border).

The surgeon again picks up the inferior (proximal) conjunctival flap with a pair of Bishop forceps carefully observing for the wisp-like adhesions that traverse vertically from the orbicularis oculi (anteriorly) to the septum (posteriorly) and that define the preseptal plane (Fig. 4-11). The dissection is carried out with the hot-tip, hand-held cautery. The authors prefer a preseptal dissection because of a more controlled and natural dissection plane than afforded by postseptal entry. The preseptal dissection plane is defined as the natural cleavage plane that separates the septum and postseptal fat posteriorly from the orbicularis-oculi muscle anteriorly (Fig. 4-12). (Conversely, a postseptal dissection involves direct entry into the postseptal fat without defining the orbital-septal plane.)

A small puncture is made in the orbital septum over the medial-fat pocket with the hot-tip cautery, and the fat is gently teased out while the other hand applies gentle pressure on the globe (Fig. 4-13). The amount of fat that protrudes is correlated with the preoperative images that should be prominently displayed in the operating suite for reference. These standardized preoperative portraits, particularly the close-up frontal view, act as indispensable guides because the supine patient reveals little information about the amount of herniated fat that is present. If any arcade of vessels traverse the fat to be removed, they can be teased back into the globe with a cotton-tipped applicator rather than clamped and

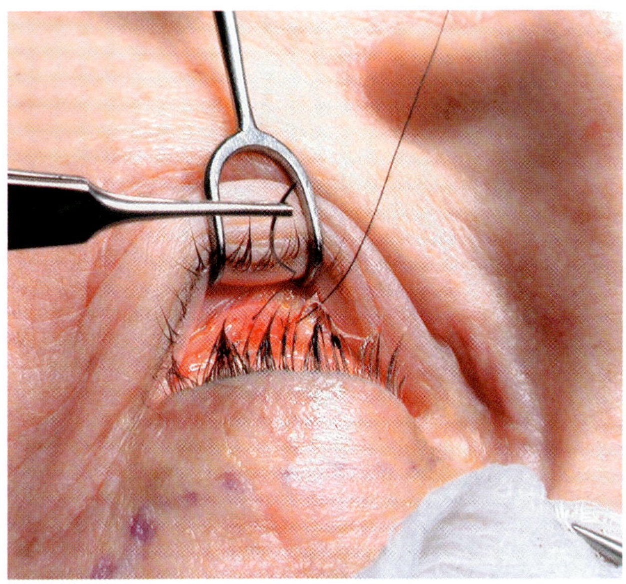

FIGURE 4-10. Lower Transconjunctival Blepharoplasty, Step 3. The Jaeger plate is removed and the inferior aspect of the transected conjunctival border (i.e., the side closest to the surgeon) is grasped with a Bishop forceps, and a 6-0 silk suture is passed through the conjunctiva so that the inferior (proximal) conjunctival flap can be retracted upward over the globe for protection and retraction. The silk loop is secured with a hemostat and placed on the patient's forehead resting on a moist 4 × 4 gauze to provide adequate tension on the conjunctival flap.

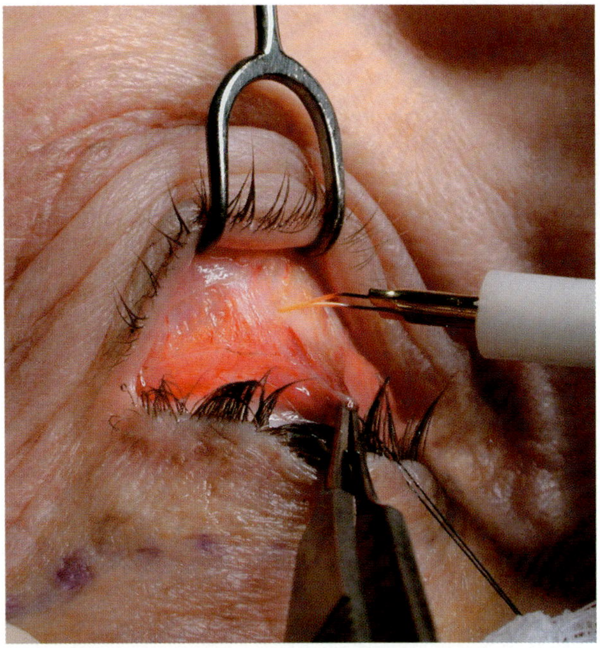

FIGURE 4-11. Lower Transconjunctival Blepharoplasty, Step 4. The surgeon again picks up the inferior (proximal) conjunctival flap with a pair of Bishop forceps carefully observing for the wisp-like adhesions that traverse vertically from the orbicularis oculi (anteriorly) to the septum (posteriorly) that define the preseptal plane.

cauterized. This maneuver may reduce the risk of postoperative retroseptal hemorrhage. No additional local anesthesia is administered to the dissected fat: The authors believe that the few seconds that transpire between anesthetic injection and fat removal do not permit sufficient time for the local

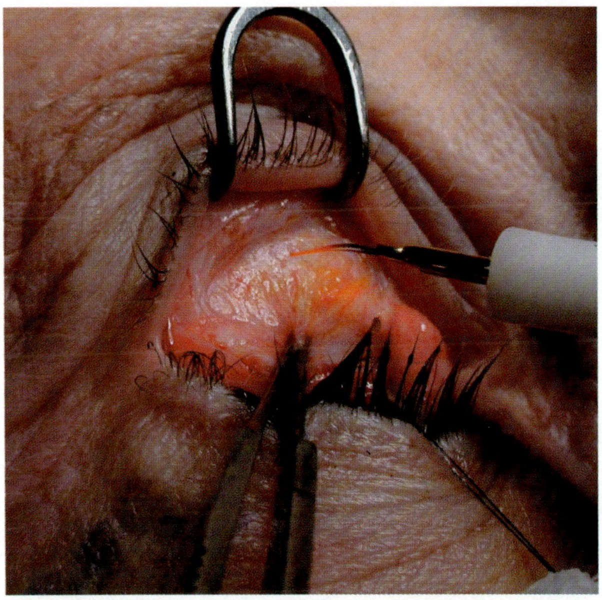

FIGURE 4-12. Lower Transconjunctival Blepharoplasty, Step 5. The dissection is carried out with hot-tip, hand-held cautery. The authors prefer a preseptal dissection because of a more controlled and natural dissection plane than afforded by postseptal entry. The preseptal dissection plane is defined as the natural cleavage plane that separates the septum and postseptal fat posteriorly from the orbicularis-oculi muscle anteriorly.

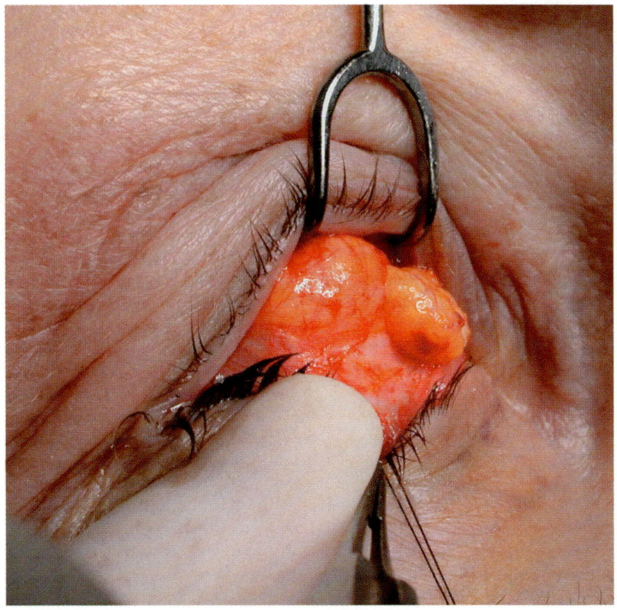

FIGURE 4-13. Lower Transconjunctival Blepharoplasty, Step 6. A small puncture is made in the orbital septum over the medial fat pocket with the hot-tip cautery, and the fat is gently teased out while the other hand applies gentle pressure on the globe. The amount of fat that protrudes is correlated with the preoperative images that should be prominently displayed in the operating suite for reference.

anesthesia to function properly. (If the reader should elect to inject local anesthesia postseptally, he or she is reminded of the necessity to use only plain lidocaine to avoid the risk of vasospasm and consequent visual loss.)

The dissected adipose then is clamped with a hemostat and held in position by the surgical assistant (Fig. 4-14). The surgeon applies bipolar cautery along the clamp (Fig. 4-15) and then excises the fat along the clamp with a pair of

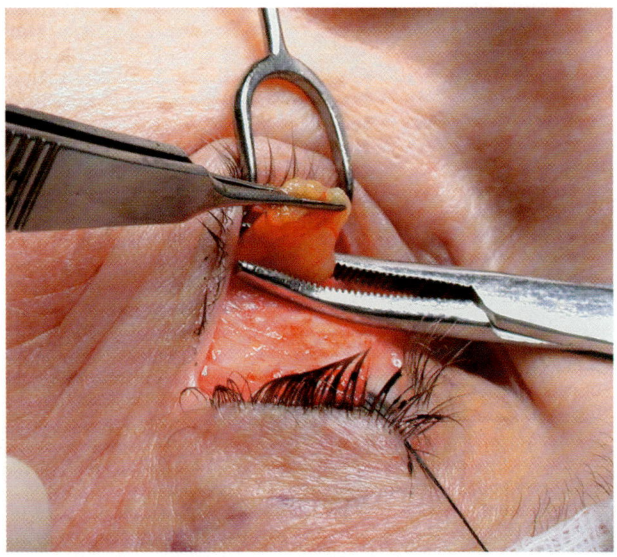

FIGURE 4-14. Lower Transconjunctival Blepharoplasty, Step 7. The dissected adipose is clamped with a hemostat and held in position (away from the skin) by the assistant.

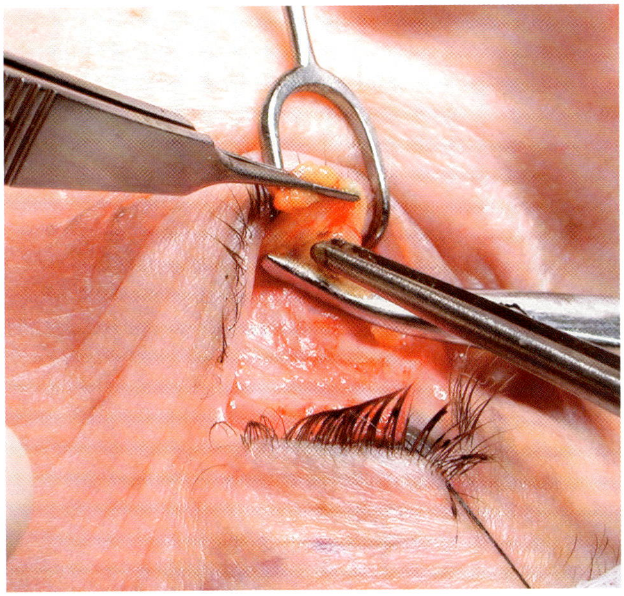

FIGURE 4-15. Lower Transconjunctival Blepharoplasty, Step 8. The surgeon applies bipolar cautery along the clamp prior to excision of the excess adipose.

tenotomy scissors (Fig. 4-16). Additional bipolar cautery is applied to the adipose cuff that remains along the hemostat after fat excision (Fig. 4-17). Prior to the assistant's release of the hemostat tines, the surgeon grasps the remaining fat below the clamp with a pair of Bishop forceps. As the clamp is released, the surgeon carefully observes for any signs of uncontrolled hemorrhage, which is promptly addressed with bipolar cautery (Fig. 4-18). The reader is also reminded about the risk of inadvertent injury to the inferior-oblique muscle, which separates the medial-fat from the central-fat pockets. The surgeon then progresses laterally to the central-

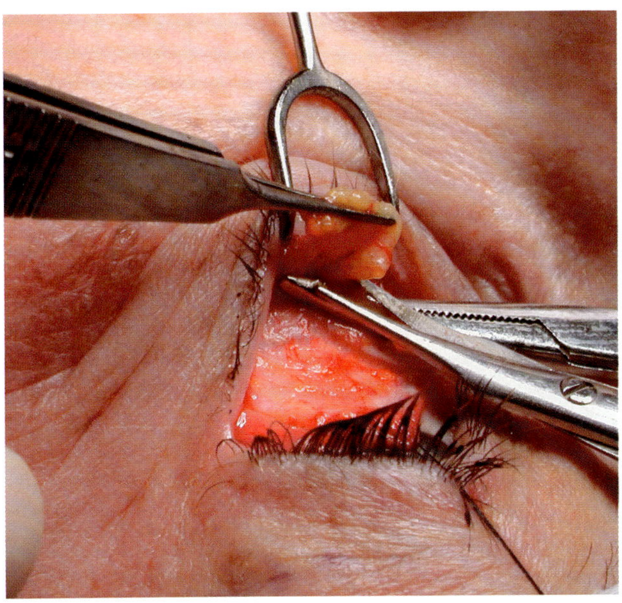

FIGURE 4-16. Lower Transconjunctival Blepharoplasty, Step 9. The excess fat is trimmed with a pair of tenotomy scissors.

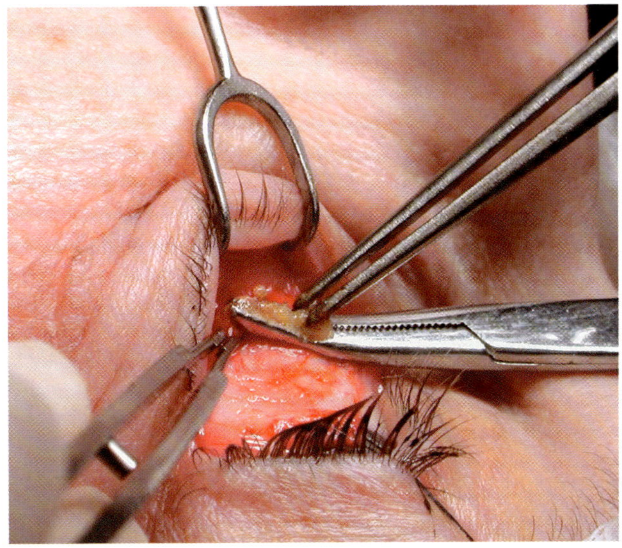

FIGURE 4-17. Lower Transconjunctival Blepharoplasty, Step 10. Additional bipolar cautery is applied to the adipose cuff that remains along the hemostat after fat excision.

fat and lateral-fat pockets in a similar fashion, as dictated by the patient's pathology. The conjunctiva is left to heal without suture closure. If any skin redundancy is evident, an Allis clamp is used to pinch the excess skin about 1 mm from the lid margin while carefully observing for eyelash eversion. The amount of skin removed is dictated by eyelash position, where the eyelashes should just begin to assume a perpendicular orientation to the skin when the skin is grasped by the Allis. The crimped excess skin then is removed with Bishop forceps and fine iris scissors. Any irregular skin edges are not rectified by additional corrective trimming, because

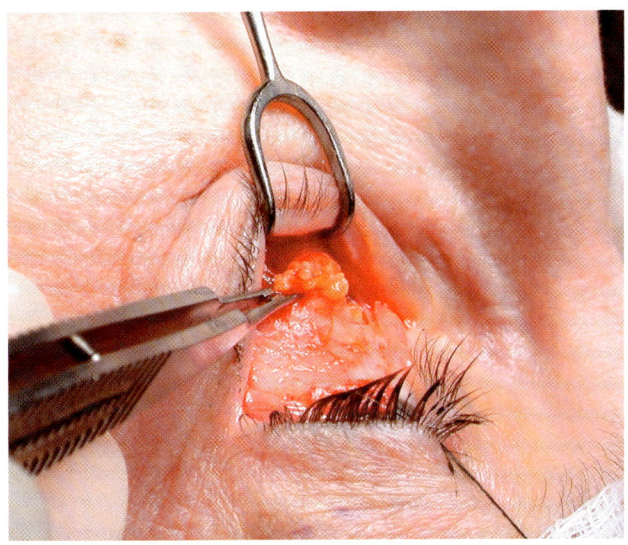

FIGURE 4-18. Lower Transconjunctival Blepharoplasty, Step 11. Prior to the assistant's release of the hemostat tines, the surgeon grasps the remaining fat below the clamp with a pair of Bishop forceps. As the clamp is released, the surgeon carefully observes for any signs of uncontrolled hemorrhage, which is promptly addressed with bipolar cautery as needed.

this predisposes to vertical lid shortening and is simply unnecessary for favorable healing. Hemostasis is obtained with hot-tip cautery, and the wound edges are approximated with a running, nonlocking 7-0 polypropylene suture with the medial extent fastened to the skin with a Steri-Strip rather than tied. Leaving the medial end untied allows edema to loosen the suture appropriately and facilitates suture removal. Sutures are removed at 6 days postoperatively.

DVD Lower Blepharoplasty (Skin–Muscle/Extended Skin–Muscle)

As mentioned, the transconjunctival approach remains the authors' mainstay for lower-lid blepharoplasty. However, a skin–muscle flap is indicated in certain select conditions that favor this technique. If excessive lower-lid laxity or frank ectropion is present, then a lower-lid shortening procedure (e.g., tarsal strip) may be required. Alternatively, a lateral-canthal fixation suture may be used to suspend the lower lid sufficiently in proper position. Although a transconjunctival blepharoplasty may prevent the onset of postoperative lower-lid malposition, preexisting lower-lid malposition requires correction with a tarsal strip or lateral-canthal suspension. If a tarsal strip or lateral-canthal plication suture is required, then a skin–muscle flap is advised. Furthermore, if the patient suffers from malar descent (festooning or malar bagging) and declines a browlift/transbrow midface lift, then an extended skin–muscle flap may be undertaken instead. For any of these reasons, a skin–muscle type flap may be the approach of choice.

If an extended blepharoplasty is to be carried out, then an extended incision that follows a natural skin crease radiating from the lateral canthus should be marked out with a surgical marking pen. One percent lidocaine with 1:50,000 epinephrine is injected along the line of incision and inferiorly over the area of dissection. The appropriate 10 minutes of hemostatic time is allowed to transpire before the initial incision is made. A No. 15 Bard–Parker blade is used to make the first few millimeters of an incision approximately 1 to 2 mm from the inferior lid margin at the most lateral extent through both skin and muscle. A pair of iris scissors then are inserted through this incipient incision and gently spread to develop the plane of dissection below the skin–muscle flap from lateral to medial. One blade of the scissors then is inserted into the incision with the other blade remaining externally, and in this way the incision is opened laterally to medially as far as required but always lateral to the medial punctum (to minimize risk of medial-canthal web formation) (Fig. 4-19). The bleeding muscle edge then is cauterized with a hot-tip hand-held electrocautery or a bipolar cautery device.

A 6-0 silk suture is passed through the superior aspect of the incision and clamped with a hemostat in order to retract the lower lid upward, protecting the globe and providing countertraction to the elevated skin–muscle flap. Bishop forceps or a wide, double-pronged retractor then is used to retract the skin–muscle flap inferiorly while the hand-held or monopolar cautery dissects the skin–muscle flap from the underlying orbital septum. This flap is carried downward onto the midface under the malar bag/festoon if an extended lower-lid blepharoplasty is intended (Fig. 4-20). If pseudo-

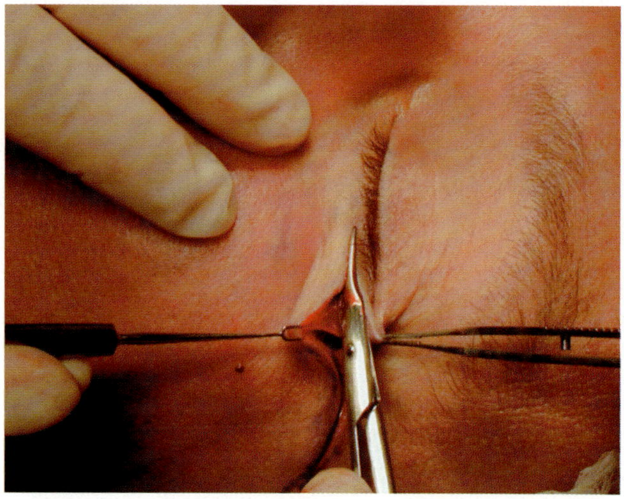

FIGURE 4-19. Lower (Extended Skin–Muscle) Blepharoplasty, Step 1. A No. 15 Bard-Parker blade is used to make the first few millimeters of an incision approximately 1 to 2 mm from the inferior lid margin at the most lateral extent through both skin and muscle. A pair of iris scissors then are inserted through this incipient incision and gently spread to develop the plane of dissection below the skin–muscle flap from lateral to medial. One blade of the scissors then is inserted into the incision with the other blade remaining externally, and in this way the incision is opened laterally to medially as far as required but always lateral to the medial punctum (to minimize risk of medial-canthal web formation).

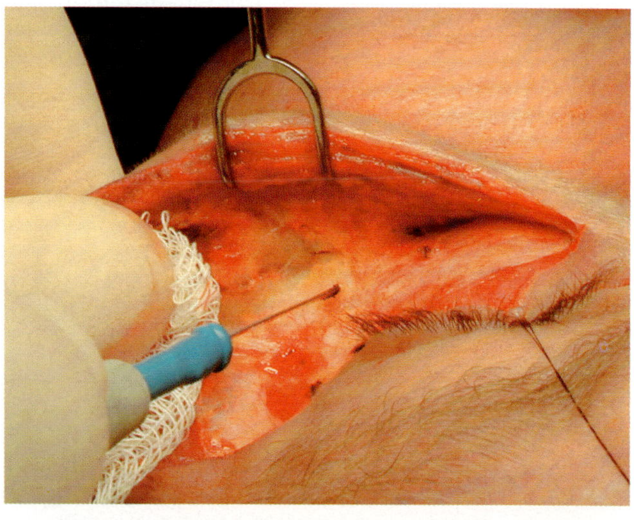

FIGURE 4-20. Lower (Extended Skin–Muscle) Blepharoplasty, Step 2. A 6-0 silk suture is passed through the superior aspect of the incision and clamped with a hemostat in order to retract the lower lid upward, protecting the globe and providing countertraction. Bishop forceps or a wide, double-pronged retractor is used to retract the skin–muscle flap inferiorly while the hand-held or monopolar cautery dissects the skin–muscle flap from the underlying orbital septum. This flap is carried downward onto the midface under the malar bag/festoon if an extended lower-lid blepharoplasty is intended.

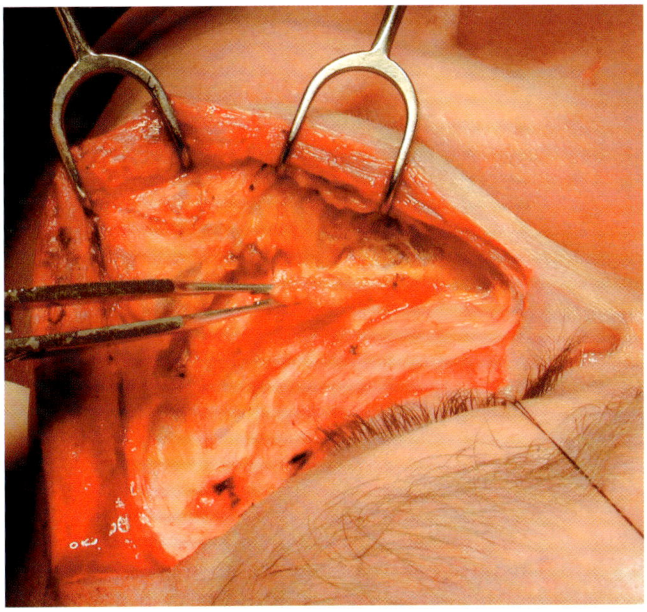

FIGURE 4-21. Lower (Extended Skin–Muscle) Blepharoplasty, Step 3. The malar fat pad is identified and grasped with fine forceps for suspension to the lateral orbital rim.

herniation of fat exists, then the orbital septum is entered and the fat clamped and removed as described earlier for the transconjunctival approach. If an extended blepharoplasty is undertaken to efface a malar bag/festoon, then the malar bag/festoon is suspended to the lateral orbital rim using a 4-0 polydioxanone (PDS [Ethicon, Cornelia, GA], Maxon [U.S. Surgical/Davis & Geck, Norwalk, CT]) or CV-4 Gore-Tex suture (Figs. 4-21, 4-22, and 4-23). A single pronged hook is placed into the lateral aspect of the incision to provide proper tension and alignment prior to skin-flap excision (Fig. 4-24). Any excessive skin–muscle flap then is trimmed with curved serrated iris scissors erring on the conservative side to avoid unintended lid eversion and vertical shortening, especially medially (Fig. 4-25). The incision line then is reapproximated with a running, nonlocking 7-0 polypropylene suture. A lateral canthal suspension suture still should be considered for a standard skin–muscle blepharoplasty to lessen the probability of postoperative lid malposition. This suture is placed in a similar fashion as described for the extended technique but often with less vertical elevation. (The midface does not require suspension in this circumstance.)

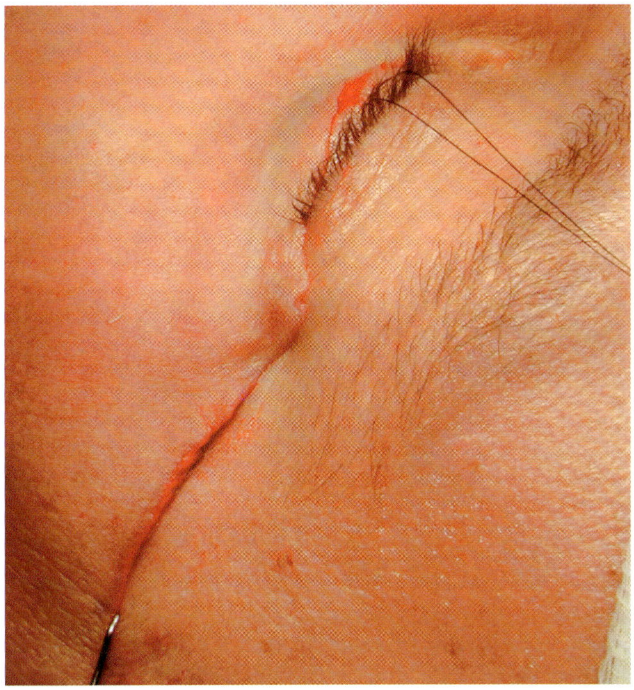

FIGURE 4-24. Lower (Extended Skin–Muscle) Blepharoplasty, Step 5. A single pronged hook is placed into the lateral aspect of the incision to provide proper tension and alignment prior to skin-flap excision.

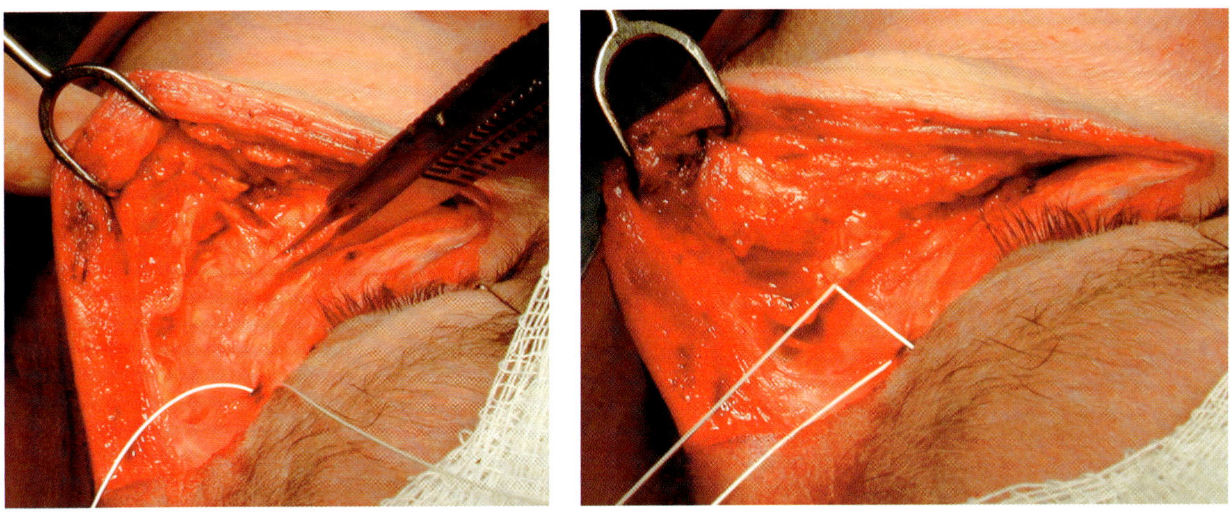

FIGURES 4-22 and 4-23. Lower (Extended Skin–Muscle) Blepharoplasty, Step 4. A 4-0 polydioxanone or 4-0 Gore-Tex suture is used to suspend the malar fat pad to the lateral orbital periosteum.

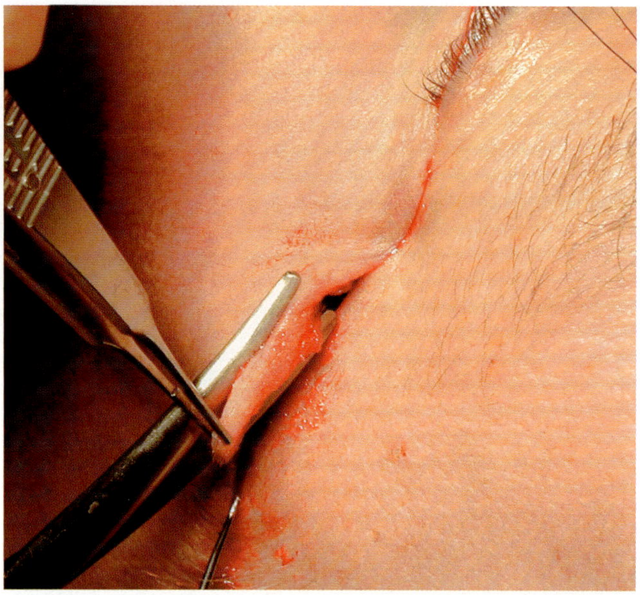

FIGURE 4-25. Lower (Extended Skin–Muscle) Blepharoplasty, Step 6. Any excessive skin–muscle flap then is trimmed with curved serrated iris scissors erring on the conservative side to avoid unintended lid eversion and vertical shortening, especially medially.

If a tarsal strip is to be conducted, then this may be performed after the skin–muscle flap has been properly elevated and in lieu of the described suspension suture. A pentagonal wedge (or Kuhnt-Szymanowski) is not preferred for risk of lid notching. The tarsal-strip procedure is briefly reviewed herein (Fig. 4-26). A lateral canthotomy is undertaken, followed by an inferior cantholysis. After an inferior cantholysis, the lower lid should be freely detached from the globe. The freed lower lid should be retracted supero-laterally so that the lower lid crosses 1 mm above the inferior limbus. The amount of lid excess can be determined with the lid retracted in this way, and the corresponding anterior lamella (orbicularis oculi and skin) should be divided sharply from the posterior lamella to expose the tarsus. The excessive conjunctiva is abraded away with the belly of the No. 15 blade to create the tarsal strip. The tarsal strip then is suspended to its physiologic locus (at Whitnall's tubercle) through the periosteum with a double-armed 5-0 white Mersilene suture in a vertical mattress configuration. The authors have noted that actual suspension to Whitnall's tubercle, located in the inner aspect of the orbital rim, causes undue prolonged eyelid distortion and may be avoided by simply tacking the tarsal strip to the anterior-medial border of the orbital rim instead. The excessive tarsal strip then is trimmed away. The lateral canthus is reapproximated to its correct anatomic location using 7-0 nylon. Excess skin and muscle are removed, principally in the lateral aspect of the wound (the same technique as advocated for an extended skin–muscle flap) tapering medially. Skin closure then is completed with a running 7-0 nylon suture.

DVD Upper Blepharoplasty (Pinch with Medial Fat Dissection)

If an upper blepharoplasty is to be performed in conjunction with a browlift, it should always be done after the browlift so that proper estimation of excess skin tissue may be assessed. Some surgeons prefer to wait for 6 weeks after a browlift so that some inevitable brow descent will not create a recurrent problem with upper-lid skin excess. However, the authors believe that this delayed return of excess lid skin is minimal to none, and this situation can be addressed with an additional skin pinch at the time it arises. The surgeon should exercise greater caution regarding skin removal if a patient has already undergone a prior upper-lid blepharoplasty and/or browlift. It may be warranted to wait several weeks before electing to remove lid skin under this circumstance.

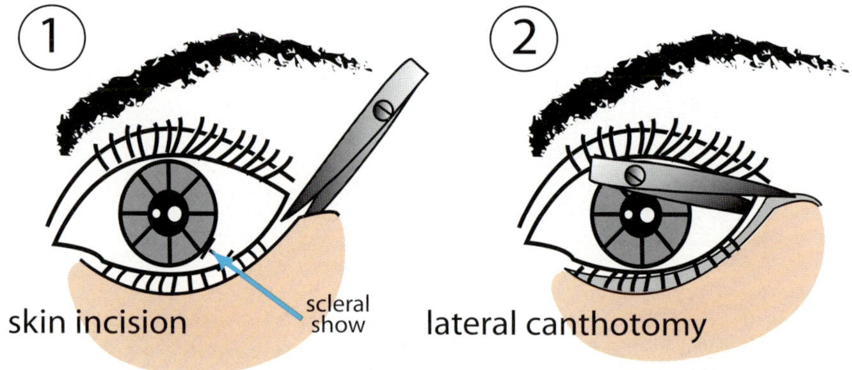

FIGURE 4-26. The illustrations show how to perform a tarsal strip. **1:** First, a skin–muscle flap is raised along the subciliary margin as undertaken in a standard lower-lid transcutaneous blepharoplasty. The skin incision extends past the lateral canthus, as undertaken in an extended lower-lid transcutaneous blepharoplasty. **2:** A lateral canthotomy is performed by severing the cutaneous junction at the lateral canthus. *(continued)*

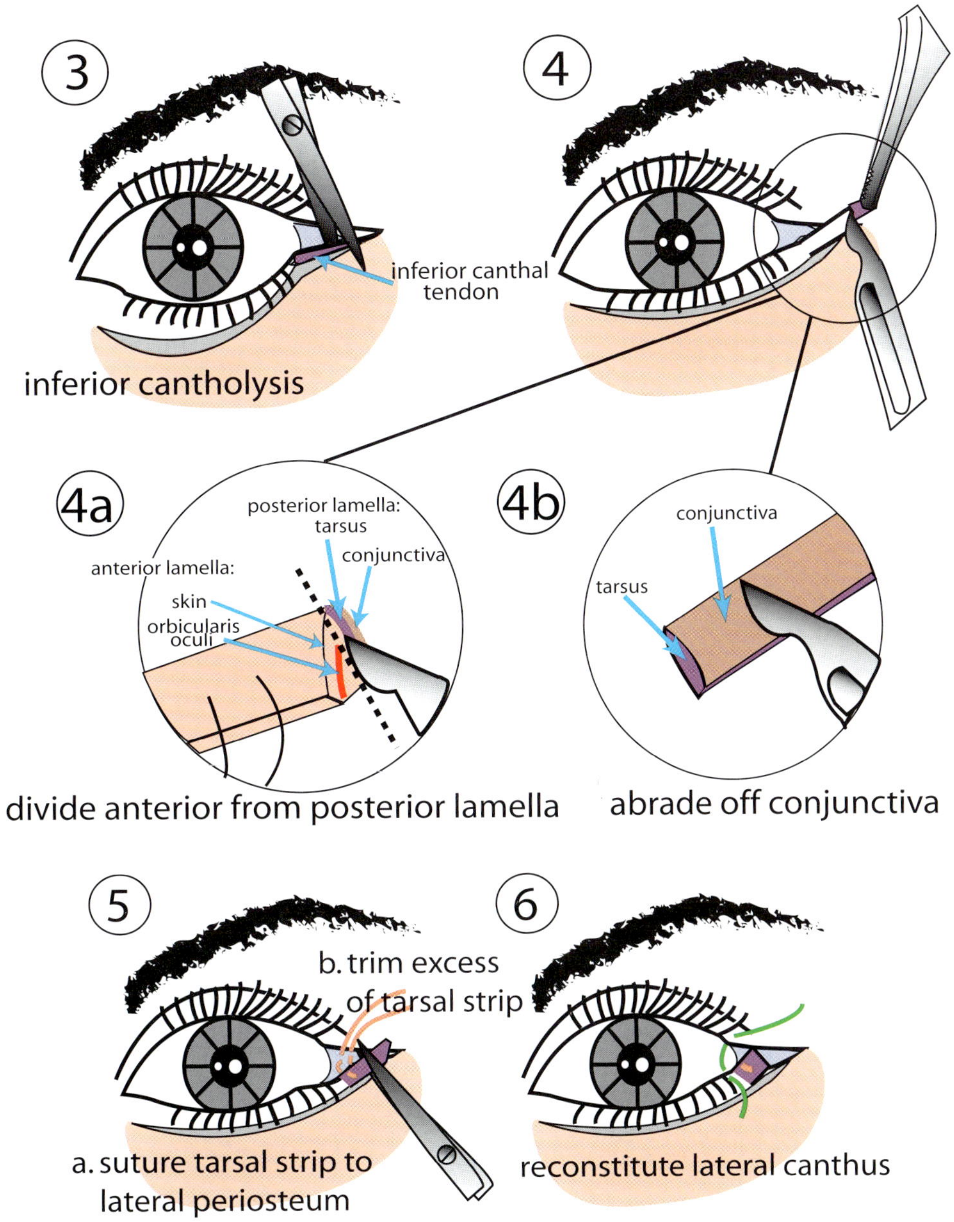

FIGURE 4-26. *(Continued)* **3:** The tines of the scissors are then directed downward to transect the inferior lateral canthal tendon (inferior cantholysis) as laterally as possible, which should be evidenced by a freely mobile lower-lid segment after transection. **4A:** The anterior lamella (composed of the skin and orbicularis-oculi muscle) is divided sharply from the underlying posterior lamella (composed of the tarsus and conjunctiva) with a No. 15 blade for a short distance so that the exposed tarsal strip can be affixed to the lateral periosteum (*in light blue*). The requisite distance of anterior lamellar resection can be estimated by holding the tarsal strip laterally so that the lid appears to override the inferior limbus by 1 mm. **4B:** The conjunctiva then is abraded from the tarsal strip for the same distance used to remove anterior lamella. Conjunctiva must be removed to avoid trapped epithelial inclusion cysts from arising. **5A:** The tarsal strip (*in purple*) is tacked to the lateral periosteum (*in light blue*) using a double-armed 5-0 white Mersilene suture in a vertical mattress configuration. **5B:** The excess tarsal strip then is trimmed away. **6:** The lateral canthus is reapproximated with 7-0 nylon suture. *(continued)*

The supratarsal crease is first marked out with a fine marking pen. The lid can be gently retracted until the crease is apparent if it cannot be readily visualized with the lid closed. One percent lidocaine with 1:50,000 epinephrine is instilled under the skin, carefully avoiding injection of the underlying muscle, which can lead to untoward ecchymosis and hematoma formation. An Allis clamp is used to pinch the excess skin so that minimal, incipient lid eversion is noted (Fig. 4-27). The inferior aspect of the skin clamped is the supratarsal crease, as all skin removed is superior to this

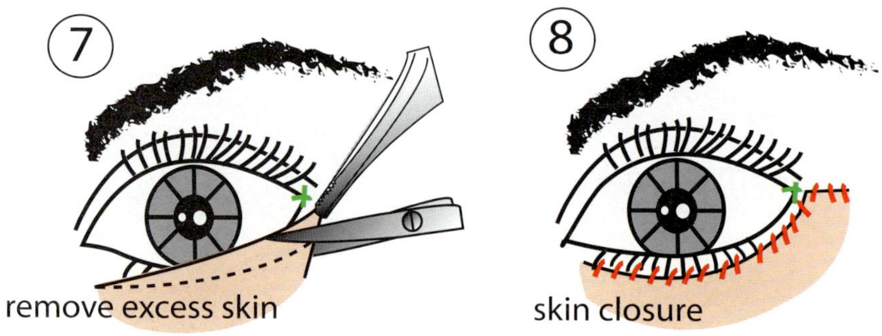

FIGURE 4-26. *(Continued)* **7:** The excess skin (and muscle) are trimmed away by holding the excess skin upward and tapering the amount of excision medially. **8:** The skin then is closed with a running, nonlocking 7-0 nylon suture.

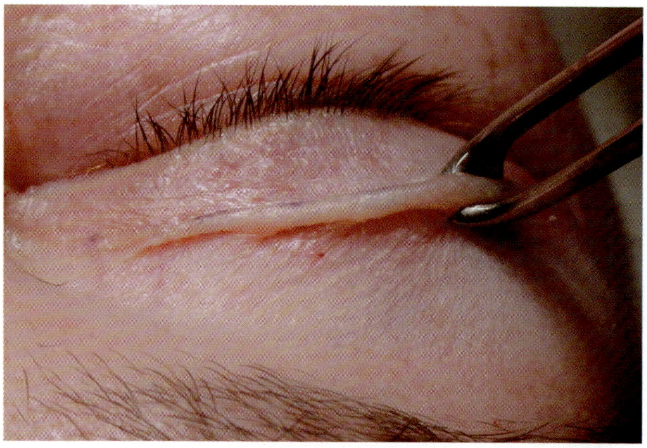

FIGURE 4-27. Upper Blepharoplasty, Step 1. After carefully marking the supratarsal crease and infiltrating 1% lidocaine and 1:50,000 epinephrine into the subcutaneous tissue, an Allis clamp is used to pinch the excess skin so that minimal, incipient lid eversion is noted. The inferior aspect of the skin clamped is the supratarsal crease, because all skin removed is superior to this line.

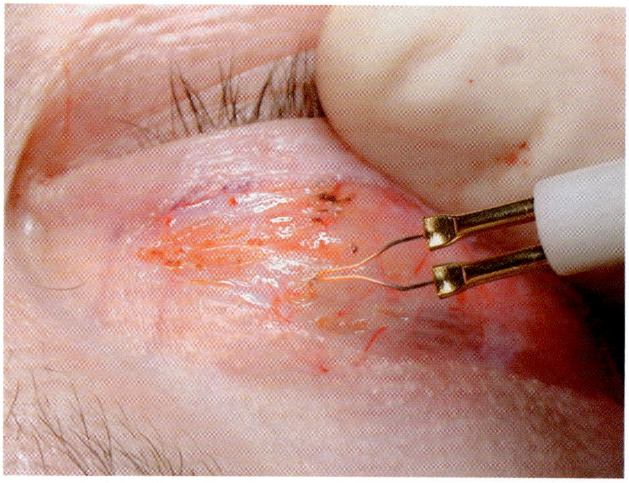

FIGURE 4-29. Upper Blepharoplasty, Step 3. Hemostasis is achieved with a hand-held, hot-tip cautery.

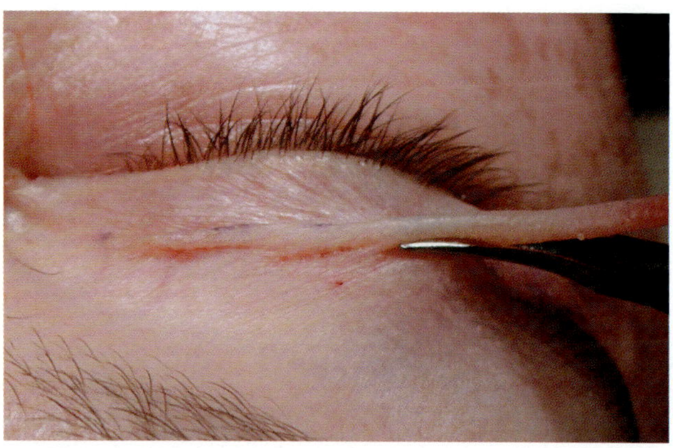

FIGURE 4-28. Upper Blepharoplasty, Step 2. The clamped skin is removed with a pair of tenotomy scissors.

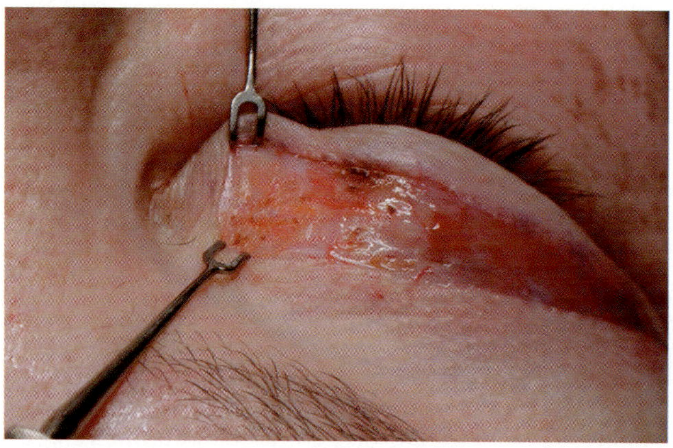

FIGURE 4-30. Upper Blepharoplasty, Step 4. Small, double-hooked forceps are used to retract opposing sides of the septum upward and away from the wound to facilitate entry into the medial-fat pocket.

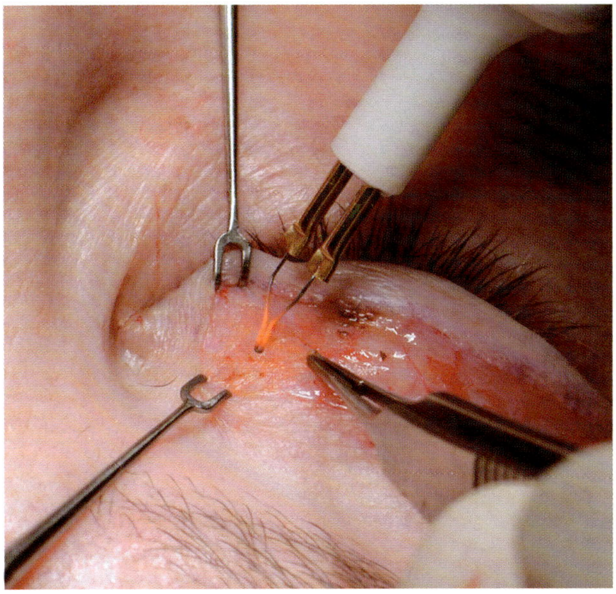

FIGURE 4-31. Upper Blepharoplasty, Step 5. A hot-tip cautery is used to transect the muscle and septum to expose the underlying medial fat pad.

line. The clamped skin is removed with a pair of tenotomy scissors (Fig. 4-28). Hemostasis is achieved with a hand-held hot-tip cautery (Fig. 4-29).

If medial fat protrusion exists (as confirmed by preoperative photographs), then the muscle and septum must be transected medially over the fat pad for exposure. Small double-hooked forceps are used to retract opposing sides of the septum upward and away from the wound (Fig. 4-30). A hot-tip cautery is used to transect the muscle and septum (Fig. 4-31), and the globe is gently balloted to determine the amount of fat to be removed. Bishop forceps are employed to tease out the excessive adipose tissue (Fig. 4-32), and the same technique as described in the preceding is enlisted to

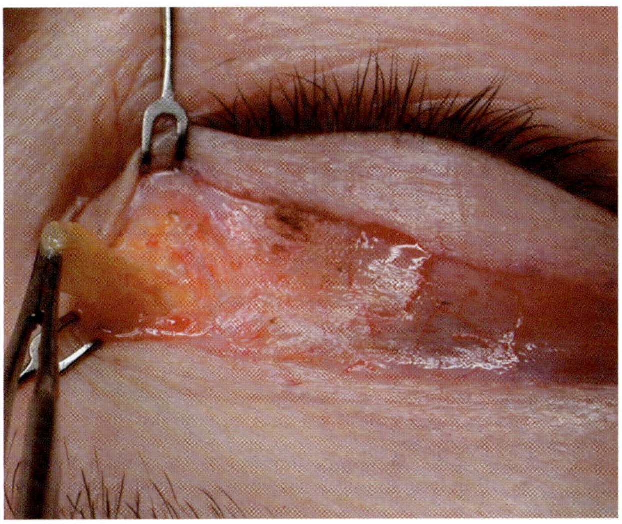

FIGURE 4-32. Upper Blepharoplasty, Step 6. The globe is gently balloted to determine the amount of fat to be removed, and Bishop forceps are employed to tease out the excessive adipose tissue.

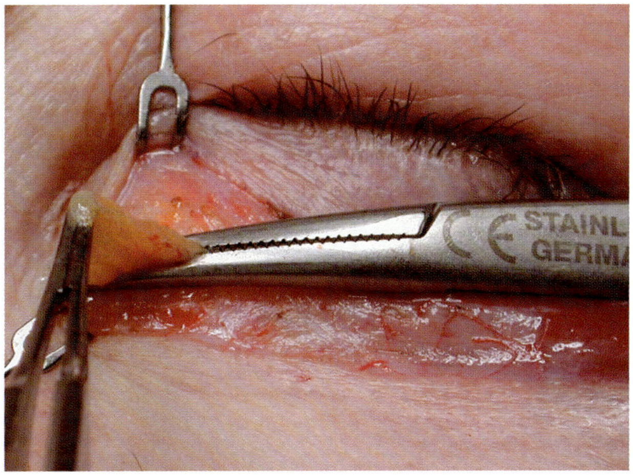

FIGURE 4-33. Upper Blepharoplasty, Step 7. The prolapsed fat pad then is clamped with a small, curved hemostat.

clamp and remove the fat (Figs. 4-33, 4-34, 4-35, and 4-36). It should be emphasized once more that irregular skin edges should not be further tailored for risk of excessive skin removal; furthermore, such action is unnecessary. Wound closure is achieved with the described running 7-0 polypropylene suture with only minimal skin purchase on both sides of the wound to avoid unwanted lid eversion (Fig. 4-37). Care should be taken to avoid violating the underlying muscle with the skin suture because of the preventable outcome of potential hematoma and added ecchymosis.

Ptosis Repair (External Approach)

Although ptosis repair may appear to be beyond the confines of expertise for the facial plastic surgeon, an external approach may be easily and effectively combined with an upper-lid blepharoplasty to affect the maximal aesthetic and functional outcome for the patient. Clearly, more advanced eyelid pathologies should be relegated to the oculoplastic colleague for advice and care. The internal (Müller resection) approach is not discussed herein in order to maintain sim-

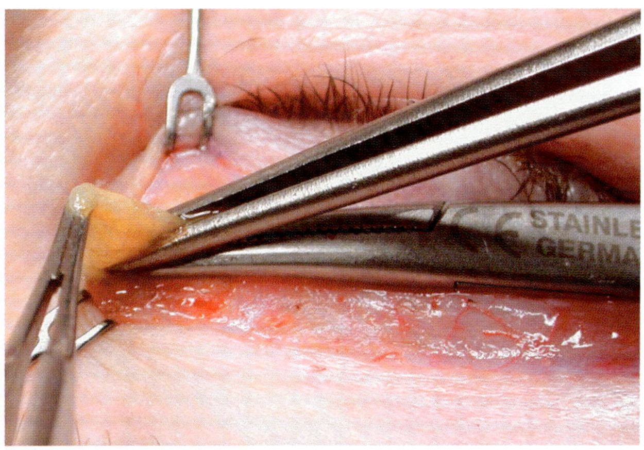

FIGURE 4-34. Upper Blepharoplasty, Step 8. Bipolar cautery is used along the base of the fat prior to excision.

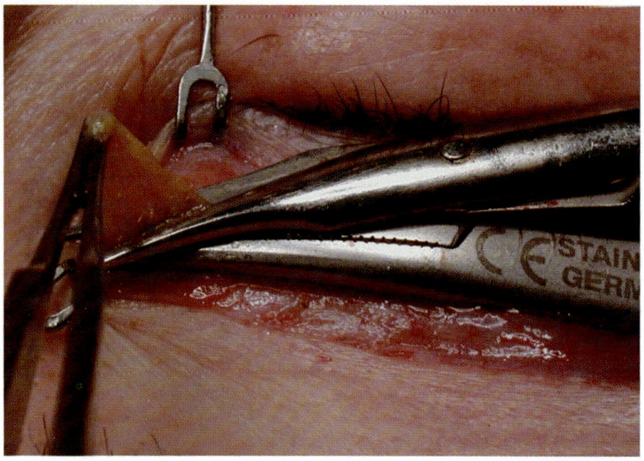

FIGURE 4-35. Upper Blepharoplasty, Step 9. Tenotomy scissors are used to transect the excess fat.

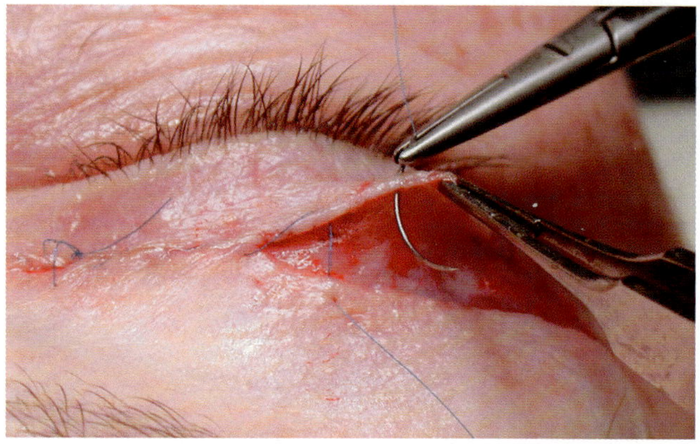

FIGURE 4-37. Upper Blepharoplasty, Step 11. Wound closure is achieved with a running, nonlocking, 7-0 polypropylene suture with only minimal skin purchase on both sides of the wound to avoid unwanted lid eversion. Care should be heeded to avoid violating the underlying muscle with the skin suture because of the preventable outcome of potential hematoma and added ecchymosis.

plicity and minimize confusion.[11] Furthermore, the internal approach has more restricted applications and is really more suited for younger patients who exhibit only a marginal degree of lid ptosis. If browlift surgery is planned, it should be undertaken several weeks before ptosis repair is considered, because brow elevation may exacerbate blepharoptosis.

The reader is advised to review the salient points of preoperative assessment described in detail in the previous section before studying the operative technique (Fig. 4-38) and should fully understand the pertinent upper-eyelid anatomy before embarking on this procedure (Fig. 4-39). First, the patient should be under minimal to no sedation so that the patient may cooperate with lid opening and closing during the procedure. The supratarsal crease is marked out with a surgical marking pen first. In addition, the superior half of the limbus may be traced out over the eyelid, when the lid is in primary gaze and fully open. The migration of this line upward after injection with local anesthesia containing epinephrine informs the surgeon how much the stimulation of Müller's muscle has contributed to lid elevation. The surgeon then needs to overcorrect the ptotic lid by this additional amount to compensate for Müller's activity. The alternative method of using plain lidocaine is less than desirable given the vascularity of the orbicularis muscle that must be transected.

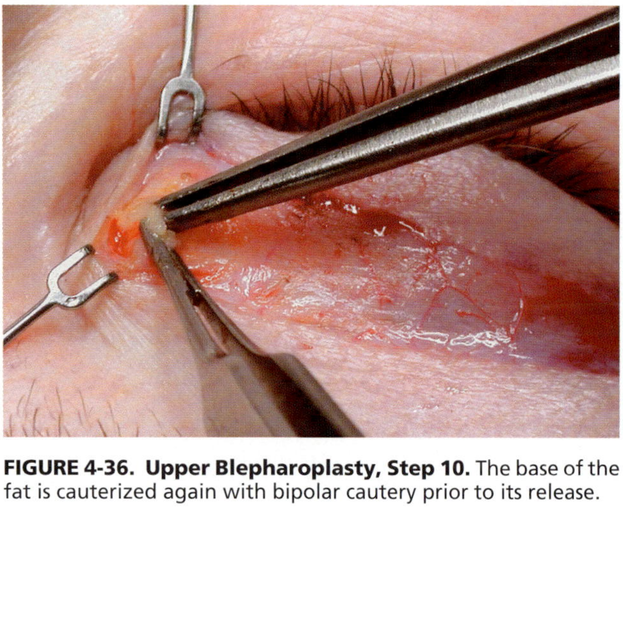

FIGURE 4-36. Upper Blepharoplasty, Step 10. The base of the fat is cauterized again with bipolar cautery prior to its release.

After the local anesthesia has achieved the desired effect, the redundant upper-lid skin is clamped in a similar fashion to that described for an upper-lid blepharoplasty. The skin and orbicularis-oculi muscle are incised through the marked supratarsal crease to expose the underlying orbital septum (Fig. 4-40). The orbital septum is widely incised with iris scissors at the midpoint of the wound. Any excessive herniated fat is clamped and removed in the fashion described for blepharoplasty (Fig. 4-41). The remaining postseptal adipose is gently swept upward to reveal the glistening white sheet of the levator aponeurosis (Fig. 4-42). If the surgeon is uncertain whether the levator is in view, then the patient may be asked to look upward and downward because the levator is noted to move in a similar fashion. If the levator is fully dehisced, then a thickened white roll may be seen that represents the separated inferior edge of the muscle. At times, the surgeon must search superiorly, as the muscle edge may have retracted upward. If the levator edge is only attenuated, then this prominent white roll will not be found. Fatty infiltration along the attenuated levator also may be visible. A strip of orbicularis-oculi muscle along the inferior wound wedge may need to be removed in order to expose the superior tarsal border (Fig. 4-43). The attenuated or dehisced levator edge then is sutured in a horizontal mattress fashion to the tarsal border at the midpupil with a 5-0 polydioxanone suture and a slipknot is used, which can be unfastened if the knot needs to be adjusted (Fig. 4-44). One should be extremely cautious not to catch any orbital septum with the suture needle owing to the risk of lagophthalmos.

The patient is inclined to a near upright position and asked to open and close the eyelid. The position of the upper lid is noted at rest with the eyes open and at primary gaze.

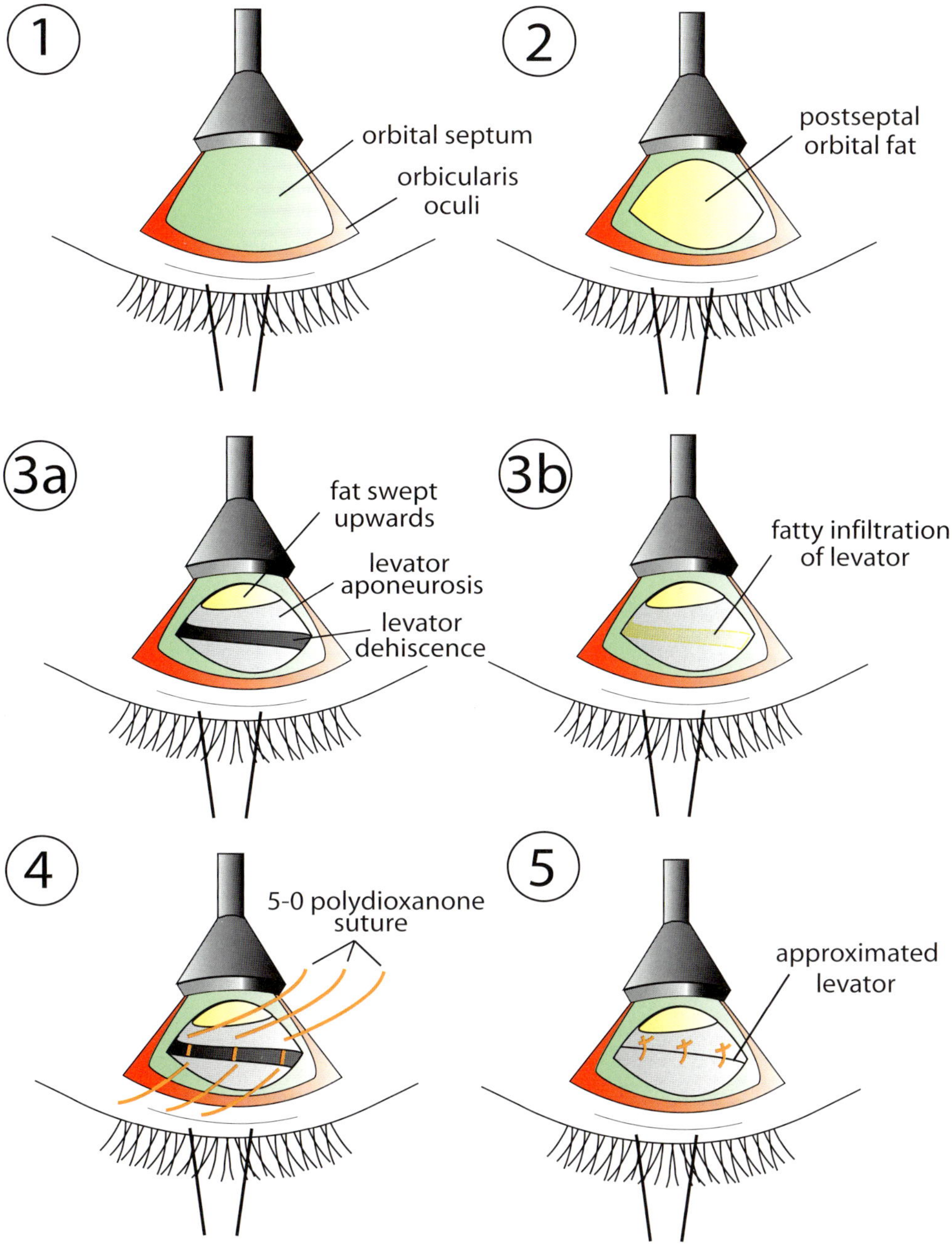

FIGURE 4-38. The series of illustrations depict the salient operative steps in blepharoptosis repair. **1:** After the skin and orbicularis oculi have been transected, the surgeon should encounter the orbital septum, through which the postseptal adipose may be visible. At times, some preseptal fat may need to be cleared before visualizing the orbital septum. **2:** The orbital septum is transected to expose the underlying postseptal adipose tissue. **3A:** The postseptal adipose tissue then is swept upward or partially removed to expose the glistening white levator aponeurosis, which may be fully dehiscent. **3B:** Alternatively, it may be only attenuated with some fatty infiltration. If the levator is completely dehisced, its superior border may be retracted upward and must be identified. **4:** The levator then is approximated to the tarsal plate using 5-0 polydioxanone suture first along its central aspect, and the eyelid height is verified to be suitable in the sitting position. The remaining sutures are placed with repeated eyelid verification in the sitting position before closure. **5:** The illustration shows the levator reapproximated to the tarsal plate.

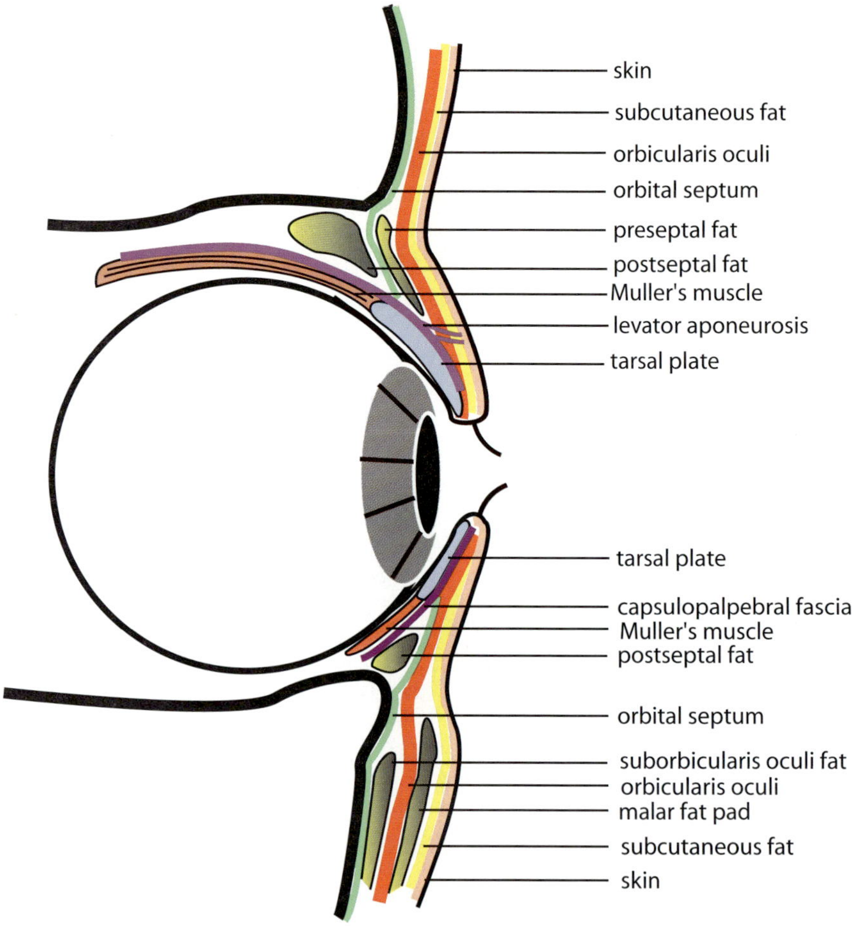

FIGURE 4-39. A lateral cross-sectional view of the eyelids that emphasizes the layers of the upper and lower eyelids that the surgeon encounters as he or she progresses through each anatomic plane of dissection. For ptosis repair, the surgeon traverses the skin, then orbicularis-oculi muscle, preseptal fat (variable), orbital septum, postseptal fat, and finally arrives at the levator complex via an incision through the supratarsal crease. The superior half of the limbus is traced out over the eyelid, when the lid is in primary gaze and fully open. The migration of this line upward after injection with local anesthesia containing epinephrine informs the surgeon how much the stimulation of Müller's muscle has contributed to lid elevation. The surgeon then needs to overcorrect the ptotic lid by this additional amount to compensate for Müller's activity. The alternative method of using plain lidocaine is less than desirable given the vascularity of the orbicularis muscle that must be transected and the brevity of the local anesthetic effect.

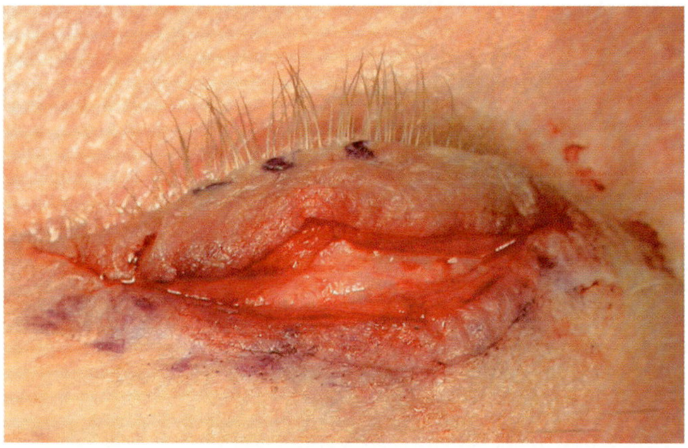

FIGURE 4-40. Ptosis Repair, Step 1. The skin and orbicularis-oculi muscle are incised through the marked supratarsal crease to expose the underlying orbital septum. Of note, the lateral, medial, and superior limbus have been marked out as three points near the lid margin. The position of the superior limbus is estimated by completing the circle of the iris on the upper lid. All these marks are undertaken before infiltration of local anesthesia, and the amount of upper lid elevation that ensues from activation of Müller's muscle by the epinephrine mixture is recorded so that overcorrection of the eyelid position can be undertaken to account for this effect. All of the measurements should be made with the patient in the sitting position with the eyes in primary gaze.

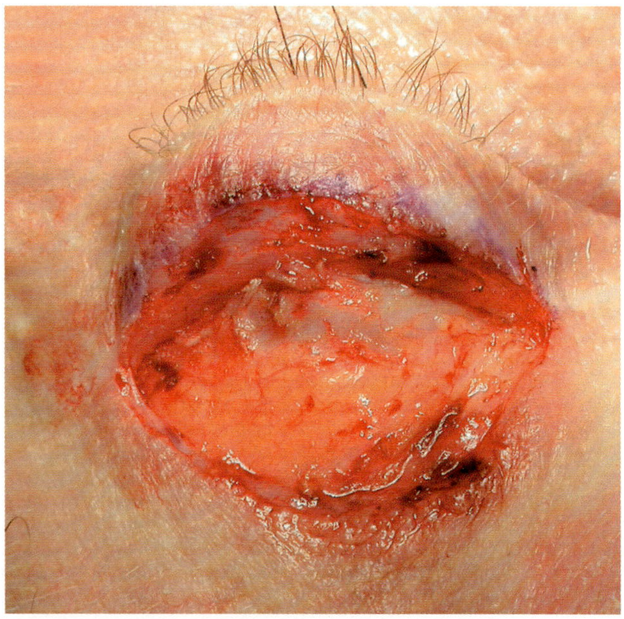

FIGURE 4-41. Ptosis Repair, Step 2. The orbital septum is widely incised with iris scissors at the midpoint of the wound to expose the underlying preaponeurotic adipose tissue. Any excessive herniated fat is clamped and removed in the fashion described for blepharoplasty.

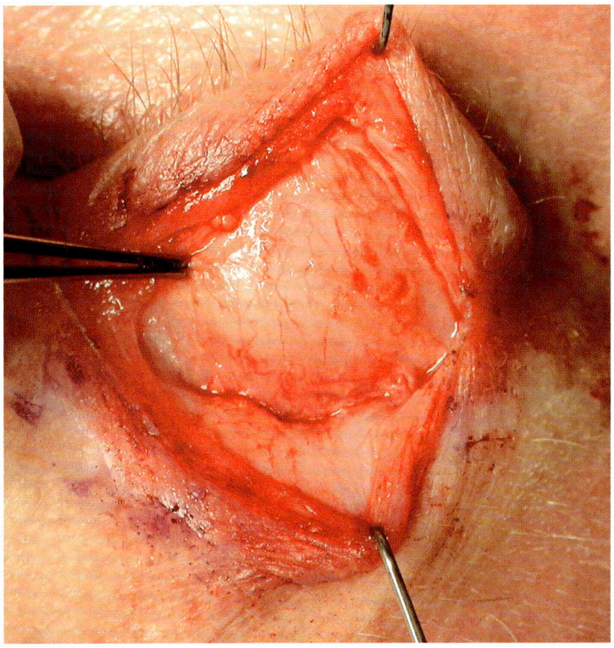

FIGURE 4-42. Ptosis Repair, Step 3. The remaining postseptal adipose is gently swept upward to reveal the glistening white sheet of the levator aponeurosis. If the surgeon is uncertain whether the levator is in view, the patient may be asked to look upward and downward because the levator is noted to move in a similar fashion. In addition, the septum remains relatively fixed when gently tugged with forceps, whereas the levator moves more freely when traction is applied. If the levator is fully dehisced, then a thickened white roll may be seen that represents the separated inferior edge of the muscle. At times, the surgeon must search superiorly, because the muscle edge may have retracted upward. If the levator edge is only attenuated (as seen), then this prominent white roll is not found.

The lid should be at the superior limbus or slightly above if overcorrection is required. Any lagophthalmos that is noted usually resolves after 1 week. The patient is returned to a fully reclined position and the slipknot is passed such that the knot is secured rather than unraveled if the surgeon is contented with the lid position. Similar technique is applied to fixation sutures temporally located (at the lateral limbus) and nasally (at the medial limbus). Surgeons have described use of only the central suture with success, but this technique may predispose the patient to an unnatural notched lid appearance. Of note, the patient may have to be evaluated several times before the suture position is deemed suitable. Because of the tedious nature of this procedure, some surgeons may elect to carry out only one side at a time if bilateral blepharoptosis is present. The upper-lid skin incision then is closed with a 7-0 polypropylene or nylon suture in the method described for blepharoplasty.

Minimally Invasive Brow and Midface Lift

The brow and midface are rejuvenated as one complex that permits a consolidated surgical rejuvenation of the upper two thirds of the face (Fig. 4-45). The patient is administered anesthesia via intravenous sedation and monitored anesthesia care as the preferred route of anesthetic delivery unless the patient is believed to require general anesthesia. With proper consultation with the anesthesiologist, the surgeon may prefer to undertake general anesthesia (with laryngeal mask or endotracheal tube) for several reasons: (a) the anesthesiologist or anesthetist is inexperienced or uncomfortable with intravenous sedation; (b) the patient expresses undue anxiety about sedation; or (c) a strong history of alcohol or narcotic usage may make maintenance of monitored sedation difficult. Unlike in rhytidectomy, the ventilating tube does not readily interfere with surgical access.

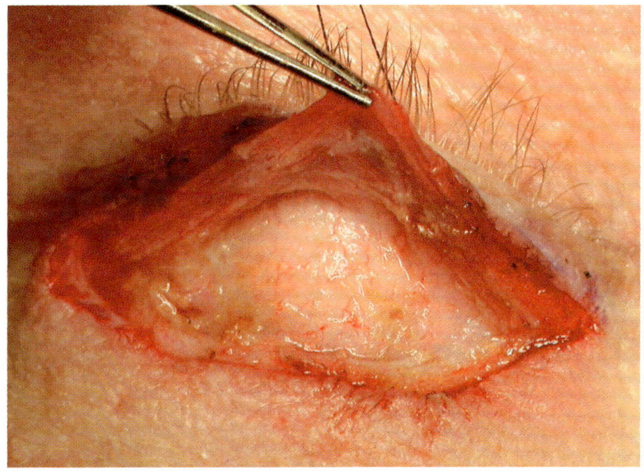

FIGURE 4-43. Ptosis Repair, Step 4. The skin–muscle flap is elevated inferiorly to expose the tarsal plate.

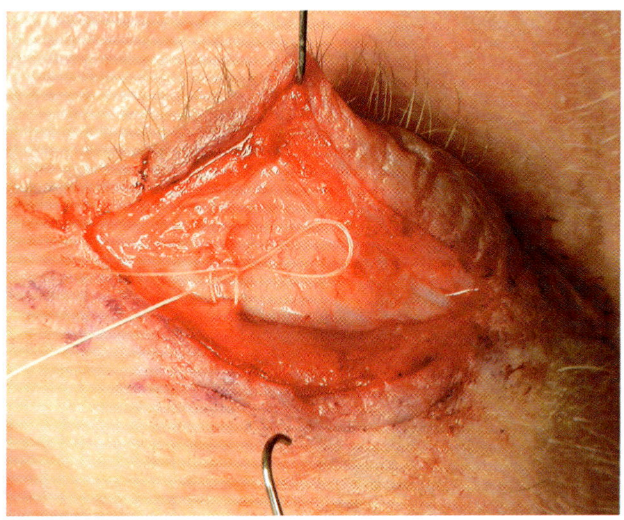

FIGURE 4-44. Ptosis Repair, Step 5. The attenuated or dehisced levator edge then is sutured in a horizontal mattress fashion to the tarsal border at the midpupil with a 5-0 polydioxanone suture and a slipknot is used, which can be unfastened if the knot needs to be adjusted. One should be extremely cautious not to catch any orbital septum with the suture needle because of the risk of lagophthalmos. Two additional sutures are placed, one nasally and one laterally. Eyelid position is confirmed after each suture with the patient seated upright.

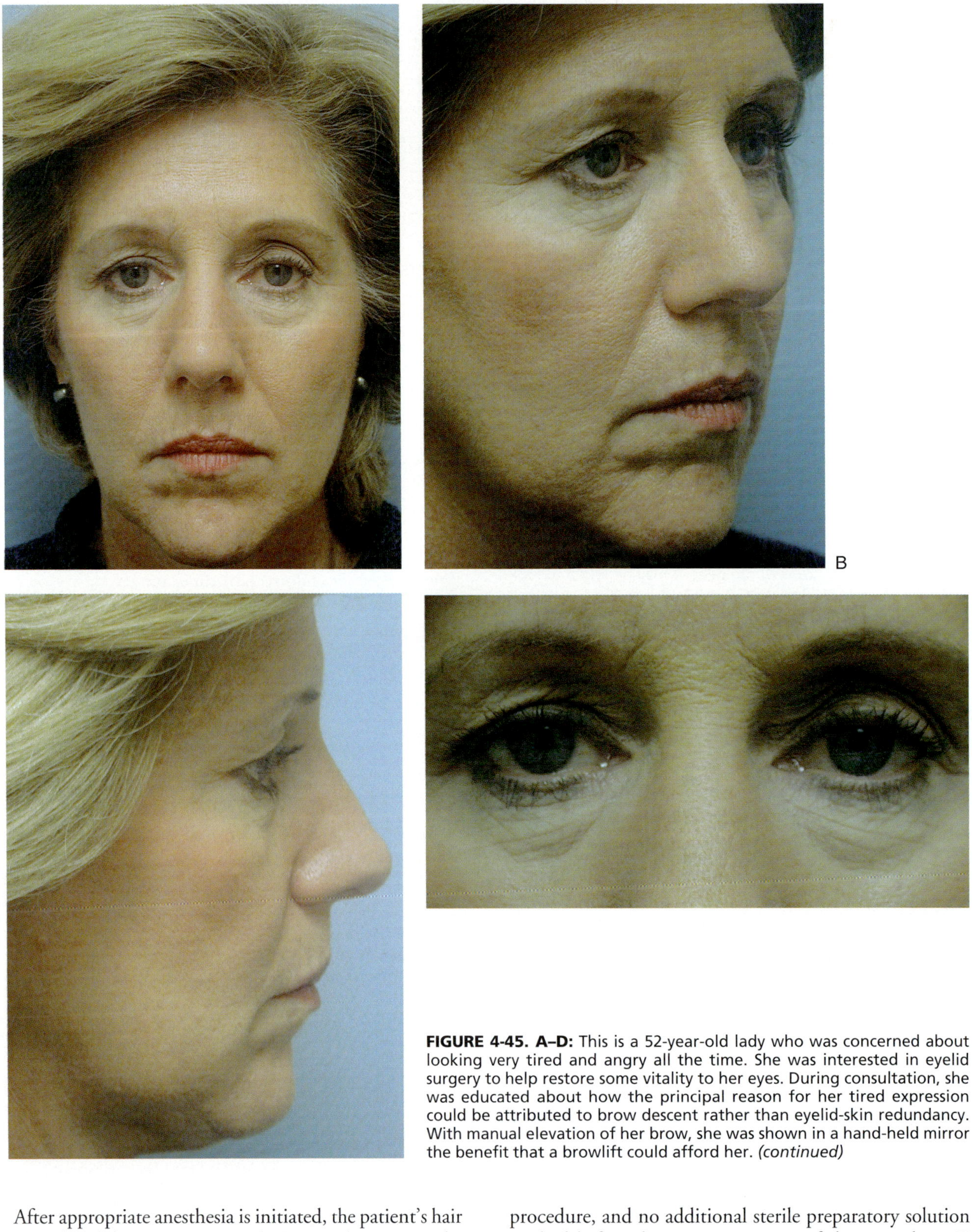

A B C D

FIGURE 4-45. A–D: This is a 52-year-old lady who was concerned about looking very tired and angry all the time. She was interested in eyelid surgery to help restore some vitality to her eyes. During consultation, she was educated about how the principal reason for her tired expression could be attributed to brow descent rather than eyelid-skin redundancy. With manual elevation of her brow, she was shown in a hand-held mirror the benefit that a browlift could afford her. *(continued)*

After appropriate anesthesia is initiated, the patient's hair is secured with brown paper tape (Micropore) to expose the planned surgical incision sites. Of note, tape is much easier and faster to apply than traditional rubber bands. Before surgery, the patient is instructed to cleanse his or her hair and scalp with an antibacterial shampoo the morning of the procedure, and no additional sterile preparatory solution is applied before the commencement of the procedure. Five standard endoscopic-browlift incisions are marked out with a surgical marking pen with one situated in the midline; two located lateral to the midline in the paramedian position (approximately at the lateral canthus) just posterior to the

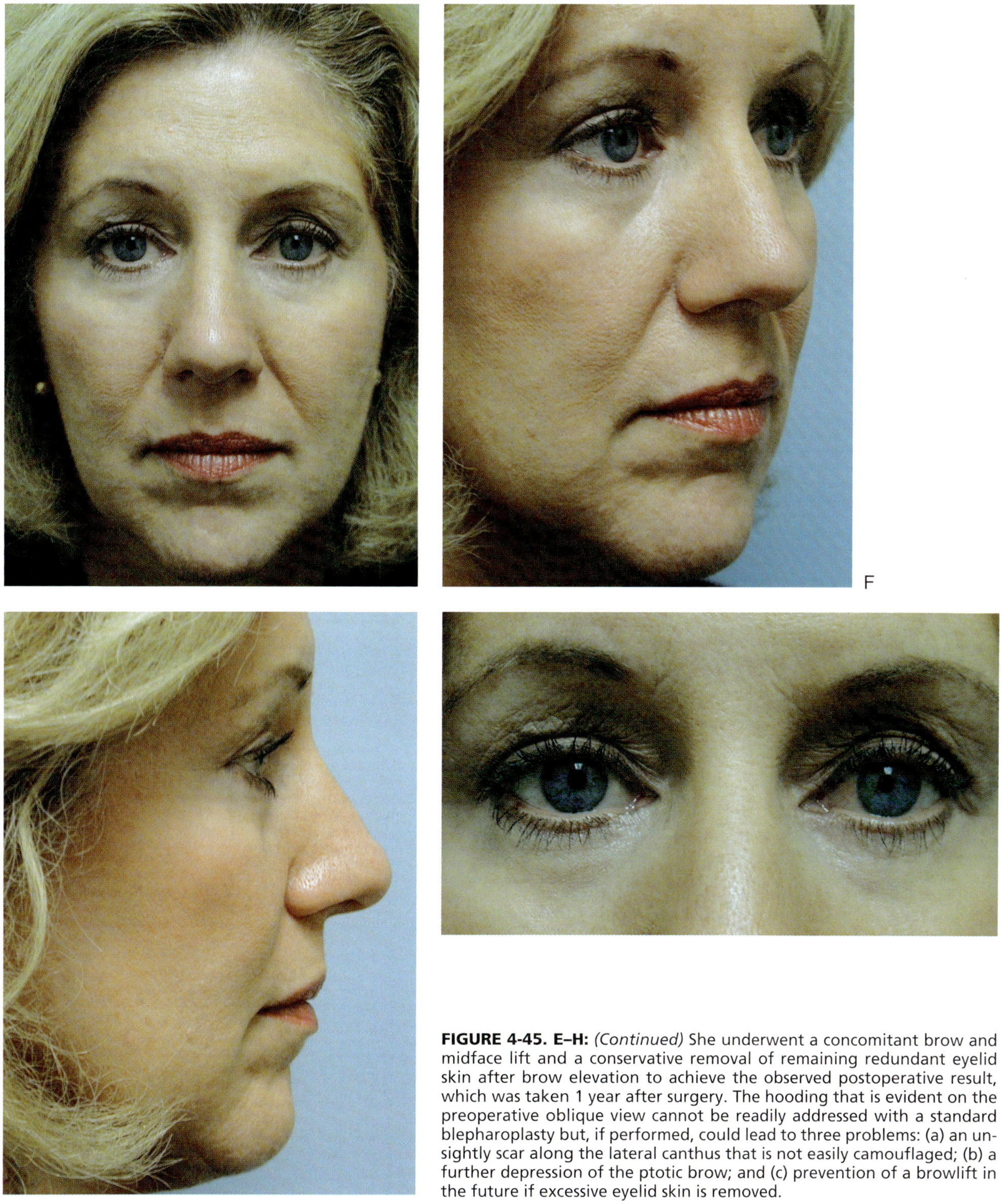

E F G H

FIGURE 4-45. E–H: *(Continued)* She underwent a concomitant brow and midface lift and a conservative removal of remaining redundant eyelid skin after brow elevation to achieve the observed postoperative result, which was taken 1 year after surgery. The hooding that is evident on the preoperative oblique view cannot be readily addressed with a standard blepharoplasty but, if performed, could lead to three problems: (a) an unsightly scar along the lateral canthus that is not easily camouflaged; (b) a further depression of the ptotic brow; and (c) prevention of a browlift in the future if excessive eyelid skin is removed.

hairline; and two additional, longer incisions located more temporally also camouflaged by the hairline and extending over a 4-cm distance above the helical crus and over the temporalis muscle and fascia (Fig. 4-46). The supraorbital notches are palpated and marked with a surgical marking pen on each side.

One percent lidocaine with 1:100,000 epinephrine then is infiltrated into the described incision sites and along the entire orbital rim, zygomatic arch, and midface bilaterally. Of note, the forehead region, lying between the orbital rim and the incision sites, is spared local anesthesia: The authors have found that this area does not require the anesthetic or

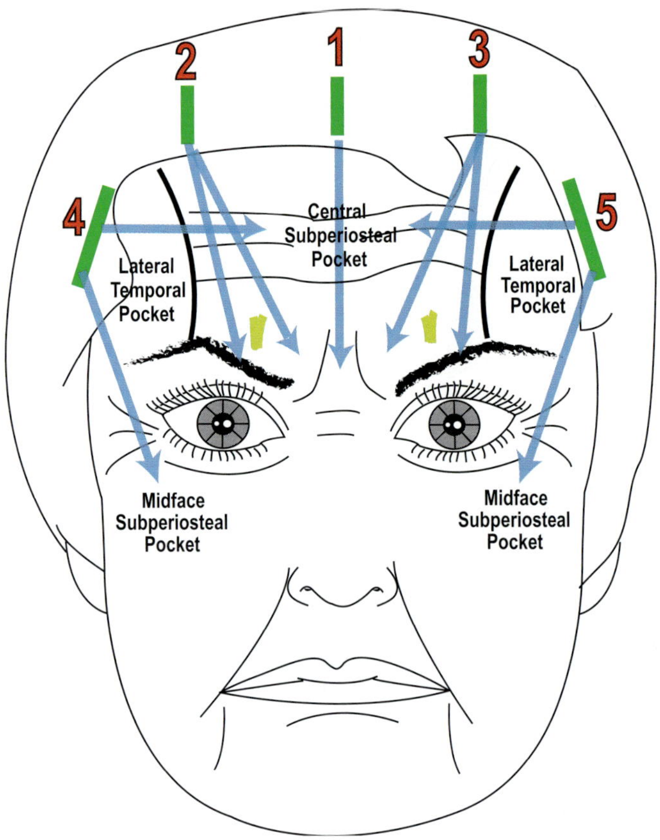

FIGURE 4-46. Illustration that shows the five standard incisions for minimally invasive brow surgery (*in green*): One incision is placed in the midline, two are located lateral to the midline in the paramedian position (approximately at the lateral canthus) just posterior to the hairline; and two, additional, longer incisions located more temporally also camouflaged by the hairline and extending over a 4-cm distance above the helical crus and over the temporalis muscle and fascia. The numbers (*in red*) indicate the order that the incisions are made and the lines and arrows (*in blue*) indicate the path of dissection from each incision. Of note, the supraorbital neurovascular bundles (*in yellow*) are avoided by dissecting around them and only lifting gently starting 1.5 to 2 cm above the orbital rim at the palpated supraorbital notch.

hemostatic properties of the lidocaine–epinephrine mixture (Figs. 4-47 and 4-48). A full 10 minutes are allowed to transpire prior to the first incision in order to ensure adequate anesthesia and hemostasis. A moistened laparotomy sponge is draped over the patient's head behind the incision sites and secured with an overlying surgical towel and clip as part of the surgical draping of the patient. A moistened pad significantly absorbs any bleeding and prevents blood from trickling back into the remaining occipital hair.

If a transconjunctival lower-lid blepharoplasty is entertained, then this procedure should be undertaken before brow and midfacial suspension. After midfacial elevation, the lower lid becomes excessively taut, restricting ease of transconjunctival entry to the lid. This increase in lower-lid tension after brow and midface suspension has been remarked by Quatela and associates (unpublished data). Conversely, an upper-lid blepharoplasty should be deferred until the brow and midface are appropriately elevated so that an accurate assessment of residual cutaneous redundancy can be made.

At the outset of the brow lift, the patient is inclined approximately 60 degrees in a semisitting position. This upward position facilitates ease of bone tunneling and visualization of the midface using the headlight and retractor (see the following). Proper patient positioning cannot be overemphasized, which permits ease of inspection and dissection.

First, the right, paramedian incision (vertically situated in the hairline approximately above the lateral canthus) is made with a No. 15 Bard-Parker blade down through the periosteum (Fig. 4-48). Monopolar electrocautery is used to achieve hemostasis along the cut edges of the wound, being careful not to apply excessive cautery to the exposed hair follicles. The cautery device is also used to ensure that the periosteum is completely incised (Fig. 4-49). A small, sharp, flat periosteal elevator is used to dissect subperiosteally for a distance of a few centimeters circumferentially around the incision site (Fig. 4-50). Little additional dissection is carried out posterior to the incision site beyond the initial few centimeters, because extensive dissection toward the occiput provides limited benefit in transposition of the brow upward. With proper wound retraction using wide-double pronged hooks, a hand drill outfitted with a 1.5-mm wide × 6-mm long drill bit is used to enter the outer calvarial table at 30 degrees (to the horizontal) and joined with an opposing entry of the drill in order to form a bone tunnel through which the brow-fixating suture may be passed at the end of the case. The drill initially should be aimed perpendicular with the skull to engage the drill for the first 1 to 2 mm before angling the instrument forward in the prescribed 30-degree angle. In addition, the bone tunnel should be made in the posterior aspect of the incision, because suspension of the brow upward will cover the bone tunnel if the tunnel is created too anteriorly relative to the incision. An expanded polytetrafluoroethylene (ePTFE, or Gore-Tex; W.L. Gore and Associates, Inc., Flagstaff, AZ) CV-3 needle is passed through the tunnel to ensure easy passage of the needle at the end of the case (Fig. 4-51A–D). The senior author has found that a 6-mm long recessed drill bit permits ease of bone-tunnel creation while minimizing inadvertent entry through the full thickness of the skull if the drill bit is angled approximately 30 degrees to the skull contour. Similarly, a 1.5-mm wide bit accommodates the desired caliber of needle.

A larger, sharp, flat periosteal elevator (Fig. 4-52A), that reduces the risk of periosteal shearing, then is introduced into the same paramedian incision where the bone tunnel was just made in order to elevate the remaining periosteum *toward* the arcus stopping short before actually breaking the arcus (Fig. 4-52B). (The smaller, sharp elevator is used to free the periosteum at the arcus marginalis.) Of note, the technique described herein has now evolved to eliminate use of endoscopic instrumentation of any kind. All dissection is

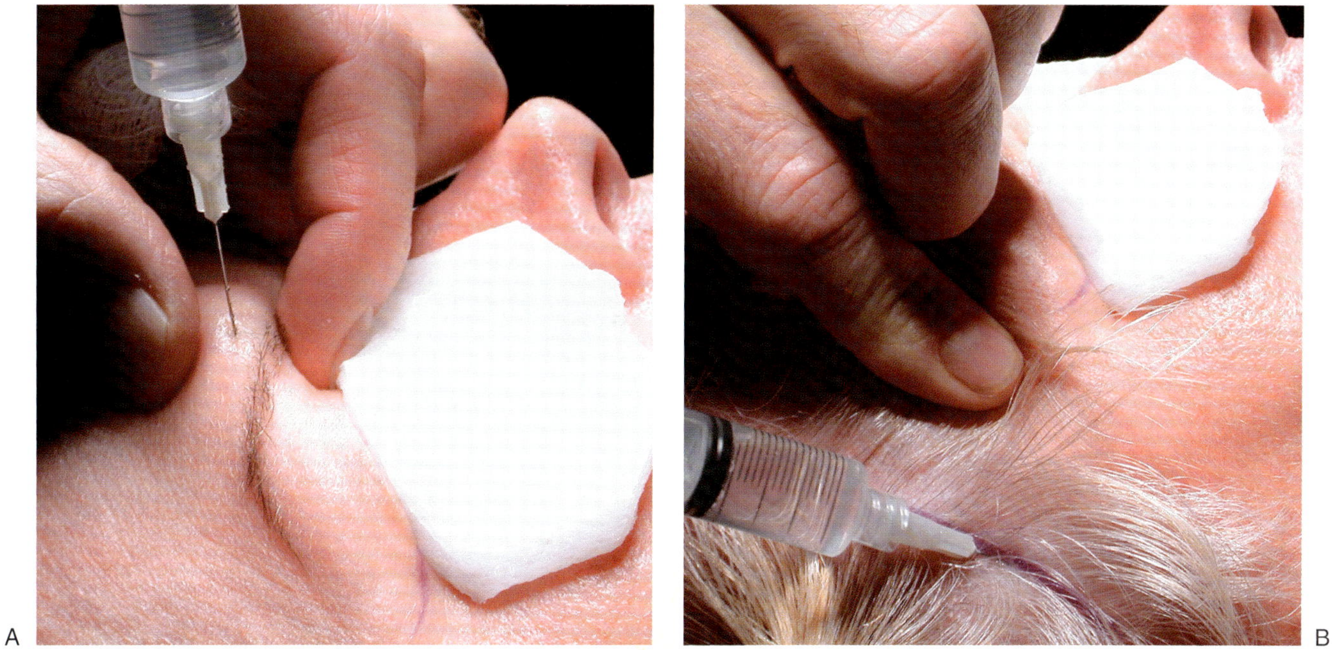

FIGURE 4-47. Brow and Midface Lift, Step 1. A,B: One percent lidocaine and 1:100,000 epinephrine is infiltrated only into the incision sites and along the orbital rim and midface. The forehead area that lies between the incision sites and orbital rim is not infiltrated with anesthesia, because this is unnecessary when dissecting in the subperiosteal plane.

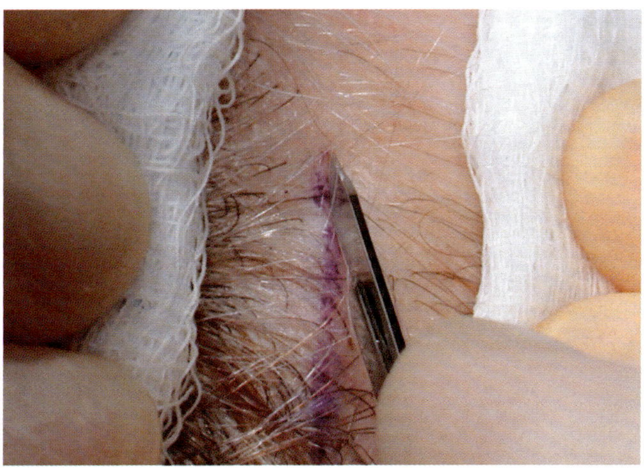

FIGURE 4-48. Brow and Midface Lift, Step 2. A No. 15 Bard-Parker blade is used to dissect down through the periosteum along the right, paramedian incision.

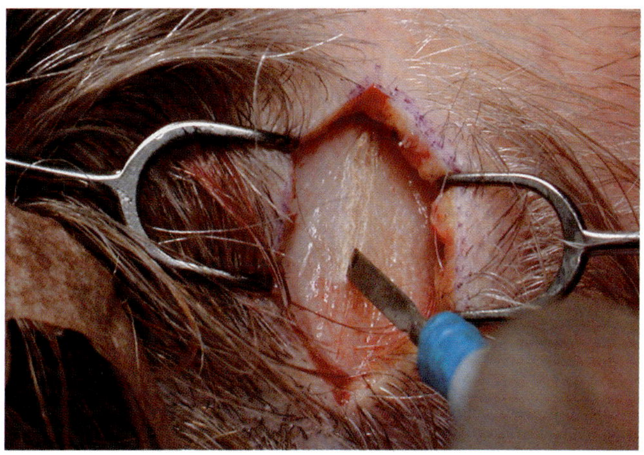

FIGURE 4-49. Brow and Midface Lift, Step 3. Monopolar electrocautery is used to achieve hemostasis along the cut edges of the wound, being careful not to apply excessive cautery to the exposed hair follicles. The cautery device is also used to ensure that the periosteum is completely incised.

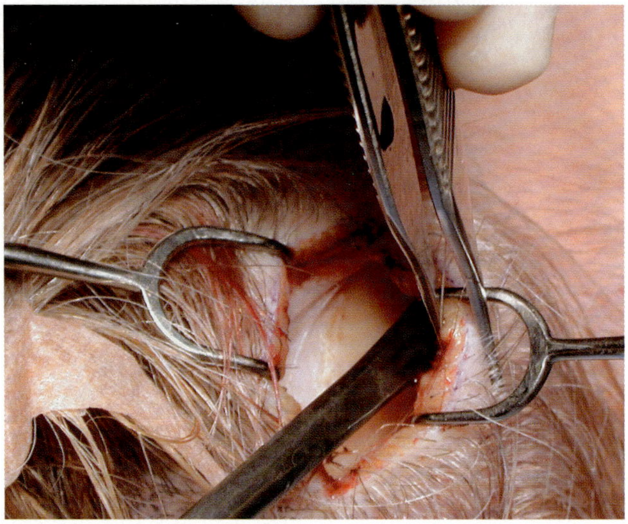

FIGURE 4-50. Brow and Midface Lift, Step 4. A small, sharp, flat periosteal elevator is used to dissect subperiosteally for a distance of a few centimeters circumferentially around the incision site. Little additional dissection is carried out posterior to the incision site beyond the initial few centimeters, as extensive dissection toward the occiput provides limited benefit in transposition of the brow upward.

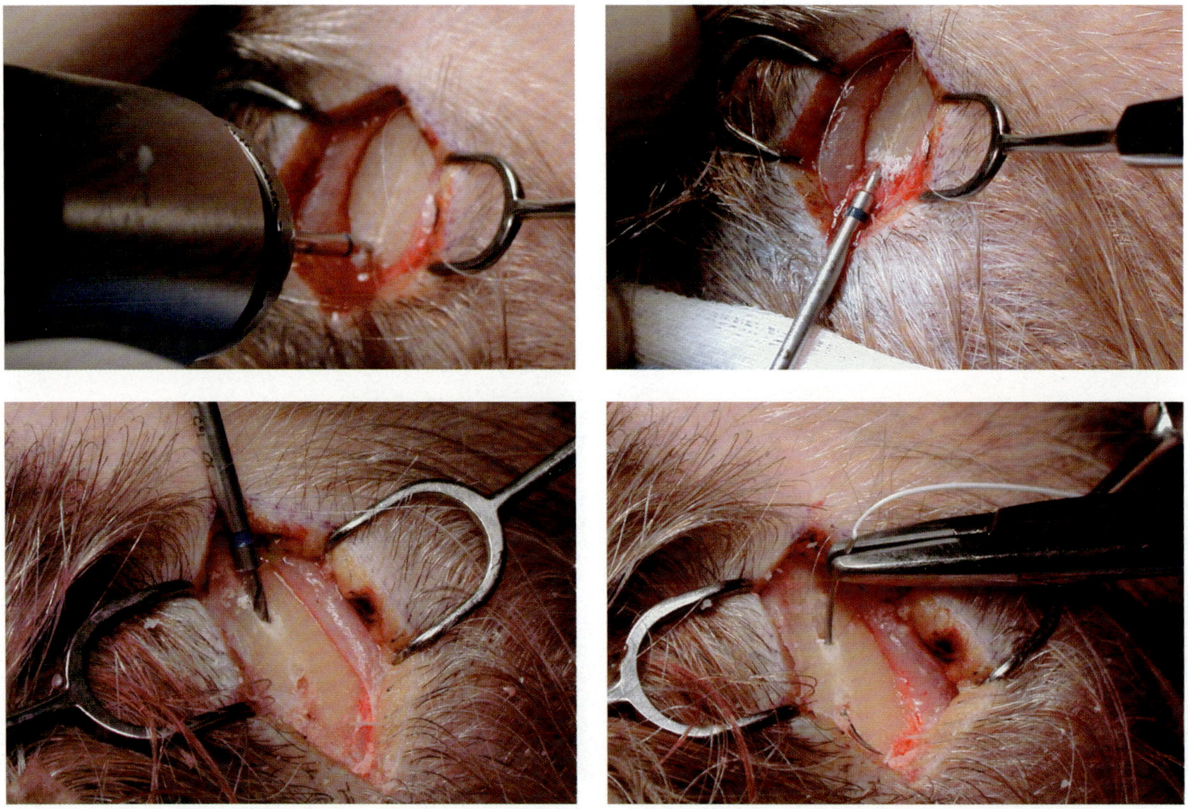

A B C D

FIGURE 4-51. Brow and Midface Lift, Step 5. A: A Stryker hand drill outfitted with a 1.5-mm wide × 6-mm long drill bit is engaged initially into the outer calvarial table in a perpendicular fashion. **B:** The drill bit then is gently (nonforcefully) turned to 30 degrees (to the horizontal) aiming anteriorly. *Of note, the patient should be seated upright at 60 degrees to facilitate ease of angling the drill; and the position of the initial drill hole should be at the posterior limit of the incision, as the brow suspension suture will move the incision posteriorly.* **C:** The contralateral tunnel is made in the same fashion (but reverse direction) so that the two bone tunnels are joined. **D:** A CV-3 Gore-Tex suture needle is passed through the tunnel to ensure easy passage of the needle when the suture is placed toward the end of the case.

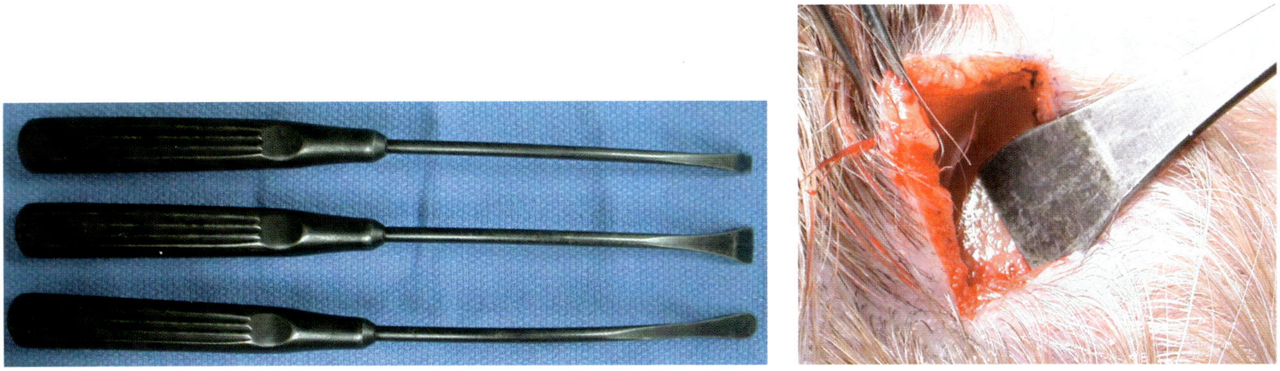

A B

FIGURE 4-52. Brow and Midface Lift, Step 6. A: Three elevators are used for dissection: a small, flat elevator; a large, flat elevator; and a round elevator. **B:** A larger, sharp, flat periosteal elevator, which reduces the risk of periosteal shearing, is introduced into the same paramedian incision where the bone tunnel was just made in order to elevate the remaining periosteum *toward* the arcus stopping short before actually breaking the arcus. (The smaller, sharp, flat elevator is used to free the periosteum at the arcus marginalis.)

conducted either blindly with tactile feedback (the so-called "smart-hand" technique) or under direct vision with a headlight and Converse retractor. The authors have found that reliance on endoscopic equipment is both an unnecessary and time-consuming endeavor. Tactile feedback is used to elevate the central pocket (i.e., the three central incisions), whereas direct vision is needed to elevate the lateral, temporal pocket and the contiguous extension of the midface. When approaching the arcus, the smaller, sharp periosteal elevator again is used in order to release the arcus more definitively than can be achieved with the larger, flat periosteal elevator. When the elevator tip approaches a 1- to 2-cm distance above the supraorbital notch (which should be marked before surgery begins), the elevator is handled only in an upward, lifting motion in order to avoid any paresthesias or neuropraxias that may ensue from violating the supraorbital neurovascular bundle (Fig. 4-53).

The midline incision then is carried out in order to access the medial-brow complex (Fig. 4-54). (If the patient has a relatively short forehead, this incision may be eliminated; and the medial brow accessed from the paramedian incisions. However, given the limited morbidity associated with this

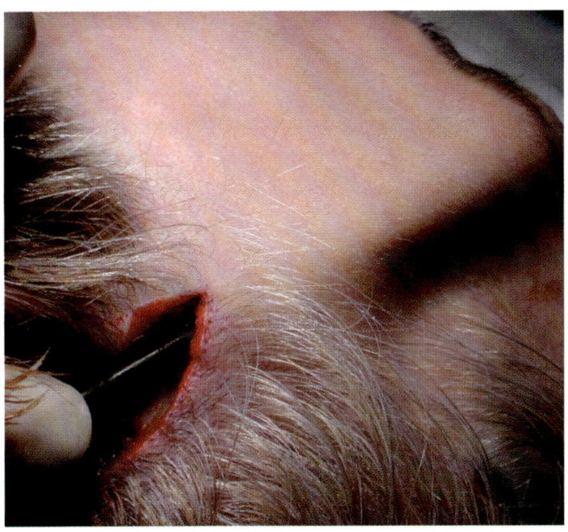

FIGURE 4-53. Brow and Midface Lift, Step 7. When approaching the arcus, the smaller, sharp periosteal elevator is again used in order to release the arcus more definitively than can be achieved with the larger, flat periosteal elevator. When the elevator tip approaches a 1- to 2-cm distance above the supraorbital notch, the elevator is handled only in an upward, lifting motion in order to avoid any paresthesias or neuropraxias that may ensue from violating the supraorbital neurovascular bundle. This method is called the "smart-hand" technique, which uses bimanual, tactile feedback to determine proper periosteal release rather than with direct, endoscopic visualization. As mentioned in the text, no endoscopic equipment is used during the procedure; however, the term "endoscopic" has been retained, because it is an established and well-known method that describes the authors' approach in large part.

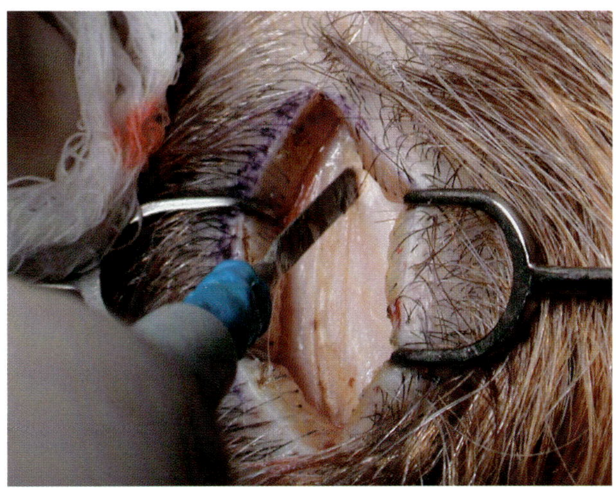

FIGURE 4-54. Brow and Midface Lift, Step 8. The midline incision is carried out in order to access the medial-brow complex in the same fashion as described for the lateral, paramedian incision. Specifically, a No. 15 blade is used to cut down through to the periosteum, followed by monopolar cautery to achieve hemostasis and ensure that the periosteum is completely transected. Then, the small sharp periosteal elevator is introduced to begin the initial circumferential dissection around the incision site, followed by the larger periosteal elevator to dissect downward toward the arcus marginalis.

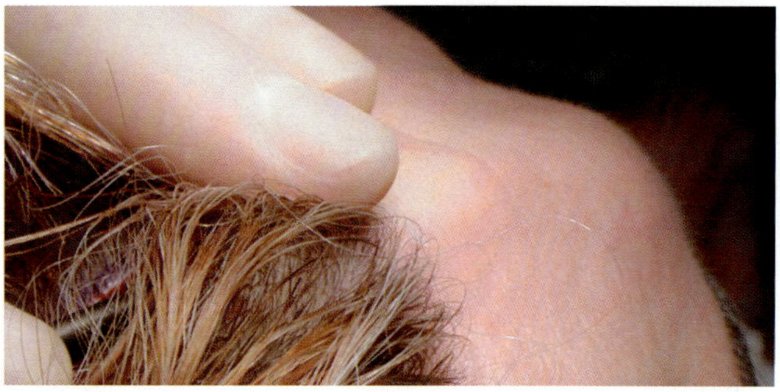

FIGURE 4-55. Brow and Midface Lift, Step 9. The small, sharp, flat periosteal elevator is introduced to free the periosteal attachment at the arcus marginalis. Of note, aggressive dissection of the musculature has been abandoned, because return of muscle function often has been observed despite the most meticulous removal of the procerus–corrugator complex. In addition, significant morbidity may arise from aggressive muscular resection, including contour irregularity, asymmetric brow depression, and the most dreaded outcome, frank cutaneous necrosis.

additional incision, the authors favor carrying out this incision for a more direct release of the medial brow in most cases.) The principal objective is release of the periosteum at the arcus in order to achieve unrestricted brow elevation (Fig. 4-55). Aggressive dissection of the musculature has been abandoned, because return of muscle function often has been observed despite the most meticulous removal of the procerus–corrugator complex. In addition, significant morbidity may arise from aggressive muscular resection, including contour irregularity, asymmetric brow depression, and the most dreaded outcome, frank cutaneous necrosis. Instead, chemical ablation with botulinum toxin type A has been the preferred method to address the medial depressor complex.

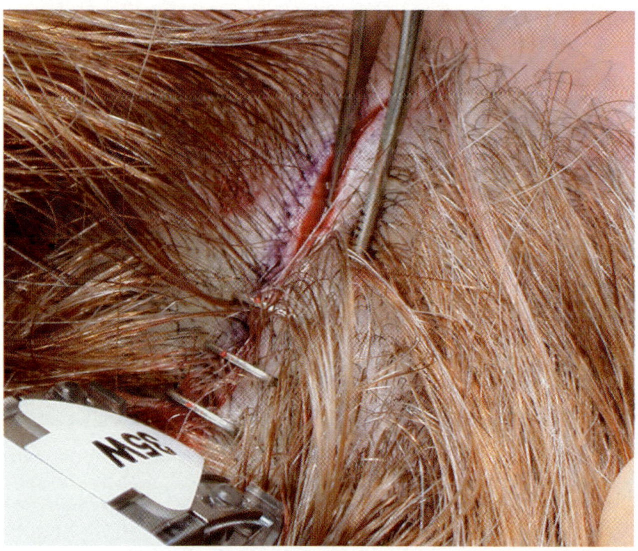

FIGURE 4-56. Brow and Midface Lift, Step 10. The midline incision is closed with surgical clips before continuing to the left side. The same technique for making the incision, subperiosteal dissection, bone-tunnel creation, and periosteal release is undertaken as described for the right, paramedian incision.

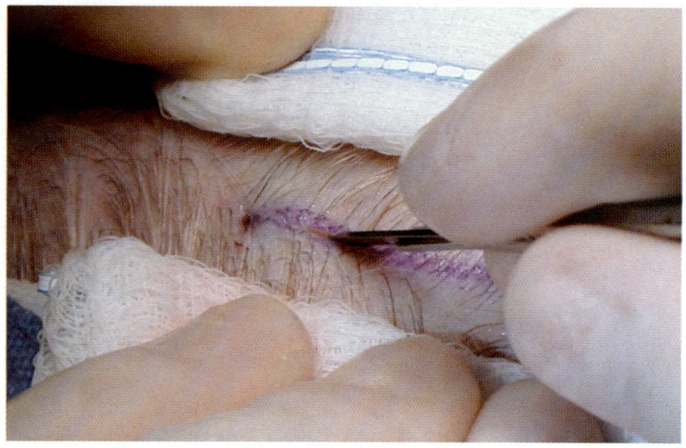

FIGURE 4-57. Brow and Midface Lift, Step 11. Next, the right temporal incision is incised with a No. 15 blade down through the subcutaneous tissue.

The midline incision is closed with surgical clips before continuing to the left side (Fig. 4-56). The left paramedian incision then is made, and the same method of bone–tunnel creation and periosteal release is carried out as previously described for the contralateral, paramedian incision.

After the surgical maneuvers have been completed in the central pocket (medial to the conjoined tendons of the temporalis muscle), the longer, lateral temporo-parietal incisions are then addressed (Figs. 4-57 and 4-58). Dissection is carried down through the temporo-parietal fascia (TPF) so that a proper tissue plane may be achieved between the TPF and the true temporalis fascia to avoid injury to the frontal branch of the facial nerve. The incision should be situated approximately 1 cm behind the hairline to lie over the temporalis muscle and not more posteriorly to avoid transection of the superficial temporal artery and to minimize the long trajectory of dissection needed to reach the midface. Initial dissection is performed with a large, blunt elevator over the true temporalis fascia (Fig. 4-59), and then the larger, flat periosteal elevator is used to break the conjoined tendon of the temporalis muscle that divides the central and lateral pockets (Fig. 4-60). It is imperative that the surgeon aim the elevator superiorly to ensure that the entire length of the conjoined tendon has been freed. Aiming up toward the right paramedian incision and passing the instrument through that incision ensure that complete release of the tendon has been accomplished. Of note, only three periosteal elevators are used for the entire case (the small, sharp, flat elevator; the large, sharp, flat elevator; and the large, rounded, blunt elevator). Further, all three instruments are coated with an ebonized finish to minimize unwanted, reflective glare off the surface.

Under direct vision with a headlight and Converse retractor, dissection is taken downward to the orbital rim with the small, sharp periosteal elevator, carefully looking for the presence of the cephalic vein (Fig. 4-61). If the vein lies in the direct path between the upper and midface, then it may be skeletonized and cauterized with a bipolar device and

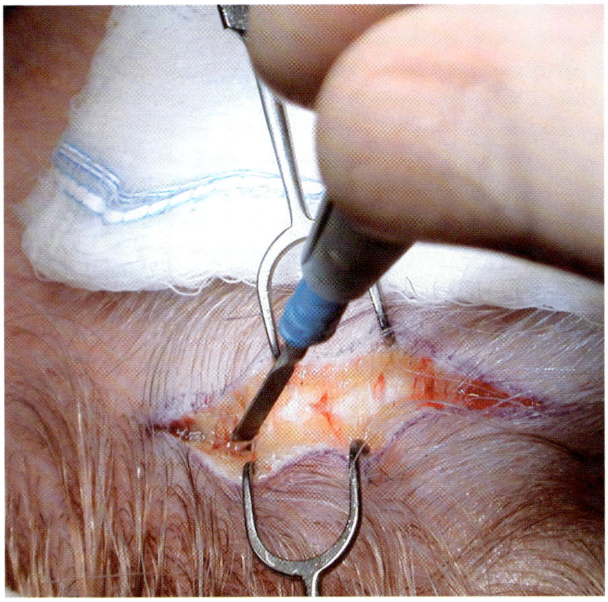

FIGURE 4-58. Brow and Midface Lift, Step 12. Hemostasis is achieved with monopolar cautery in the subcutaneous plane before continuing on with the dissection down through the temporo-parietal fascia.

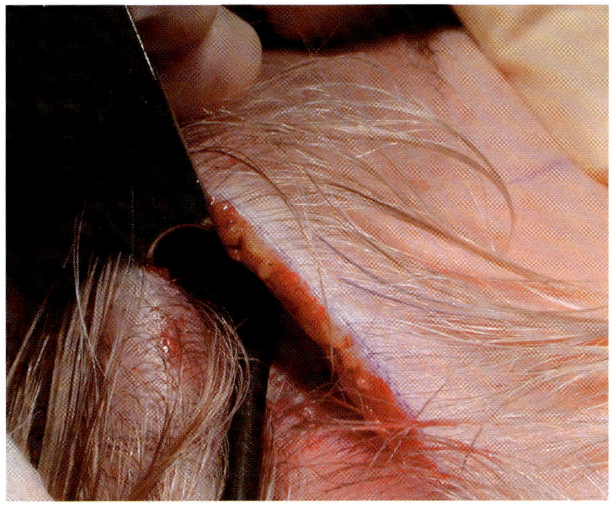

FIGURE 4-60. Brow and Midface Lift, Step 14. Under continued direct visualization, the blunt elevator is exchanged for the small, sharp, flat elevator that is used to free the conjoined tendon of the temporalis muscle that divides the central and lateral pockets. It is imperative that the surgeon aims the elevator superiorly to ensure that the entire length of the conjoined tendon has been freed. Aiming up toward the right paramedian incision and passing the instrument through that incision ensures that complete release of the tendon has been accomplished.

transected with scissors in order to permit entry into the midface. Injudicious cautery of the cephalic vessel, especially if the bipolar cautery tips are aimed superficially, may jeopardize the frontal branch of the facial nerve. The arcus marginalis then is released from the supero-lateral orbital rim near the lateral canthus with the periosteal elevator. The assistant places a finger along the lateral margin of the orbital rim to limit the surgeon's dissection and to avoid excessive release of periosteum from the lateral canthus, which may otherwise contribute to undesirable, lateral-canthal elevation (Fig. 4-62).

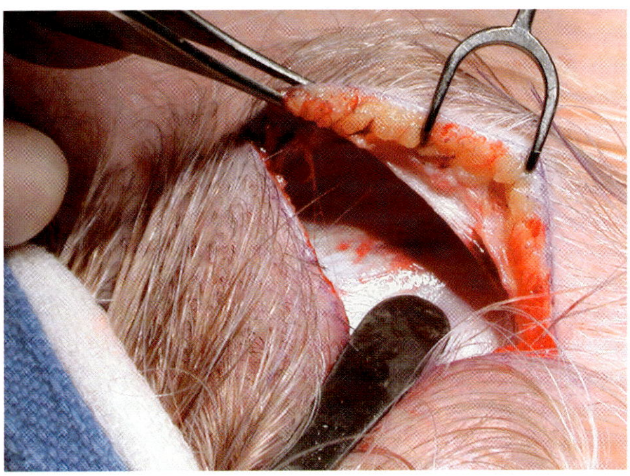

FIGURE 4-59. Brow and Midface Lift, Step 13. The round elevator is used to confirm that the filmy temporo-parietal fascia has been entirely elevated off of the shiny true temporalis fascia. If there is any doubt, the No. 15 blade should be used to incise the temporalis fascia to confirm that the naked temporalis muscle resides below. As the temporal branch of the facial nerve lies within the temporo-parietal fascia, it is critical to ensure that this layer has been elevated off the true temporalis fascia before continuing with the dissection. Dissection over the temporalis fascia should be performed with direct headlight visualization and assisted with a Converse retractor.

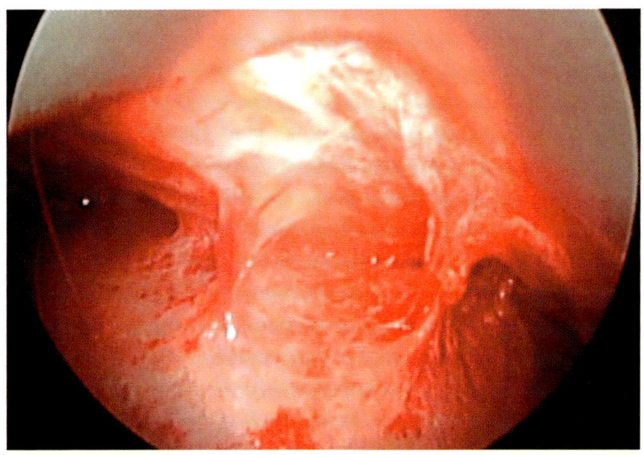

FIGURE 4-61. Brow and Midface Lift, Step 15. Under direct vision with a headlight and Converse retractor, dissection is taken down to the orbital rim with the small, sharp periosteal elevator, carefully looking for the presence of the cephalic vein. If the vein lies in the direct path between the upper and midface, then it may be skeletonized and cauterized with a bipolar device and transected with scissors in order to permit entry into the midface. Injudicious cautery of the cephalic vessel, especially if the bipolar cautery tips are aimed superficially, may jeopardize the frontal branch of the facial nerve. (*Note:* Although this image shows an endoscopic view, no endoscope is usually used during the procedure. The endoscope is only used here for illustrative purposes.)

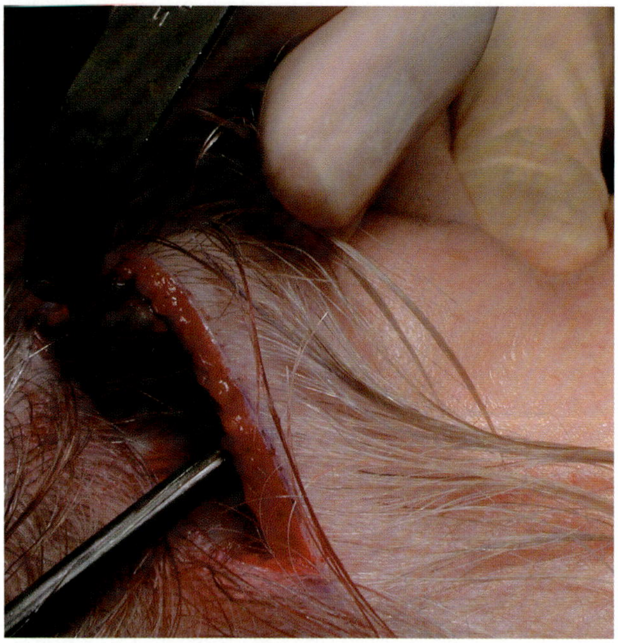

FIGURE 4-62. Brow and Midface Lift, Step 16. The arcus marginalis is released from the supero-lateral orbital rim near the lateral canthus with the periosteal elevator. The assistant places a finger along the lateral margin of the orbital rim to limit the surgeon's dissection and avoid excessive release of periosteum from the lateral canthus, which may otherwise contribute to undesirable, lateral-canthal elevation.

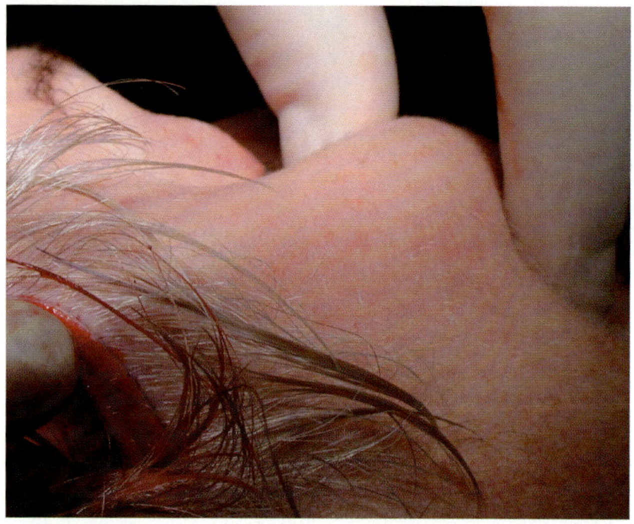

FIGURE 4-63. Brow and Midface Lift, Step 17. Again under direct view, the large, sharp periosteal elevator is guided downward to enter the temporal fat pad and then release the periosteal attachments overlying the zygomatic arch itself. This technique offers the surgeon direct access to the midfacial structures. Next the periosteal elevator is continued inferiorly over the malar eminence to release the zygomaticus major and minor muscular attachments and malar fat pad from the underlying malar bone using the smart-hand technique (as seen in the photograph).

Again under direct view, the large, sharp periosteal elevator is guided downward to enter the temporal fat pad and then to release the periosteal attachments overlying the zygomatic arch itself. This technique offers the surgeon direct access to the midfacial structures. Next the periosteal elevator is continued inferiorly over the malar eminence to release the zygomaticus major and minor muscular attachments and malar fat pad from the underlying malar bone (Fig. 4-63). Although minimal, medial dissection limits both lateral-canthal distortion and potential facial-nerve injury, the dissection is continued until the midfacial structures are adequately released. Once the zygomatic muscular attachments have been severed, the surgeon should be wary of further inferior dissection and unintended masseteric elevation that may result in trismus. A CV-3 Gore-Tex suture is passed through the temporalis fascia and muscle just antero-inferior to the temporo-parietal incision (Fig. 4-64) and then passed through the malar fat pad with a long needle driver (Fig. 4-65). This maneuver is technically difficult to perform and requires a learning curve to be proficient. The suture is pulled superiorly to test if sufficient release of the midfacial tissues has been achieved (Fig. 4-66). If not, then further dissection medially and inferiorly is carried out until appropriate release of the midface is observed. The paramedian suture on the same side is tied down before the suture is fastened superiorly to the temporalis muscle. The paramedian suture is fixated first in order to relieve any tension on the suture that elevates the midface and permit better brow positioning by suspending the most superior suture initially. The CV-3 Gore-Tex suture is used to secure the overlying frontalis muscle through the bone tunnel in the paramedian incision. A technical consideration that should be observed is a generous bite of frontalis muscle needs to be grasped with the suture needle to achieve a secure and adequate suspension (Fig. 4-67). The suture is secured using a square knot tied in the air, which then is fastened down: Unlike most other sutures, Gore-Tex permits sliding a square knot down into place. After the paramedian suspen-

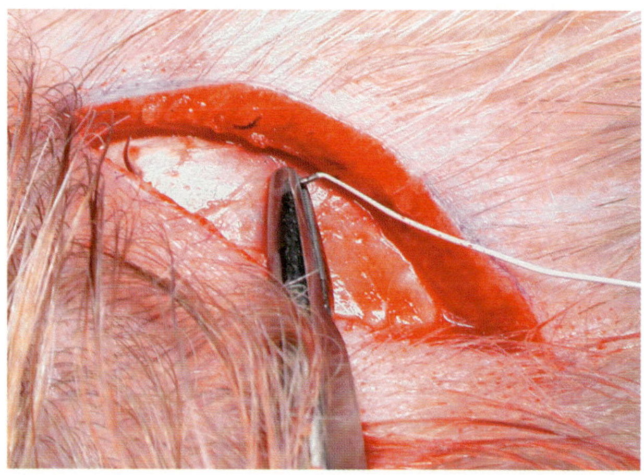

FIGURE 4-64. Brow and Midface Lift, Step 18. A CV-3 Gore-Tex suture is passed through the temporalis fascia and muscle just antero-inferior to the temporo-parietal incision, which will serve as the proximal anchoring point for the midfacial suture.

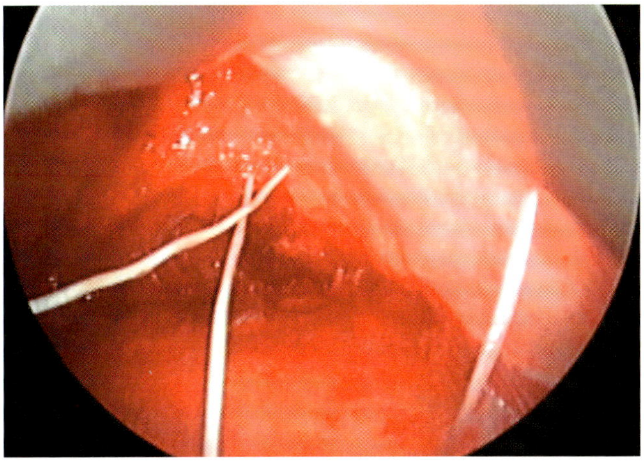

FIGURE 4-65. Brow and Midface Lift, Step 19. An endoscopic view shows the same suture anchored proximally in Figure 4-64 placed distally through the malar fat pad.

sion has been completed and the incision closed (Fig. 4-68), the surgeon should return to the lateral temporal incision to suspend the already distally placed suture through the malar fat pad to the proximal temporalis muscle and fascia at the incision site (Fig. 4-69). The vector of suspension should be vertically oriented, and the suture through the malar fat pad should be situated more laterally over the malar prominence—both of which minimize untoward distortion of the lateral canthus. Next, the TPF just anterior to the temporoparietal incision is sutured to the temporalis muscle and fascia more superiorly with the CV-3 Gore-Tex suture to pull the overlying brow and soft tissue supero-laterally (Fig. 4-70A,B). This suture placement is undertaken twice. All incisions are then closed with surgical clips. Suturing in the hair-bearing scalp is both unnecessarily laborious in place-

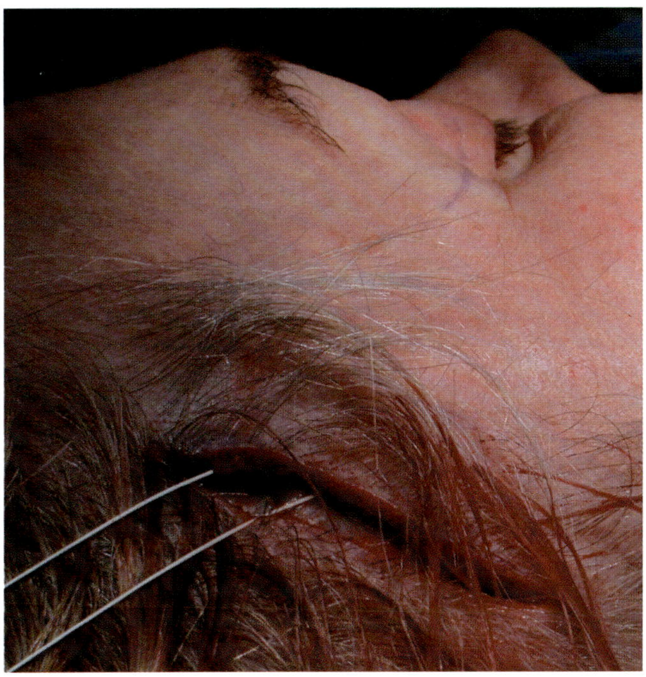

FIGURE 4-66. Brow and Midface Lift, Step 20. The suture then is pulled superiorly to test if sufficient release of the midfacial tissues has been achieved. The knot is not tied until the frontalis muscle has been suspended to the bone tunnel in the paramedian incision.

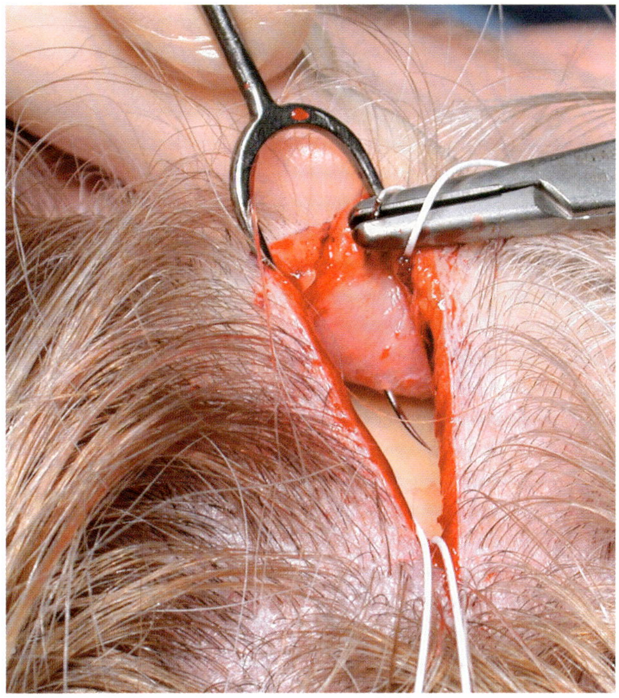

FIGURE 4-67. Brow and Midface Lift, Step 21. As mentioned, the surgeon should then direct his or her attention to the right paramedian port. A generous bite of frontalis muscle is taken at the anterior margin of the paramedian incision (as shown) and suspended through the bone tunnel. The knot then is fastened before returning to secure the midfacial suture.

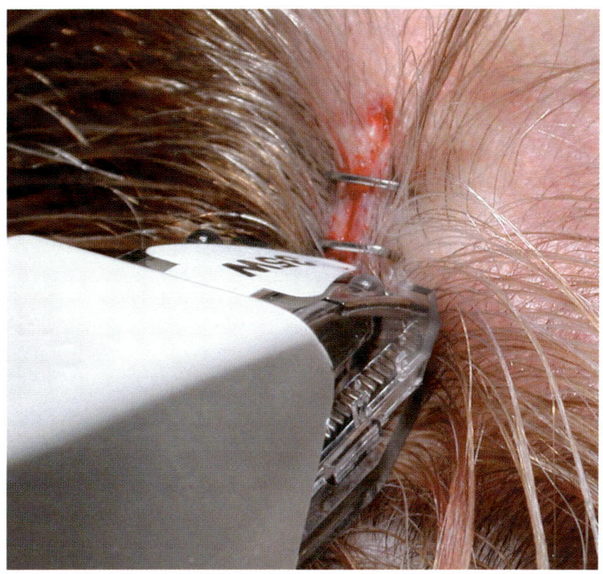

FIGURE 4-68. Brow and Midface Lift, Step 22. The right, paramedian incision is closed with surgical clips.

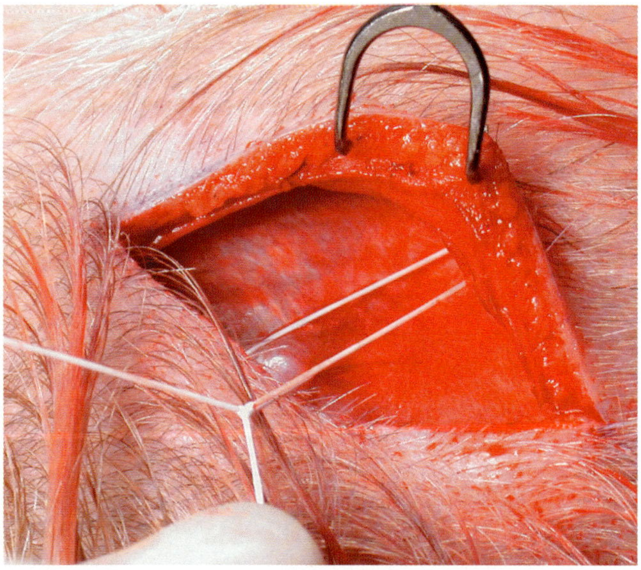

FIGURE 4-69. Brow and Midface Lift, Step 23. The midfacial suspension suture is tied down, while observing the elevation of the midfacial tissue.

ment and removal, and the senior author has achieved a very favorable cosmetic result with surgical-staple closure. Therefore, surgical staples are recommended to close the hair-bearing scalp. Bacitracin ointment is applied to the external incisions, and a pressure dressing is fashioned into place. Stepwise approach to the brow and midface ensures consistent, reproducible results (Figs. 4-71A,B and 4-72).

Of note, if cutaneous resurfacing is entertained to efface deep horizontal rhytids (which are usually not amenable to surgical correction with brow elevation alone), the surgeon may carry out resurfacing with impunity as far as vascular integrity to the underlying flap is concerned because the plane of dissection is subperiosteal. Jessner's solution followed by 35% TCA is preferred for mild to moderate rhytidosis, and carbon dioxide laser is reserved for deeper rhytidosis (especially glabellar) and more severe actinic damage. All resurfacing is undertaken before performing the preceding brow and midface lift.

Alloplastic Malar Augmentation

The cheek complex can be restored with an alloplastic malar implant as well. As one ages, skeletal support is lost and the bony malar prominence may become less so. If significant malar soft-tissue ptosis is evident, however, then an alloplast usually is insufficient to buttress the ptotic tissue, and a midface lift is necessary. The primary goal of a malar implant is to achieve a more youthful bony cheek structure.

The surgical technique begins with adequate anesthesia. The authors prefer general endotracheal anesthesia to achieve the desired level of sedation. Hemostasis is obtained with 1% lidocaine and 1:100,000 epinephrine infiltrated into the gingiva-buccal sulcus bilaterally. The malar implant then is placed on the cheek skin where the desired position is and outlined with a marking pen. Generally speaking, the implant should reside ideally with approximately two thirds of its body on the malar eminence and the remaining one

A

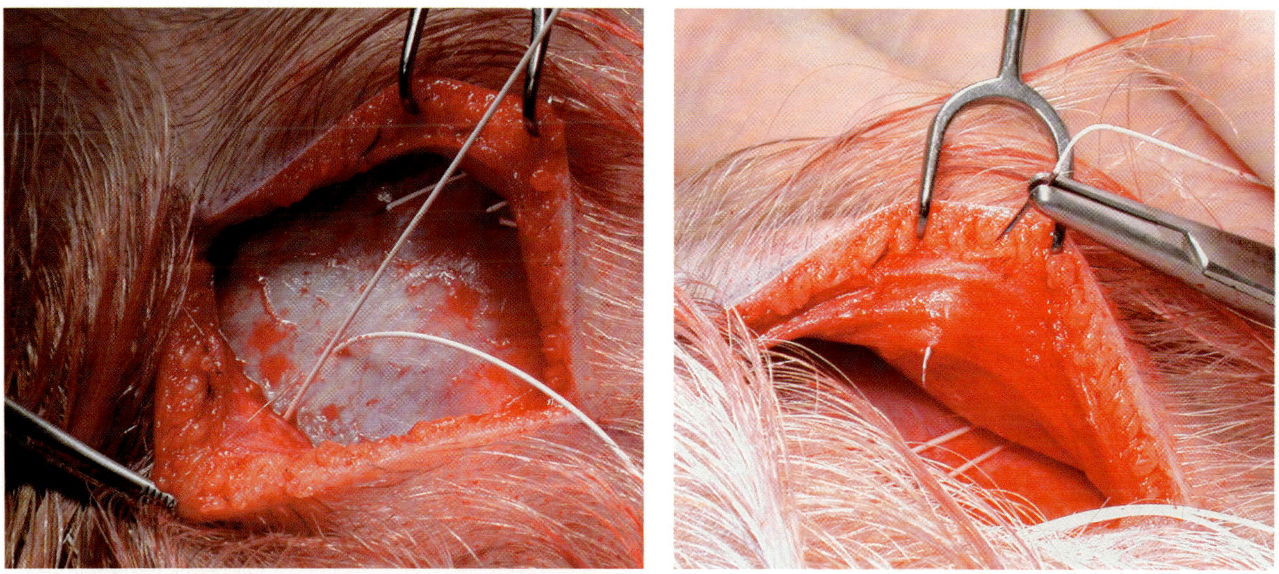

B

FIGURE 4-70. Brow and Midface Lift, Step 24. A,B: Next, the temporo-parietal fascia just anterior to the temporo-parietal incision is sutured to the temporalis muscle and fascia more superiorly with the CV-3 Gore-Tex suture to pull the overlying brow and soft tissue supero-laterally. This suture placement is undertaken twice on each side of the head. All incisions are then closed with surgical clips. The same procedure is carried out on the contralateral side of the head.

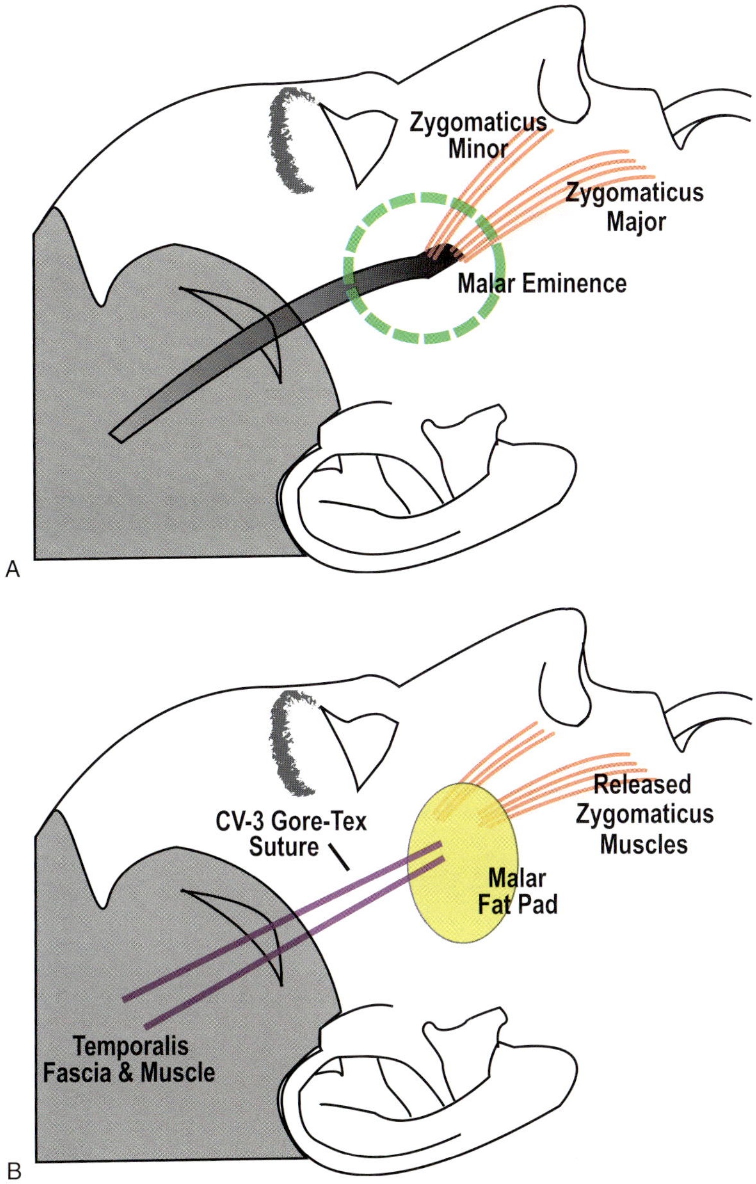

FIGURE 4-71. A: The illustration shows the dissection of the zygomaticus muscles (*in red*) off of the malar bony eminence (*circumscribed in dashed green circle*). **B:** The malar fat pad (*in yellow*) can be suspended to the temporalis muscle and fascia with a CV-3 Gore-Tex suture (*in purple*) after release of the lateral zygomaticus muscles (*in red*).

third more inferiorly over the submalar space. The more superiorly the implant is placed near the zygomatic arch and inferior orbital rim, the more technically difficult it is to position accurately, and resulting asymmetry may ensue. Although many shapes of implants have been advocated as well as different locations for these respective implants, the authors have relied principally on a standard ePTFE malar implant placed according to the prescribed anatomic parameters for consistently satisfactory to very good results. In the majority of cases, the authors rely on a medium-sized implant for malar augmentation. However, the patient's aesthetic desires and the surgeon's judgment ultimately should contribute to the decision for the proper implant size. Of note, ePTFE has been the most reliable material used for malar implantation for several reasons. Although silicone has been used successfully in many experienced hands, the senior author contends that the lack of tissue ingrowth with silicone predisposes toward implant mobility. Also, the tissue ingrowth that arises with ePTFE implants does not make implant removal a burdensome task, as hydroxyapatite or other materials may engender.

The surgical procedure can commence 10 minutes after injection of local anesthesia. Army–Navy retractors are used to elevate the lip away from the gingiva. A monopolar cautery is used to enter the gingiva-buccal sulcus, leaving a generous 1-cm cuff of buccal mucosa to the attached gingiva in order to facilitate easy mucosal approximation at the end of the case (Fig. 4-73). Dissection is taken straight down to the anterior face of the maxilla through the periosteum. A large periosteal elevator is used to dissect an adequate pocket

Salient Technical Points

Transconjunctival Lower-Lid Blepharoplasty

1. A chemical peel may serve to remove fine rhytidosis that could not be achieved with skin removal. The peel always should be done first when the patient is still awake and in the semiinclined position so that inadvertent entry of peel solution can be reported to the physician and promptly irrigated out.
2. Additional skin should only be cautiously removed if concurrent resurfacing is undertaken.
3. Transconjunctival blepharoplasty always should precede a brow/midface lift because the tightening of the lid secondary to brow/midface suspension does not permit easy entry through the conjunctiva.
4. A 6-0 silk is used to retract the conjunctival flap and protect the globe. No corneal shield is used, which would otherwise make the surgery more difficult and prevent easy ballottement of the globe when assessing fat herniation.
5. No monopolar cautery should be used near the eye because of the risk of eyelid incineration.
6. A preseptal plane of dissection (between the orbital septum and orbicularis-oculi muscle) is favored.

Skin–Muscle Lower-Lid Blepharoplasty

1. Although a transconjunctival approach is preferred in the majority of cases, a skin–muscle flap is indicated if:
   a. A lower lid shortening procedure is planned.
   b. A lateral canthal plication suture is required.
   c. Extension to the midface is desired.
2. If a lid-shortening procedure is planned, the authors advocate that a lateral tarsal strip be undertaken rather than a central-lid pentagonal wedge to minimize risk of lid notching. For tarsal-strip suspension, the suture should be placed through the anterior-medial aspect of the orbital-rim periosteum rather than the more physiologic inner aspect (Whitnall's tubercle) because of protracted lid malposition.

Upper-Lid Blepharoplasty

1. The supratarsal crease should be delineated with a surgical marking pen at the outset and should define the lower extent of skin removal.
2. Local anesthesia should remain superficial to the orbicularis-oculi muscle to minimize hematoma formation and added ecchymosis.
3. Upper-lid blepharoplasty always should follow a browlift.
4. The amount of skin excision should only just begin to evert the lid margin.
5. Any irregular skin edges that remain after removal of the excess skin should not be trimmed, because this is both unnecessary and predisposes to lagophthalmos.
6. Only the skin edges should be taken with the suture needle to avoid inadvertent lagophthalmos.

Ptosis Repair

1. If a browlift is required, it should be performed first and the ptosis repair deferred until at minimum several weeks later because brow elevation may exacerbate blepharoptosis. Therefore, ptosis elevation may be more accurately assessed only after brow elevation.
2. Local anesthesia with minimal to no sedation is required for patient cooperation during the procedure.
3. The remaining portion of the limbus may be traced out over the eyelid so that after anesthesia is infiltrated the effect of Müller's muscle may be observed. Accordingly, the amount of overcorrection can then be assessed.
4. No orbital septum should be sutured.
5. The levator may be identified by the glistening white quality of its surface and its mobility on the patient's upward and downward gaze.
6. A slipknot may facilitate easy removal of the fixation suture if it is not properly positioned.

Brow and Midface Lift

1. No endoscopic equipment is used. Instead the "smart-hand" technique relies on tactile feedback and a lifting rather than shearing motion near the supraorbital bundle to avoid neurapraxia. Direct vision with a headlight and Converse retractor permit visualization of the lateral temporo-parietal pocket, which avoids injury to the cephalic vessel. The smart-hand technique is again used to enter the midface and to dissect the zygomaticus musculature off the malar eminence.
2. Only the cephalic vessel that obstructs passage to the midface should be cauterized. Bipolar cautery should be aimed low (or deep) away from the superficial fascia where the facial nerve lies in proximity. Before the vessel is cauterized, all surrounding soft-tissue should be freed from the vessel to minimize transmission of cautery to the nearby soft tissue.
3. To ensure that a natural lift occur with minimal lateral-canthal distortion:
   a. The vector of pull should be primarily directed vertically rather than diagonally for the midfacial suspension suture.
   b. The periosteum at the lateral canthus should not be fully detached. The assistant's finger along the orbital rim at the lateral canthus can restrict the surgeon's overzealous elevation of the periosteum in this area.

c. Only sufficient dissection should be carried over the midface to release the zygomaticus muscle and ligamentous structures and further medial dissection should be minimized.

4. All suspension sutures (midfacial, temporo-parietal [2], frontal) are placed laterally. No medial suspension is attempted to avoid an unnatural, startled appearance.

Alloplastic Malar Augmentation

1. The principal purpose of this procedure is to restore skeletal loss of the malar eminence and has less impact on buttressing ptotic soft tissue.
2. The implant is outlined with a surgical marking pen first on the cheek skin to determine proper position.
3. A 1-cm gingival–buccal cuff of mucosa is left intact so that mucosal closure may be facilitated.
4. Dissection is carried out subperiosteally, first medially and superiorly then directed laterally so that the implant is well secured in its pocket.
5. The implant should be positioned with approximately two thirds of its body on the malar eminence, with the remaining one third situated over the submalar space. Positioning the implant too superiorly near the inferior orbital rim or zygomatic arch can result in likely asymmetry.
6. A medium-sized ePTFE implant is used in the majority of cases, but a smaller or larger implant may be used as aesthetically indicated.
7. The implant is secured with a 2- × 12-mm screw after drilling a suitable hole with a 1.5- × 10- to 12-mm hand drill against the zygomatico-maxillary buttress.
8. Symmetry is ensured by bilateral palpation and observation before closure.

to accommodate the implant. Generally, the direction of dissection should commence medially and be aimed upward while inspecting for the infraorbital nerve that may come into view. The dissection then is aimed laterally until the lateral zygomatico-maxillary (ZM) buttress is encountered. The implant is placed into the pocket and the overlying skin outline is used to confirm proper position (Fig. 4-74). A drill hole then is created through the implant and the ZM buttress using a 1.5- × 10- to 12-mm hand drill. A 2- × 12-mm screw is secured into position so that the malar implant is fixated at this point. The screw should be inserted such that the screw head is recessed into the malar implant; that is, the head remains buried below the outer contour of the implant (Fig. 4-75). The same technique is used for the contralateral placement of the implant. Symmetry is confirmed by simultaneous, bilateral palpation and observation before closure (Fig. 4-76). The gingiva-buccal incision is closed with a running 3-0 chromic suture.

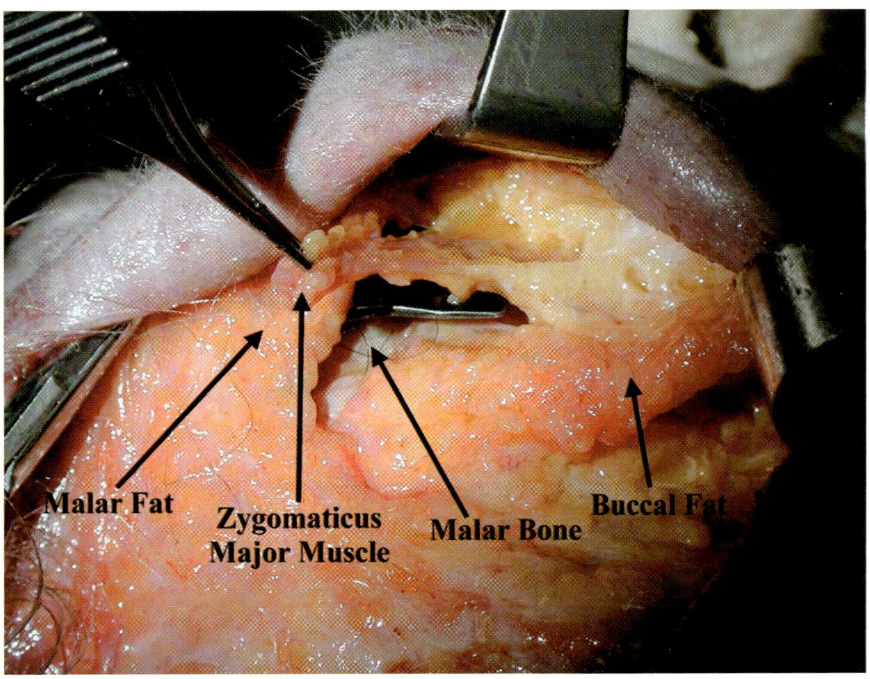

FIGURE 4-72. A photograph of the right side of a fresh cadaver's head viewed through a right-sided rhytidectomy incision that shows the elevator passed in a subperiosteal plane lifting the zygomaticus muscles free from their attachments. In addition, the qualitative difference in appearance and location of the malar- and buccal-fat pads may be noted.

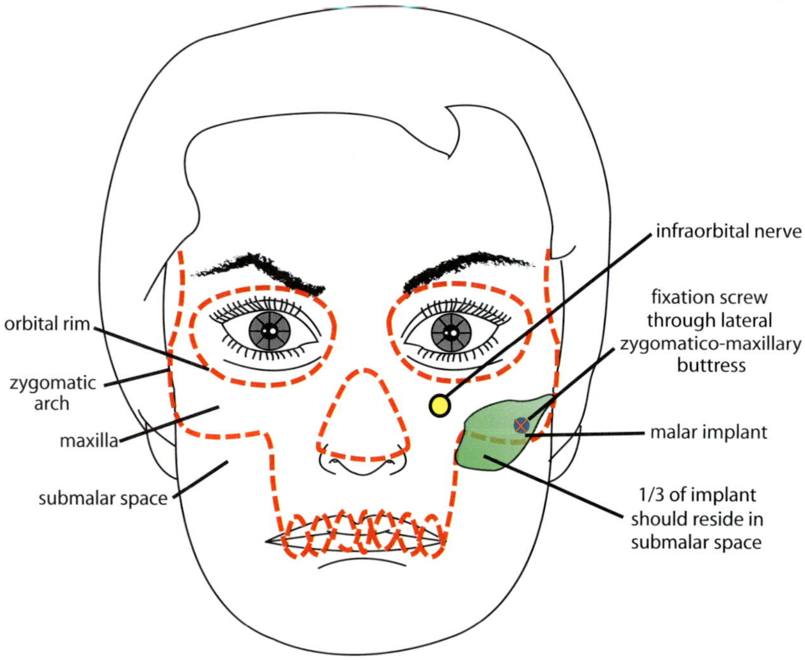

A

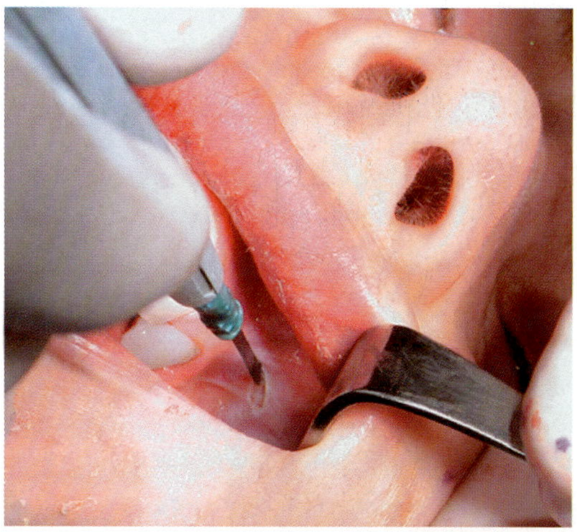

B

FIGURE 4-73. Alloplastic Malar Augmentation, Step 1. A: Illustration shows the relationship of the bony landmarks vis-à-vis the position of the malar implant. Note that the implant should be positioned with approximately one third of its body over the submalar space. The closer that the implant resides near the inferior orbital rim or zygomatic arch, the proportionately higher risk that exists for potential, postoperative asymmetry. **B:** A monopolar cautery is used to enter the gingiva-buccal sulcus leaving a generous 1-cm cuff of buccal mucosa to the attached gingiva in order to facilitate easy mucosal approximation at the end of the case.

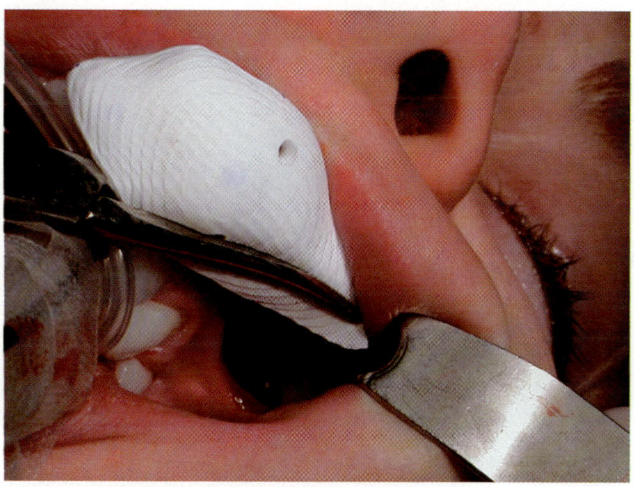

FIGURE 4-74. Alloplastic Malar Augmentation, Step 2. The implant is placed into the pocket and the overlying skin outline is used to confirm proper position.

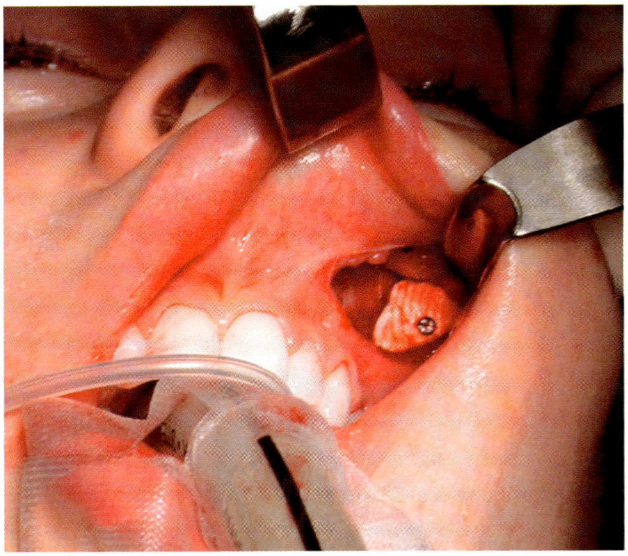

FIGURE 4-75. Alloplastic Malar Augmentation, Step 3. A drill hole then is created through the implant and the ZM buttress using a 1.5 × 10- to 12-mm hand drill. A 2- × 12-mm screw is secured into position so that the malar implant is fixated at this point. The screw should be inserted such that the screw head is recessed into the malar implant (i.e., the head remains buried below the outer contour of the implant). The same technique is carried out for the contralateral side.

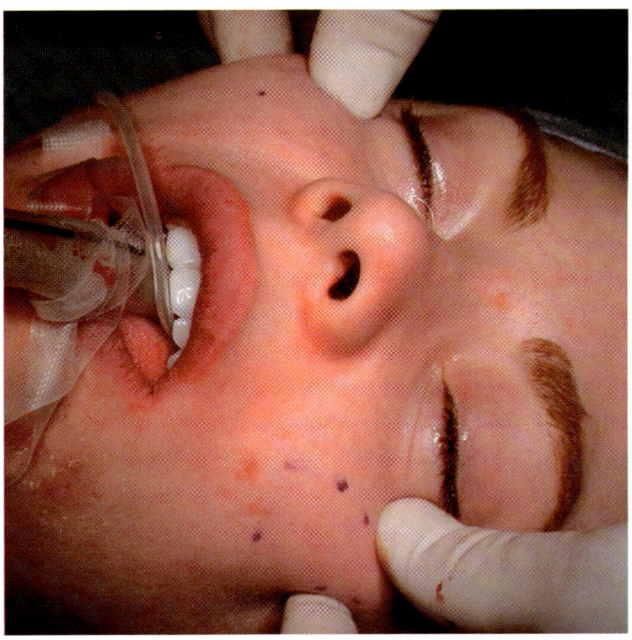

FIGURE 4-76. Alloplastic Malar Augmentation, Step 4. Symmetry is confirmed by simultaneous, bilateral palpation and observation before closure with a running 3-0 chromic suture.

POSTOPERATIVE CONSIDERATIONS: CARE, FOLLOW-UP, AND COMPLICATIONS

Postoperative Care and Follow-Up

Unlike the more labor-intensive care that is required for the resurfacing patient, postoperative management of the patient who has undergone upper and midfacial restorative procedures is rather more straightforward.

1. Blepharoplasty. Patients are advised neither to wear contact lenses nor to manipulate their eyes very much for risk of wound dehiscence. As usual, the suture line is gently cleansed with hydrogen peroxide and kept moist with Bacitracin ointment, both of which are applied with a cotton-tipped applicator, until the sutures are removed. (Refer to Chapter 3 for postoperative instructions.) Usual postoperative care is followed if resurfacing is performed. (Refer to Chapter 9 for details.) The patients are seen 6 days postoperatively for suture removal.
2. Ptosis Repair. The patient is seen at 1 week postoperatively, and eyelid position is assessed. If the eyelid appears ptotic or asymmetrical at this time, the suture(s) may be removed and repositioned in the office setting. It is not entirely unexpected if some suture replacement may be required at this time, and the patient should be properly counseled prior to surgery about this possibility.
3. Brow and Midface Lift. The patient is seen on postoperative day 1, and the wounds are inspected and cleaned with peroxide. A lighter dressing is applied that the patient will remove himself or herself the following day. Mild serous collection occasionally develops under the forehead flap, which is natural and expected to resolve. The patient returns on postoperative day 6, and all surgical clips (staples) are removed at that time.

Complications and Management

This section does not endeavor to cover every complication that can arise but reviews basic management strategies for important and common complications that may occur after a particular procedure.

Blepharoplasty

Postseptal Hemorrhage

The most dreaded complication that may occur is a postseptal hemorrhage with the attendant risk of visual loss. Fortunately, this complication remains a rare entity but deserves review herein. The surgeon must expeditiously determine the patient's visual status (whether intact, impaired, light perception only, or complete anopsia) as well as confirm extraocular movements, pupillary response, and palpable induration of the globe relative to the other eye. During this initial assessment, the assistant or nurse should be in an effort to contact the most available ophthalmologist, who can be available immediately for evaluation and further care.

The wound should be opened and carefully explored for any obvious bleeding points. However, typically the source of bleeding already has retracted back into the orbit and is not readily apparent. The patient should remain calm and not unduly agitated, because equanimity will reduce the likelihood of hypertension-exacerbated hemorrhage. Correspondingly, the anesthesiologist should be instructed to monitor blood pressure closely and medicate the patient appropriately if the pressure is deemed too high. Intravenous steroids are of equivocal benefit, because the time required for onset of action is on the order of hours, but may be enlisted nevertheless as an adjunct in this desperate situation. Similarly, mannitol, or an equivalent diuretic agent, does little to abate the increased ocular pressure but may be attempted all the same.

If the patient demonstrates any evidence of visual loss or ballotable tension, the surgeon should not hesitate to execute a lateral canthotomy and inferior cantholysis as a vital temporizing maneuver. A lateral canthotomy involves placing one blade of the tenotomy scissors into the lateral canthus down to the orbital rim and the other external to the skin to transect the skin down to the bony rim. Then an inferior cantholysis is completed by placing one blade of a tenotomy scissors under the inferior canthal tendon near the lateral canthus and transecting it fully. (A lateral canthotomy/inferior cantholysis is shown as part of the tarsal-strip sequence in Figure 4-26.) An immediate release of pressure should be evidenced on severing the tendon.

If the patient experiences further deterioration despite this maneuver, the surgeon is obligated to undertake more aggressive orbital decompression with or without ophthalmologic assistance. Similar to orbital decompression for Grave's orbitopathy, the surgeon should perform a bony reduction to reduce ocular pressure. The surgeon should perform the type of decompression with which he or she is most comfortable; for example, a medial wall or floor decompression. As mentioned, the surgeon rarely encounters this disturbing misfortune and even more seldom does this occurrence mandate the implementation of the entire algorithm described.

Corneal Abrasion

Although uncommon, corneal abrasion should be readily identified and promptly treated. The most defining symptom that should alert the physician that the patient might have sustained a corneal abrasion is a foreign-body sensation that is remarked on opening and closing the eye. The patient should be treated presumptively for a corneal abrasion if he or she complains of this symptom. The eye should be lubricated with a thick ophthalmic ointment and bandaged closed with two eye pads that are held in position with adhesive tape. The patient also should be prescribed a topical ophthalmologic ointment (e.g., tobramycin) without a steroid component, to minimize an infectious complication, most commonly *Pseudomonas aeruginosa.* The bandage should be retained for 3 days, and the patient reevaluated at that time for improvement. If the patient has improved somewhat, the bandage should be maintained for another 3 days until complete resolution of symptoms. However, if no improvement is witnessed, then he or she should seek prompt ophthalmologic consultation for slit-lamp evaluation and further care.

Lower-Lid Malposition

Perhaps one of the most common and distressing complications that occur after blepharoplasty is lower-lid malposition, whether mild lateral rounding or frank ectropion. Usually this complication arises because of poor preoperative lid tone that worsens after transection of the lower-lid retaining mechanisms, which occurs whether a transconjunctival or transcutaneous approach is implemented.

The patient should begin active and frequent massage of the distorted lateral canthal region, sweeping upward and laterally to encourage the lid to heal in that position. Squinting exercises several times daily also strengthen the orbicularis-oculi sling, especially if it has been violated by a transcutaneous approach. Taping the lower lid up to the temple region so that the lower-lid position is restored also serves as an effective treatment for this malady: all day long if tolerated otherwise only at night. If the patient exhibits some lagophthalmos, then an ocular lubricant at night and artificial tears during the day should provide adequate protection against exposure keratitis. Early and prompt treatment of this condition expedites favorable healing and avoids permanent scarring and contraction of the orbital septum, or middle lamella, to the anterior lamella, resulting in vertical lid shortening. The lid position should return to normal after several weeks of compliant treatment but may require several months in unusual cases for full resolution.

Persistence of this condition may result from overly ambitious removal of lid skin and represent an anterior-lamellar deficiency or middle-lamellar scarring. If the patient's lower-lid malposition is exclusively caused by poor lid tone, then one finger that the surgeon applies to the lateral canthus should restore the lid to normal position. If the malposition is caused by anterior- or middle-lamellar deficiency, then a second finger must be placed at the midpupillary region of the lower lid to restore the lid to a normal configuration. If insufficient lid tone is the etiology for the malpositioned lid, then a lid-shortening procedure (e.g., tarsal strip) may resolve the problem. However, if true vertical lid shortening exists, then the patient will require a skin graft from the contralateral upper lid or preauricular skin or, interestingly, as Dr. Schorr reports, a posterior lamellar graft (e.g., hard palate).[12,13] Grafting procedures lie beyond the scope of this textbook, and ophthalmologic expertise may be warranted to address this problem.

Milia

Milia develop several weeks after blepharoplasty and represent epidermal inclusion cysts or pustules that form because of local irritation. They should be differentiated from suture tract marks that may manifest at the time of suture removal. The preferred suture for closure is 7-0 polypropylene; even if retained longer than a week, it rarely results in noticeable tract marks.

Milia are rather common sequelae postblepharoplasty and usually resolve without incident. However, if the patient is troubled by the presence of these lesions, the surgeon can unroof them with a No. 11 blade and express the contents with opposing cotton-tipped applicators. If they persist, tretinoin (Retin-A) may expedite resolution.

Hypertrophic Scar/Keloid

Although frank keloid formation on the face is quite rare, hypertrophic scarring may be more prevalent, especially in patients with dark complexions. Prophylactic, intraoperative triamcinolone acetonide injection (10 mg/mL) with 0.1 mL total per eyelid may be advisable in Fitzpatrick IV–VI patients, especially along the medial extent of the wound. If this complication should arise, then triamcinolone should be directly injected into the scar not more frequently than every 3 weeks to avoid dermal atrophy. Adjuvant treatment with the pulsed-dye laser also has been proved efficacious as a management option. As mentioned, an extended skin–muscle blepharoplasty incision can be visible because of the disparity between the thicker cheek and thinner eyelid skin (Fig. 4-77A–D). Subsequent dermabrasion may be required to address this conspicuous line if it does not resolve after several months of expectant observation.

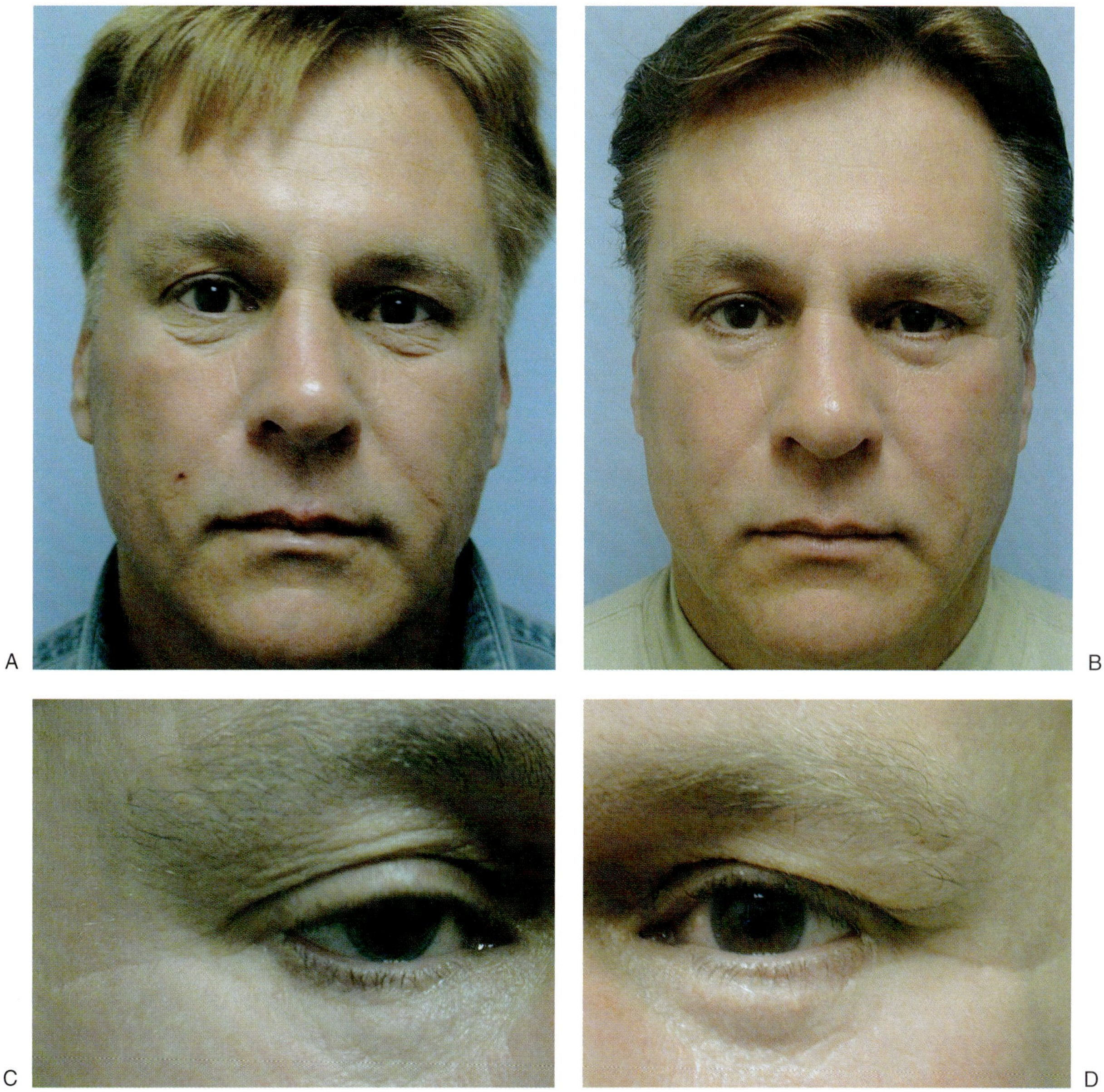

FIGURE 4-77. A: This patient is shown preoperative to a midface lift using an extended lower-lid incision. **B:** The postoperative photograph shows the obvious incision lines present 1 year after surgery because of the disparity in skin thickness between the thicker, cheek and thinner, eyelid skin. **C,D:** Close-up, oblique views confirm the noticeable incision line.

Ptosis Repair

Lagophthalmos

Lagophthalmos usually is a transient phenomenon that resolves by the first postoperative week. However, lagophthalmos may result from inadvertent suture placement through the orbital septum during levator fixation and may be corrected by replacing the fixation suture during the first postoperative visit in the office setting. Attentive surgery should avoid the more dreaded etiology of lagophthalmos, which arises because of excision of too much lid skin.

Asymmetry/Improper Lid Position/Notched Lid

Insufficient, excessive, or asymmetric lid elevation may be corrected by replacement of the fixation suture during the first postoperative visit. The patient should be properly counseled during the preoperative visit that correction may be required postoperatively and should not signify any ominous complication. Also, an unnatural notched lid appearance may result from overtightening and suspension of the midpupillary fixation suture, which should be removed and replaced.

Brow and Midface Lift

Asymmetry

Symmetry is perhaps the most difficult aesthetic result to achieve in facial plastic surgery, partly because of the patient's natural disposition to resume any preoperative tendency toward asymmetry. Patients who present with an asymmetric brow during the preoperative consultation should be admonished as to the limitation of the surgery to create a symmetric countenance. If gross asymmetry exists postoperatively that was not present preoperatively, technical error may be the source of this outcome (e.g., incomplete release of the periosteal arcus marginalis, suture dehiscence, or facial nerve paresis).

Facial Nerve Neuropraxia

Albeit uncommonly encountered, any facial nerve neurapraxia will most likely engender considerable trepidation on the part of surgeon and patient alike. The most likely causes for this outcome are indiscriminate bipolar cautery near the cephalic vessel,[14] improper plane of dissection in the temporo-parietal region (which may cause injury to the frontal branch of the facial nerve), or injury during midfacial dissection (which may cause injury to the zygomatico-buccal branches) (Fig. 4-78A,B). The few cases that the authors have encountered have uniformly resolved after a period of 3 to 6 months, which may seem interminable to all parties involved. Frequent and amiable reassurance should be maintained throughout the postoperative course to ensure good patient rapport and provide much-needed patient support. Ocular protection with lubrication is an integral component to proper care. Otherwise, expectant care

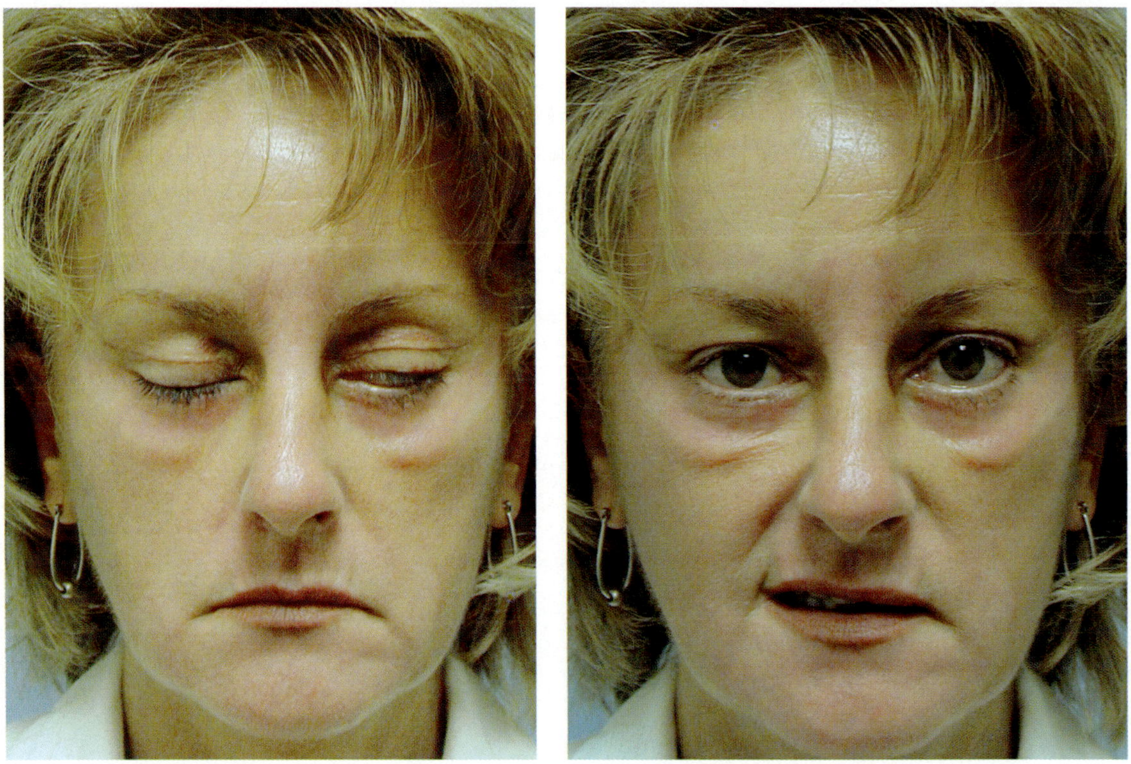

A B

FIGURE 4-78. A,B: This patient demonstrates left-sided zygomatico-buccal facial neurapraxia after an uneventful brow and midface lift. The patient's neuropraxia fully resolved by 6 months postoperatively.

is warranted in all cases. The authors have noted that aggressive midfacial dissection medially toward the nasolabial sulcus has been associated with a greater likelihood for buccal-branch paresis.

Alopecia/Scar

Incision alopecia may be avoided by adhering to the following three tenets:

1. Bevel the knife blade according to the pattern of the hair follicles: perpendicularly at the three medial incisions and postero-anteriorly for the two temporal incisions. The follicles should be attentively observed for inadvertent transection as the surgeon is cutting through the skin.
2. Limit excessive monopolar cautery at the wound edges.
3. Avoid tension along the incision line at the time of wound closure. The authors have noted no further evidence of alopecia, or scarring, because modification of technique from screw suspension to bone-tunnel suture suspension technique, which may result from the fact that the erstwhile screw held the brow suspended by the skin rather than the frontalis muscle.

If any wound alopecia or scarring should develop, simple excision and revision of the wound should ameliorate the appearance.

Alloplastic Malar Augmentation

Infection

Prophylactic, perioperative oral antibiotics are administered to patients for the first postoperative week in all cases of alloplastic implantation. However, no attempt is made to prepare the implant or the surgical site with povidone-iodine, or an equivalent solution because ePTFE is hydrophobic and the oral flora are not easily sterilized. If an infection should arise, the patient is administered a dose of intravenous broad-spectrum antibiotics (e.g., ampicillin/sulbactam) and maintained on a 10-day course of amoxicillin/clavulanic acid. Warm pads are applied locally to the infected site three times daily, and the patient is closely followed. If frank abscess forms, the wound is opened, cultured, and thoroughly irrigated. An infection usually results in implant removal, and an abscess almost definitely does. If the infection does not resolve or recurs, then the implant should be removed and another implant placed after a 3-month quiescent period. Albeit not obligatory, return of the infected implant to the manufacturer may be advisable to detect any unlikely flaw in implant integrity that might have predisposed to contamination.

Malposition

Use of a fixation screw has virtually eliminated the occurrence of implant malposition. However, if this complication should arise, return to the operating room to reposition and secure the implant is the only recourse to resolve the problem.

CLINICAL PRESENTATIONS: A SYNTHESIS OF APPROACH

Case #1 (Fig. 4-79A–H)

This 49-year-old patient stated that she had a lifelong adult history of looking tired. She stated that she always had bags under her lower eyelids as long as she can recall and that she was becoming more self-conscious of her appearance. She expressly stated that she was not interested in significant facial rejuvenation and was very explicit about only having her lower eyelids addressed. On examination, she was noted to have blue eyes and a Fitzpatrick II skin classification. She presented with fine to moderate rhytids that traversed her lower eyelids and exhibited significant pseudoherniation of the medial, middle, and lateral fat pockets in her lower lids. Additionally, this patient demonstrated moderate to moderately severe laxity of her lower eyelids, as evident by a two-finger snap test.

Procedure

This section describes transconjunctival lower-eyelid blepharoplasty with a Jessner's/35% TCA peel to the lower eyelids.

Discussion

This patient was first treated with Jessner's/35% TCA chemical peel to her lower eyelids. The authors prefer to apply a chemical peel to the lower eyelids with the patient in a sitting position so that the chemical-peeling solution would less likely enter the eye. The patient was also asked to fix her gaze upward to keep the lower eyelids more taut. Once the chemical peel was completed, a transconjunctival lower-eyelid blepharoplasty was performed in the preseptal plane (see text) in order to remove a moderately conservative amount of fat in all three pockets. Of note, given the significant laxity to her lower eyelids, any skin excision would have predisposed her to postoperative scleral show, or worse yet, vertical shortening of the lower lid. Although a chemical peel can give rise to some temporary postoperative lower-lid rounding, the likelihood for inadvertent vertical shortening is unlikely. Further, the finer rhytids are more optimally effaced with a chemical peel than with simple skin excision. The peel also promotes skin contracture, which is beneficial to draw in the skin previously distended by fat.

Case #2 (Fig. 4-80A,B)

This is a 73-year-old gentleman who was concerned with the appearance of his lower eyelids, which had been worsening over the past 15 years. He denies any ocular irritation related to his condition (e.g., dry eye symptoms, epiphora, or burning). He has not sought prior ophthalmologic or cosmetic consultation for this problem and has never undergone or entertained any cosmetic surgery in the past. On physical ex-

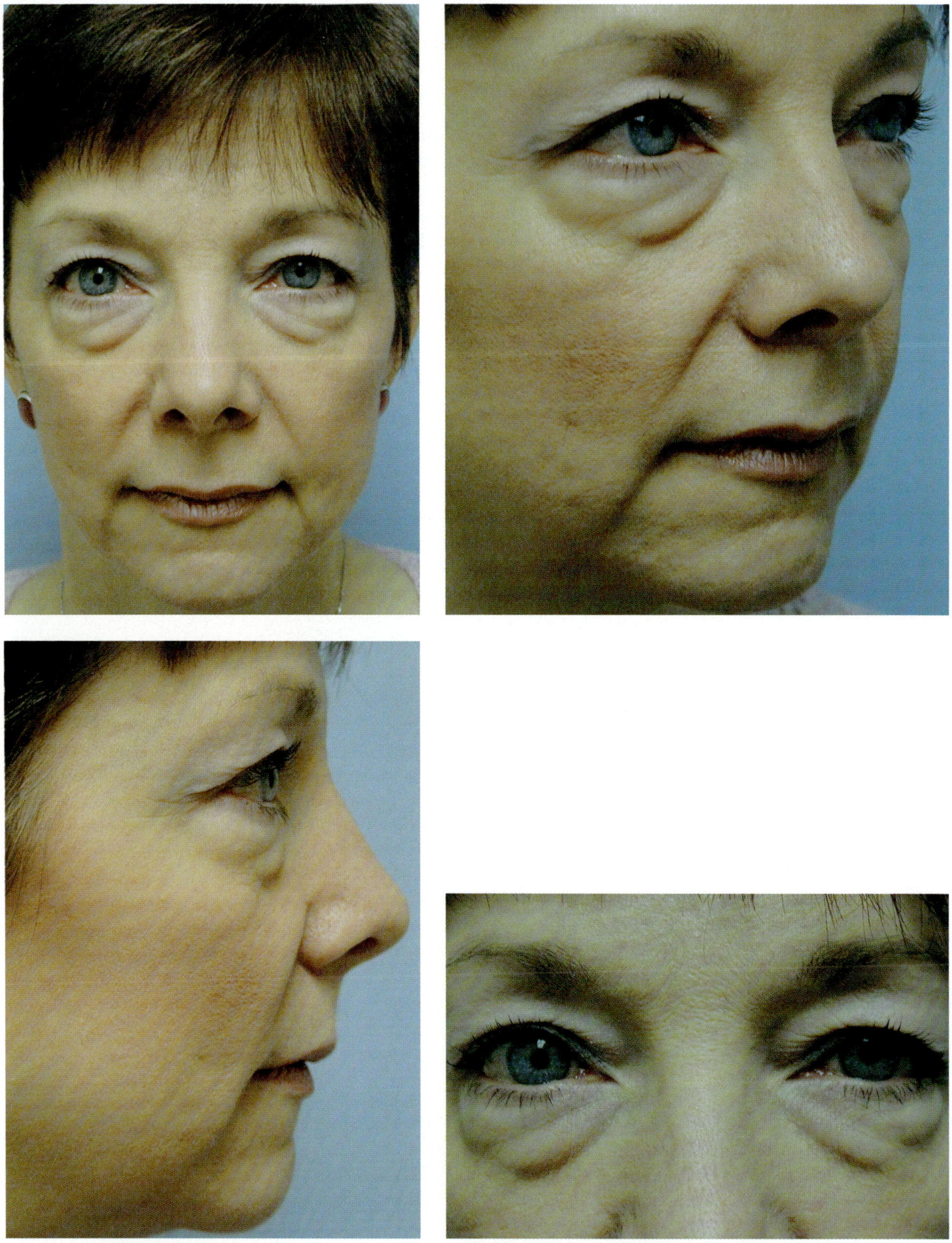

A B C D

FIGURE 4-79. A–D: This is a 49-year-old lady who presents with disproportionate aging in her lower eyelid region and only wanted treatment of this area. She exhibited significant pseudoherniation of fat with visible delineation of her fat pockets. She also demonstrated moderately severe laxity to her lower eyelids. *(continued)*

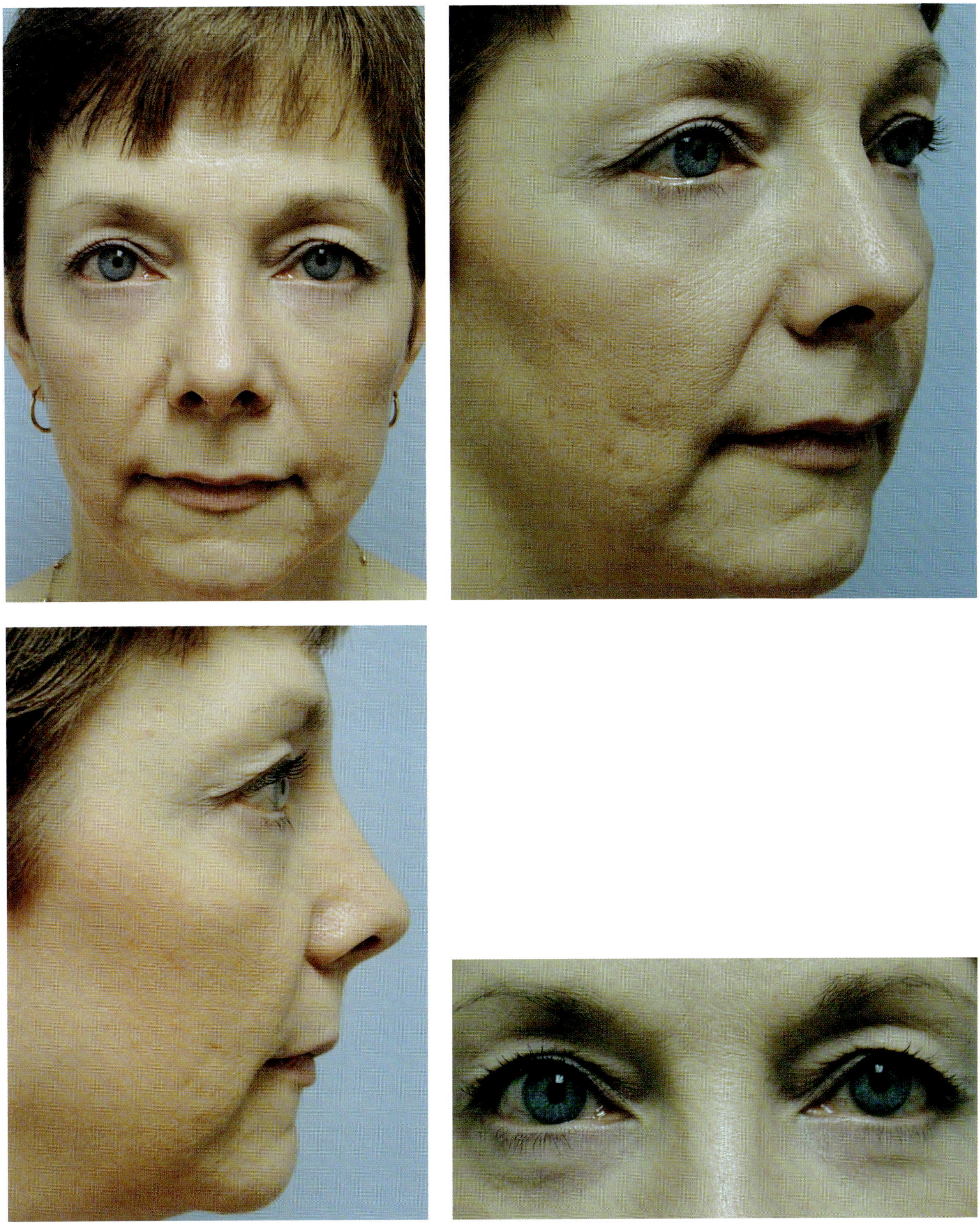

E F G H

FIGURE 4-79. *(Continued)* **E–H:** This is a 49-year-old lady who presents with disproportionate aging in her lower eyelid region and only wanted treatment of this area. She exhibited significant pseudoherniation of fat with visible delineation of her fat pockets. She also demonstrated moderately severe laxity to her lower eyelids. She underwent transconjunctival blepharoplasty and lower-lid resurfacing with Jesssner's/35% TCA peel. The chemical peel provides tightening of her lower-lid skin without the added risk of vertical-lid shortening and ectropion that would accompany skin excision in this higher risk patient. She is noted to have significant improvement of her lower-eyelid region after the combined blepharoplasty and TCA peel at 6 months postoperatively.

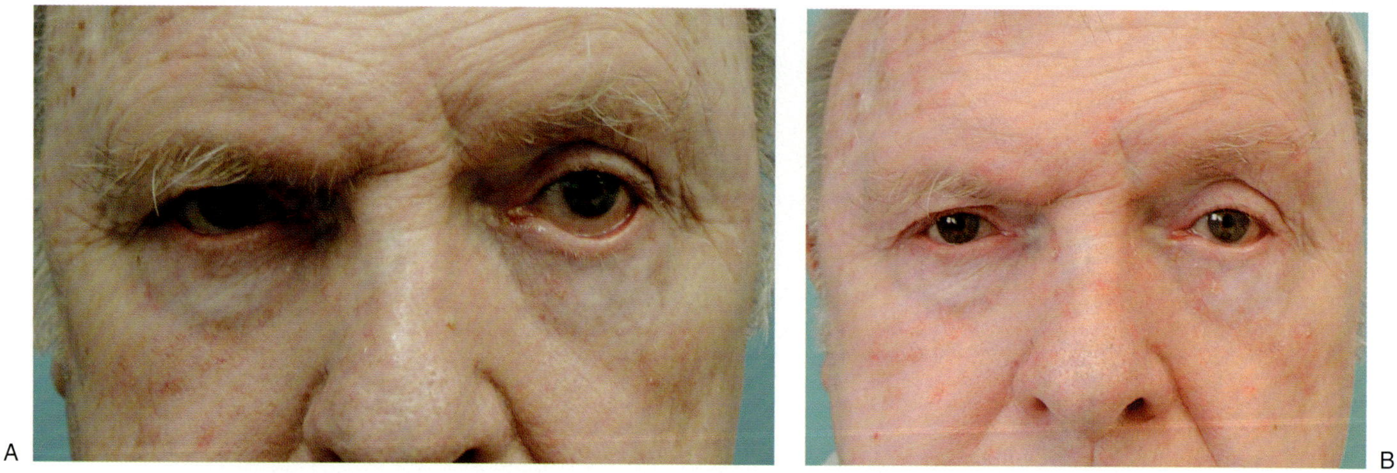

FIGURE 4-80. A,B: This is a 73-year-old gentleman who presents with bilateral (left worse than right) ectropion without any symptoms of ocular irritation. The patient has not had a history of any prior blepharoplasty and has a fully functioning facial nerve. He underwent a bilateral tarsal strip with notable improvement in his aesthetic appearance. He is shown 3 months after the operation.

amination, he exhibits frank ectropion on the left side without any punctal eversion and only some lateral scleral show on the right side. He has a poor snap test on both the right and left sides. His facial nerve is completely intact bilaterally. His Schirmer's test is also normal. The patient exhibits right greater than left brow ptosis and some pseudoherniation of lower-lid fat without significant lower-lid dermatochalasis. The patient does not want his brow or eyelid areas rejuvenated other than repairing his lower-lid laxity.

Procedure

This section describes a bilateral tarsal strip procedure.

Discussion

The major distinction that must be discerned concerning lower-lid ectropion is whether vertical shortening of the lower lid is the causative factor. On history taking, prior blepharoplasty or cicatricial injury may lead to the diagnosis of vertical lower-lid shortening, which can be confirmed on physical examination. Unlike senile lower-lid laxity, vertical shortening presents without any notable laxity but the lid appears more taut against the globe. Management of vertical shortening is a complicated topic and lies beyond the scope of this textbook.

In regard to ectropion that results from senility or paralysis, the lower-lid tone is reduced, and a tarsal strip typically addresses the problem. The patient should always receive a detailed history and physical examination that pertains to the orbital region before undertaking any kind of eyelid surgery. In particular, the amount of lower-lid laxity should be carefully delineated; that is, the presence of mild scleral show laterally to frank punctal and medial-eyelid eversion. This text has outlined a simple, straightforward approach to management of lower-lid laxity when it affects the lateral aspect of the lower lid via a tarsal-strip procedure. The surgical steps to correct medial lower-lid laxity represent an advanced topic that is better relegated to an oculoplastic textbook.

Case #3 (Fig. 4-81A–D)

This is a 54-year-old operating-room nurse who presented for possible facial rejuvenation. The patient stated that she had never been motivated cosmetically. However, over the past 2 to 3 years, she has felt that she appeared much older than her stated age. She declared that the youth and vitality of her grandchildren have inspired her to seek cosmetic rejuvenation of her face. Being an operating-room nurse, she expressed fear of "having an operated-on look." On clinical examination, she was noted to exhibit fair skin and significant periorbital rhytids. In addition, she demonstrated moderate to severe brow ptosis, malar festoons, and a double-contour configuration of her lower eyelids.

Procedure

This section describes a transconjunctival lower-eyelid blepharoplasty, CO_2-laser resurfacing of the lower eyelids and periorbital area, minimally invasive browlift, subperiosteal upper and midface lift, and upper-eyelid blepharoplasty.

For the patient undergoing a minimally invasive brow and midface lift, it is important to perform the transconjunctival lower-eyelid blepharoplasty first, as elevation of the midface and periorbital complex results in increasing the tension of the lower eyelid, making transconjunctival entry technically more difficult. Additionally, edema that arises af-

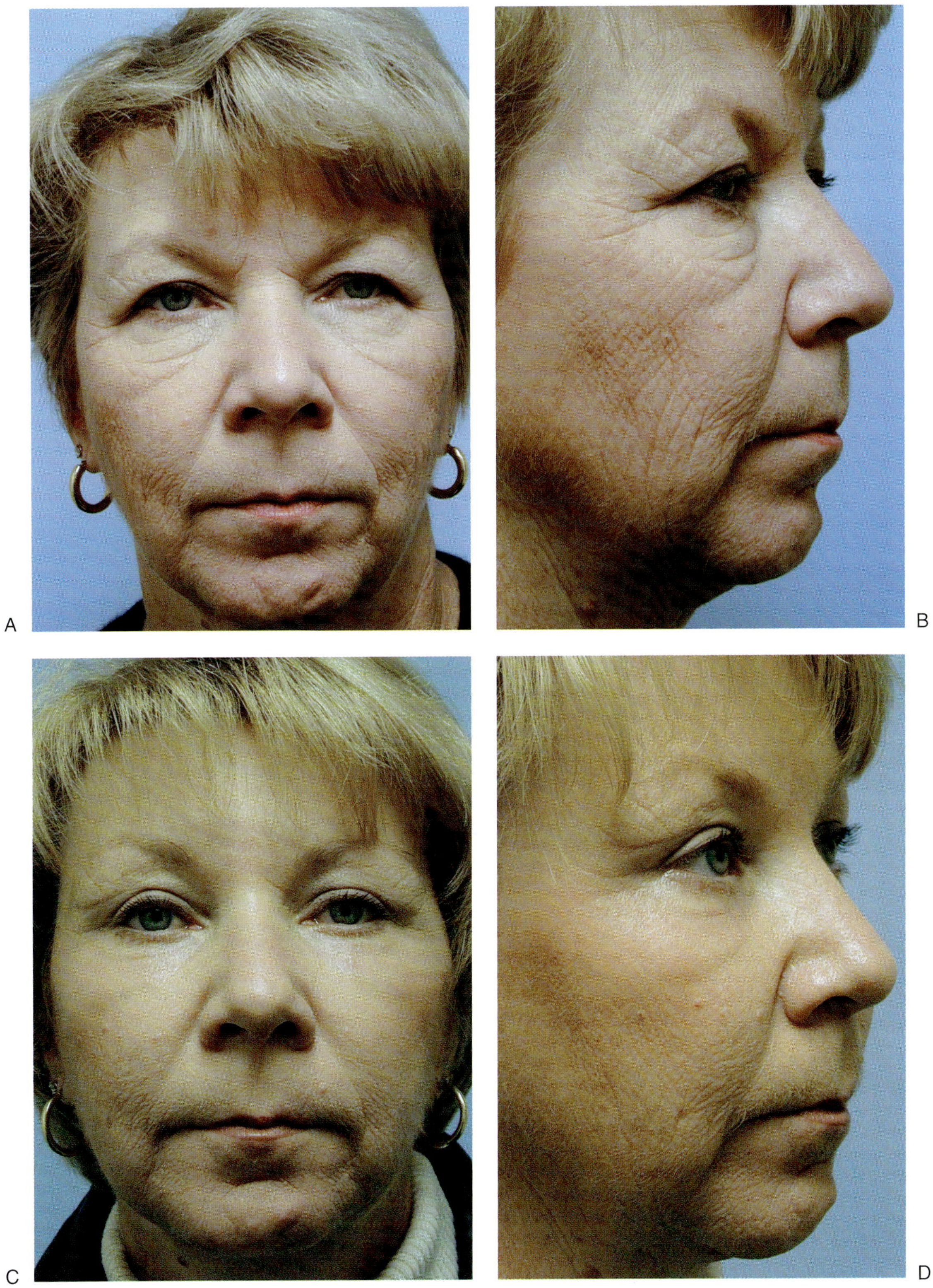

FIGURE 4-81. A–D. This is a 54-year-old lady who desires facial rejuvenation but is quite fearful of "having an operated-on look." She demonstrates moderate to severe brow ptosis, malar festoons, and a double-contour configuration of her lower eyelids. She underwent transconjunctival lower-eyelid blepharoplasty, CO_2 laser resurfacing of the lower eyelids and periorbital region, brow and midface lift, and upper-eyelid blepharoplasty. She shows remarkable resuspension of her descended mid- and upper-facial soft tissues as well as a rejuvenated skin appearance in the periocular region at 1 year postoperatively.

ter subperiosteal midfacial dissection may render lower-eyelid surgery more demanding. The browlift was performed using the "smart-hand" technique in lieu of endoscopic guidance after the transconjunctival lower-eyelid blepharoplasty and laser resurfacing were completed. After dissection over the true temporalis fascia and under the temporo-parietal fascia, the subperiosteal plane was entered over the zygomatic arch to enter the malar region for proper zygomaticus release. As per routine, a cuff of periosteum near the lateral canthus was kept intact to minimize any untoward lateral canthal elevation. Midfacial dissection should stop short of the masseteric muscle to avoid inadvertent trismus but be sufficiently aggressive to release the zygomaticus ligaments.

Discussion

This patient suffers from as much cutaneous pathology as gravitational tissue descent. Rejuvenation of either aspect alone would only be partly successful and leave a somewhat unbalanced and incomplete cosmetic benefit. Her principal rhytids circumscribe the eye and appear to be very coarse and deep in nature. Although a TCA peel is effective, CO_2-laser resurfacing provides the optimal rejuvenation for this more recalcitrant type of rhytidosis. The lower-lid region tends to be very tolerant of CO_2-laser resurfacing. Conversely, extensive, full-facial, CO_2-laser resurfacing is quite aggressive for the majority of patients except the few who exhibit a very deep, crevicelike rhytidosis. Even in these patients, a combined technique is useful in which a TCA peel can be applied more universally across the face and the CO_2 laser reserved for more severe areas. Also, it is important to note that concurrent resurfacing is a safe proposition for a patient who undergoes a brow and midface lift, because the plane of dissection remains in the subperiosteal level medially and the subtemporo-parieto-fascial level laterally (i.e., below the vascular supply of the overlying flap). Cutaneous resurfacing will not compromise the integrity of the flap because the vascular supply to the dissected flap is preserved. This stands in contradistinction to lower-facial lifting surgery (e.g., rhytidectomy), which partially severs the flap's blood supply, and concurrent resurfacing in this case should be avoided or used with great caution. As mentioned, the authors strongly contend that the most natural result for midfacial rejuvenation is derived from a brow approach rather than an extended lower-lid or facelift incision.

Case #4 (Fig. 4-82A–D)

This 43-year-old self-employed lady complained of looking increasingly more tired. According to the patient, she noticed that over the past 2 to 3 years she has acquired a tired, drawn expression all the time despite adequate rest at night. She desired eyelid surgery but adamantly expressed her fear of looking "operated." On physical examination, she was found to exhibit slight asymmetry of both upper and lower eyelids with a minimal amount of pseudoherniation present in the lower, medial orbital fat pockets. Some fine rhytids of the lower eyelids and dermatochalasis of the upper eyelids are evident. The patient has a fair complexion with light-colored eyes and shows moderate hooding of the lateral-brow area. A recommendation was made first to review options for a lower-eyelid blepharoplasty and then turn the attention to the upper-eyelid and brow region. Care was taken in this particular case to educate the patient about the difference in pathology between the upper-eyelid versus the brow-periorbital complex. The patient was informed that a conservative upper-eyelid blepharoplasty could be performed with only a minimal amount of skin excision. She was admonished that it was ill advised to remove a significant amount of skin in the attempt to compensate for brow descent.

Procedure

This section describes a transconjunctival lower-eyelid blepharoplasty, 35% TCA chemical peel of the lower eyelids, and minimally invasive brow and midface lift.

Discussion

A conservative lower-eyelid transconjunctival blepharoplasty was performed by removing only a small amount of fat from the medial pocket of the lower eyelid. It was felt in this patient that the double contour of the lower eyelid resulted not from pseudoherniation of the lower-eyelid fat laterally but rather from a descent of the malar fat pad. With a midface lift, the descended cheek fat is restored to a more youthful height without need for removal of excessive lower-lid fat. To reiterate, elevation of the midface via an extended lower-lid incision is not preferred for several reasons:

1. The more that the midface must be elevated, the longer the lower-eyelid incision must be carried laterally. Further, a greater degree of soft-tissue elevation mandates a proportionate amount of skin removal. Because the thicker, brow skin does not match the thinner, eyelid skin, the disparity between the skin edges often manifests as a more conspicuous scar. This entrenched line of demarcation may persist for several months but may last indefinitely, requiring dermabrasion to camouflage the line.
2. Because the brow and midface often descend as a unit, restoration of the midface without concomitant brow elevation often can look unnatural. Suspension of the midface via a brow incision permits rejuvenation of the two regions as one unified complex.

Case #5 (Fig. 4-83A,B)

This is a 48-year-old lady who had undergone a minimal-incision brow and midface lift. Before her upper and midfacial rejuvenation, she was noted to have some minimal ble-

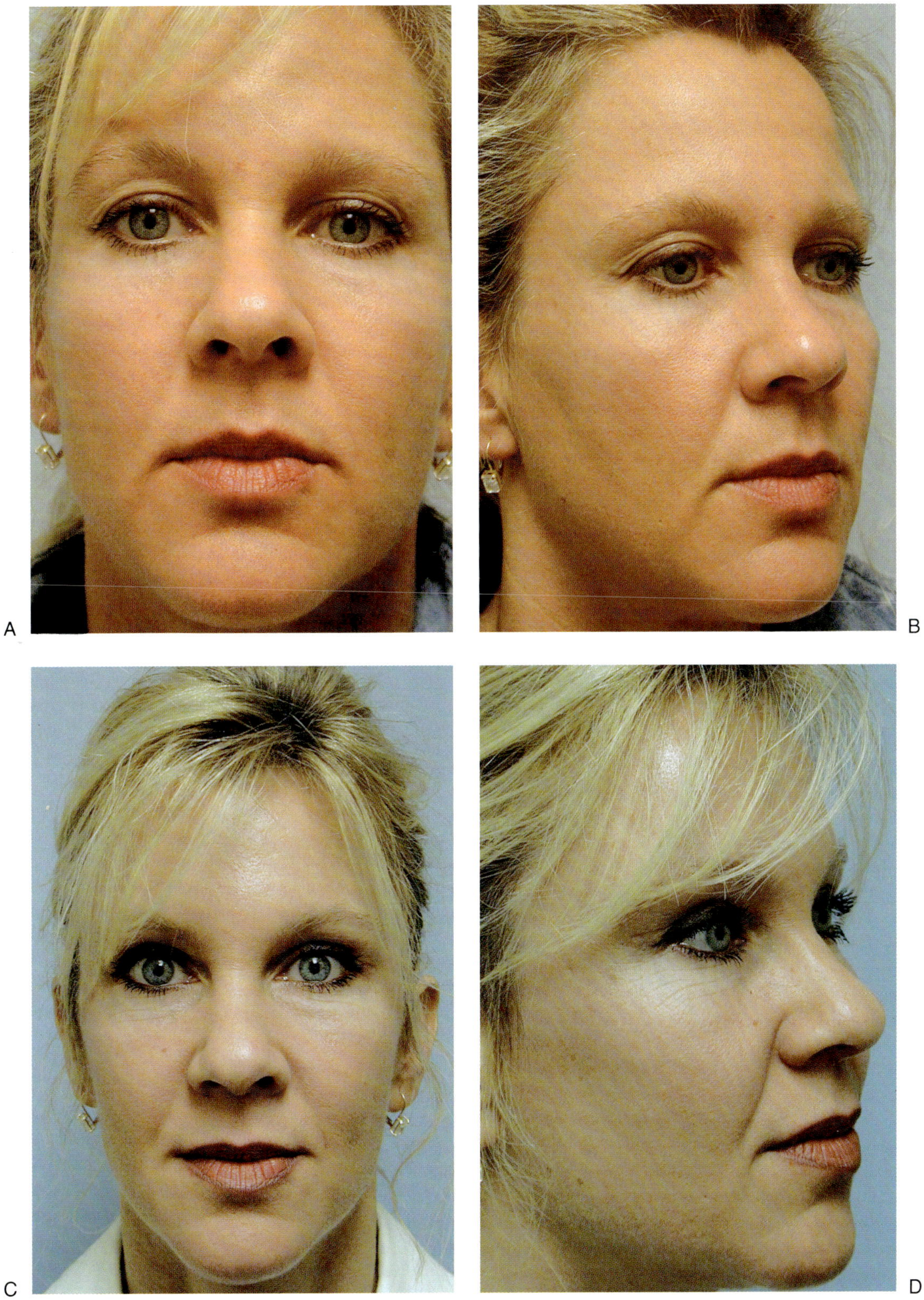

FIGURE 4-82. A–D: This is a 43-year-old lady who complained of looking more tired lately. The patient declared interest in eyelid surgery but was counseled on the benefits that a browlift would offer her in terms of optimal rejuvenation. The patient underwent a transconjunctival lower-eyelid blepharoplasty, 35% TCA peel of her lower eyelids and brow and midface lift. She is shown 1 year postoperatively with notable improvement in her upper and midface.

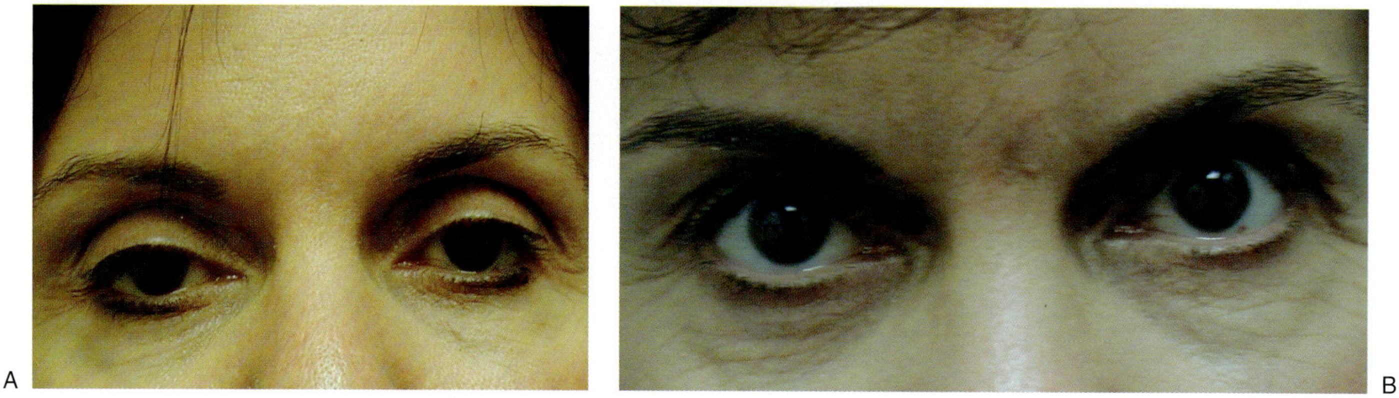

FIGURE 4-83. A,B: This is a 48-year-old lady who had undergone a prior browlift and whose blepharoptosis became worse after her browlift. She was counseled regarding this possibility prior to her browlift surgery. She underwent bilateral blepharoptosis repair approximately 6 months after her initial browlift surgery with notable functional and aesthetic improvement.

pharoptosis bilaterally, but the patient expressed more concern about the descent of her brow tissue. She was informed that her blepharoptosis could be exacerbated by her browlift surgery. She is shown several months after her initial browlift with more notable blepharoptosis, right worse than left, and concomitant functional visual-field compromise, which was confirmed by formal testing. The patient elected to proceed with bilateral blepharoptosis repair.

Procedure

This section describes a bilateral blepharoptosis repair.

Discussion

Any patient who entertains browlift surgery may have a subclinical blepharoptosis unmasked. If the patient exhibits some mild ptosis preoperatively, he or she should be advised that this condition might be exacerbated by brow-rejuvenation surgery. If the patient requires both a browlift and a ptosis repair, the browlift always should be completed before the ptosis repair. Obviously, if the ptosis is repaired first, the patient's condition may return after a browlift. If subclinical or minimal blepharoptosis becomes more clinically apparent postoperatively, the surgeon should patiently wait a minimum of 3 to 6 months before considering ptosis repair for two reasons. The patient should have complete resolution of edema and have the brow position settle to its ultimate position. More important, the patient should be afforded adequate time to recover from the first procedure, both physically and psychologically, before embarking on the next procedure. If the patient has only unilateral ptosis present, the reader is reminded that the ptotic lid should be held up manually to observe whether the contralateral lid will fall because of release of tonic inhibition (Hering's Law).

Bilateral (simultaneous or staged) ptosis repair should be elected if this is the case.

Case #6 (Fig. 4-84A–F)

This is a 51-year-old lady who had undergone a previous cervico-facial rhytidectomy and transconjunctival blepharoplasty with lower-lid CO_2-laser resurfacing 3 years earlier. She now complains that she is unsatisfied with the hypoplastic appearance of her malar region. She says that she has always had a very shallow cheek contour but has only been aesthetically troubled by this feature since her facelift. She states that prior to her facelift, she was only focused on her aged neck. Now that the cervical region had been addressed, she has become more attentive to the other aesthetic deficiencies of her face, notably her underprojected malar region.

Procedure

This section describes bilateral malar augmentation with medium-sized ePTFE implants.

Discussion

A patient who presents with midfacial complaint can be managed via two principal approaches: midfacial suspension (via an extended lower-lid blepharoplasty or temporal browlift incision) or midfacial augmentation with a malar implant. The patient who complains of some cheek descent (prominent malar bag or festoon) should be managed by a midface lift. However, the patient who complains of a shallow-appearing midface should be offered a malar implant instead. A patient who is focused on his or her midfacial hypoplasia often is not satisfied with the aesthetic result from a midface lift alone even if considerable midfacial descent is evident. The reader is referred to the principal text for the technical details regarding proper implant placement to ensure a successful outcome.

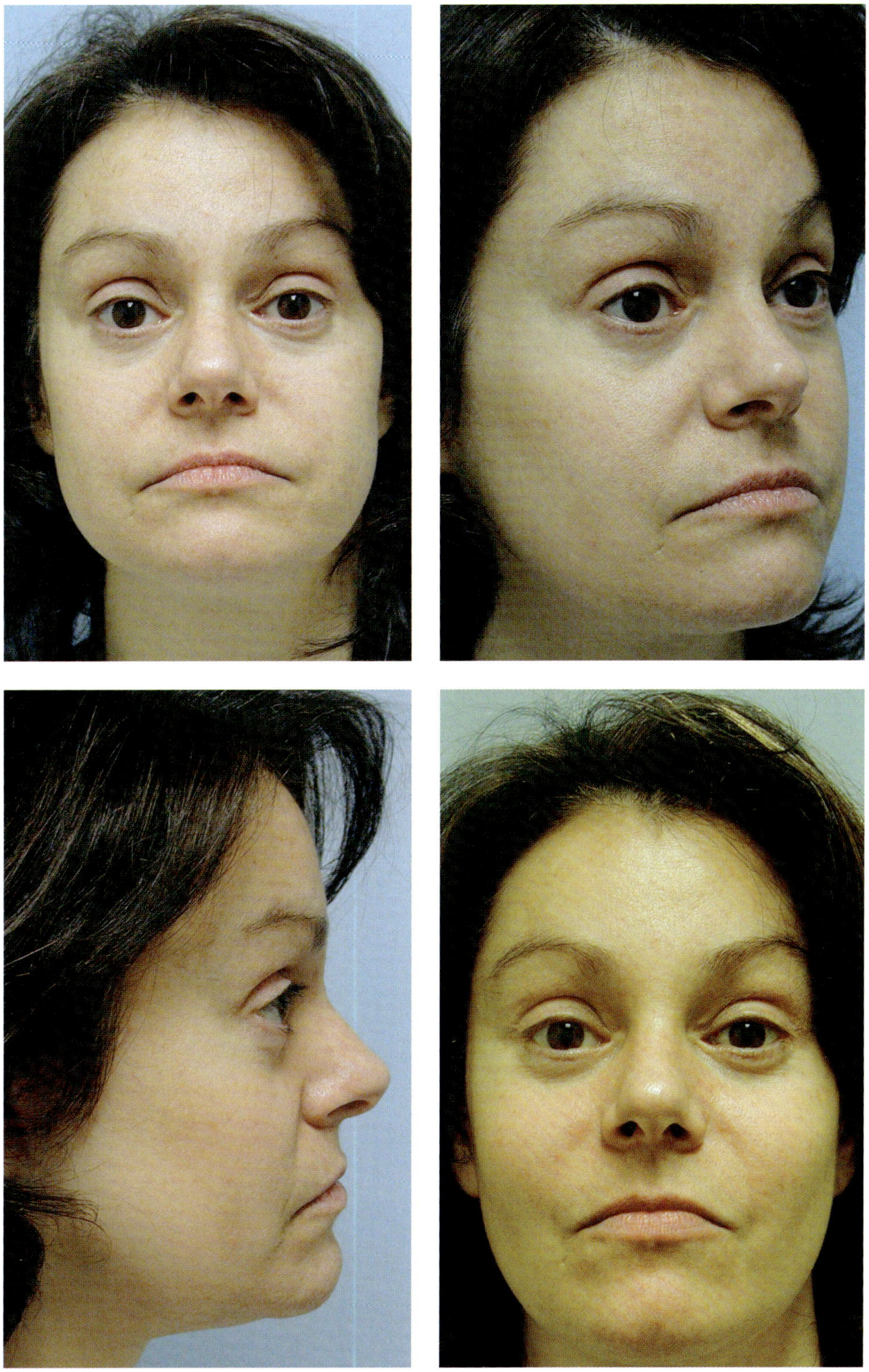

A B C D

FIGURE 4-84. A–D: This is a 51-year-old lady who had undergone a prior facelift 3 years earlier and who now complains of malar hypoplasia—a condition that she has had all of her life but that has troubled her more recently. *(continued)*

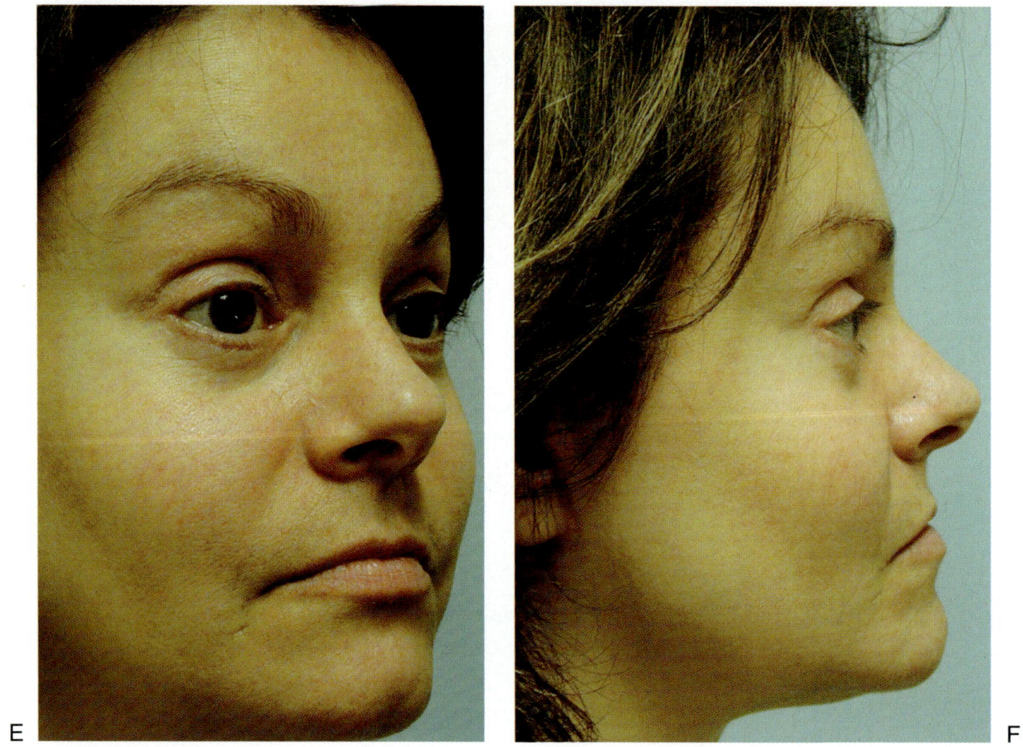

FIGURE 4-84. *(Continued)* **E–F:** She underwent bilateral malar augmentation with medium-sized ePTFE implants with notable improvement in the malar region.

REFERENCES

1. Knize DM: An anatomically based study of the mechanism of eyebrow ptosis. Plast Reconstr Surg 1996;97:1321–1333.
2. Cook BE Jr, Lucarelli MJ, Lemke BN: Depressor supercilii muscle: anatomy, histology, and cosmetic implications. Ophthal Plast Reconstr Surg 2001;17:404–411.
3. Lemke BN, Stasior OG: The anatomy of eyebrow ptosis. Arch Opthalmol 1982;100:981–986.
4. Dempsey PD, Oneal RM: Subperiosteal brow and midface lifts. Aesthetic Plastic Surg 1995;19:59–68.
5. Ramirez OM: The subperiosteal approach for the correction of the deep nasolabial fold and the central third of the face. Clin Plast Surg 1995;22:341–355.
6. Hinderer UT: Vertical preperiosteal rejuvenation of the frame of the eyelids and midface. Plast Reconstr Surg 1999;104: 1482–1499.
7. Yaremchuk MJ: Subperiosteal and full-thickness skin rhytidectomy. Plast Reconstr Surg 2001;107:1045–1056.
8. Psillakis JF, Rumlay TO, Comargo A: Subperiosteal approach as an improved concept for correction of the aging face. Plast Reconstr Surg 1988;82:383–389.
9. Maillard GF, Cornette de St Cyr B, Scheflan M: The subperiosteal bicoronal approach to total facelifting. The DMAS, deep musculoaponeurotic system. Aesthetic Plast Surg 1991;15:285–289.
10. Williams EF, Lam SM: Midfacial rejuvenation via an endoscopic browlift approach: a review of technique. Facial Plast Surg 2003; 19:147–156.
11. Putterman AM, ed: Cosmetic oculoplastic surgery: eyelid, forehead, and facial techniques, 3rd ed. Philadelphia: WB Saunders, 1999.
12. Schorr N: "Madame Butterfly" procedure with hard palate graft: management of postblepharoplasty round eye and scleral show. Facial Plast Surg 1994;10:90–118.
13. Schorr N, Fallor MK: "Madame Butterfly" procedure: combined cheek and lateral canthal suspension procedure for post-blepharoplasty, "round eye," and lower eyelid retraction. Ophthal Plast Reconstr Surg 1985;1:229–235.
14. Trinei FA, Januszkiewicz J, Nahai F: The sentinel vein: an important reference point for surgery in the temporal region. Plast Reconstr Surg 1998;101:27–32.

5

LOWER FACIAL REJUVENATION

SAMUEL M. LAM
EDWIN F. WILLIAMS III

The rhytidectomy, or facelift, procedure has remained synonymous with facial rejuvenation in the lay public's mind. The term "facelift" entered the lexicon to signify any reparative endeavor ("The dilapidated edifice underwent a much-needed facelift"). In the past, a cervico-facial rhytidectomy represented the principal, if not sole, method by which the facial plastic surgeon could achieve global restoration for the aging face. The midface was uncharted terrain; and traditional options for brow rejuvenation often were judged too invasive to merit routine implementation. For these reasons, the facelift was (and often still is) undertaken to lift the midface and temporal brow region in an effort to provide a complete full facial rejuvenation through one procedure. This ambitious surgical enterprise may not always bear the best aesthetic result because of unnatural vectors of suspension and violation of the temporal hair tuft, a stigma of aging and surgical manipulation. Furthermore, the overly pulled (so-called "windswept" look) of a poorly executed facelift has traumatized the public psyche and dispirited many prospective patients from venturing any further into the realm of cosmetic surgery.

Another obstacle that has potentially hampered public enthusiasm concerns the confusing array of facelift types that are advocated, including the tri-plane facelift, the deep-plane facelift, the composite facelift, the superficial musculoaponeurotic system (SMAS) lift, the subperiosteal lift, the endoscopic facelift, the S-lift, the vertical facelift, the "weekend" facelift, the "lunch-time" facelift, and so on in endless thematic permutations. Clearly, some of these surgical techniques reflect ensconced ideologies based on empiricism and scientific inquiry, whereas others testify to unrepentant marketing strategies. Unfortunately, the public is often at the mercy of the Internet and other prejudicial mass media resources and unable to distinguish between sham and untrammeled science.

This chapter does not purport to offer a wholly impartial perspective on lower facial rejuvenation but rather espouses a philosophy and strategy that have emerged from significant clinical experience. Although deeper-tissue (sub-SMAS, extended sub-SMAS, deep-plane, and composite) rhytidectomy procedures have their proponents, the authors have noted a trend toward more conservative restorative modalities in the United States.[1] The protracted healing time and potential for higher morbidity may not always translate into a notable clinical improvement; an opinion that has been borne out by the authors' clinical experience.[2,3] Further, the authors contend that this return to a more conservative operative technique represents a paradigm shift that matches the present minimal-invasive Zeitgeist. Nevertheless, this controversy undoubtedly will be sustained for quite some time as advocates of deep-plane and SMAS techniques continue to debate the issue.

This chapter offers the reader a systematic appraisal of the aging lower face and a host of therapeutic options. For instance, the younger patient who presents with exclusive submental adipose accumulation without notable platysmal diastasis requires only a localized liposuction or lipectomy. These diagnostic deliberations are explored in more depth in the section on preoperative considerations. The reader is reminded that not all techniques for lower facial rejuvenation are reviewed in this chapter (e.g., collagen injection and alloplast implantation, for which a chapter dedicated to adjunctive procedures has been allocated). These less invasive procedures may be used in conjunction with or independent of the procedures described in this chapter in a strategy for global facial rejuvenation. Accordingly, these adjunctive procedures are reviewed in the section on preoperative considerations so that the surgeon can determine when and how these procedures can be implemented or combined. However, operative detail may be found in Chapter 8. Thoughtful reflection and open dialog will ensure that the surgeon and patient arrive at the optimal tactical treatment plan.

PREOPERATIVE CONSIDERATIONS: PATIENT SELECTION AND RELEVANT ANATOMY

As stressed in the preceding and elsewhere, the surgeon must venture to grasp the aesthetic flaw that concerns the patient before the surgeon proffers his or her own independent management agenda. After the patient has declared the specific locus or loci of concern, the surgeon must determine whether the patient desires a more limited, targeted approach (adjunctive procedures such as collagen, botulinum toxin, etc.) or a more extensive rejuvenative protocol (e.g., submentoplasty, chin augmentation, rhytidectomy, etc.). However, patients often look toward the surgeon for his or her informed and educated opinion, and the surgeon should help organize for the patient the procedures that will offer the most return on investment. For example, the surgeon can proclaim, "If you could only do one thing, this would give you the most bang for your buck (*pardon the colloquialism*); and two things I recommend, etc." Obviously, the surgeon should recommend only those procedures that are in alignment with the patient's declared interest; that is, the surgeon should not dwell on a perceived correctable nasal flaw if the patient presents for neck rejuvenation. The reader is advised to review the section on the dynamics of an effective consultation in Chapter 3 for more cogent remarks. The remainder of this section outlines a systematic approach the surgeon can apply when contemplating the optimal treatment strategy for the patient. The two principal areas that are discussed are the lower face (dependent jowl as well as prominent labiomandibular and nasolabial folds) and the neck region (platysmal banding, excessive submental adipose, redundant skin, and underprojected chin). Because these two regions are confluent and overlap, certain topics are covered in both sections by necessity. In addition, the revision or "tuck-up" rhytidectomy patient deserves special consideration during the preoperative evaluation. Although the lip constitutes part of the lower face, this particular specialized anatomic region is thoroughly investigated in Chapters 8 and 9 and is not repeated here.

The Neck and Chin Region

The central neck region is the area of principal concern for most patients. In this area, platysmal banding, submental adipose, and redundant skin can be readily apparent. A hypoplastic mentum can exacerbate these conditions and make surgical intervention less successful. As mentioned, submental adipose tissue may be an unsightly feature that appears even in early age, particularly in the White race. Submental fullness is usually more a problem only in the mature Asian patient. Conversely, platysmal diastasis is twice as prevalent in the White than the Asian race (60% versus 30%).[4] Nevertheless, individual variations mandate that the surgeon tailor the specific surgical plan according to each patient's anatomy.

The younger patient (in the thirties) often presents with submental fullness caused by adipose accumulation at times disproportionately greater than the corporal distribution (e.g., thighs and abdomen). Fortunately, a full rhytidectomy is a premature and unwarranted procedure, because redundant skin and platysmal definition have yet to occur. In addition, the favorable fibrosis induced by cervical dissection permits contraction of the overlying skin sleeve, which is still relatively elastic in the younger patient. An augmentation mentoplasty may enhance the surgical outcome by better defining the cervico-mental angle. A profile view taken in the correct Frankfort horizontal plane with appropriate preoperative and postoperative digital manipulation often is a helpful adjunct in convincing the patient of the projected improvement. Satisfaction among younger patients with confined submental adipose tissue who have undergone targeted liposuction has been uniformly high.

Augmentation mentoplasty is a marvelous adjunct to lower facial rejuvenation for several reasons. First because mentioned, when combined with submental liposuction, cervico-mental definition is increased. Second, an extended alloplast that traverses the prejowl region can diminish a heavy jowl appearance, especially when combined with a rhytidectomy. Accordingly, success of a rhytidectomy is partly contingent on the presence of a bony, angular face: The more projected mentum serves as a focal point over which the SMAS may be suspended and the skin redraped. Third, some bony resorption of the mentum occurs as a patient matures, which contributes in part to the loss of structural support and consequent platysmal separation. Alloplastic augmentation restores the more youthful prominence of the chin. Fortunately, added dissection time is minimized when combined with a submental liposuction or platysmal approximation because the same incision is used for all the preceding procedures. A sliding-type osseous genioplasty is a viable alternative for augmentation mentoplasty and is particularly versatile in that the chin may be augmented, reduced, vertically shortened, or laterally repositioned.[5] However, the authors have less extensive experience with this technique and do not elaborate on the technical specificities entailed with this procedure.

Dedo's renowned thesis on neck classification is worthy of review, because distinctive anatomic configurations and dispositions dictate surgical intervention and potentially limit surgical success—a fact that must be conveyed to the patient during the preoperative phase (Fig. 5-1).[6] A class I deformity exhibits only minimal cosmetic deficiency that may or may not warrant surgical intervention. A class II deformity presents with only skin laxity. This condition is usually quite rare because concomitant submental fat accumulation and platysmal diastasis are usually present to a varying extent. Submental liposuction alone may induce sufficient favorable skin contraction if minimal skin laxity is present. Alternatively, a limited rhytidectomy incision that only extends under the ear lobule in a lazy S configuration may provide enough exposure for dissection and adequate skin excision. However, cervical skin redundancy usually requires the standard postauricular incision for proper adjustment (*vide infra*). A class III deformity refers to excessive submandibular and submental adipose, surgical correction of which has been described above. A class IV deformity refers to anterior banding of the platysma, which is addressed in the following paragraph. Class V deformity describes the condition of retrognathia or microgenia* that can be improved with alloplas-

*Although the terms retrognathia and microgenia have been used interchangeably in the scientific literature, each word denotes a different condition. Retrognathia refers to an Angle's class II occlusion in which the hypoplastic and retruded mandible leads to an overbite and dental malocclusion. Microgenia simply refers to an underprojected chin independent of occlusal considerations.

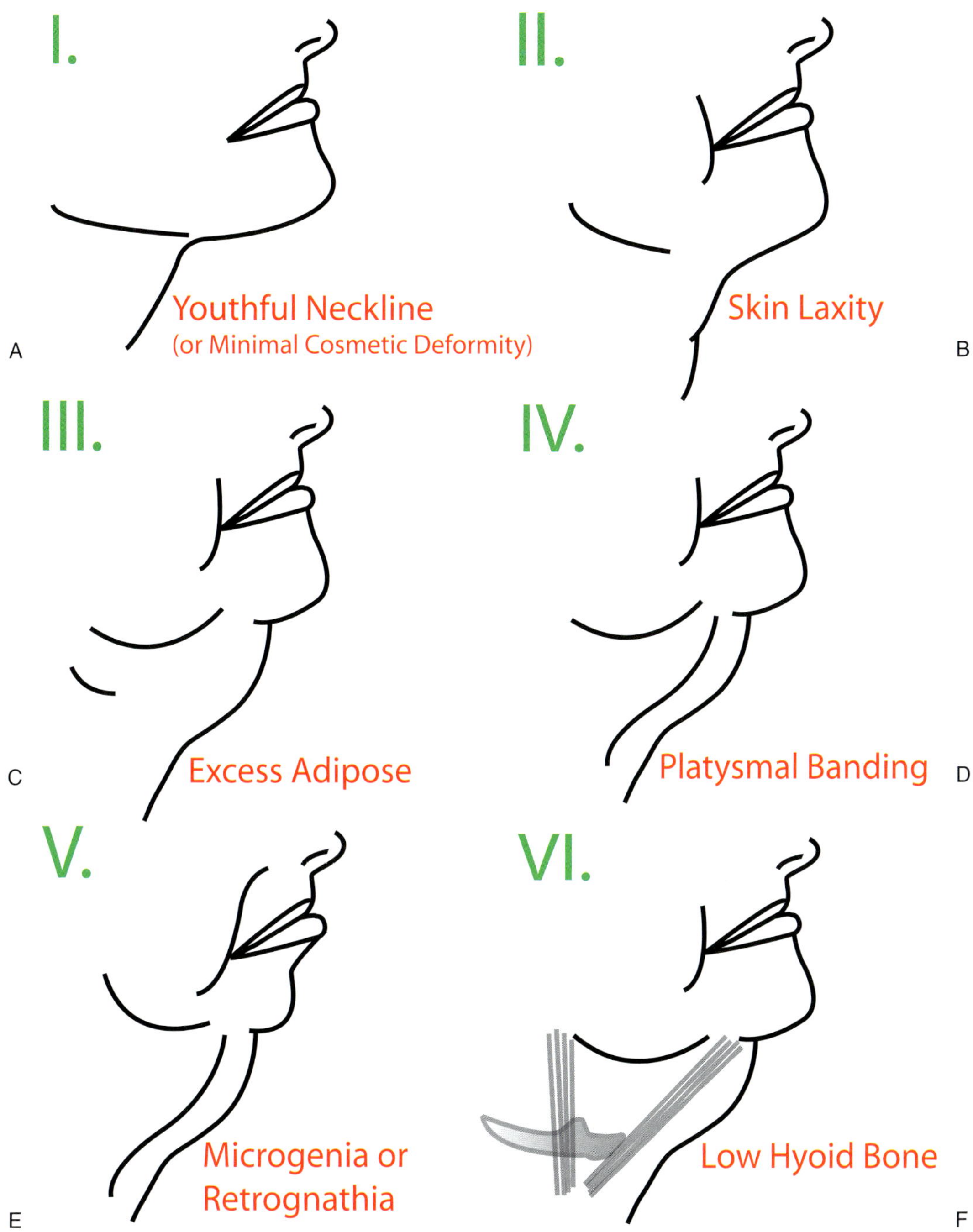

FIGURE 5-1. Illustration showing Dedo's original classification of neck laxity. **A:** Class I deformity describes only minimal cosmetic deformity. **B:** Class II deformity describes only skin laxity. **C:** Class III deformity refers to excessive submandibular and submental adipose. **D:** Class IV deformity refers to anterior banding of the platysma. **E:** Class V deformity describes the condition of retrognathia or microgenia. **F:** Class VI deformity describes a low-riding hyoid bone.

tic implantation, as outlined in the preceding. Finally, a class VI deformity describes a low-residing hyoid bone that can interfere with optimal cervical rejuvenation. Ideally, the hyoid should be situated at the fourth vertebra, near the cervical–mental interface. Although not included in the original classification schema, a ptotic submandibular gland should be carefully observed in the preoperative evaluation because this condition may limit improvement with a rhytidectomy; further correction should not be indicated for an aesthetic objective alone.

The anterior platysmal border becomes more accentuated over time because of loss of skeletal support and atrophy of the muscle. The anterior platysmal fibers insert into the mandibular periosteum and demonstrate the greatest variability in distribution. Posteriorly, the muscle fibers blend with the risorius muscle and the SMAS. Therefore, the combination of suturing the anterior platysmal bands with suspension of the posterior platysma and SMAS affects a hammocklike sling that restores definition to the neck. At times, men seek the most expedient remedy for anterior platysmal banding while refusing a rhytidectomy at all costs because of societal stigma and desire for limited surgery. Jowling and lower facial descent are of secondary concern to many men. If the male patient cannot be convinced that a rhytidectomy is the preferred route, the alternative of direct skin excision, open lipectomy, and platysma suturing can be entertained.[7] The major drawback, of course, with this approach is a noticeable incision in the midline of the neck, which can be camouflaged with multiple cutaneous z-plasties or geometric broken-line repair. The former type of repair is favored because of the alacrity of this closure and minimization of scar contracture. If the patient understands this potential (but low) risk, then a direct excision can be undertaken.

Skin redundancy of the neck can be effectively eliminated by a standard rhytidectomy in most cases. The described technique of direct excision is an alternative method in the select patient. The severity of cervical skin excess may mandate an adjunctive posterior neck lift in rare circumstances.[8] This procedure employs a T-shaped incision in which the horizontal limb resides just within the hair-bearing area near the hair–hairless interface and in which the vertical limb falls principally in the non–hair bearing area (Fig. 5-2). Therefore, the patient must be aware that a vertical scar in

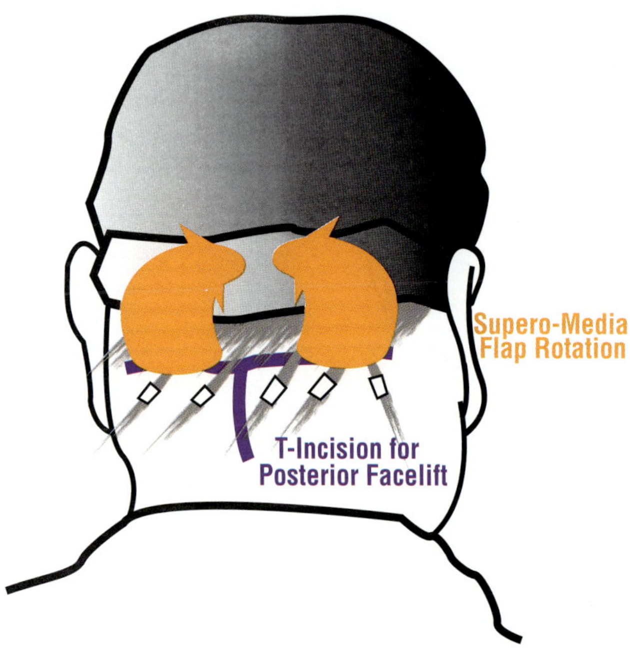

FIGURE 5-2. The posterior neck lift is a rare adjunctive procedure that may help efface lower or posterior cervical rhytidosis that is not easily addressed with the standard rhytidectomy. This procedure employs a T-shaped incision in which the horizontal limb resides just within the hair-bearing area near the hair–hairless interface and in which the vertical limb falls principally in the non–hair bearing area (*in blue*). After the flaps are undermined, they are rotated supero-medially (*in orange*) and the excess is trimmed.

the occipital midline may be evident postoperatively. Dissection is carried in the subcutaneous, supramuscular plane until adequate elevation permits sufficient skin redraping. Often, dissection must be carried out near the cervical rhytids to achieve enough skin mobility for complete effacement of the rhytidosis. Redundant skin is excised and the wound edges approximated to each other and tacked to the underlying occipital musculature. A posterior neck lift should be undertaken at a minimum of several months after initial rhytidectomy in order to determine accurately whether this procedure is needed and how much skin excision is required, as well as to minimize the risk of flap necrosis. *It should be emphasized again that this procedure is only rarely indicated.* Of note, any skin resurfacing in the neck region should be undertaken with great caution because the pilosebaceous density is markedly attenuated compared with that of the face (see Chapter 9). Clearly, cervical flap elevation should delay any resurfacing for a minimum of 6 months, at which time resurfacing should be carried out with even greater conservatism.

The Lower Facial Region

The component regions of the lower face embrace the jowl, which continues upward as the labiomandibular fold (or marionette line), and the nasolabial fold (or smile line). The lower face can be only partly (and somewhat arbitrarily) delineated from the neck region, but is done so herein in order to provide a rational framework for the reader's preoperative assessment. Although the jowl may be conceived of as an extension of the labiomandibular fold, this structure represents a unique surgical entity. Unlike the upper aspect of the labiomandibular fold that requires a soft-tissue filler, the jowl region can be effectively effaced only with a cervicofacial rhytidectomy. In fact, if the patient is principally concerned with the labiomandibular and nasolabial depressions, then he or she should be dissuaded from rhytidectomy. Instead, soft-tissue augmentation may provide the best solution to address the patient's concerns.

The labiomandibular fold is defined superiorly by the cutaneous insertion of the depressor anguli oris muscle. At rest, the labiomandibular fold is only visible along the upper one third to one half of its distance by virtue of the action of the depressor anguli oris muscle on the overlying skin. The fold is tethered specifically at two points: the aforementioned depressor muscle superiorly and the mandibular ligament along its entire length (Fig. 5-3).[9] During animation, the zygomaticus and platysma muscles exert their pull at these two points of fixation, thereby causing a bowstring effect and forming a continuous fold. These unique properties of the labiomandibular fold inform the most suitable course of labiomandibular effacement. Because the inferior aspect of the crease is absent at rest, the surgeon is advised to concentrate his or her efforts at soft-tissue augmentation only along the superior aspect of the fold. Soft-tissue injectables (tem-

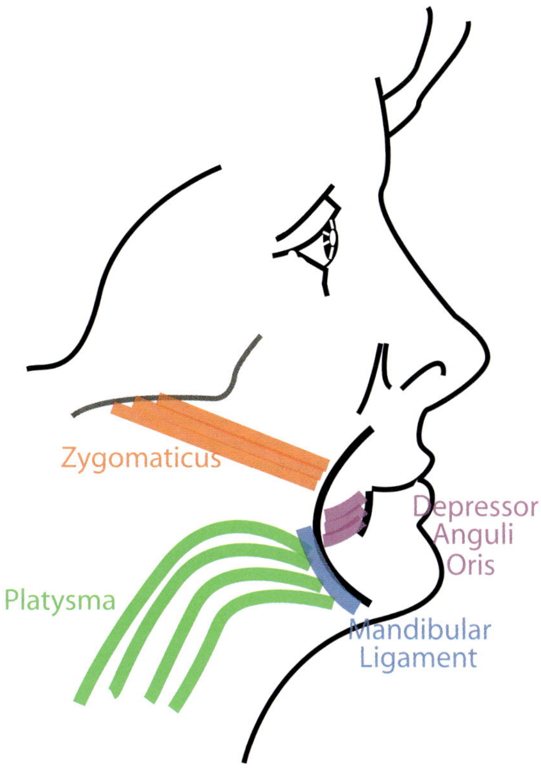

FIGURE 5-3. The labiomandibular fold is defined superiorly by the cutaneous insertion of the depressor anguli oris muscle (*in purple*). At rest, the labiomandibular fold is only visible along the upper one third to one half of its distance by virtue of the action of the depressor anguli oris muscle on the overlying skin. The fold is tethered specifically at two points: the aforementioned depressor muscle superiorly and the mandibular ligament along its entire length (*in blue*). During animation, the zygomaticus (*in red*) and platysma (*in green*) muscles exert their pull at these two points of fixation, thereby causing a bowstring effect and forming a continuous fold.

porary) or solid implants (permanent) are both acceptable methods of augmenting the superior labiomandibular fold. For a more detailed description of preoperative, intraoperative, and postoperative management of the nasolabial and labiomandibular folds, the reader is directed to Chapter 8. As mentioned, the inferior portion of the labiomandibular fold that is accentuated by the jowl should be addressed with a rhytidectomy rather than augmentation materials.

The nasolabial fold is defined by the cutaneous insertion of four principal muscles: the two levator muscles (anguli oris and alaeque nasi) as well as the paired zygomaticus muscles (major and minor).** Unlike the labiomandibular fold, the nasolabial fold may be apparent along its entire length at rest and during animation. The nasolabial fold may be thought of as a lateral mountain and a medial valley, the latter of which should be elevated with augmentation materials to soften the transition between the two areas. Some authors have also advocated direct, transcutaneous microliposuction of the lateral raised aspect to soften the transition further. However, liposuction in this area may be less forgiving than in the cervical region. If a concomitant rhytidectomy is planned, the SMAS may be excised before imbrication and used as soft-tissue filler. Unfortunately, the nasolabial and labiomandibular folds are recalcitrant to effacement via traditional rhytidectomy, regardless of whether a deep-plane or SMAS technique is undertaken.[2]

The Revision Rhytidectomy Patient

When a patient inquires in the preoperative period whether a facelift will endure for perpetuity, the surgeon can respond affirmatively. The surgical result will persist; however, the patient will continue to be subjected to both extrinsic (smoking, diet, exercise, stress, sun exposure, etc.) and intrinsic (continued aging and a genetic predisposition toward aging) forces that will slowly erode the once-stellar outcome. An example often illuminates the situation in a more concrete fashion for the patient: If the patient had a twin sibling, the patient would always appear younger than his or her twin if all extrinsic factors were negated. Based on multiple variables, the patient may return as soon as 3 years after the initial surgery for a tuck-up procedure or even a decade or more later. It may be worthwhile to introduce to the patient that a tuck-up facelift may be needed at some later interval, even as short as 2 years, so that the patient will be more accepting of this need when the time comes.

What constitutes the difference between a tuck-up and a revision facelift? A tuck-up procedure is one in which the surgeon is revisiting his or her own work, and revision surgery entails that the surgeon is operating on his or her colleague's previous surgery. Although this distinction is meant to be facetious to a certain extent, it accurately encapsulates a notable truism. When a surgeon must reoperate on another surgeon's facelift, he or she encounters a potential host of problems. First and foremost, the type of incisions that the other surgeon elected to undertake often does not parallel one's own choices. Therefore, when very little redundant skin is already present (a fact that is discussed in greater detail in the intraoperative section), the surgeon must make deliberate choices as to where he or she should create the new incisions. These incisions, which are often less than ideal in terms of exuberant scarring and location, mandate excision of the existing incision and relocation (if possible) to a more favorable site. In addition, if the facelift result is suboptimal, the surgeon must aim to correct his or her colleague's work. All of these factors often make "revision" surgery more arduous than a "tuck-up" of one's own work. Furthermore, this semantic distinction offers the surgeon a favorable language in which to couch the new surgical enterprise.

**The histological constituents of the nasolabial fold have been a subject of fierce debate over the past two decades as to whether the structure represents an extension of the SMAS, partly so, or not at all. This pedantic dispute remains outside the scope of this book, which is concerned with only pragmatic considerations.

At times, a secondary rhytidectomy may prove difficult for another reason: The patient may have unrealistic expectations of the rejuvenative potential because the degree of improvement may be more limited than in the primary setting. In the rare circumstance in which the patient demands further neck tightening than the surgeon can realistically achieve with a conventional tuck-up procedure, a rhytidectomy with an expanded polytetrafluoroethylene (ePTFE) or Gore-Tex (W.L. Gore and Associates, Inc., Flagstaff, AZ) sling may be indicated. However, the authors tend to be reluctant to use alloplasts on a frequent basis for the attendant problems that may arise with foreign materials. In addition, the patient should be counseled that the implant may be palpable and require adjustment if it feels too constrictive. The ePTFE sling should be offered as a surgical option only to the most fastidious patient who already has an established rapport with the surgeon. Therefore, the ePTFE sling should almost never be performed in the primary setting according to the senior author's experience. It should be reiterated that only a very select patient qualifies for placement of an ePTFE sling.

Psychological Aspects of the Facelift Patient

Apart from the anatomic considerations already elaborated, the surgeon always should be mindful of the psychological dynamics that inform the patient's motivation for facelift surgery.[10] Edgerton classified four subtypes of patients who seek facial rejuvenation by age and sex.[11,12] The first three categories refer to women; the fourth category is reserved for men. The first category concerns the woman aged 29 to 39 who desires surgical rejuvenation: She is viewed as an emotionally dependent personality who seeks constant approbation from her spouse and may not have fully transitioned from adolescence to adulthood in terms of psychological maturity. Given the little adjunctive procedures (e.g., collagen, botulinum toxin, chemical peels, etc.) that are available today, this categorization may be a bit outdated. The second category is defined by the woman aged 40 to 50 ("the worker group") who desires to maintain her productivity in the workplace and wishes a countenance to match her energetic lifestyle. Often, these patients only seek one to two procedures that can improve their look. The third category refers to the woman over 50 years old ("the grief group") who has lost support from her spouse either through divorce or death and is looking for a major lifestyle change through cosmetic surgery. These patients tend to pursue plastic surgical intervention with sustained fervor, demanding additional procedures but infrequently being fully satisfied with the outcome. The final, and fourth, group describes the male facelift patient and is further subdivided into two types. One subcategory refers to the male patient over 50 who is secure in his occupation and is happily married but desires to remain competitive at work: He believes that a facelift may offer him a competitive advantage in a work environment increasingly populated by younger faces. The second type of male facelift patient is the man who is recently widowed or divorced and maintains a relationship with a much younger partner: He desperately wants to retain approbation from his more junior companion and believes that a facelift may narrow the age difference. Clearly, these broad categories are not universally applicable to all patients but are only intended to serve as a framework by which the surgeon may evaluate the prospective rhytidectomy patient in a systematic fashion.

INTRAOPERATIVE CONSIDERATIONS: TECHNIQUE AND SALIENT TECHNICAL POINTS

Submentoplasty with Liposuction

A submentoplasty may be effectively combined with a rhytidectomy or chin augmentation for the optimal aesthetic result. It consists of two principal components: submental liposuction and anterior platysmaplasty. The former may be all that is required for a younger patient, whereas both elements may be necessary for the more mature patient as part of a rhytidectomy. The submentoplasty is always performed at the outset before a rhytidectomy, because the approximated anterior border of the platysma is difficult to unite after the lateral pull of the rhytidectomy has been completed. Similarly, submental liposuction always precedes anterior platysmaplasty because the removal of adipose and concomitant undermining permit visualization of the skeletonized platysma. Chin augmentation should always follow a submentoplasty but precede a facelift because the submentoplasty incision is used as the point of entry for chin implantation. Further, vigorous submentoplasty may disturb the position of the implant if performed after implant insertion.

Submentoplasty should be considered practically part of a complete rhytidectomy but is discussed herein as a separate procedure for the sake of clarity and to emphasize the versatility of it as an independent procedure (Fig. 5-4). Submental dissection should precede a rhytidectomy in most circumstances, even in the leanest necks that may not otherwise appear by intuition to warrant this intervention. Uniform submental or submandibular flap undermining promotes favorable skin contraction that largely enhances a rhytidectomy result. Undoubtedly, aggressive liposuction should be avoided in a very thin neck for risk of producing an overskeletonized appearance. Instead, sharp scissor dissection only (i.e., undermining alone) may be sufficient in these circumstances. Similarly, a platysmaplasty is justified in most cases when a rhytidectomy is also planned because the combined effect can be beneficial for the neck contour. However, if a patient presents with only minimal jowl formation correctable with an S-lift, or short-incision, rhytidectomy, then a submentoplasty of any kind may not be a requisite step.

The submentoplasty begins with a straight incision about 1 mm posterior to the submental crease that extends typically

Instrumentation and Equipment for Submentoplasty and Rhytidectomy

Prep Stand:

Nonsterile gloves
10-cc syringe (2), 27-gauge (1¼-inch long) needle (2) with lidocaine 1% and 1:100,000 epinephrine
Surgical marking pen

Instruments:

Basic soft-tissue instrument set (Chapter 4)
Bovie hand piece and tip

Sutures:

2-0 Silk FS (C-15, CE-6) [C8] <ED-3> needle (to retract the ear)
CV-3 Gore-Tex[†] Th-26 needle (for SMAS suspension)
5-0 chromic P-3 (P-13, PRE-2) <RE-3> needle (2) (for postauricular skin closure)
6-0 polypropylene P-3 (PRE-2, P-13) <RE-3> needle (2) (for preauricular and submental skin closure)
5-0 Nylon P-3 (PRE-2, P-13) <RE-3> needle (for closure of temporal skin area)
4-0 polydioxanone PS-3 (P-11, PRE-3) [PC-34] <RE-6>[‡] (for approximation of platysmal bands)
CV-4 Gore-Tex, PT-17 needle (only to suture an ePTFE sling into place for revision cases)

Other Supplies:

Skin stapler
Laparotomy pads
Earplugs
Two 8-French red rubber catheters (as postauricular drains)
Wall suction, suction tubing, liposuction cannula (for submentoplasty)
10-cc syringe (2), 27-gauge (1¼-inch long) needle (2) with lidocaine 1% and 1:100,000 epinephrine
2 × 30 cm ePTFE sling (only for revision cases that require an ePTFE sling)

Dressing:

4 × 4 gauze, two of which should have a partial curvilinear incision to accommodate the shape of the ear
3″ Conforming gauze bandage, or Kling (3)
Cotton padding
Bacitracin ointment in 5-cc syringe
1″ clear tape
Heavy Scissors

[†]The trade name Gore-Tex is employed in the text to refer to the suture material for the sake of clarity because the needle sizes used refer to those manufactured by W.L. Gore & Associates (Flagstaff, AZ). All other references to Gore-Tex material in the text are made to the generic name, expanded polytetrafluoroethylene, or ePTFE. The authors emphasize that they do not hold any financial arrangements or obtain any direct or indirect gain from the manufacturer.

[‡]The first needle size refers to the Ethicon code. The second parenthetical code refers to the equivalent needle size manufactured by US Surgical/Davis & Geck. Of note, the first code within the parentheses refers to new US Surgical code, and the second number within the parentheses refers to the older Davis & Geck code. The third bracketed code refers to the equivalent needle size made by Look. The fourth code in brackets refers to the Deknatel needle equivalent.

about 2 cm in breadth. The incision always should fall slightly posterior to the submental crease because placement of the incision directly in the crease will deepen over time so that the line will become lamentably conspicuous. After the initial incision through the skin to the underlying subcutaneous adipose is accomplished, wide double-hooked retractors are placed into the superior and inferior aspects of the wound for proper tension and retraction: The assistant retracts the superior flap while the surgeon retracts the inferior flap. The surgeon then performs wide undermining of the flap from just inferior to the jaw line (1 to 2 cm below) across the submental region to the contralateral jaw line using a pair of Metzenbaum scissors in the subcutaneous plane (Fig. 5-5A). Dissection should not pass directly over the jaw line in order to minimize risk of marginal mandibular nerve injury. Although the nerve should be protected under the platysma in most cases, an attenuated or dehiscent platysmal layer may predispose the nerve to inadvertent harm. Furthermore, dissection with a pair of Metzenbaum scissors is preferred to blunt tunneling dissection with the liposuction cannula because the former permits a more uniform undermining and thereby reduces the chance of uneven contour to the skin. The depth of dissection should leave approximately a 3- to 4-mm thick skin subcutaneous flap so as to avoid an uneven contour that may develop after liposuctioning and ensure vascularity to the overlying skin flap.

After the submental region has been widely undermined, a liposuction cannula can be introduced with the aperture always facing deep, away from the flap (Fig. 5-5B). The aperture of the cannula should be directed away from the flap in order to avoid the development of an irregular skin contour from suctioning the overlying flap. Furthermore, the vascular supply of the flap emanates from its deep surface, and liposuction under the flap may lead to vascular compromise. The liposuction canister pressure should match the ideal setting of 29" Hg before beginning the procedure. The surgeon should ensure that the instrument is evenly passed over the entire expanse of the undermined submental region, with perhaps additional treatment centrally where a greater adi-

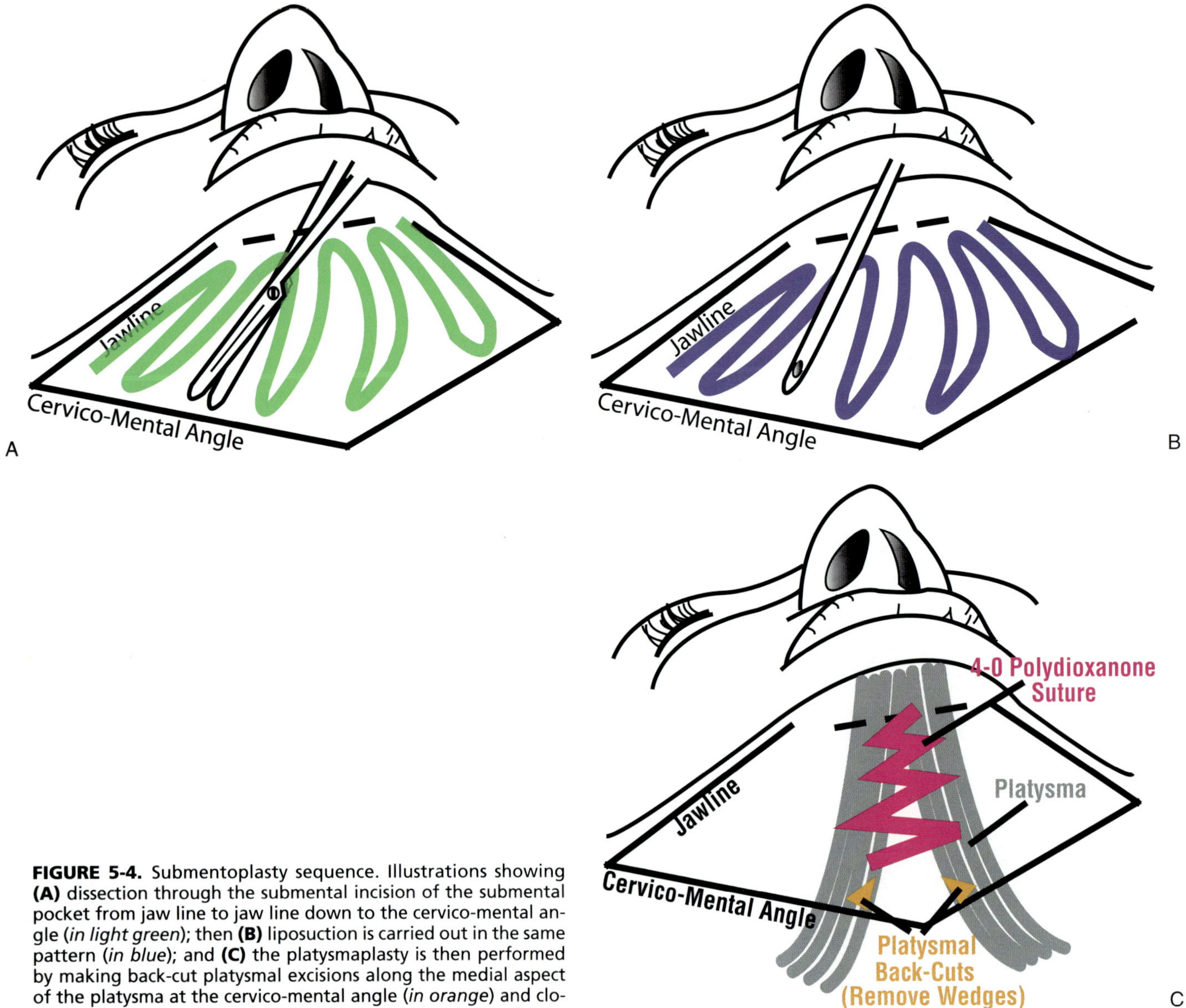

FIGURE 5-4. Submentoplasty sequence. Illustrations showing **(A)** dissection through the submental incision of the submental pocket from jaw line to jaw line down to the cervico-mental angle (*in light green*); then **(B)** liposuction is carried out in the same pattern (*in blue*); and **(C)** the platysmaplasty is then performed by making back-cut platysmal excisions along the medial aspect of the platysma at the cervico-mental angle (*in orange*) and closure with a running 4-0 polydioxanone suture (*in magenta*).

pose deposit may be observed. The authors discourage routine use of open lipectomy only because direct excision alone tends to be limited to the midline of the neck, leading to an uneven cervical contour, or worse yet a "cobra" deformity. Certainly, a cobra deformity may arise after liposuction (like lipectomy) of the neck if it is conducted in an aggressive fashion only in the central cervical compartment. A cobralike deformity may be further accentuated if the anterior platysmal bands are not united after a central lipectomy.[13] However, a central lipectomy may be a useful adjunct in select cases. First, a central lipectomy may be conducted to remove discrete adipose pockets that remain in the midline *after* a broad liposuction has been carried out. Second, a central lipectomy may be required in order to visualize the anterior platysmal bands obscured by exuberant fat deposition. In select cases, a central lipectomy alone is justified (e.g., a patient who exhibits a discrete submental fat pad), but this task should be carried out in a conservative fashion.

The authors would like to stress a few more remarkable operative considerations concerning liposuction technique. Because the submental incision has already been made and the submental or cervical region undermined before liposuction is begun, it should be noted that "open" versus "closed" liposuction is a superfluous technical distinction. The liposuction aperture is in direct apposition to the adipose bed, thereby forming a sealed, or closed, environment despite the open nature of the wound at the time of liposuction. Recent reports have suggested that other liposuction techniques (e.g., tumescent, liposhaving, ultrasound assisted), may be superior to traditional liposuction. Tumescent technique, which has been applied with success for body liposuction, is less than ideal for the cervico-facial region because the dis-

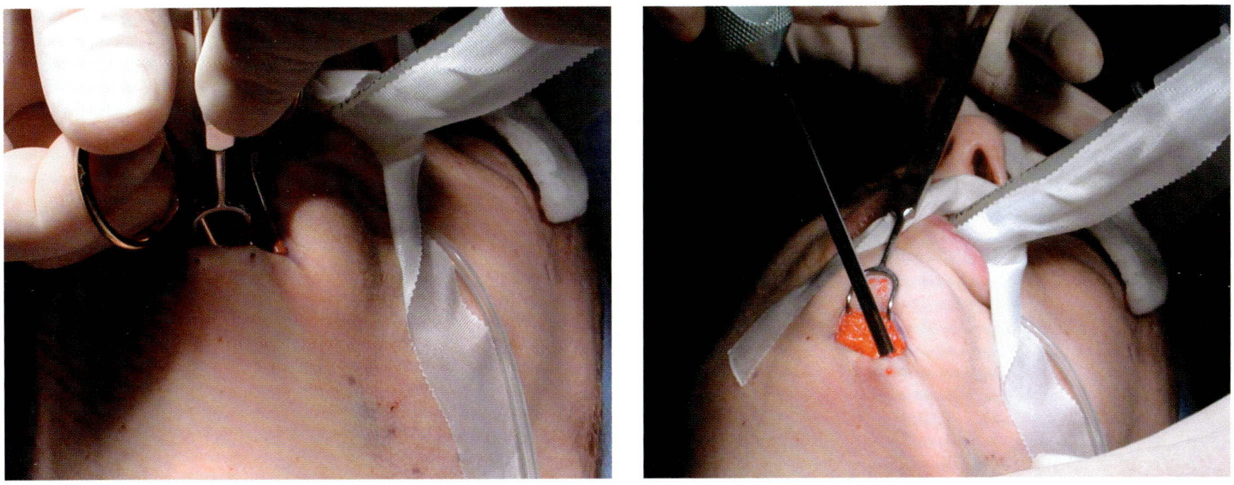

A B

FIGURE 5-5. Submentoplasty, Steps 1 and 2. A: Submentoplasty begins with wide undermining of the skin flap from just inferior to the jaw line (1 to 2 cm below) across the submental region to the contralateral jaw line using a pair of Metzenbaum scissors in the subcutaneous plane. Dissection should not pass directly over the jaw line in order to minimize risk of marginal mandibular nerve injury. Although the nerve should be protected under the platysma in most cases, an attenuated or dehiscent platysmal layer may predispose the nerve to inadvertent harm. Furthermore, dissection with a pair of Metzenbaum scissors is preferred to blunt tunneling dissection with the liposuction cannula because the former permits a more uniform undermining and thereby reduces the chance of uneven contour to the skin. **B:** After the submental region has been widely undermined, a liposuction cannula can be introduced with the aperture always facing deep, away from the flap. The aperture of the cannula should be directed away from the flap in order to avoid the development of an irregular skin contour from suctioning the overlying flap. Use of the nondominant hand can help guide the passage of the liposuction cannula.

tortion engendered renders assessment difficult and the persistent edema that arises an unwarranted drawback. The risk of third-space volume shifts further compounds the problem with the tumescent method. Although safety with the liposhaver has been documented in a multi-institutional review,[14] the hazard of higher seroma and hematoma rate has not been disproved entirely. The ultrasound method suffers from the attendant risk of increased thermal injury (if internally applied) and neural and cutaneous flap injury. These adverse outcomes are not definitively established because no controlled studies exist, but they remain of concern nevertheless. In all surgical endeavors, the authors advocate that the surgeon strive to undertake the procedure with the most straightforward, yet safest, technique without the crutch of unneeded gadgetry, which may in fact encumber the surgeon and unnecessarily add to overhead cost and intraoperative labor.

The platysmaplasty may be undertaken after the liposuction has exposed the anterior platysmal border (Fig. 5-6). With headlight illumination and a Converse retractor, the surgeon should properly visualize the anterior terminal fibers of the platysma. If the platysma appears obscured by a wealth of overlying adipose, the surgeon can perform a selective lipectomy with scissor dissection or with the liposuction cannula, as mentioned. The surgeon may elect to resect a narrow strip along the anterior border of the platysma to promote better adherence. Although the efficacy of this step has not been rigorously validated, the authors routinely undertake it unless the platysma is determined to be minimally redundant and the consequent tension of closure would be too great if additional platysmal resection is performed. If the platysmal borders appear widely separated, which would preclude a relaxed closure, then sufficient undermining is carried out to facilitate closure. However, significant subplatysmal dissection increases both the likelihood of poorly controlled and visualized hemorrhage and the risk to the marginal mandibular branch of the facial nerve. Before the platysma may be approximated, the inferior extent of the platysmal closure should be identified (the cervico-mental angle, typically located at the thyroid notch). Small (1- to 2-cm) back cuts with Metzenbaum scissors into each side of the platysma at this level are executed for two reasons: (a) Tension of the closure may effectively be reduced; and (b) the neck profile appears more natural with a graduated break at the cervico-mental angle. The reader is reminded that any platysmal dissection, resection, or transection will lead to some hemorrhage, which should be managed with bipolar cautery at the time the bleeding is encountered. If several areas of hemorrhage are allowed to propagate unabated before electrocautery control, the surgeon will encounter the dubious task of extinguishing these bleeding sites under limited visualization in the confined cervical space illuminated only by headlight. After the platysmal borders have been properly exposed and dissected, the task is then to approximate the anterior free edges with 4-0 polydioxanone (PDS, Ethicon, Somerville, NJ; Maxon, US Surgical/Davis & Geck, Norwalk, CT), or

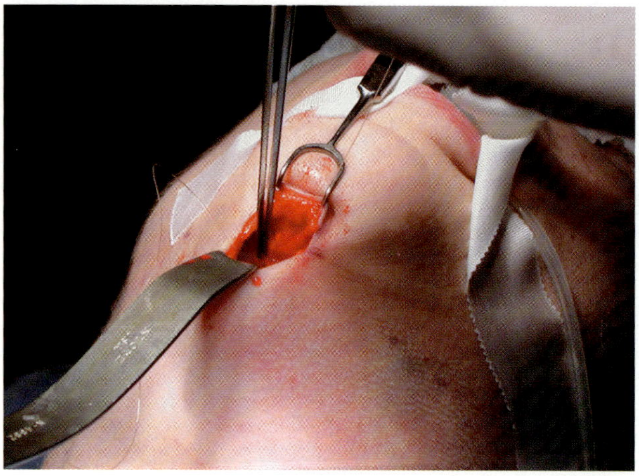

FIGURE 5-6. Submentoplasty, Step 3. After the liposuction has exposed the anterior platysmal border, the platysmaplasty may be undertaken. With headlight illumination and a Converse retractor, the surgeon should properly visualize the anterior terminal fibers of the platysma. If the platysma appears obscured by a wealth of overlying adipose, the surgeon can perform a selective lipectomy with scissor dissection or the liposuction cannula. If the platysmal borders appear widely separated, which precludes a relaxed closure, then sufficient undermining is carried out to facilitate closure. Before the platysma may be approximated, the inferior extent of the platysmal closure should be identified (the cervico-mental angle, typically located at the thyroid notch). Small (1- to 2-cm) back cut wedge excisions are carried out with Metzenbaum scissors on each side of the platysma at this level. After the platysmal borders have been properly exposed and dissected, the task is then to approximate the anterior free edges with 4-0 polydioxanone, or equivalent, suture in a running, nonlocking fashion (as shown in the photograph). It is important to suture these edges together loosely to avoid postoperative bunching.

equivalent, suture in a running, nonlocking fashion. The suture should not be tied very tightly to avoid the complication of a bunched appearance in this area after resolution of edema. To reiterate, the suture should be started approximately at the thyroid notch, or cervico-mental angle, immediately superior to the back cuts that were executed in that region. If a chin implant is not planned, then the submental skin incision is closed with a 6-0 running, locking polypropylene suture alone without the deeper 4-0 polydioxanone subcutaneous retention suture.

DVD Chin Augmentation

As mentioned, chin augmentation should be carried out after submentoplasty and prior to rhytidectomy. The intended objective for mentoplasty should be kept in mind when deciding on the type of implant to be used. If a hypoplastic mentum requires projection, then a standard implant that is thicker in the middle should be employed. However, if the labiomandibular fold, or prejowl region, requires correction, then a longer implant that extends over the jowl with less central projection should be implemented. An ePTFE or silicone implant can be shaved in the central aspect in order to achieve this desired profile for the prejowl implant, whereas a proper Mersilene mesh implant (Ethicon) may be fashioned with a longer base segment and fewer shorter central segments (*vide infra*). Although many types of implants have been used successfully for augmentation mentoplasty, the authors have relied on either ePTFE or Mersilene mesh as the two major methods for alloplastic insertion. Both materials offer long-term stability, low morbidity, and a natural appearance. Decision as to which implant to employ is a matter of surgical preference. Expanded polytetrafluoroethylene exhibits the favorable qualities of good biocompatibility, especially in the chin region, ease of insertion and removal, and limited postoperative edema. Mersilene mesh is also very well tolerated, costs considerably less than ePTFE, and may be deemed more versatile as the surgeon can create different sizes of the implant at the time of surgery. However, Mersilene mesh requires additional preparatory time for creation of the implant both preoperatively and intraoperatively (*vide infra*), is more difficult to insert and remove, and shows more exuberant postoperative edema that resolves over a 1- to 2-week period. Because of these reasons, the authors have shifted away from Mersilene somewhat despite the added expense of ePTFE.

If an ePTFE, or silicone, implant is used, then no preliminary work need be done during the preoperative phase. On the other hand, a Mersilene mesh sheet must be rolled and sutured into precise, prescribed shapes before use. Dr. Perkin's article provides an excellent defense and review of technique for Mersilene mesh chin augmentation, and the reader is referred there for more details about the background, rationale, safety, and surgical implementation.[15] However, this book provides a summary of the major technical points in fabrication of a Mersilene mesh implant with some important modifications of the technique that have worked well for the senior author (Figs. 5-7 and 5-8). All the implants are derived from a single 30- × 30-cm sheet of Mersilene mesh. A 10- × 1-cm cardboard template is used to guide construction of the Mersilene-mesh implant: The sheet is rolled over the cardboard template nine times in order to obtain an implant that is 10 layers thick. The cardboard template is then removed from one end of the roll, and the roll is suture fixated together using a 4-0 polydioxanone suture. A smaller-size implant is created that measures 5- × 1-cm in dimensions using another cardboard template in the same fashion as in the preceding. The smaller 5- × 1-cm segment is suture fixated to the anterior, central aspect of the larger implant (10 × 1 cm) during surgery as needed. Before surgery, all of these individual rolls are packaged and sterilized for intraoperative use. During surgery, the size of augmentation is determined, and the number of tiers that are required to achieve proper chin projection is assessed. At the time of surgery, the segments are sutured together as a stack to achieve the desired height (Figs. 5-7 and 5-8) and the edges are tapered for ease of insertion (Fig. 5-8C). Generally speaking, a medium-sized

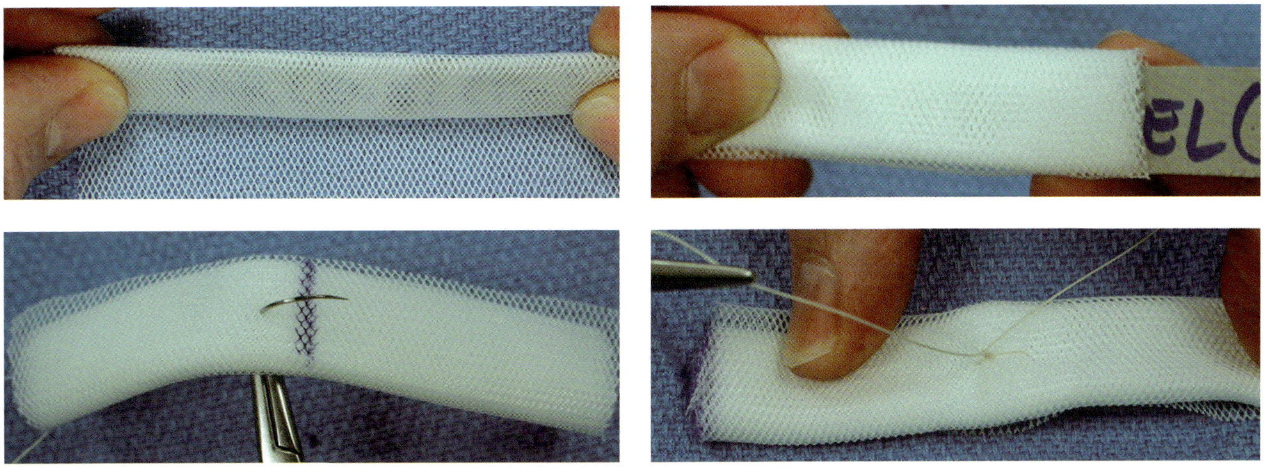

FIGURE 5-7. Mersilene Chin Implant Preparation (Preoperative Sequence). A: A 30- × 30-cm sheet of Mersilene mesh is cut to 10 × 10 cm and rolled over a cardboard template (10 × 1 cm in size) nine times to achieve a 10-layered implant. **B:** The cardboard template is removed. **C,D:** The rolled implant is held together using a 4-0 polydioxanone suture at the marked midline and both ends of the implant. The same method is used to fashion the smaller 5- × 1-cm sized implants. Each of these created segments are individually sterilized to be used for insertion at time of surgery.

implant that approximates the size of a medium-sized extended ePTFE chin implant requires one 5- × 1-cm implant sutured atop a 10- × 1-cm base segment. This configuration constitutes the most common clinical scenario. A larger implant can be made using two 5- × 1-cm segments on top of a single 10- × 1-cm segment. However, this amount of augmentation is rarely indicated. Conversely, a smaller amount of augmentation can be achieved with a single 10- × 1-cm implant. Two 10- × 1-cm implants may be sutured together for increased lateral augmentation in patients with a very pointed chin. Again, this indication is infrequent. Further, insertion of two 10- × 1-cm implants into the lateral, subperiosteal pockets may be quite difficult.

As far as the ePTFE implant is concerned, the implant is typically manufactured in three extended sizes: small, medium, and large. In the great majority of cases (approxi-

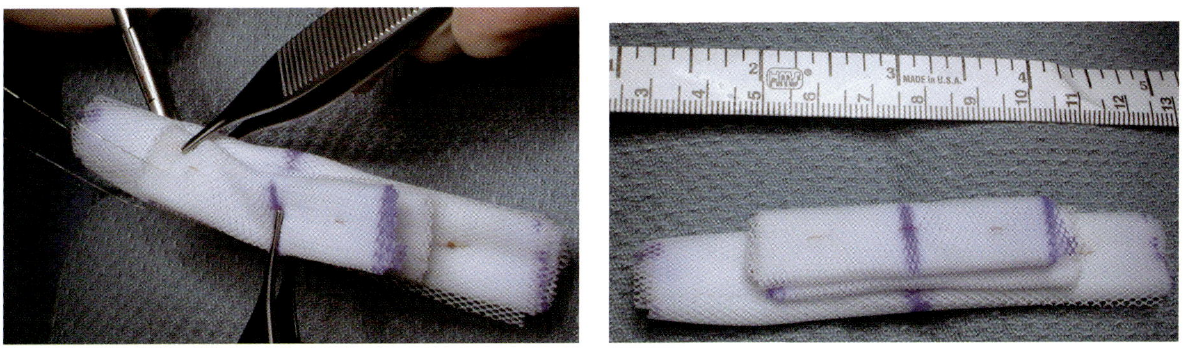

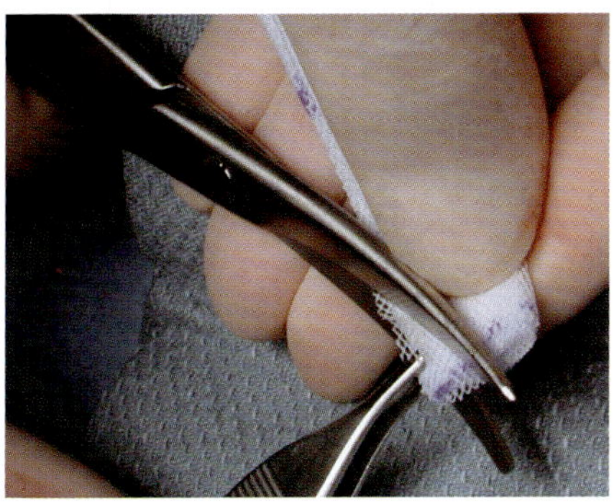

FIGURE 5-8. Mersilene Chin Implant Preparation (Intraoperative Sequence). A–C: At the time of operation, the sterilized 10- × 1-cm base segment can be combined with the sterilized 5- × 1-cm base segment to achieve a medium-sized augmentation. A smaller amount of augmentation can be obtained with a single 10- × 1-cm implant, whereas large augmentation is accomplished with two 5- × 1-cm segments affixed to a 10- × 1-cm base segment. For the pointed chin, two 10- × 1-cm implants may be used to create a fuller lateral dimension to the chin. The implant segments are sutured together using 4-0 polydioxanone sutures in an interrupted fashion. **C:** The lateral edges of the 10- × 1-cm implant are trimmed to a tapered point for ease of insertion.

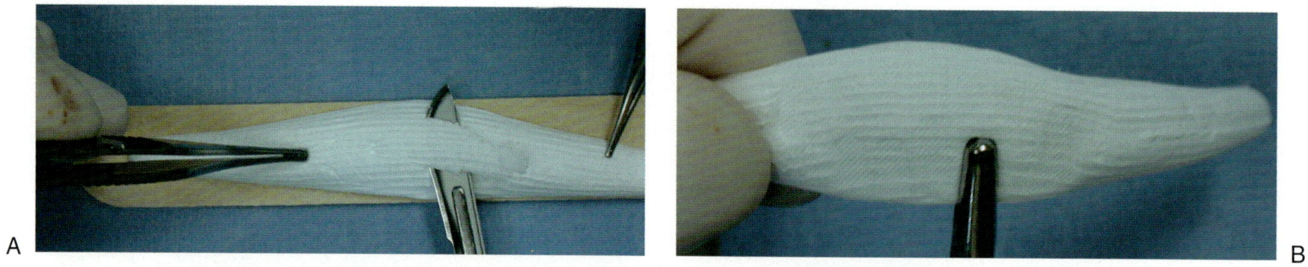

FIGURE 5-9. ePTFE Chin Implant Preparation (Intraoperative Sequence). A: A larger expanded polytetrafluoroethylene implant can be reduced in profile by shaving down the central prominence with a No. 10 blade. **B:** A needle holder can be used to compress the implant to assume an even flatter profile. Gently crushing the implant after shaving down the central aspect permits a smoother, less abrupt, transition at the interface of the cut edge. In addition, crushing the implant permits reducing the profile further without compromising the integrity of the implant that would occur if it were overly thinned by resection alone.

mately 80%), a medium-sized implant is sufficient for adequate projection or to soften the prejowl fullness, whereas the remaining 20% of the time is equally divided between use of a small and large implant. The small implant is really designed for the minority of patients who only want very subtle augmentation. Because most patients who elect to undergo chin augmentation are willing to incur the extra expense, they typically desire a little more noticeable augmentation than can be afforded by a small-sized implant. In addition, the medium-sized implant is more versatile because it can be sculpted to be smaller in size: Carving the central aspect down with a No. 10 blade followed by crushing the implant with a needle holder along the central aspect can reduce the projection of the implant (Fig. 5-9A,B). Crushing the implant after carving also helps to soften the transition along the transected edge. With the large implant, the reader is reminded to assess the patient's occlusion before electing to place this implant. Often, the patient who has a significant recession of the chin exhibits concomitant occlusal disharmony, usually a class II occlusion, or "overbite." Obviously, placement of a large implant will do nothing for the occlusal problem, and the patient should be counseled about that fact.

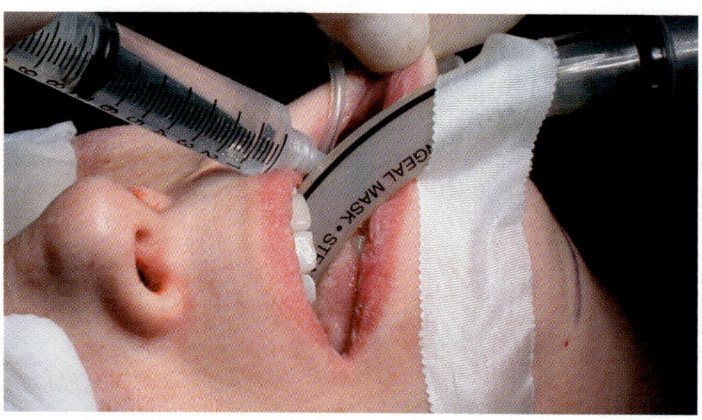

FIGURE 5-10. Mersilene Chin Implantation, Step 1. Appropriate local anesthesia of 1% lidocaine with 1:100,000 epinephrine is infiltrated directly into the submental incision as well as transorally for a mental-nerve block.

Appropriate local anesthesia of 1% lidocaine with 1:100,000 epinephrine is infiltrated directly into the submental incision as well as transorally for a mental-nerve block (Fig. 5-10). The procedure is begun with a submental incision, as described in detail in the preceding section on submentoplasty. With proper headlight illumination and retraction on the superior wound edge, dissection is carried out over the anterior aspect of the chin in the plane below the mentalis muscle but above the periosteum. The implant is seated in a supraperiosteal plane centrally and in a subperiosteal plane laterally in order to ensure maximal fixation (Fig. 5-11). A Converse retractor should be used to inspect the

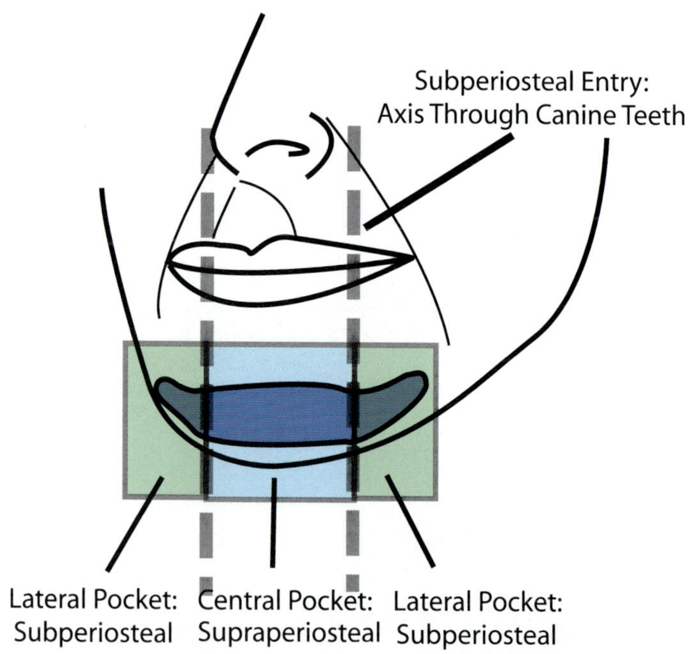

FIGURE 5-11. Illustration showing the ideal position of a chin implant (*in dark blue*), subperiosteal lateral pockets (*in light green*), and a supraperiosteal central pocket (*in light blue*) to ensure maximal fixation and projection along with minimal bone resorption. The point of entry into the subperiosteal plane should be carried out at a point along the axis through the canine teeth.

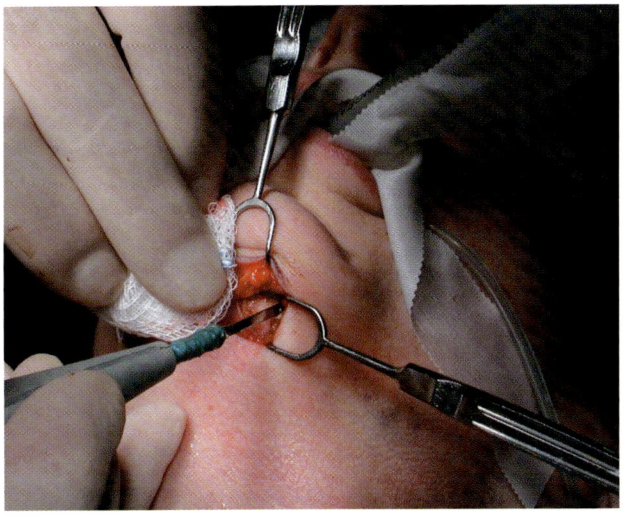

FIGURE 5-12. Mersilene Chin Implantation, Step 2. A monopolar cautery is used to score the periosteum in a vertical direction in a parasagittal line running through the canine teeth.

pocket laterally as the surgeon prepares to enter the subperiosteal plane. A monopolar cautery is used to score the periosteum in a vertical direction in a parasagittal line running through the canine teeth (Fig. 5-12), and a Joseph elevator is then inserted into this subperiosteal plane to dissect the pocket laterally (Fig. 5-13). The ePTFE implant tends to be easier to insert, and a tighter lateral, subperiosteal pocket can be fashioned. A slightly more generous pocket is often necessary for the Mersilene-mesh implant, which tends to resist easy insertion into the subperiosteal pocket. The midline of the implant itself should be marked before placement by excising a small, vertical wedge in the presumed midline along the inferior aspect of the implant, if not already inscribed in some fashion by the manufacturer. Any further trimming of the implant should then be completed prior to

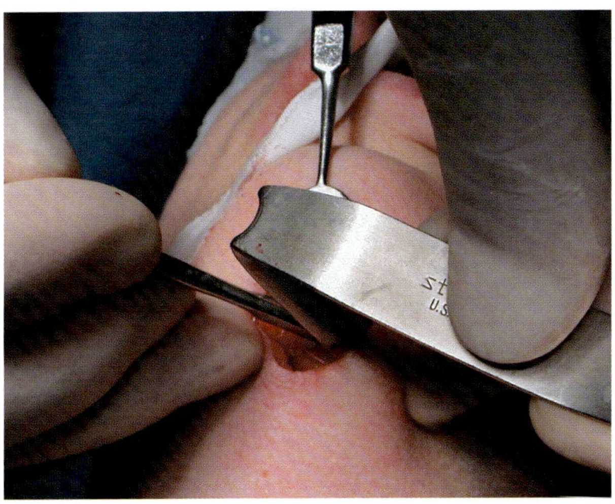

FIGURE 5-13. Mersilene Chin Implantation, Step 3. A Joseph elevator is then inserted into this subperiosteal plane to dissect the lateral subperiosteal pockets.

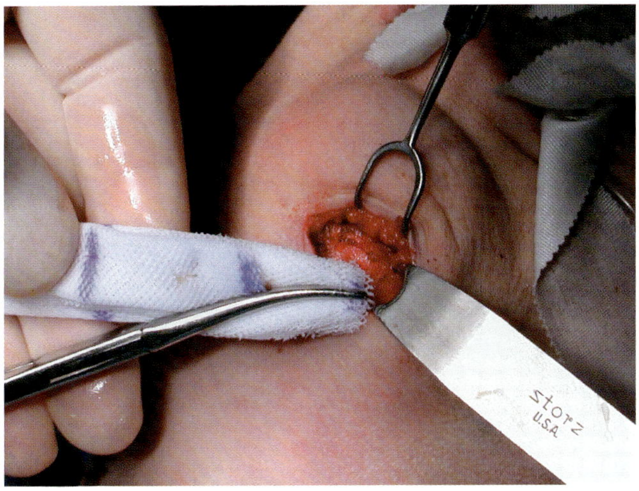

FIGURE 5-14. Mersilene Chin Implantation, Step 4. A curved, tonsil hemostat is used to grasp one end of the implant with the tines extending to the end of the implant to ensure that the implant does not fold back onto itself and to facilitate ease of placement. (It is important to mark the midline of the implant prior to insertion.)

insertion. A tonsil, or equivalently large and curved hemostat is used to grasp one end of the implant with the tines extending to the end of the implant to ensure that the implant does not fold back onto itself and to facilitate ease of placement (Fig. 5-14). With a Converse retractor and headlight, the implant is gently delivered into the subperiosteal pocket (Fig. 5-15), and the same maneuver is conducted on the contralateral side (Fig. 5-16A,B). Before the incision is closed, the implant should be noted to be in the midline (according to the designated mark) and completely residing over the anterior aspect of the mentum. At times, the distal end of the implant may buckle, particularly with the Mersilene mesh implant; and the surgeon is advised to palpate the distal aspect carefully before closure of the incision. The inferior aspect of the implant should be suture fixated with a 4-0 polydioxanone suture to the mentalis and the periosteum to avoid the risk that the central aspect of the implant should migrate inferiorly over the mandibular border. Unlike in a

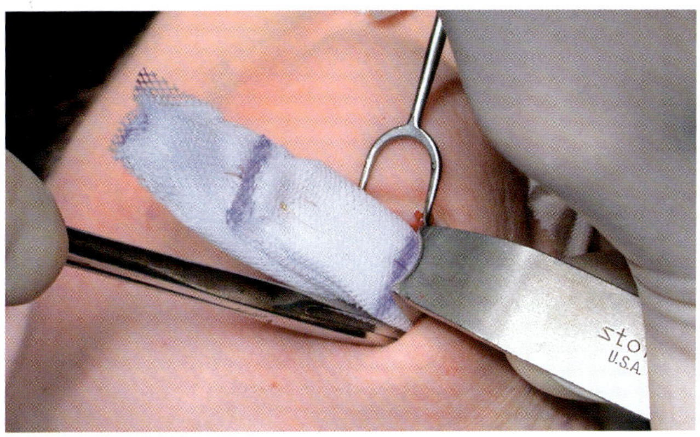

FIGURE 5-15. Mersilene Chin Implantation, Step 5. With a Converse retractor and headlight, the implant is gently delivered into the lateral, subperiosteal pocket.

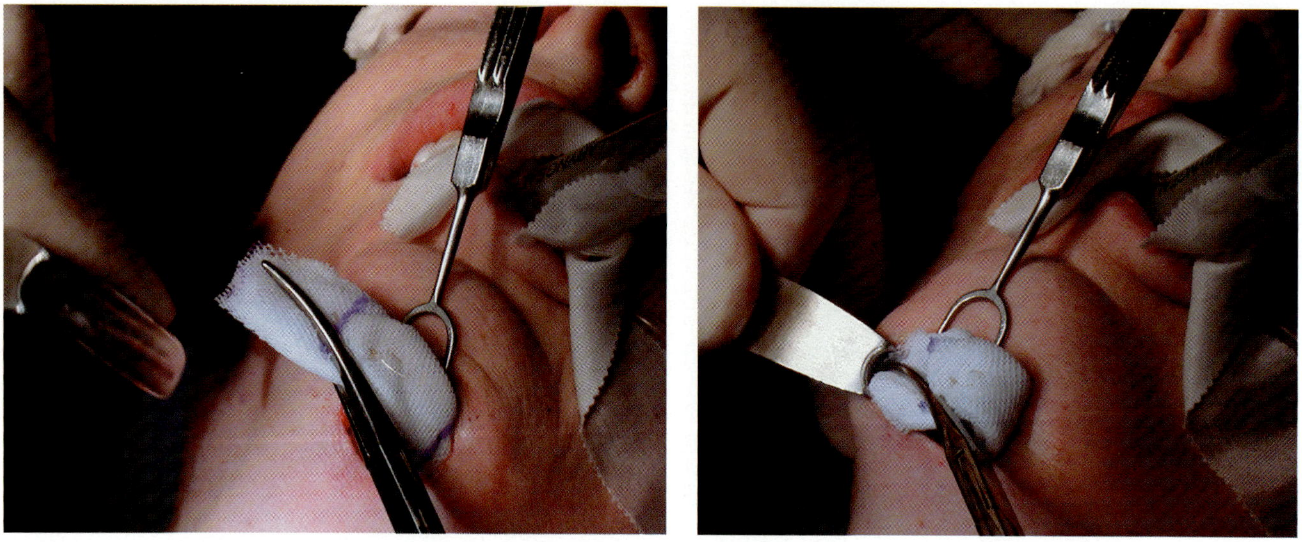

A B

FIGURE 5-16. Mersilene Chin Implantation, Step 6. A,B: The same technique is used to insert the implant into the contralateral subperiosteal pocket.

straightforward submentoplasty, a subcuticular closure with a 4-0 polydioxanone suture is also warranted: The violated mentalis muscle can be reapproximated to secure the implant further in position and to prevent a "witch's chin" deformity (Fig. 5-17A). The skin incision is then closed with a running, locking 6-0 polypropylene suture as described for a standard submentoplasty (Fig. 5-17B).[§]

[§]The figure references in this section refer to the technique for Mersilene-mesh chin augmentation. Although the insertion technique for Gore-Tex implant does not differ from Mersilene mesh, a separate sequence showing Gore-Tex insertion has been included for clarity (Fig. 5-19A–O).

Primary Rhytidectomy

Cervico-facial rhytidectomy provides rejuvenation of the lower one-third of the face as well as the neckline (Fig. 5-18). Like in all facial plastic procedures, infiltration of sufficient and well-timed local anesthesia containing epinephrine is a critical first step for success. One percent lidocaine mixed with 1:100,000 epinephrine should be placed into the postauricular, preauricular, and cheek areas on the right side of the face toward the close of the submentoplasty. Similarly, the left side of the face should be injected toward the completion of the right side of the face. Judicious timing with a 10-minute delay ensures maximal hemostasis and adequate

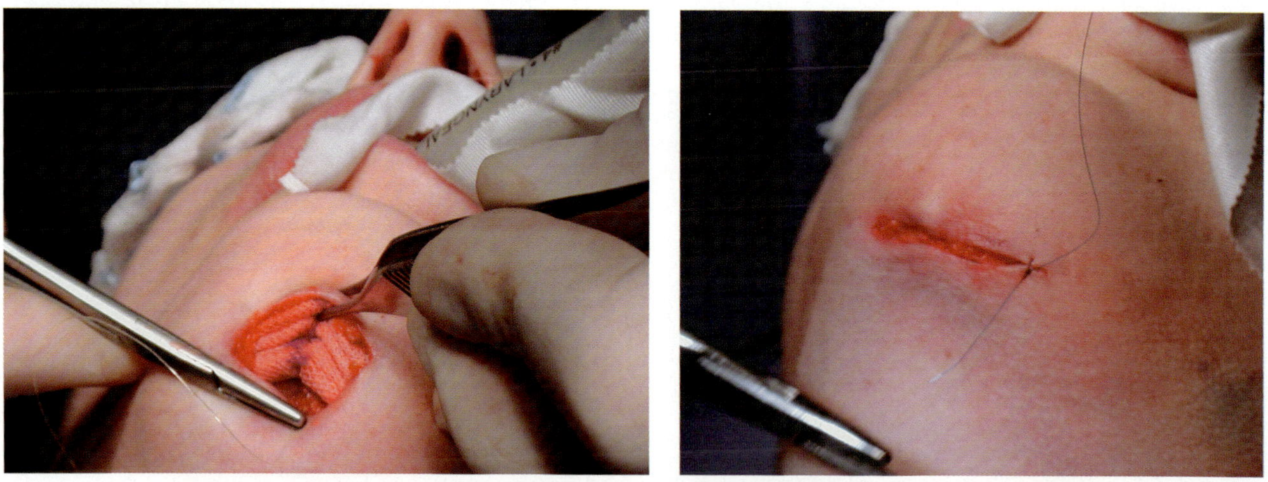

A B

FIGURE 5-17. Mersilene Chin Implantation, Step 7. A: The inferior aspect of the implant should be suture fixated with a 4-0 polydioxanone suture to the mentalis and the periosteum to avoid the risk that the central aspect of the implant should migrate inferiorly over the mandibular border. Then, a 4-0 polydioxanone suture should be used to close the mentalis muscle: The violated mentalis muscle can be reapproximated to secure the implant and prevent a "witch's-chin" deformity. **B:** The skin incision is then closed with a running, locking 6-0 polypropylene suture as described for a standard submentoplasty.

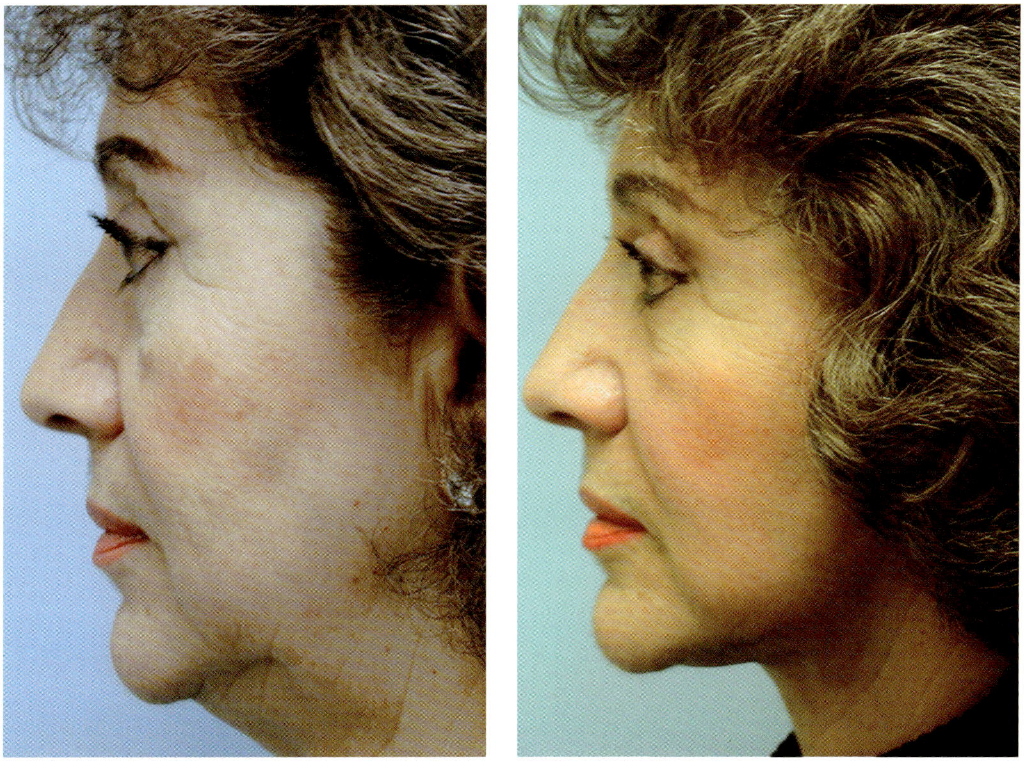

A B

FIGURE 5-18. A, B: This is a 65-year-old lady who complains only of her aged neck line and would like aesthetic rejuvenation. She underwent a cervico-facial rhytidectomy with submental liposuction with notable improvement in her cervico-mental angle and restoration of her jawline. She is shown 6 months postoperatively.

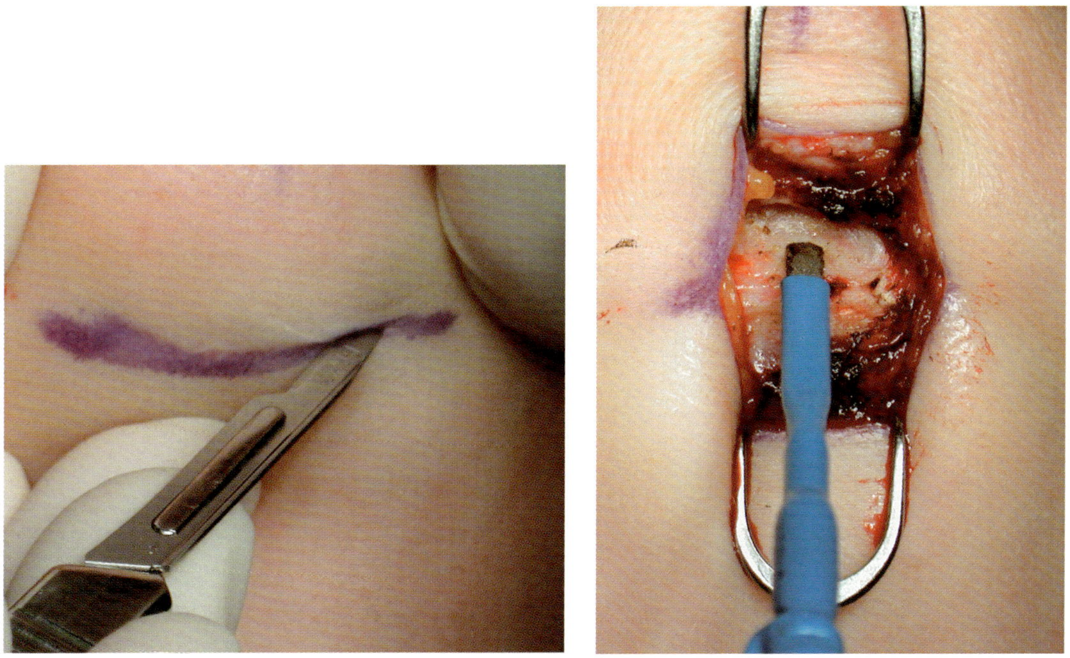

A B

FIGURE 5-19. ePTFE Chin Implantation Sequence. A: The submental incision is made with a No. 15 blade about 1 to 2 mm behind the submental crease. **B:** Monopolar cautery is used to dissect down through the subcutaneous tissue and the mentalis muscle to the level of the periosteum. *(continued)*

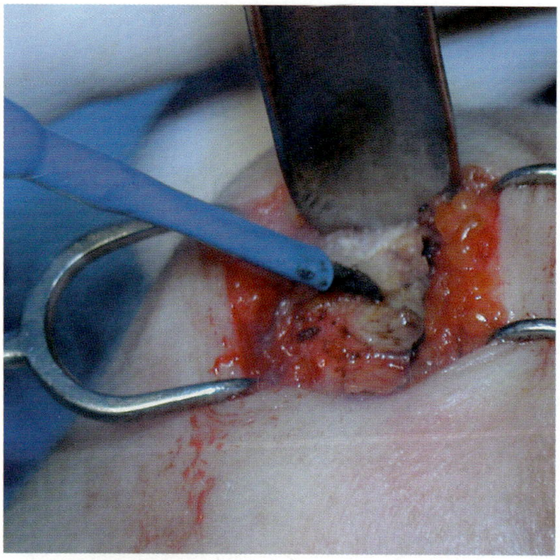

C

FIGURE 5-19. *(Continued)* **C:** A monopolar cautery is used to score the periosteum in a vertical direction in a parasagittal line running through the canine teeth. **D:** Then, a Joseph elevator is used to dissect the lateral subperiosteal pocket from the entry point created by the monopolar cautery. **E:** The same technique of subperiosteal dissection is carried out in the contralateral side. **F:** The implant is placed in the midline, and the midline registered on the skin with a surgical marking pen and registered on the implant using a small V-wedge cut out along the inferior aspect of the implant for alignment. **G:** The implant is then inserted into the lateral subperiosteal pocket with a curved tonsil clamp that is placed all the way to the tip of the implant to prevent buckling. A Converse retractor is used to expose the subperiosteal pocket during insertion. *(continued)*

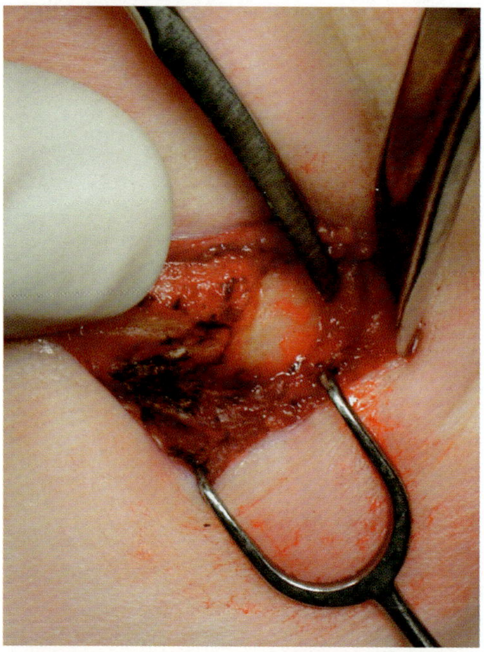

D

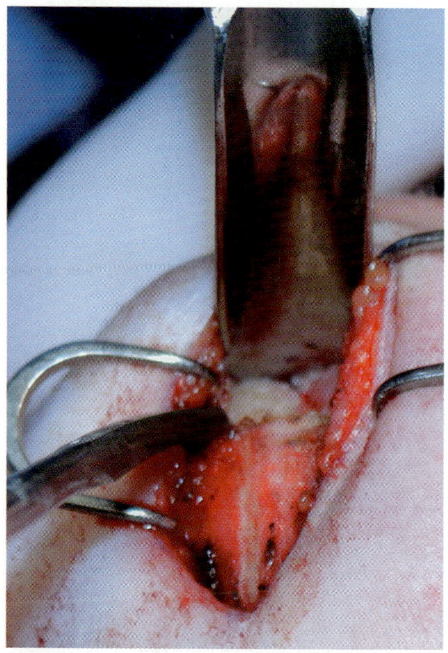

E

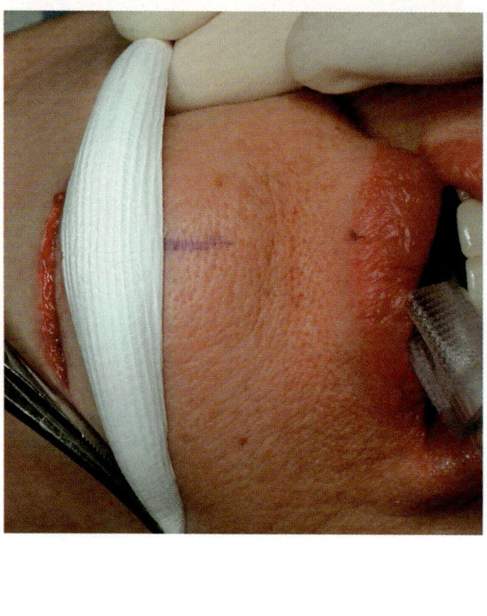

F

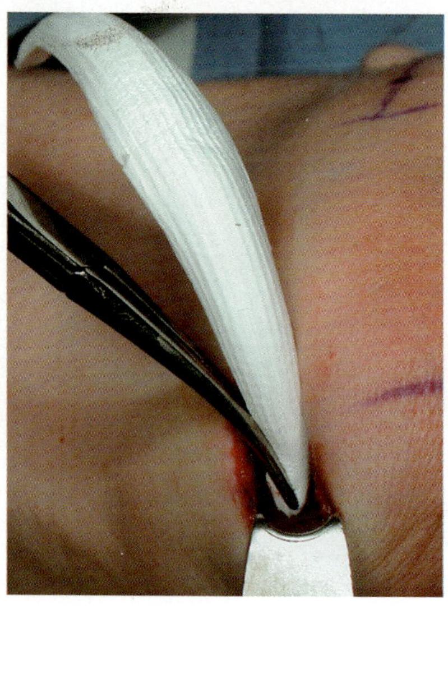

G

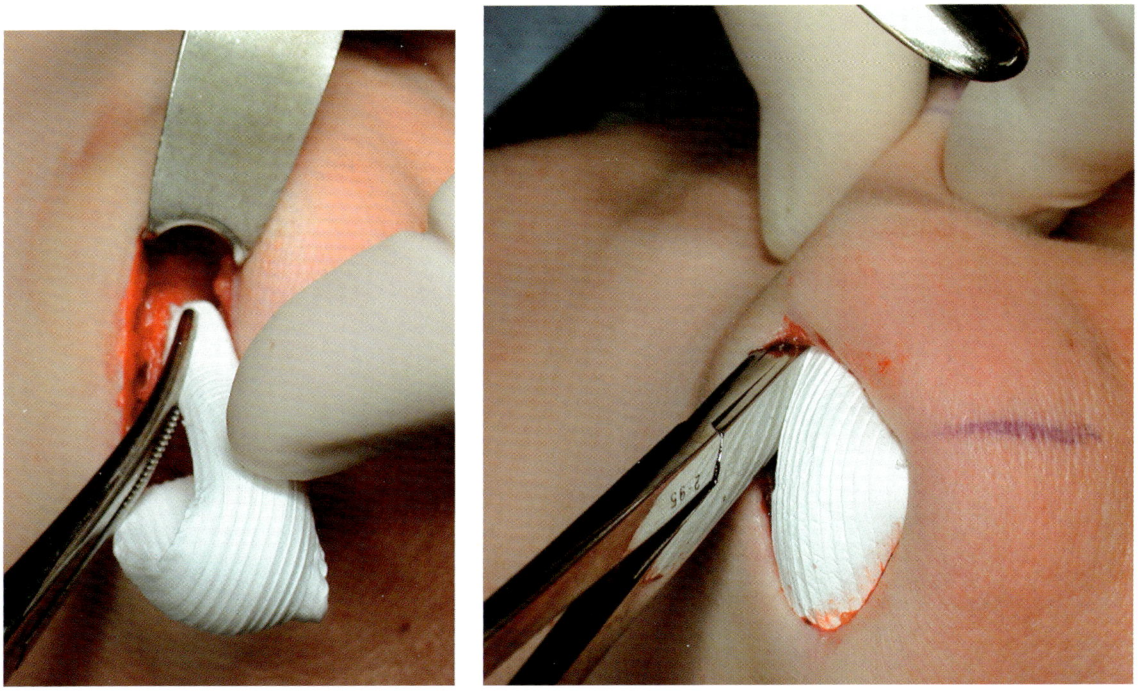

H I

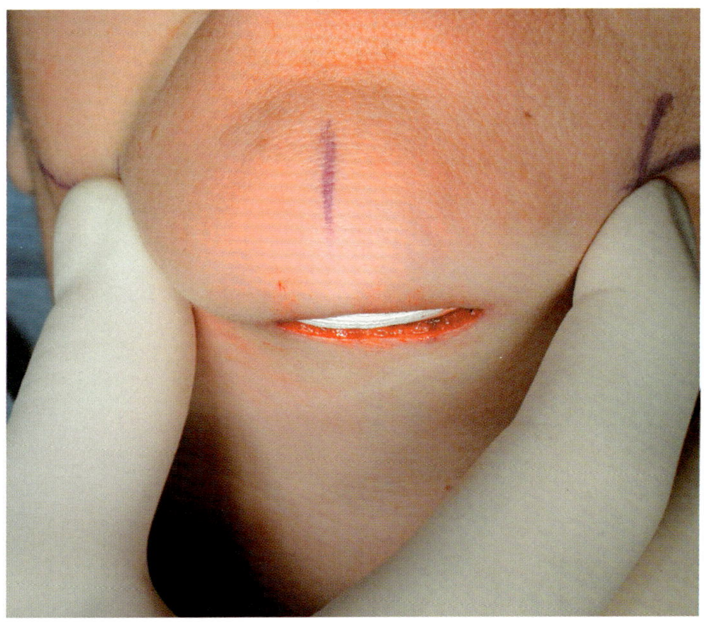

J

FIGURE 5-19. *(Continued)* **H,I:** With the implant securely positioned in one subperiosteal pocket, the contralateral side is approached in the same manner. **J:** Both ends of the implant are palpated to ensure that the lateral edges have not buckled or rotated in an unfavorable attitude (too high, asymmetrically, or below the mandibular border). Also, the central aspect of the implant is confirmed to be in the midline by ensuring that the small V-wedge created at the inferior border of the implant aligns with the marked midline on the skin. *(continued)*

anesthesia for the intended operative time. Of note, the effects of the lidocaine and epinephrine markedly diminish after one and a half hours, making diligent and expeditious surgery mandatory for an optimal result.

In order to minimize postoperative edema, an ice pack should be placed along each area that has just been dissected. For instance, immediately after the submentoplasty, an ice pack can be placed under the chin while the right side of the face is dissected. Similarly, an ice pack should be placed along the right side of the face and held in place with the blue towel that circumscribes the head while the left side of the face is being completed. An easy and inexpensive option for creation of a suitable ice pack is pouring water into a surgical glove, which in turn is then tied off at the wrist and placed into the freezer overnight.

Before actual surgery commences, a cotton tampon consisting of either a Kitner sponge or the cottony central portion of an eye pad should be inserted into the entrance of the external ear canal to absorb any blood. In addition, a liberally moistened laparotomy sponge is opened lengthwise to circumscribe the hair-bearing scalp, and a surgical towel is applied exterior to this laparotomy pad—both are held in place

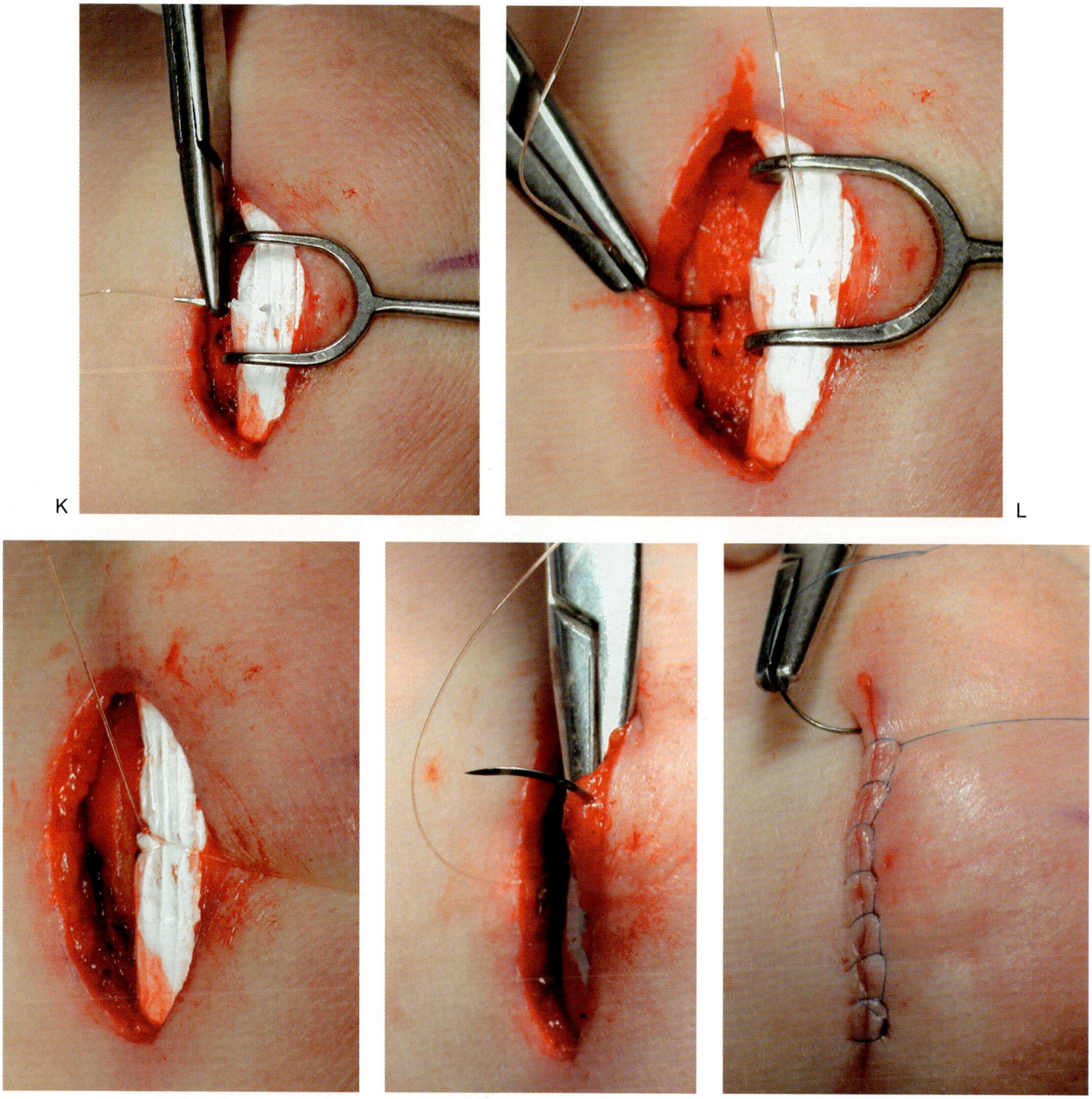

K L M,N O

FIGURE 5-19. *(Continued)* **K–M:** The implant is then secured inferiorly to the periosteum and mentalis muscle with a 4-0 polydioxanone suture to avoid the central aspect of the implant from rotating freely over the mandibular border. **N:** The mentalis muscle is then closed as a separate layer using a 4-0 polydioxanone suture. **O:** The skin is closed with a running, locking 6-0 polypropylene suture. In addition, a single, interrupted suture can be placed in the midline as insurance against the incision from opening up.

with a towel clamp. This dressing serves to absorb the majority of any excessive blood during the operation and thereby minimize the need for labor-intensive cleaning of the hair at the end of the procedure.

Although many variations of skin incisions have been proposed for a rhytidectomy, the authors advocate the formula described herein for the best aesthetic outcome. The following guidelines stress the philosophical underpinnings that have informed the authors' chosen pattern of incisions. Beginning postauricularly, the surgeon should strive to follow the incision along the hairline rather than traverse the naked skin into the hairline at the midauricular level (Fig. 5-20). Many mature women who desire rhytidectomy prefer a shorter hairstyle that precludes the more readily visible

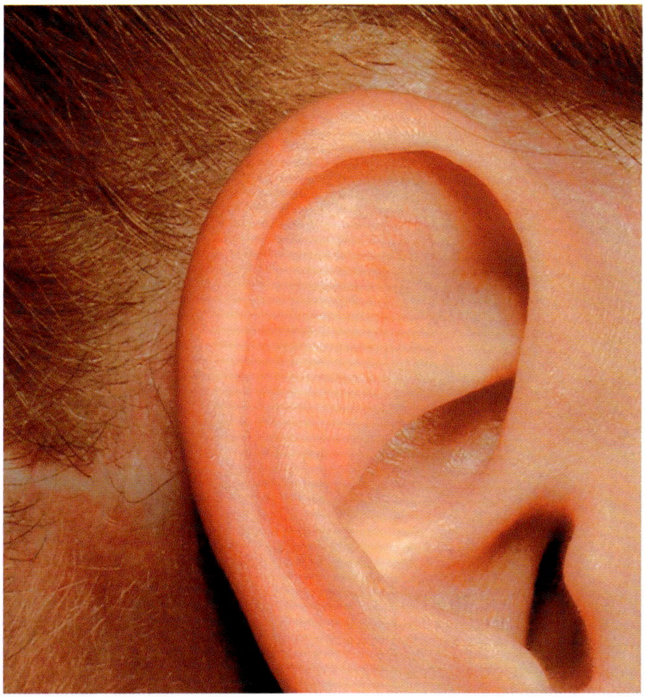

FIGURE 5-20. Primary rhytidectomy sequence. This photograph shows the type of facelift incisions that are not favorably located in the authors' opinion. Superiorly, the incision violates the temporal hair tuft, which removes precious hair, and will be evident as a temporal hair recession if another facelift is undertaken. The preauricular incision can be more visible than the preferred postauricular incision because it forms a continuous, almost straight line that stands in contradistinction to the principles of good scar camouflage. The lobular region shows a widened scar, which may result from tension at the time of incision closure. The straight, postauricular incision into the hairline has three unfavorable qualities: (a) an unsightly, conspicuous location of the scar, especially if the hair should be worn short or tied up; (b) potential hair loss from this type of incision, owing to trimming of hair, cautery of hair follicles, or tension at closure; and (c) difficult dissection in the vascular, hair-bearing tissue.

lower postauricular incision. In the preauricular region, the surgeon should strive to follow the natural curvature around the lobule, behind the tragus, and again around the helical crus superiorly: Straight or pretragal incisions may be more conspicuous, particularly in individuals with dark complexions and in those prone to exuberant scar formation. Whether to use a pretragal or posttragal incision remains controversial. However, the authors strongly contend that the latter serves to camouflage the incision more discreetly and has unequivocally resulted in a natural appearance. Finally, the temporal hair tuft should not be violated because the recessed position after surgery is a glaring stigma of advanced aging. After repeated rhytidectomy in this manner, the alopecia may be serious enough to justify a tedious (and often unsatisfactory) hair transplantation to correct this problem.

To begin the rhytidectomy, the posterior aspect of the auricle is pierced with a 2-0 silk suture toward the base of the ear and further superiorly so that the entire length of the ear may be retracted with the suture pulled anteriorly to expose the postauricular skin. A hemostat should be clamped to the suture to facilitate the assistant's retraction of the ear. The second maneuver in a rhytidectomy is a directed stab incision at the base of the lobule and insertion of a single-pronged hook for proper retraction inferiorly (Fig. 5-21). The postauricular region is always initially incised in a complete rhytidectomy for the simple, perhaps obvious, fact that any prior preauricular incisions will trickle blood into the postauricular site, obscuring ease of dissection. The postauricular incision should be begun along the inferior hairline using a No. 15 Bard-Parker blade and carried superiorly until the hairline meets the posterior surface of the ear but should be notched in a V configuration immediately prior to this junction to avoid unfavorable scar contracture (Fig. 5-22). The incision is continued onto the actual postauricular surface of the ear (about 1 to 2 mm anterior to the auricular–postauricular interface and situated on the cartilaginous portion of the ear) in order to facilitate ease of closure and resist the tendency toward deepening of the postauricular sulcus over time. The postauricular incision terminates at the aforementioned lobular stab incision.

A tiny, double-hooked retractor is inserted into the superior aspect of the postauricular incision (near the hairline–auricular junction), and sharp dissection is undertaken of the postauricular flap with a No. 15 Bard-Parker blade (Fig. 5-23). Transillumination of the flap with one overhead operative light directed through the flap from above and the other over the surgeon's right shoulder aimed under the flap provides the best visualization of the dissection plane. A headlight, on the other hand, may interfere with this type of

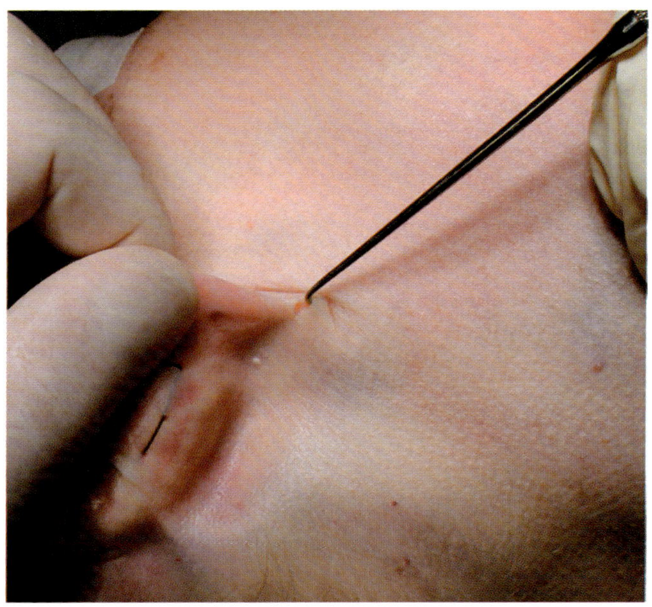

FIGURE 5-21. Primary Rhytidectomy, Step 1. After a 2-0 silk suture is placed to retract the ear forward, a directed, stab incision is made at the base of the lobule, and a single-pronged hook is inserted for proper retraction inferiorly.

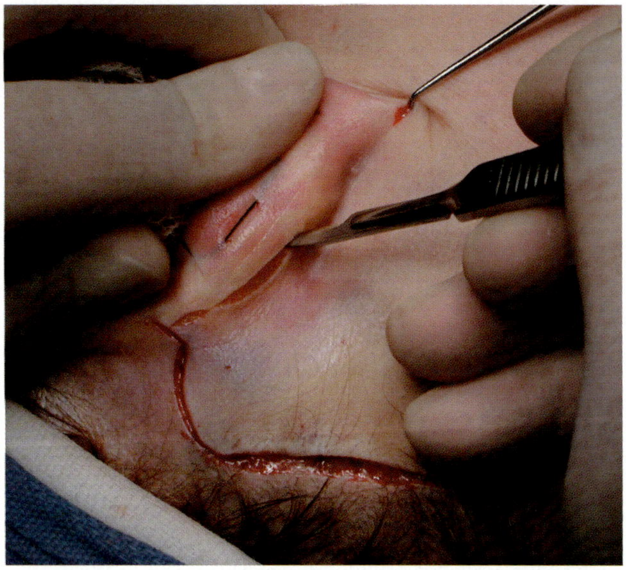

FIGURE 5-22. Primary Rhytidectomy, Step 2. The postauricular region is always initially incised in a complete rhytidectomy for the simple, perhaps obvious, fact that any prior preauricular incisions will trickle blood into the postauricular site obscuring ease of dissection. The postauricular incision should be begun along the inferior hairline using a No. 15 Bard-Parker blade and carried superiorly until the hairline meets the posterior surface of the ear but should be notched in a V-configuration immediately prior to this junction to avoid unfavorable scar contracture. The incision is continued onto the actual postauricular surface of the ear (about 1 to 2 mm anterior to the auricular–postauricular interface and situated on the cartilaginous portion of the ear) in order to facilitate ease of closure and resist the tendency toward deepening of the postauricular sulcus over time.

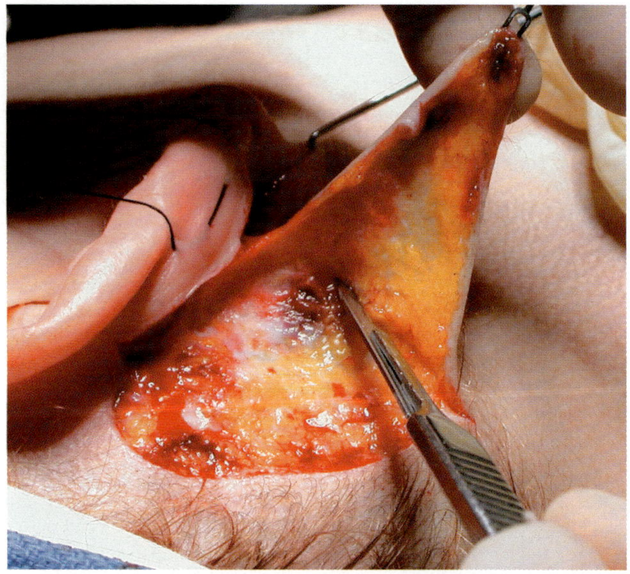

FIGURE 5-23. Primary Rhytidectomy, Step 3. A tiny, double-hooked retractor is inserted into the superior aspect of the postauricular incision (near the hairline-auricular junction), and sharp dissection is undertaken of the postauricular flap with a No. 15 Bard-Parker blade. Transillumination of the flap with one overhead operative light directed through the flap from above and the other over the surgeon's right shoulder aimed under the flap provides the best visualization of the dissection plane. All postauricular dissection is conducted sharply with the No. 15 blade because the plane of dissection over the sternocleidomastoid muscle is somewhat ill defined. The surgeon should strive to elevate the flap, leaving the glistening sternocleidomastoid fascia intact on the muscle surface. This surgical plane prevents inadvertent injury to the major branch of the great auricular nerve and undue hemorrhage from muscle transection.

illumination technique. All postauricular dissection is conducted sharply with the No. 15 blade because the plane of dissection over the sternocleidomastoid muscle is somewhat ill defined. The surgeon should strive to elevate the flap, leaving the glistening sternocleidomastoid fascia intact on the muscle surface: This surgical plane prevents inadvertent injury to the major branch of the great auricular nerve and undue hemorrhage from muscle transection. As the cervical pocket is approached, the surgeon may elect to continue the dissection with sharp Metzenbaum scissors to expedite completion of postauricular flap elevation (Fig. 5-24).

After the postauricular flap has been successfully completed, the surgeon should turn his or her attention to the preauricular region. The described curvilinear, posttragal incision should be initiated with the No. 15 blade. The exception to this rule is the male patient who requires a preauricular incision to avoid translocation of hair-bearing skin onto the tragus, making daily shaving a treacherous exercise (Fig. 5-25). The incision is carried around (i.e., inferior to the temporal tuft of hair, or sideburn) with the knife blade beveled slightly away from the hair to prevent follicular transection. Two tiny, double-pronged hooks should be placed on either side of the tragus to retract the skin forward and assist in initial flap elevation (Fig. 5-26). As the flap is developed, larger double-pronged retractors may be substituted for the smaller versions to facilitate flap elevation (Fig. 5-27A,B). The same orientation of the two overhead lights as described for the postauricular dissection should be used for the preauricular region. Sharp Metzenbaum or dedicated facelift scissors are used to elevate the preauricular flap: The flap should be elevated by advancing the scissors forward under the flap with tines held slightly ajar rather than opening and closing them in a traditional manner: This method helps to establish the proper plane of dissection to lessen the chance of flap transection ("button-holing") (Fig. 5-28A,B). After several of these passes have been made and the dissection plane is identified, the surgeon can elect to connect these pockets by gentle spreading of the scissor tines or by opening and closing the tines as usual.

The length of the cutaneous flap is dictated by several factors. Most important, the distance of flap elevation should depend on the ease with which the SMAS can be retracted and suspended, which can be assessed by tugging on the SMAS with a pair of Brown-Adson forceps (Fig. 5-29A). If any resistance is met or if the skin appears to drape poorly, then additional undermining of the skin flap is recommended. Generally, a "medium"-length flap that terminates near the midcheek, just medial to the lateral canthus, is a rea-

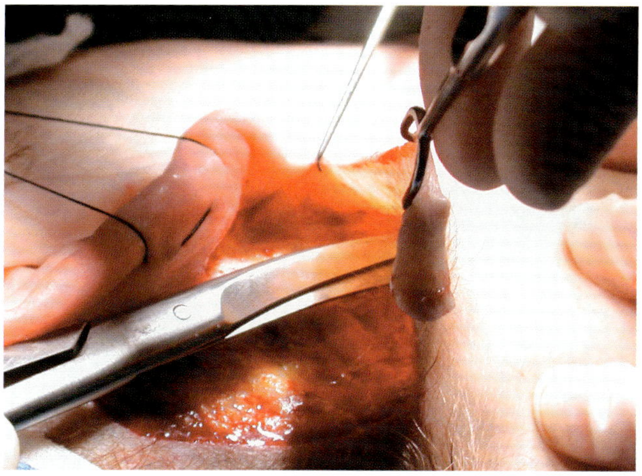

FIGURE 5-24. Primary Rhytidectomy, Step 4. As the cervical pocket is approached, the surgeon may elect to continue the dissection with sharp Metzenbaum scissors to expedite completion of postauricular flap elevation.

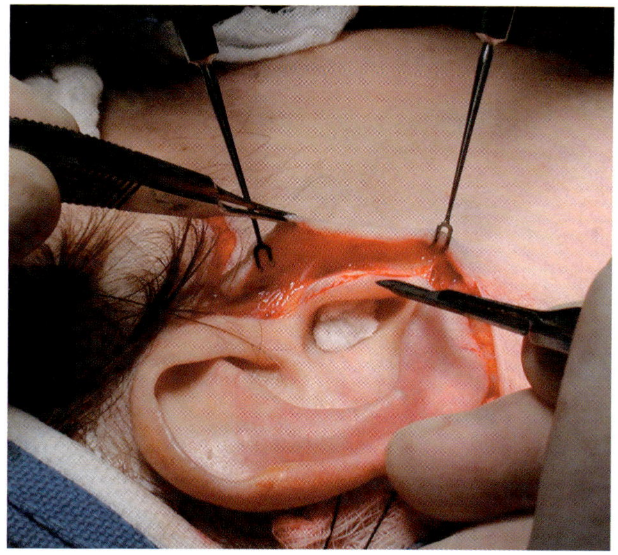

FIGURE 5-26. Primary Rhytidectomy, Step 5. The preauricular incision is initiated and carried around (i.e., inferior, to the temporal tuft of hair, or sideburn), with the knife blade beveled slightly away from the hair to prevent follicular transection. Two tiny double-pronged hooks should then be placed on either side of the tragus to retract the skin forward and to assist in initial flap elevation.

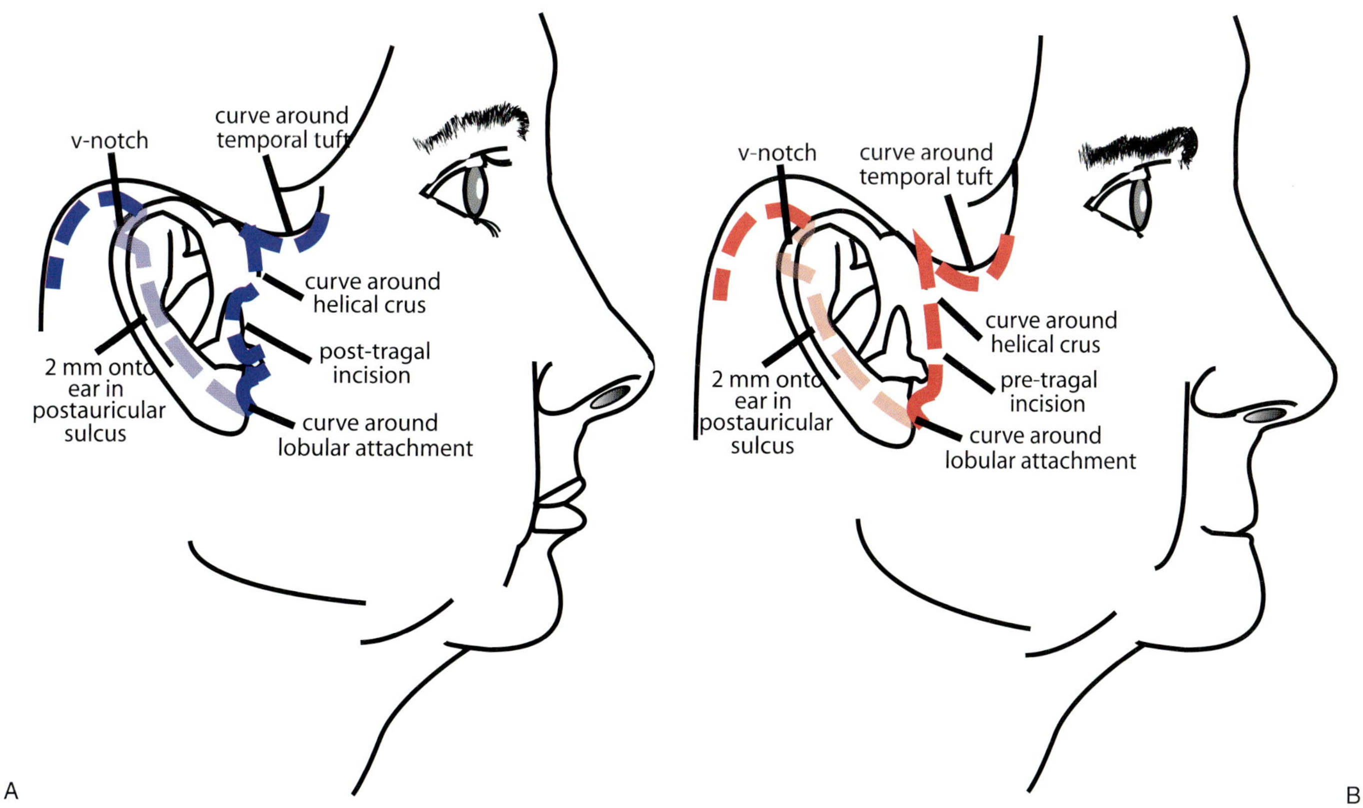

FIGURE 5-25. Illustration showing the ideal incisions for a female patient **(A)** (posttragal) and a male patient **(B)** (pretragal).

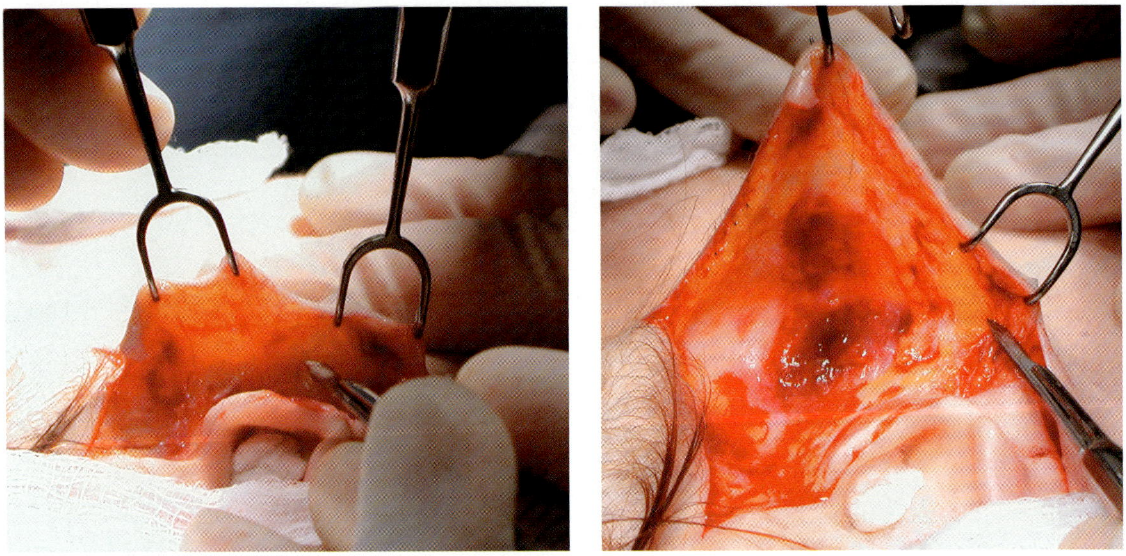

A B

FIGURE 5-27. Primary Rhytidectomy, Step 6. A,B: As the flap is developed, larger double-pronged retractors may be substituted for the smaller versions to facilitate flap elevation.

sonable first attempt. Another factor that may inhibit the surgeon from extensive flap elevation is the fear of flap necrosis secondary to tobacco usage, diabetes mellitus, or other impediments of a vascular or healing nature. The authors have not made it a strict policy to abstain from surgery in chronic, habitual smokers because they almost never obey instructions and more conservative flap elevation generally protects against any flap compromise. However, the patient is asked to cease all forms of tobacco for a 2-week period before and after surgery (total of 1 month), knowing well that this request most likely will be breached despite stern admonition to refrain.

Subcutaneous dissection also should be limited along the jaw line to avoid any injury to the marginal mandibular branch of the facial nerve. The marginal mandibular branch becomes vulnerable approximately halfway along the mandibular body, where it attains a more superficial position because the SMAS-fascia becomes more attenuated in this region. The area at risk is defined as 2 cm behind the oral commissure in a circle whose radius extends from the mandible

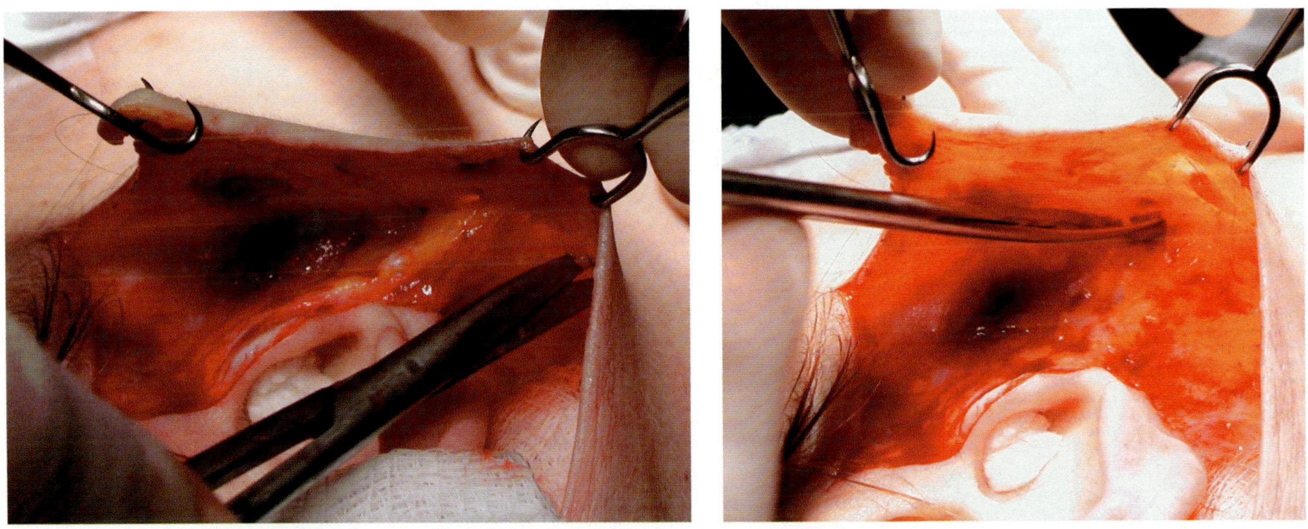

A B

FIGURE 5-28. Primary Rhytidectomy, Step 7. A,B: Sharp Metzenbaum or dedicated facelift scissors are used to elevate the preauricular flap: The flap should be elevated by advancing the scissors forward under the flap with tines held slightly ajar rather than opening and closing them in a traditional manner: This method helps to establish the proper plane of dissection to lessen the chance of flap transection ("button-holing"). After several of these passes have been made and the dissection plane identified, the surgeon can elect to connect these pockets by gentle spreading of the scissor tines or by opening and closing the tines as usual.

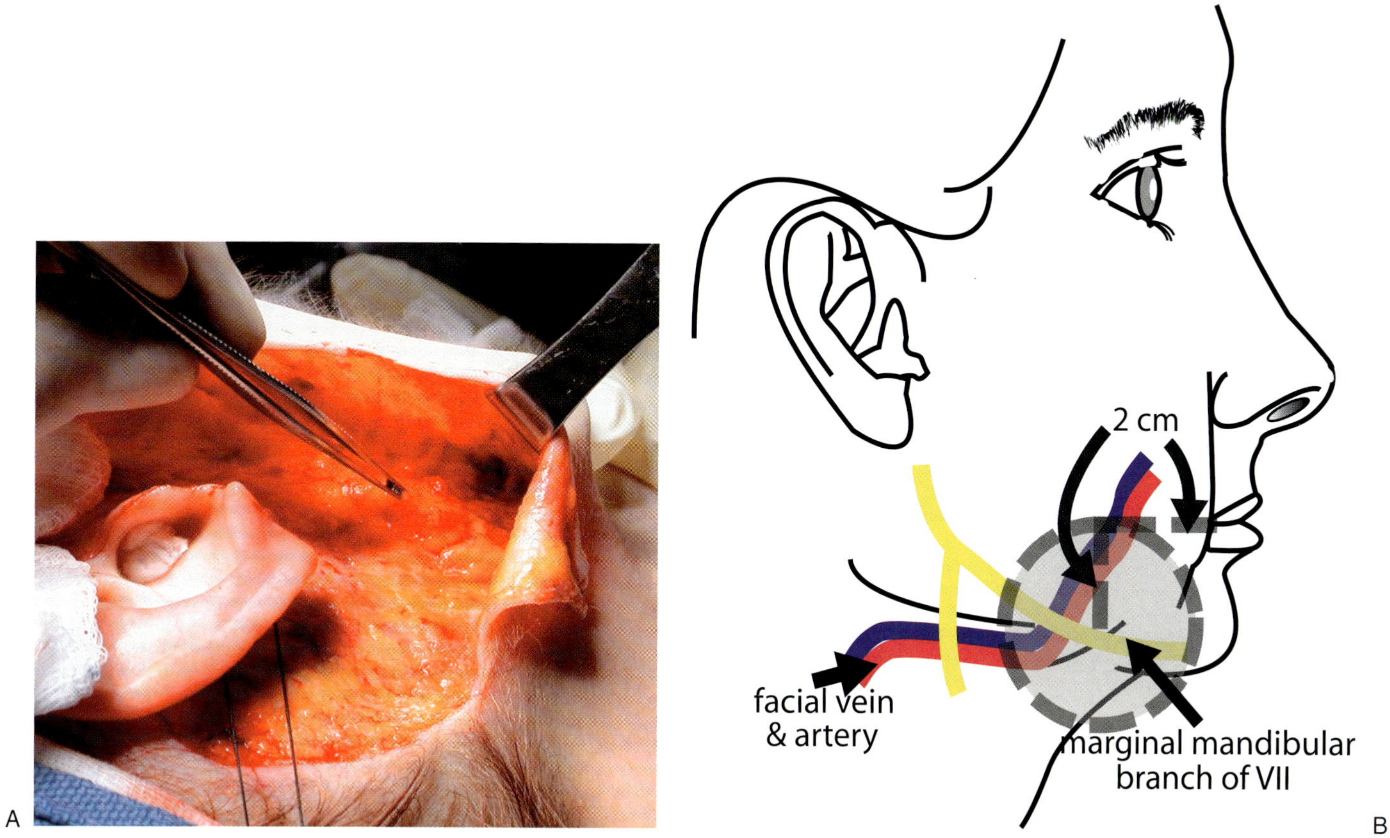

FIGURE 5-29. Primary Rhytidectomy, Step 8. A: The length of the cutaneous flap is dictated by several factors. Most important, the distance of flap elevation should depend on the ease with which the superficial musculoaponeurotic system (SMAS) can be retracted and suspended, which can be assessed by tugging on the SMAS with a pair of Brown-Adson forceps. Care should be taken not to pass the midportion of the mandible to avoid injury to the marginal-mandibular branch of the facial nerve. **B:** This illustration shows the area of risk for injury to the marginal mandibular branch of the facial nerve. The subcutaneous dissection should not pass an area that is located 2 cm behind the oral commissure circumscribed for a distance of 2 cm radius from this point along the mandible.

for a distance of 2 cm (Fig. 5-29B).[16] Also, at this point the facial artery and vein traverse the mandible and lie immediately deep to the facial nerve. Hence, injudicious cautery of these vessels may lead to temporary or permanent damage to the marginal mandibular branch. Accordingly, if bleeding is noted in this area, then careful bipolar cautery should be undertaken only very selectively with good headlight illumination and retraction as the surgical assistant observes for any facial movement during cauterization. Clearly, facial movement may not be present because of lidocaine infiltration in this region; therefore, this is not always a reliable indicator.

Superficial musculoaponeurotic system suspension is accomplished with either imbrication (SMAS-ectomy, or SMAS excision, followed by suture fixation of the exposed edges) or plication (folding the SMAS onto itself without excision). Imbrication is the favored technique because it typically permits a more even, less buckled, contour of the lateral cheek. Furthermore, the excised strip of SMAS tissue can be harvested for nasolabial or labiomandibular soft-tissue augmentation.[§§] Approximately a 2-cm width of SMAS adjacent to the anterior border of the ear extending inferiorly to just around the lobule but terminating superiorly before the temporal region (to avoid temporal-branch neuropraxia) should be excised as part of an SMAS imbrication (Fig. 5-30). However, in a very gaunt patient, the surgeon may prefer to undertake an SMAS plication instead to restore some youthful fullness to the face.

A very important principle should be stated at this point: The SMAS provides all suspension of descended tissue, whereas the skin is simply redraped after SMAS suspension. The skin should support no tension for two reasons: (a) a widened scar may develop; and (2) a "windswept" appearance of a poorly executed facelift often results. Conversely,

[§§]Please refer to the following section for further technical details as to the insertion of SMAS for augmentation of the nasolabial and labiomandibular regions. Insertion of SMAS soft tissue is identical to the method used for Gore-Tex and acellular dermis as described in Chapter 8.

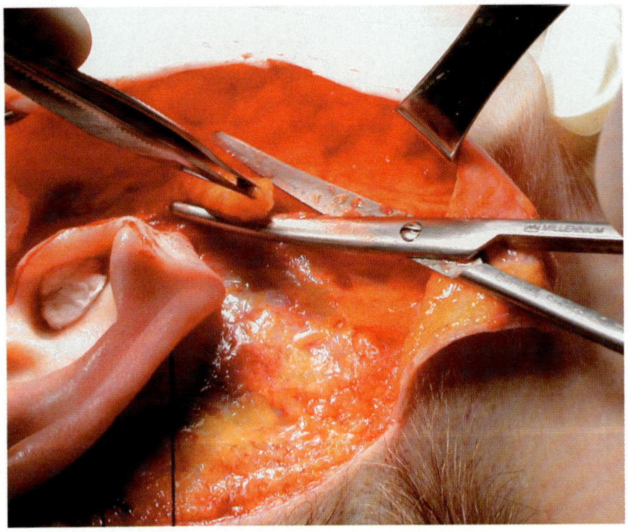

FIGURE 5-30. Primary Rhytidectomy, Step 9. Approximately a 2-cm width of superficial musculoaponeurotic system (SMAS) adjacent to the anterior border of the ear extending inferiorly to just around the lobule but terminating superiorly before the temporal region (to avoid temporal-branch neuropraxia) should be excised as part of an SMAS imbrication.

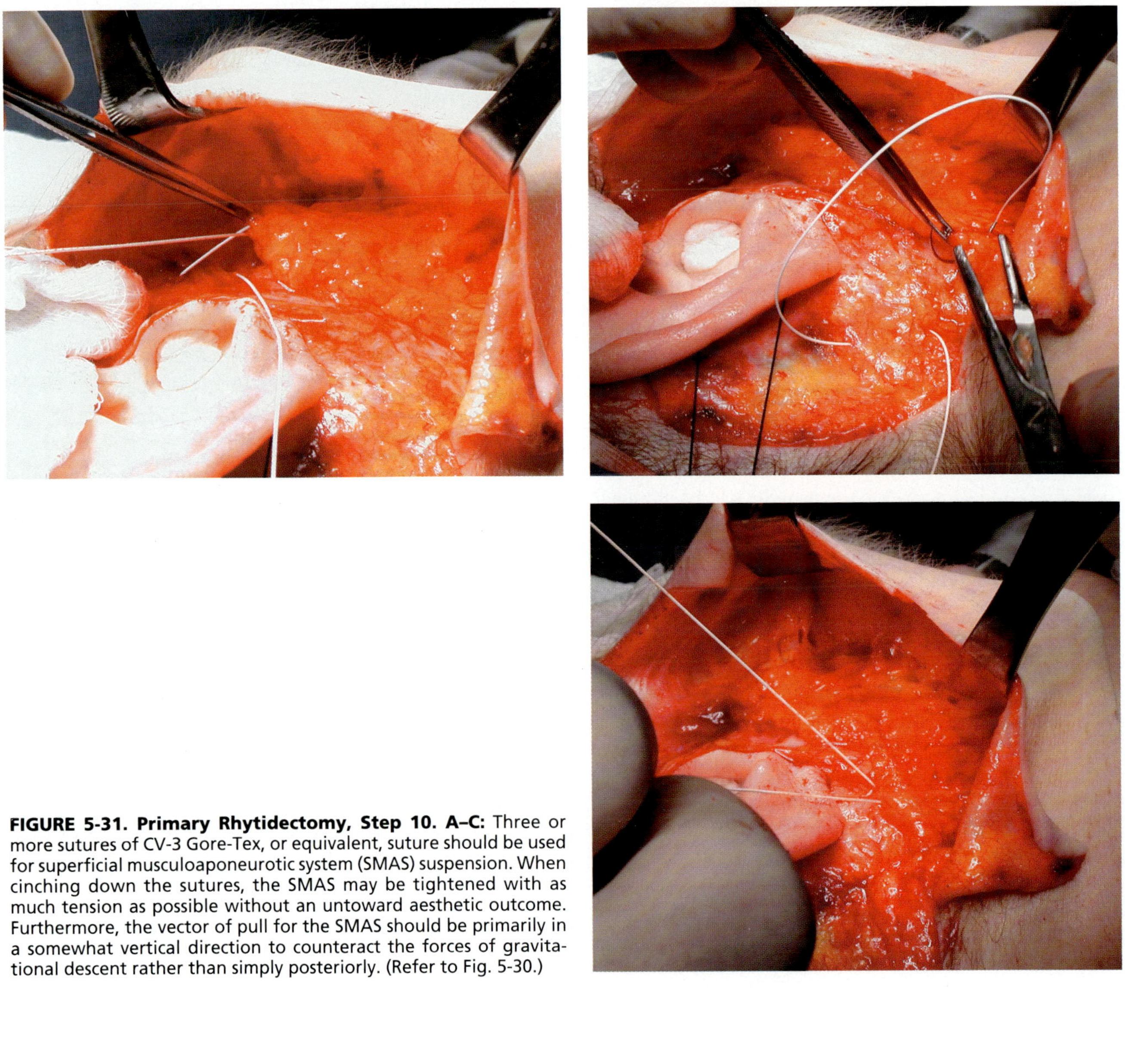

A B C

FIGURE 5-31. Primary Rhytidectomy, Step 10. A–C: Three or more sutures of CV-3 Gore-Tex, or equivalent, suture should be used for superficial musculoaponeurotic system (SMAS) suspension. When cinching down the sutures, the SMAS may be tightened with as much tension as possible without an untoward aesthetic outcome. Furthermore, the vector of pull for the SMAS should be primarily in a somewhat vertical direction to counteract the forces of gravitational descent rather than simply posteriorly. (Refer to Fig. 5-30.)

the SMAS may be tightened with as much tension as possible without an untoward aesthetic outcome. Furthermore, the vector of pull for the SMAS should be primarily in a postero-superior direction to counteract the forces of gravitational descent rather than simply posteriorly—which is more precisely delineated. Three or more sutures of CV-3 Gore-Tex, or equivalent, suture should be used for SMAS suspension (Fig. 5-31A,B,C). (If Gore-Tex suture is used, then a minimum of seven knots should be thrown per suture knot: the first three to four knots are not tied down extremely tightly because of the tendency for the suture to continue to slide when tightened down.) Only the last two to three knots should be cinched very tightly to avoid unraveling. Despite additional expense, ePTFE offers the unique ability to fasten a square knot in the air and to slide that knot down to the desired position and adjust the degree of tightness without slippage. The first suture should be placed at the jaw line and the vector of suspension should follow the jaw line posteriorly. However, the next two suspension sutures should follow the prescribed formula of one half vertical and one half posterior pull. The second suture should be placed approximately at the level of the inferior third of the face, and the next suture positioned somewhat higher at the level of the tragus (Fig. 5-32).

Finally, a suture should be placed that draws the neck tissue back and upward to provide an aesthetically pleasing, well-defined cervico-mental angle. The placement of this suture should be carefully understood so as to avoid injury to the greater auricular nerve. Placement of the suture from the upper cervical region to the postauricular area can bowstring across the greater auricular nerve and cause a painful neuroma to arise. (Refer to the Complications section for proper treatment if this complication should manifest.) A thick layer of SMAS should remain over the sternocleidomastoid and upper cervical region to provide tissue for suspension. The suture should be placed ideally anterior to the sternocleidomastoid muscle to avoid injury to the greater auricular nerve. If the posterior throw of the suture lies near or is directly over the sternocleidomastoid, the suture should be placed more vertically to avoid crossing the greater auricular nerve. Also, if the nerve can be identified visually, then injury to its structure can be more readily avoided.

The precise location of the SMAS-suspension sutures and any additional sutures are dictated by circumstance. In addition, the order in which these sutures are placed is not absolutely critical, but the reader is advised to follow a systematic pattern in all surgical endeavors. Generally, however, this method should suit the novice surgeon well until greater clinical experience is accumulated.

The next task is to redrape the skin and excise any excess. As stated, if the skin is noted to drape poorly at this point, additional undermining may be needed. However, some contour irregularity at the site of the SMAS suspension suture is commonly present and does not warrant any concern because time tends to remove these apparent imperfections. The proper sequence for skin excision and redraping should be as follows: (a) temporal region; (b) postauricular hairline; (c) ear lobule; (d) postauricular sulcus; and (e) preauricular incision. This point deserves reiteration and elaboration: *The temporal (anterior to the ear) and hairline (posterior to the ear) are always suture fixated prior to lobule adjustment* so as to prevent undue traction on the lobule with resultant pixie, or devil's ear, deformity (Fig. 5-33). First, a single hook retractor is positioned into the anterior aspect of the temporal incision and *gently* retracted anteriorly by the assistant, with almost no significant traction. The edges of the temporal skin flap are held with hemostats and pulled supero-posteriorly, while the surgeon estimates how much temporal skin to excise based on this vector (Fig. 5-33B). The excess of skin in the temporal region is excised, and the temporal incision

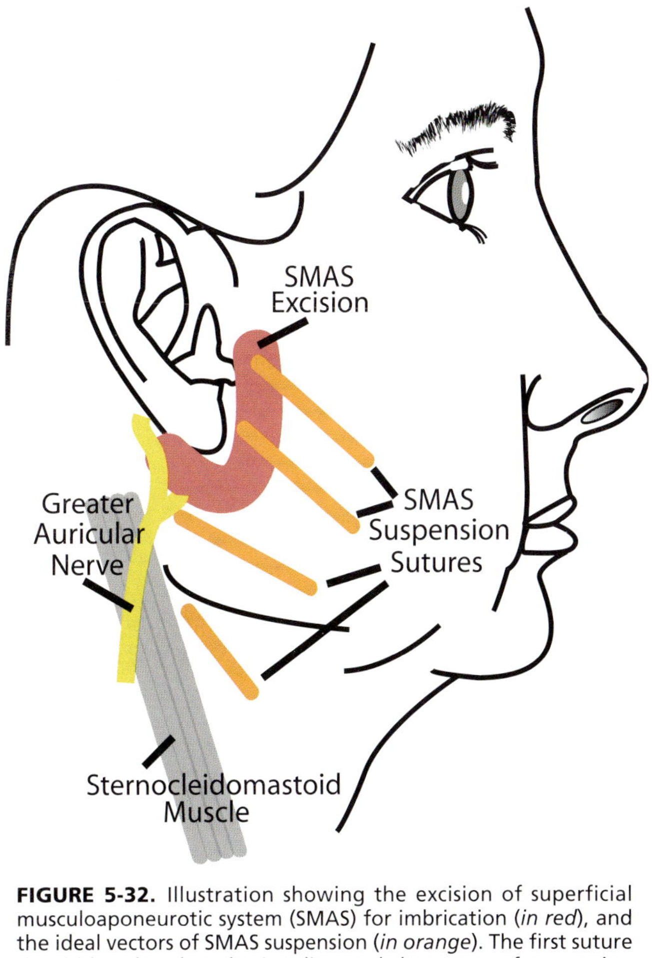

FIGURE 5-32. Illustration showing the excision of superficial musculoaponeurotic system (SMAS) for imbrication (*in red*), and the ideal vectors of SMAS suspension (*in orange*). The first suture should be placed at the jaw line and the vector of suspension should follow the jaw line posteriorly. However, the next two suspension sutures should follow the prescribed formula of one half vertical and one half posterior pull. The second suture should be placed approximately at the level of the inferior third of the face, and the third suture positioned somewhat higher at the level of the tragus. A suture in the cervical SMAS should be placed anterior to the sternocleidomastoid muscle to avoid ensnaring the greater auricular nerve (*in yellow*). The precise location of these sutures and the need for additional sutures are dictated by circumstance.

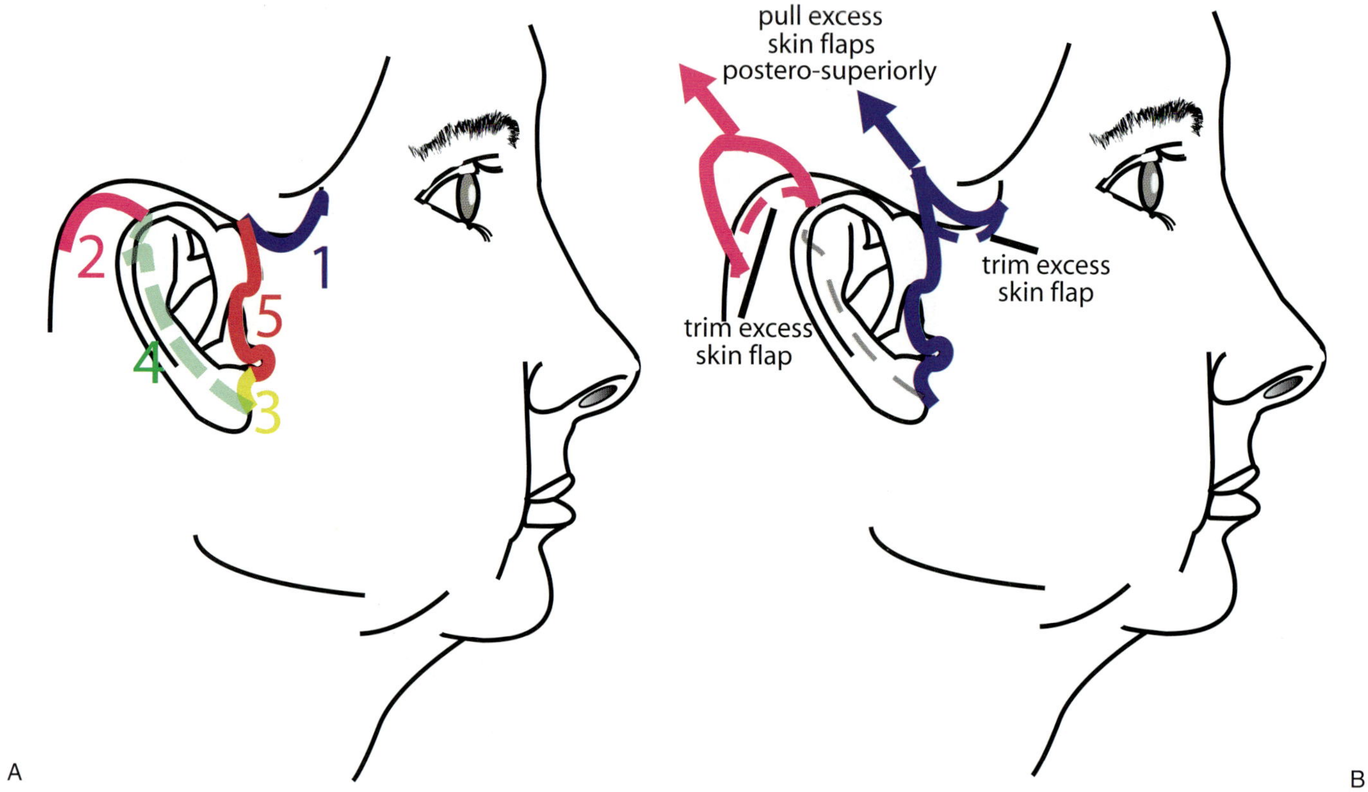

FIGURE 5-33. **A:** Illustration showing the proper sequence for skin redraping, excision, and closure. Skin of temporal region is redraped, excised, and closed *(1)*. Skin of the hairline region is redraped, excised, and closed *(2)*. The redundant lobule skin is excised *(3)*. The postauricular skin is trimmed, a drain is inserted, and the incision closed *(4)*. The preauricular or posttragal incision is trimmed and closed *(5)*. Resection of redundant skin around the lobule always should be carried out after temporal and hairline suspension in order to avoid a pixie ear deformity caused by excessive traction at this point. **B:** The temporal flap should be turned supero-posteriorly and then trimmed. Similarly, the postauricular or hairline flap should be turned supero-posteriorly and trimmed.

closed with a 5-0 Nylon suture in a running, locking fashion (Fig. 5-34). The skin along the hairline then is carefully redraped in a postero-superior vector (Fig. 5-33B) with no tension, and the excess skin is trimmed along the hairline and tacked into place with 5-0 chromic sutures (superiorly where the incision departs the hairline and approaches the ear) and surgical staples more posteriorly along the hairline (Fig. 5-35). At this point, the skin has been redraped and secured anteriorly and posteriorly to the ear with the remaining excess of skin obscuring the inferior aspect of the ear (Fig. 5-36). Before continuing, the surgeon should infiltrate local anesthesia to the other side of the face to allow for sufficient time to achieve hemostasis and adequate anesthesia. The surgeon can now safely trim the redundant skin covering the lower auricle with a pair of serrated Metzenbaum scissors down to expose the lobule (Fig. 5-37A). The surgeon should always aim toward a conservative trimming, especially during the initial pass of the scissors, to avoid tension on closure of the lobule (Fig. 5-37B). If the surgeon believes that he or she has trimmed too far past the lobule, then he or she can reapproximate the transected skin to the desired point. Similarly, if a patient presents with a pixie ear deformity, the surgeon can correct this problem with a V-to-Y advancement. (Refer to the following section for further details.)

Postauricularly, the V-shaped notch that was created at the time of initial skin incision between the postauricular sulcus and hairline (to prevent scar contracture) is recreated in the newly redraped flap and suture fixated with several interrupted 5-0 chromic sutures. Remaining excessive skin along the postauricular sulcus is trimmed and closed with a running 5-0 chromic suture (Fig. 5-38A). Prior to complete closure with the 5-0 chromic suture postauricularly, an 8-French red rubber catheter should be inserted at the midpoint of the incision to provide drainage (Fig. 5-38B). The excess skin that now remains anteriorly should be trimmed to match the curvilinear preauricular incision with careful attention to thin the tragal region appropriately (Fig. 5-39A,B,C). The preauricular skin is then closed with a 6-0 polypropylene suture in a running, nonlocking fashion: The suture is not locked for ease of closure and to permit cutting

(text continues on page 135)

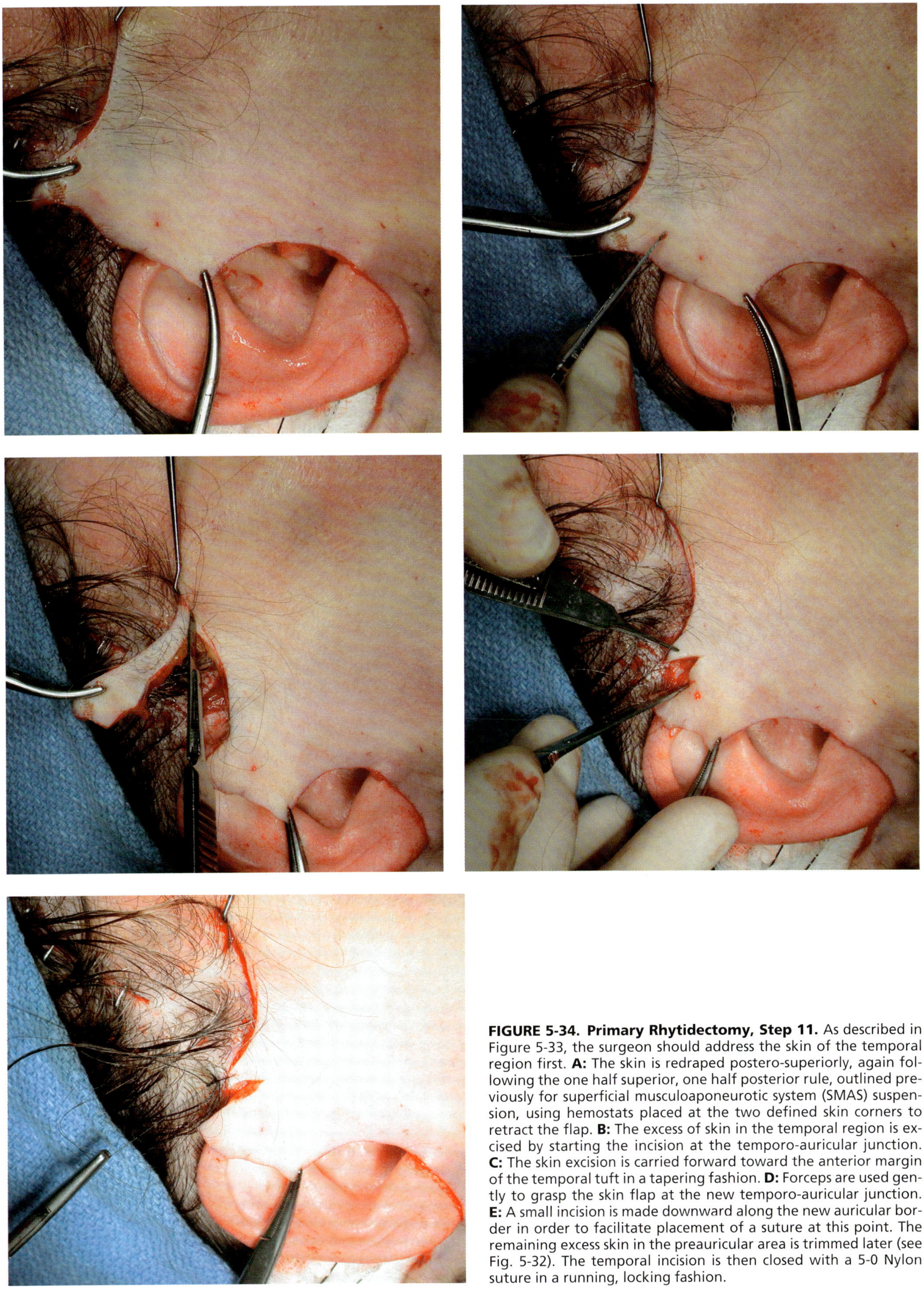

A B C D E

FIGURE 5-34. Primary Rhytidectomy, Step 11. As described in Figure 5-33, the surgeon should address the skin of the temporal region first. **A:** The skin is redraped postero-superiorly, again following the one half superior, one half posterior rule, outlined previously for superficial musculoaponeurotic system (SMAS) suspension, using hemostats placed at the two defined skin corners to retract the flap. **B:** The excess of skin in the temporal region is excised by starting the incision at the temporo-auricular junction. **C:** The skin excision is carried forward toward the anterior margin of the temporal tuft in a tapering fashion. **D:** Forceps are used gently to grasp the skin flap at the new temporo-auricular junction. **E:** A small incision is made downward along the new auricular border in order to facilitate placement of a suture at this point. The remaining excess skin in the preauricular area is trimmed later (see Fig. 5-32). The temporal incision is then closed with a 5-0 Nylon suture in a running, locking fashion.

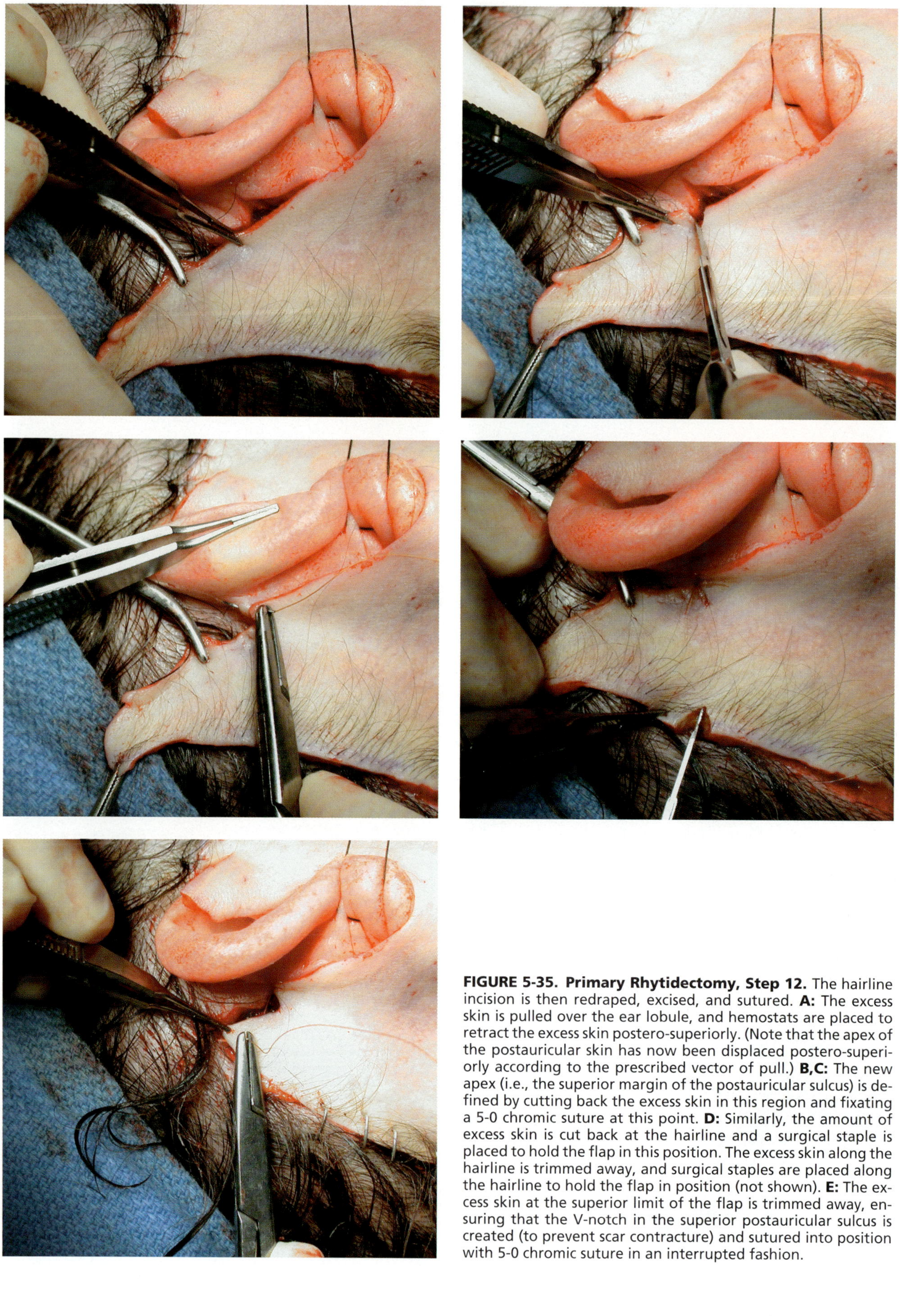

A B C D E

FIGURE 5-35. Primary Rhytidectomy, Step 12. The hairline incision is then redraped, excised, and sutured. **A:** The excess skin is pulled over the ear lobule, and hemostats are placed to retract the excess skin postero-superiorly. (Note that the apex of the postauricular skin has now been displaced postero-superiorly according to the prescribed vector of pull.) **B,C:** The new apex (i.e., the superior margin of the postauricular sulcus) is defined by cutting back the excess skin in this region and fixating a 5-0 chromic suture at this point. **D:** Similarly, the amount of excess skin is cut back at the hairline and a surgical staple is placed to hold the flap in this position. The excess skin along the hairline is trimmed away, and surgical staples are placed along the hairline to hold the flap in position (not shown). **E:** The excess skin at the superior limit of the flap is trimmed away, ensuring that the V-notch in the superior postauricular sulcus is created (to prevent scar contracture) and sutured into position with 5-0 chromic suture in an interrupted fashion.

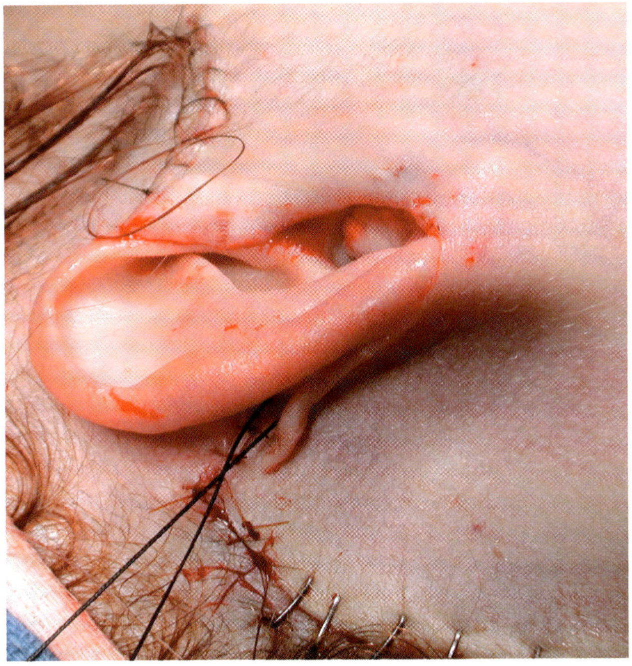

FIGURE 5-36. Primary Rhytidectomy, Step 13. At this point, the skin has been redraped and secured anteriorly and posteriorly to the ear with the remaining excess of skin obscuring the inferior aspect of the ear.

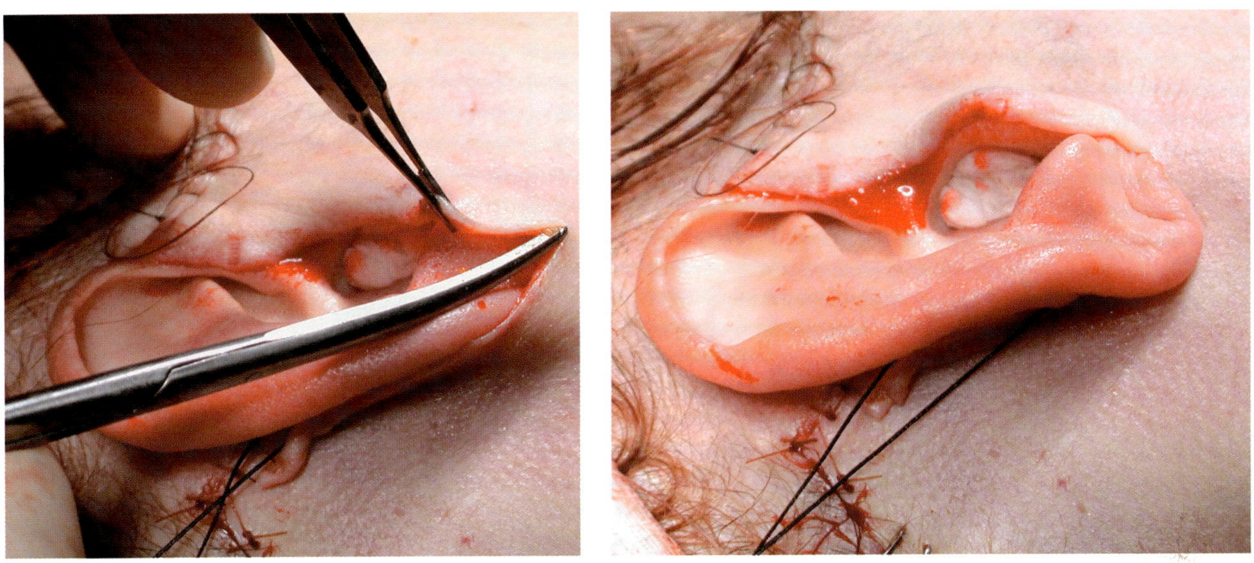

A B

FIGURE 5-37. Primary Rhytidectomy, Step 14. A: The surgeon can now safely trim the redundant skin covering the lower auricle with a pair of serrated Metzenbaum scissors down to expose the lobule. **B:** The surgeon should always aim toward a conservative trimming, especially during the initial pass of the scissors, to avoid tension on closure of the lobule.

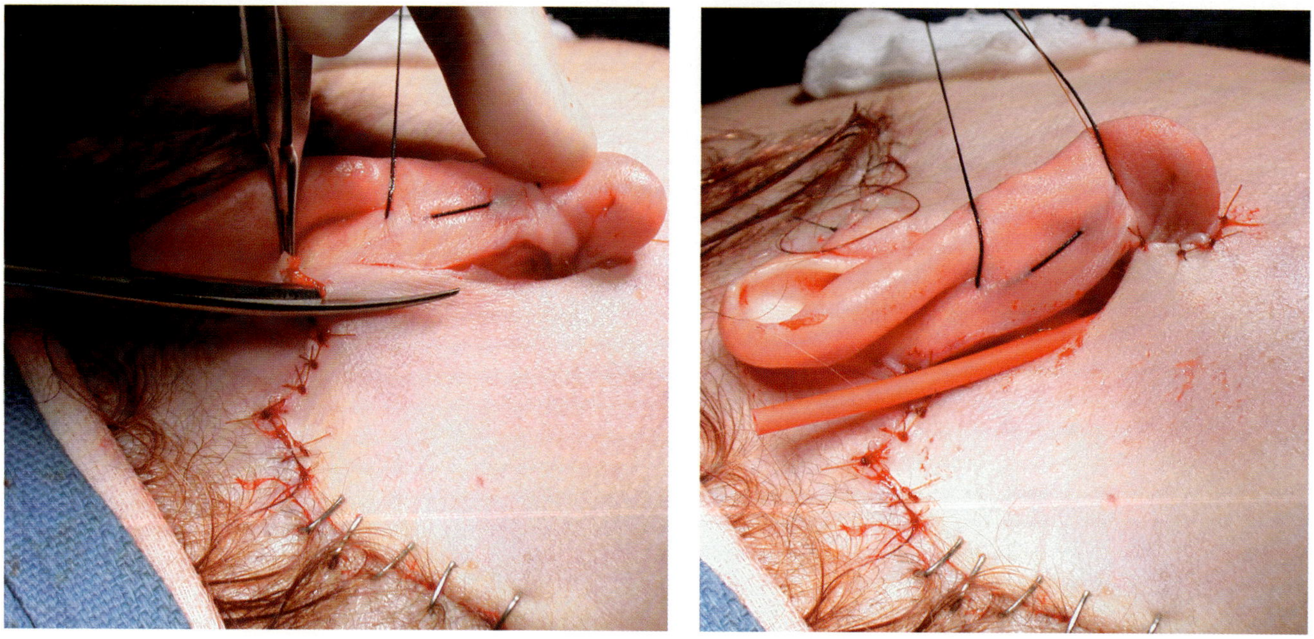

A B

FIGURE 5-38. Primary Rhytidectomy, Step 15. A: Remaining excessive skin along the postauricular sulcus is trimmed and closed with a running 5-0 chromic suture. **B:** Prior to complete closure with the 5-0 chromic suture postauricularly, half of a red rubber catheter should be inserted at the midpoint of the incision to provide drainage (which is removed the following day.)

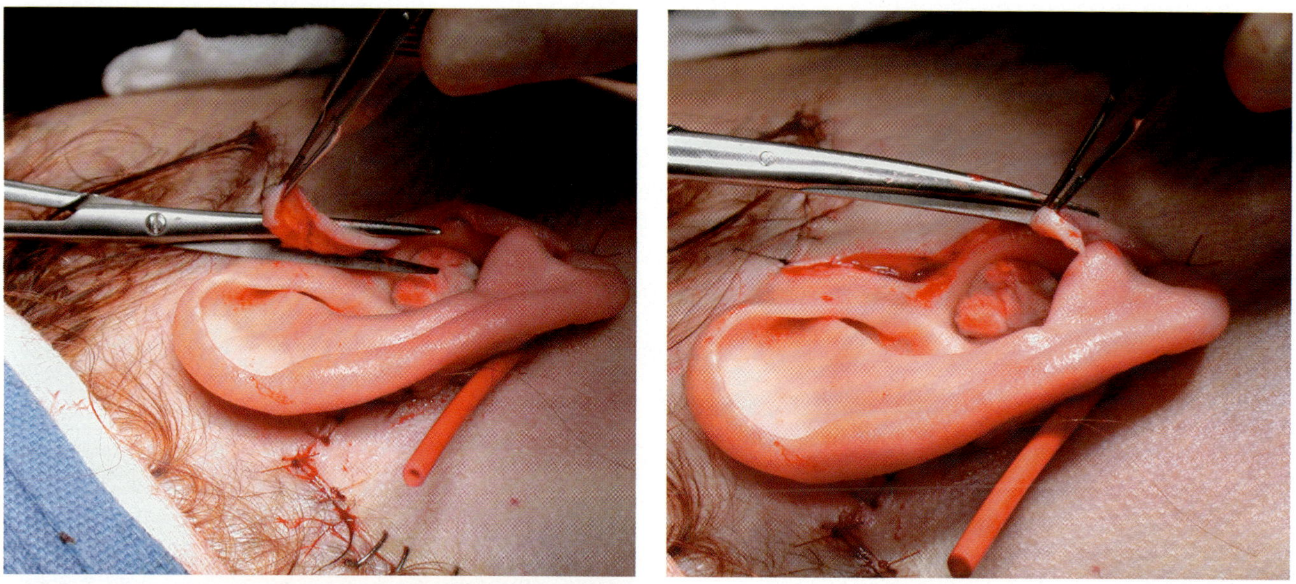

A B

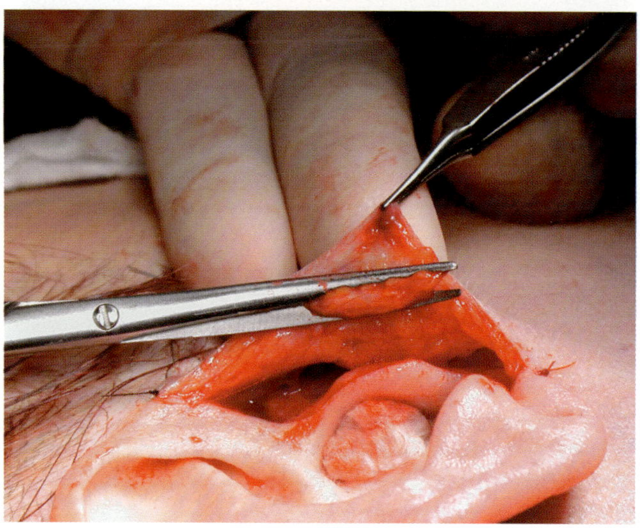

C

FIGURE 5-39. Primary Rhytidectomy, Step 16. A–C: The excess skin that now remains anteriorly should be trimmed to match the curvilinear preauricular incision, with careful attention to thin the tragal region appropriately.

every other suture at 7 days postoperatively, as described in the postoperative section.

The contralateral side of the face is completed in the same manner as described in the preceding. By convention, the authors complete the right side of the face prior to the left side: Whatever progression the reader ultimately decides to follow, he or she is encouraged to remain consistent in that order. Also, the reader is reminded that local anesthesia for the contralateral face always should be infiltrated 10 to 15 minutes prior to actual incision on that side for ideal anesthesia and hemostasis. The hair should not be cleaned with peroxide unless the hair color is already white for risk of unintended bleaching. Placement of a heavily moistened laparotomy pad around the hair-bearing head absorbs most of the blood during the operation and usually eliminates the need for any painstaking cleaning. At the end of the case, a pressure dressing is fashioned in the following manner. Bacitracin ointment is applied to all incision sites before the placement of the dressing. A 4 × 4 gauze with a curvilinear incision to accommodate the shape of the ear is placed over each ear, followed by several uncut 4 × 4 gauze sponges on top (Fig. 5-40A). Additional 4 × 4 gauze dressings are placed

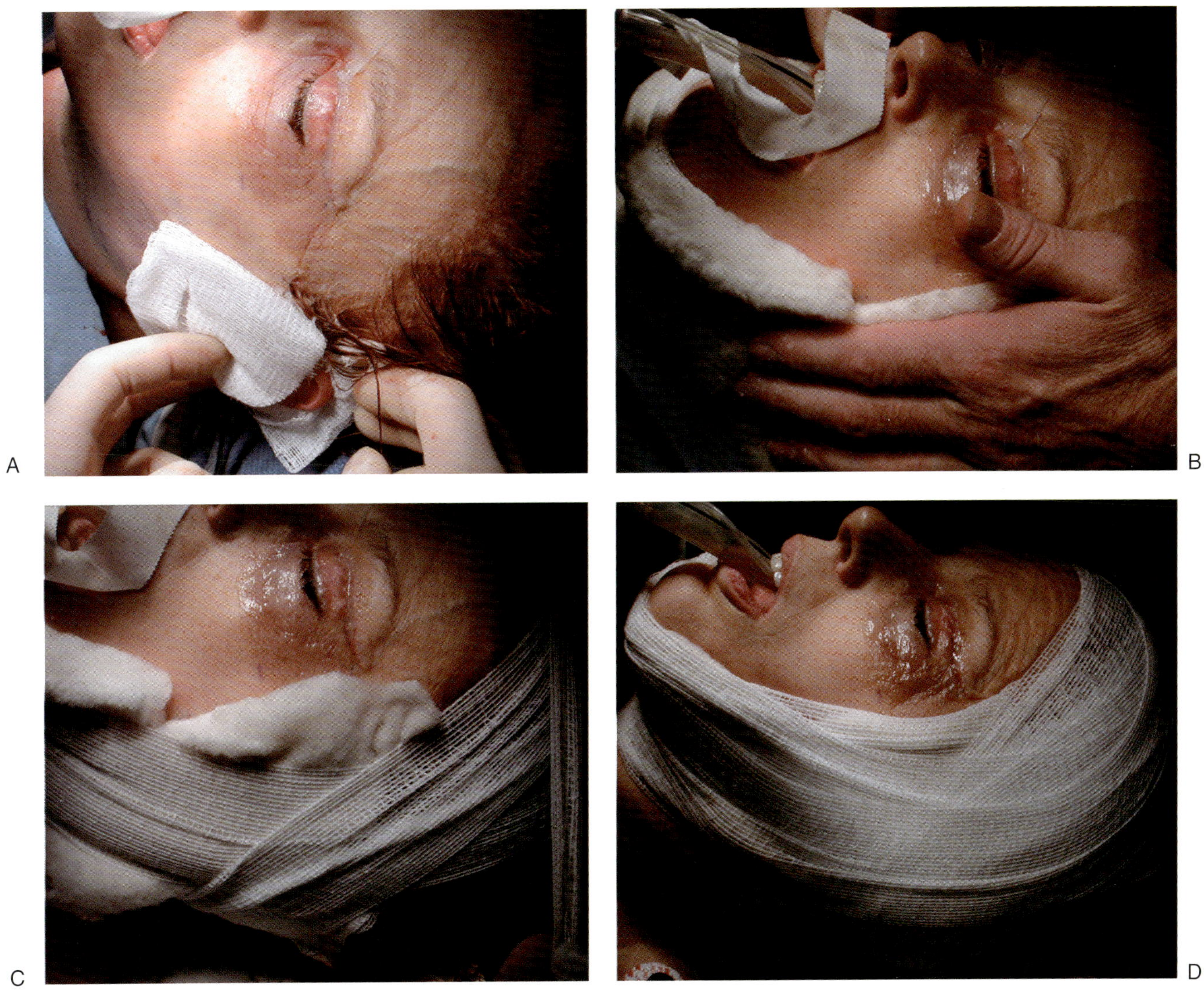

FIGURE 5-40. Primary Rhytidectomy, Step 17. A–D: At the end of the case, a pressure dressing is fashioned in the following manner. Bacitracin ointment is applied to all incision sites prior to the placement of the dressing. **A:** A 4 × 4 gauze with a curvilinear incision to accommodate the shape of the ear is placed over each ear, followed by several uncut 4 × 4 gauze sponges on top. Additional 4 × 4 gauze dressings are placed in the postauricular area. A folded 4 × 4 gauze is placed immediately over the submental incision site. **B:** Thick cotton dressing is applied over the 4 × 4 gauze along the jaw line and over the postauricular site for additional reinforcement. The cotton dressing always should rest superficially to the 4 × 4 gauze and not make direct contact with the skin or hair because it tends to adhere tenaciously, making its removal tedious. **C,D:** Finally, a 3-in. conforming bandage (Kling) is secured over the dressing in two vectors: (1) from the submental area to the superior aspect of the head, like a Barton's bandage; and (2) from occiput to forehead.

in the postauricular area. Folded 4 × 4 gauze is placed immediately over the submental incision site. Thick cotton dressing is applied over the 4 × 4 gauze along the jaw line and over the postauricular site for additional reinforcement (Fig. 5-40B). The cotton dressing should always rest superficially to the 4 × 4 gauze and not make direct contact with the skin or hair because it tends to adhere tenaciously, making removal of it a tedious exercise. Finally, a 3" conforming gauze bandage, or Kling, is secured over the dressing in two vectors: (a) from the submental area to the superior aspect of the head, like a Barton's bandage; and (b) from occiput to forehead (Fig. 5-40C,D). The reader is advised not to overtighten the Kling wrap but to exert only enough force to circumscribe the head. Although the above text appears to be self-explanatory, proper application of dressing is not always intuitive and can avoid needless headaches.

Superficial Musculoaponeurotic System Insertion for Augmentation of the Nasolabial and Labiomandibular Folds

For the sake of clarity, insertion of SMAS tissue to augment the nasolabial and labiomandibular folds is separately presented from primary rhytidectomy. Clearly, this adjunctive procedure can only be performed during a rhytidectomy when the tissue is harvested during resection of SMAS for imbrication. Rather than discarding this extra tissue, it can be used to augment the nasolabial and labiomandibular folds. The technique is the same as that described for acellular dermis (Alloderm, Lifecell Corp., Branchburg, NJ) and ePTFE in Chapter 8.

This section presents precisely how to insert the SMAS tissue to augment the labiomandibular folds. As expected, the same technique applies to augmentation of the nasolabial folds. The lips should not be augmented with SMAS for several reasons. The amount of SMAS is generally insufficient to augment the nasolabial, labiomandibular, and labial regions. More important, SMAS is typically too irregular in contour to be acceptable for lip augmentation. Also because the SMAS is more tenuous than acellular dermis or ePTFE, it may break off during insertion and leave only half of the lip augmented. For all these reasons, SMAS insertion should be reserved only for the nasolabial and labiomandibular folds. For more detail about nasolabial fold or lip augmentation, the reader is referred again to Chapter 8.

The SMAS is harvested in the manner prescribed previously (Fig. 5-41). The excised SMAS tissue is then measured to determine the proper length needed to augment the desired fold, and an 0 silk suture is tied to one end of the implant while the other end of the suture is affixed to a long Keith needle (Fig. 5-42).¶ A stab incision is placed at both ends of the labiomandibular fold, and the introducer that resembles a Freer elevator with a central groove is used to create a subcutaneous pocket to receive the implant (Fig. 5-43). The aforementioned needle is then passed into the central groove of the introducer device (Fig. 5-44), and the introducer is then removed with the needle still in position. Tiny, double hooks are used to retract the wound edges while the needle is pulled through in order to draw the implant into the recipient pocket (Fig. 5-45). A hemostat is placed onto the free end of the SMAS to prevent pulling the SMAS too far through the incision. The excess tissue is trimmed to leave an excess of 1 cm on either end (Fig. 5-46), and fine-toothed forceps are used to tuck the excess 1 cm of both ends distal to the incision by this length (Fig. 5-47). (The rationale for this technique is further elaborated in Chapter 8.) The stab inci-

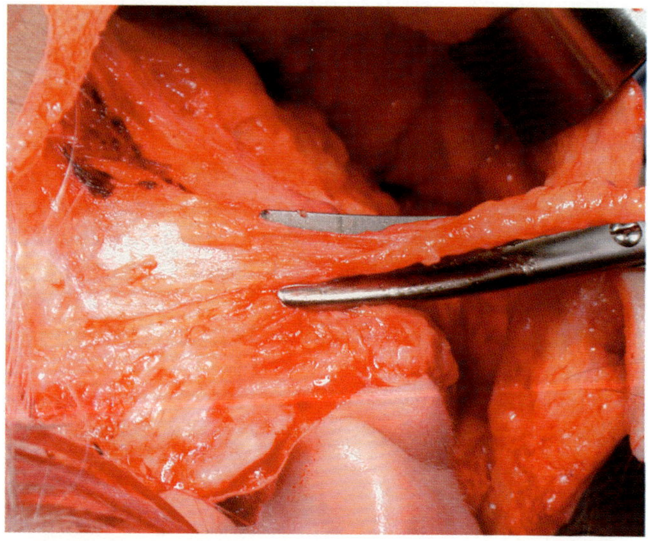

FIGURE 5-41. SMAS Insertion, Step 1. Superficial musculoaponeurotic system tissue is harvested during standard imbrication rhytidectomy and used for augmentation of the nasolabial and labiomandibular folds.

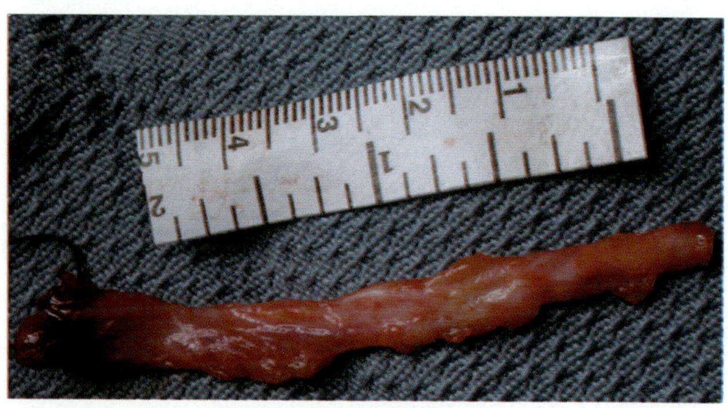

FIGURE 5-42. SMAS Insertion, Step 2. The excised superficial musculoaponeurotic system tissue is then measured to determine the proper length needed to augment the desired fold, and a 0 silk suture is tied to one end of the implant while the other end of the suture comes attached to a 60-mm Keith needle.

¶The introducer that the authors use resembles a Freer elevator with a central groove that accommodates a long Keith-type needle. Rather than use the needle that comes with the kit, the authors use an 0 silk that is already attached to a 60-mm disposable Keith needle.

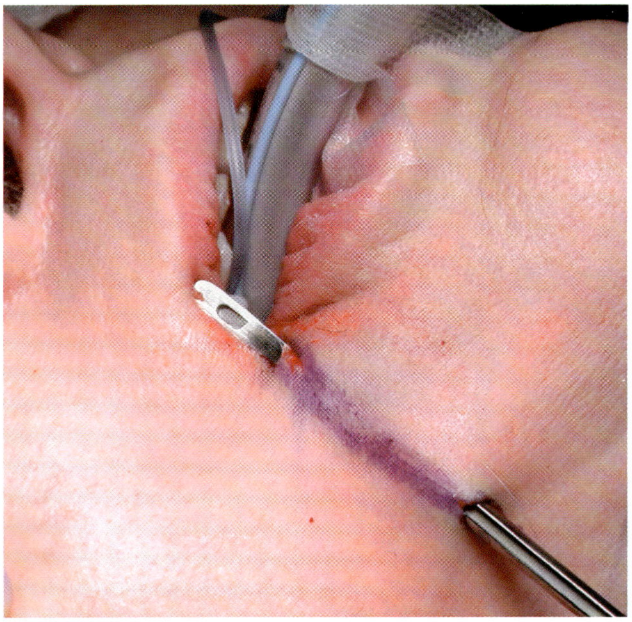

FIGURE 5-43. SMAS Insertion, Step 3. A stab incision is placed at both ends of the labiomandibular fold, and the introducer that resembles a Freer elevator with a central groove is used to create a subcutaneous pocket to receive the implant.

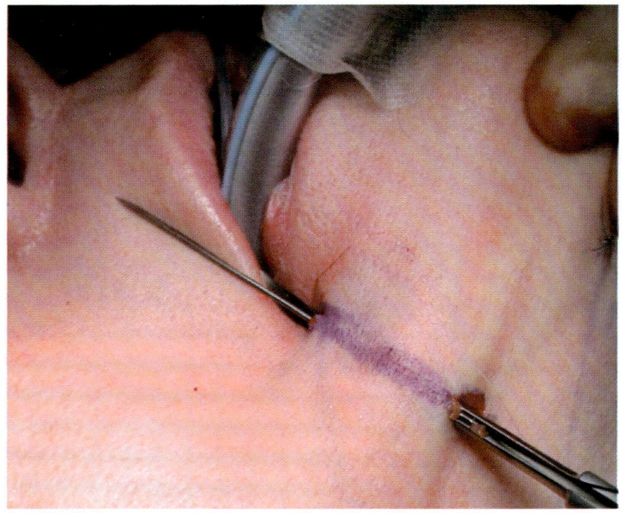

FIGURE 5-44. SMAS Insertion, Step 4. The needle is then passed into the central groove of the introducer.

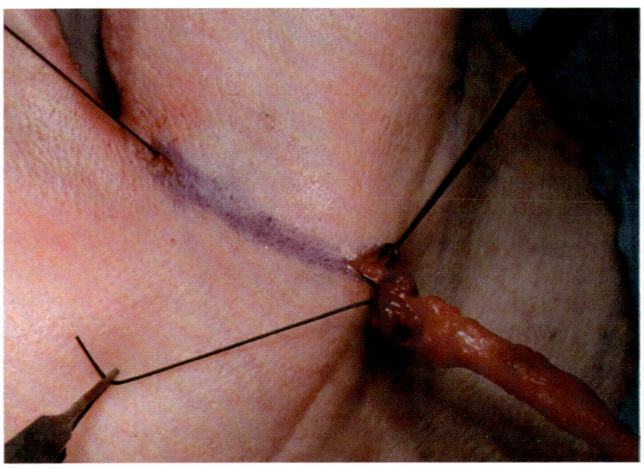

FIGURE 5-45. SMAS Insertion, Step 5. After the introducer is withdrawn, tiny double hooks are used to retract the wound edges as the needle is pulled through in order to draw the implant into the recipient pocket.

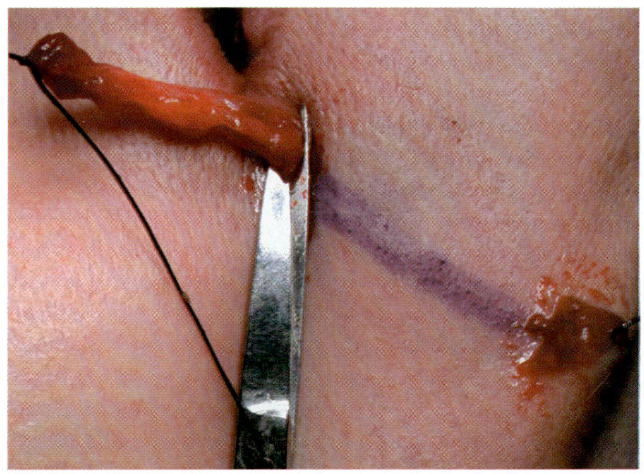

FIGURE 5-46. SMAS Insertion, Step 6. The excess tissue is trimmed leaving an excess of 1 cm of superficial musculoaponeurotic system tissue on both ends.

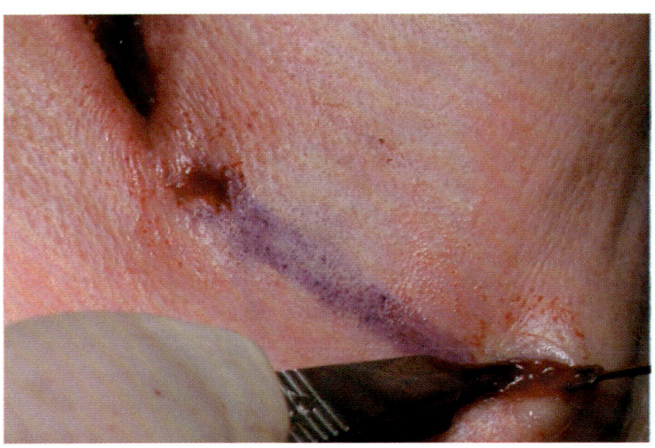

FIGURE 5-47. SMAS Insertion, Step 7. Fine-toothed forceps are used to tuck the excess 1-cm tails further distal to the incision sites.

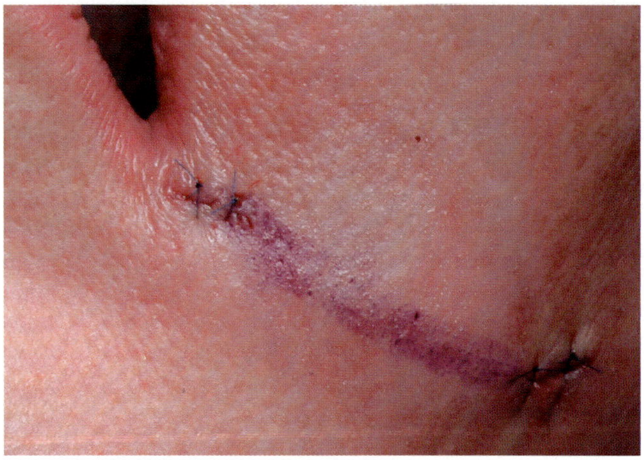

FIGURE 5-48. SMAS Insertion, Step 8. The incisions are then closed with interrupted 6-0 polypropylene sutures.

sions are closed with interrupted 6-0 polypropylene sutures (Fig. 5-48). Usually two sutures per incision should suffice.

Secondary Rhytidectomy

A secondary rhytidectomy is inevitable because all individuals continue to mature and require additional surgery later to maintain their rejuvenative appearance. The timing and extent of surgery is predicated on the combined extrinsic and intrinsic factors that lead to further aging. The procedure can be a straightforward or complicated affair, often depending on whether the surgeon is operating on his or her own handiwork or someone else's. This practical distinction has already been addressed in the preoperative section of this chapter. However, it is worthwhile to reiterate two important principles: (a) *very little if any skin need usually be excised in a secondary rhytidectomy;* and (b) decision to revise the placement of unfavorable incisions is determined in part by the laxity of skin that will permit translocation of the incision (e.g., movement of an incision from a pretragal to a posttragal position).

The next factor that should be determined, just as in a primary rhytidectomy, concerns the intended area for rejuvenation (e.g., submental, jowl, etc.). If the anterior platysmal bands were already sutured together during primary rhytidectomy and no visible platysmal cords are evident, then this procedure need not be repeated. However, even in the most assured previous platysmal closure, the returning patient may exhibit platysmal diastasis that mandates repeat muscular approximation. Alternatively, submental undermining followed by liposuction or lipectomy may be all that is necessary to achieve the desired objective in the cervical region. Often, the submental area may not require any intervention at all. Nevertheless, the submental incision with undermining should be carried out in order to facilitate ePTFE sling placement if this is to be performed. Unlike a primary rhytidectomy, which often necessitates a full-length incision from the anterior temporal region to posterior hairline, a secondary rhytidectomy incision may be more abbreviated and tailored to the precise anatomic area that warrants rejuvenation. Typically, an S-lift type of incision is all that is needed: This S-shaped incision line begins at the superior aspect of the tragus, descends and curves around posttragally, then curves around the base of the lobule to terminate a short distance postauricularly (Fig. 5-49A,B,C). Extensions of this incision anteriorly may be necessary to address any standing-cone deformity that arises. This S-lift incision combined with a submental incision is designed to accommodate an ePTFE sling. The reader is referred to the preoperative considerations section of this chapter for further detail regarding the appropriate candidate for this type of surgery.

Although many types of incisions and techniques exist for secondary rhytidectomy, the following operative description describes an S-lift incision with placement of an ePTFE sling. Recounting the myriad permutations of incisions possible for a secondary rhytidectomy is not a meaningful exercise. Instead, the S-lift incision is described because it is the most common method to achieve improvement in the lower face and cervical regions in a secondary setting, and this limited incision can facilitate ePTFE sling placement. Although an ePTFE sling is an uncommon technique in the authors' practices (accounting for less than 10% of all secondary rhytidectomies), description of this procedure may prove instructive to the reader. Without mention of an ePTFE sling, the following operative narrative would reflect nothing more than an abbreviated primary rhytidectomy that is not worthy of reiteration.

Unlike a formal, primary rhytidectomy, which may require a few hours of labor, a secondary rhytidectomy may only require an hour or so to complete—if no significant revision work is required to reposition the existing incisions. For this reason, the patient may not need deep anesthesia but rather tolerate lighter intravenous midazolam sedation instead. Prior to sedation, if an ePTFE sling is to be undertaken, the precise location of the cervico-mental angle should be marked out with the patient in the sitting position so that the ePTFE sling can be properly situated at this level. Because of the shorter time frame, the surgeon should elect to infiltrate the local anesthesia into the submental region and both sides of the face at the outset if the projected time should be an hour or less. As per routine, the submental incision (refer to the section on submentoplasty for further detail) is undertaken initially, and submental undermining and liposuction carried out. The extent of undermining should be sufficient to visualize and pass the ePTFE sling. Therefore, the submental incision is not closed until the sling already has been passed through, secured, and verified.

Next, the aforementioned S-lift incision is executed on the right side of the face that extends along posttragally around the lobule to expose the mastoid periosteum, where the ePTFE sling will be anchored. As explained for primary rhytidectomy, the dissection is begun sharply with a No. 15

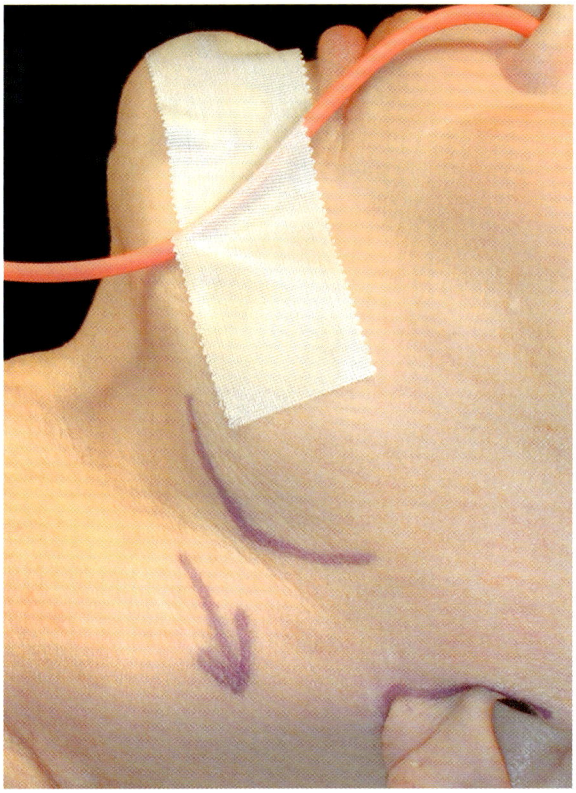

A

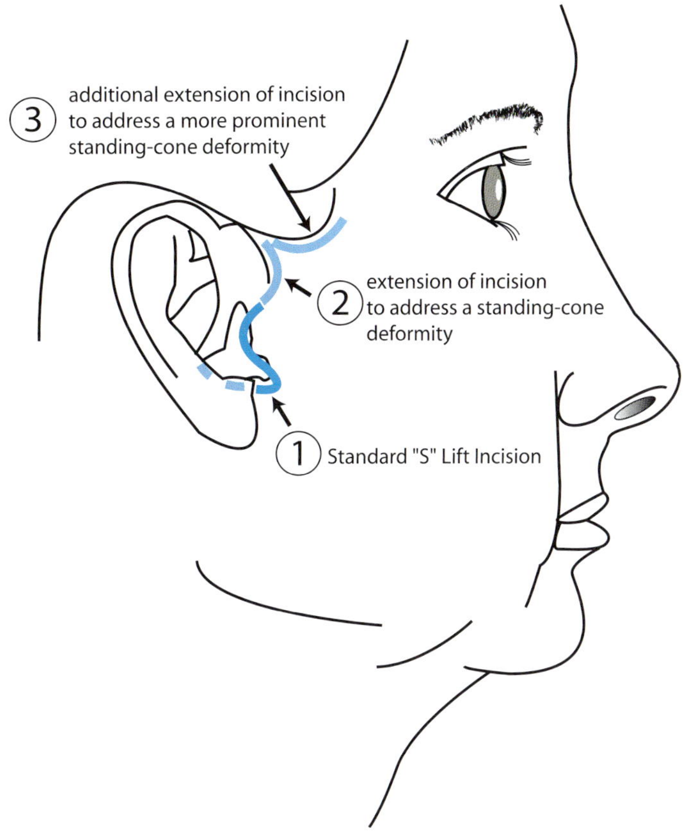

C

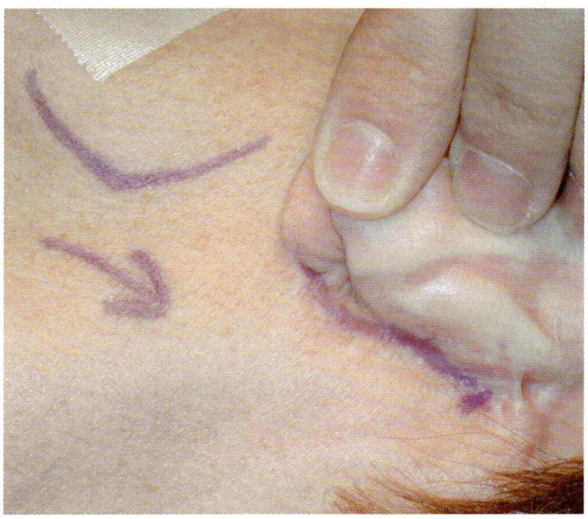

B

FIGURE 5-49. Secondary Rhytidectomy with ePTFE Sling Sequence. A,B: The length of the incision for a secondary rhytidectomy can be more abbreviated in length whether an expanded polytetrafluoroethylene sling is performed or not. **C:** The configuration resembles an S-shape, hence the name S-lift. This abbreviated length is also suitable for younger patients who do not have significant skin redundancy but only some incipient jowling. To address a standing-cone deformity that may arise, the anterior skin incision can be extended up to or all the way around the temporal tuft as needed.

Bard-Parker blade and continued with Metzenbaum or facelift scissors. Flap undermining should be adequate for placement of SMAS suspension sutures and to pass the ePTFE sling around to the other side. SMAS suspension sutures are placed along the jaw line in the plication method described for primary rhytidectomy; only one to two sutures usually can be completed because of the more limited size of the incision. An imbrication of the SMAS (i.e., SMAS excision) often is unnecessary and difficult to execute through the shorter incision.

The size of the ePTFE sling preferred is 2 × 30 cm; and it should be prestretched using two heavy clamps affixed to both ends so that the original 2-cm width is approximately narrowed by one third (Fig. 5-50). Although stretching of the ePTFE sling and all subsequent manipulation of the implant are undertaken on the sterile field, any preparation of the implant with povidone-iodine, or equivalent sterilizing solution is a superfluous task because ePTFE is hydrophobic by nature. After the sling has been stretched, it is then secured with several (four to five) buried sutures of CV-4

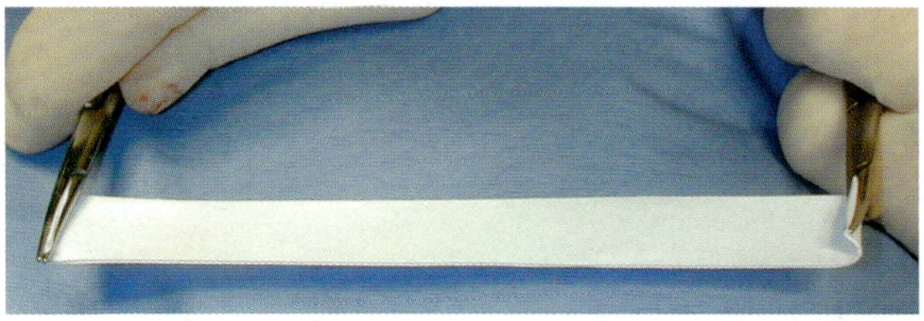

FIGURE 5-50. Secondary Rhytidectomy with ePTFE Sling Sequence. The size of the expanded polytetrafluoroethylene sling should be 2 × 30 cm; and it should be pre-stretched using two heavy clamps affixed to both ends so that the original 2-cm width is approximately narrowed by one third.

Gore-Tex to the mastoid periosteum (Fig. 5-51) and then passed through the submental incision with a long hemostat. The contralateral S-incision and SMAS suspension are carried out in the same manner. After that, the ePTFE sling is passed back through the submental incision to the other side of the face, and its position should be verified through the submental incision (i.e., the contour should be flat and situated at the cervico-mental angle).

The length of the sling should be trimmed so that the distance extends to the mastoid periosteum without significant tension or lack thereof. Overtightening of the sling results in difficulty swallowing and breathing, as well as persistent discomfort. However, the patient routinely experiences some constrictive sensation for several weeks postoperatively, about which he or she should be properly informed. The sling is then secured to the mastoid periosteum with four to five buried sutures of CV-4 Gore-Tex, as described for the contralateral side of the face. Again, the position of the sling should be verified by visual inspection through all three incisions and confirmed by palpation before closure. The postauricular incisions are closed with 4-0 chromic suture in a running, nonlocking fashion, and a red rubber catheter should be placed at the midpoint of the incision during closure. The preauricular skin is carefully inspected for any redundancy and excess skin is trimmed: The reader is reminded that more often than not no skin at all is excised. The preauricular incisions are then approximated with 6-0 polypropylene in a running, nonlocking fashion. Finally, the submental incision is closed with 6-0 polypropylene in a running, locking manner. Bacitracin is applied to all incision sites before a pressure dressing (as described in detail in the primary rhytidectomy section) is placed.

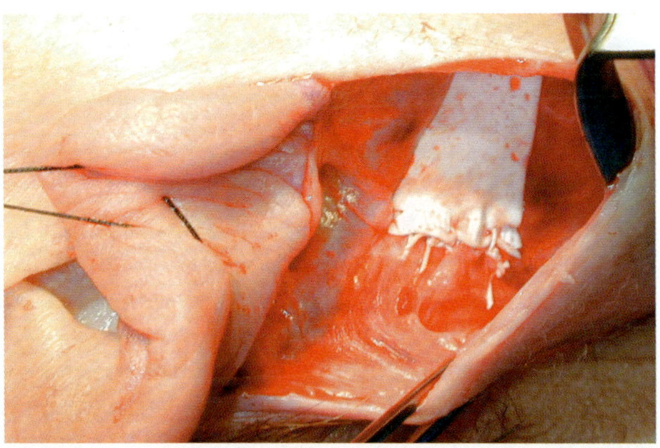

FIGURE 5-51. Secondary Rhytidectomy with ePTFE Sling Sequence. After the sling has been stretched, it is then secured with several (four to five) buried sutures of CV-4 Gore-Tex to the mastoid periosteum and then passed through the submental incision with a long hemostat.

Lobule Reduction

Although lobule reduction is an infrequent surgical request, its technical aspects are worth a brief discussion. Several techniques exist to correct the descended lobule; which technique, or combination thereof, is selected depends in part on the principal pathology. If the unattached, fleshy portion is too large and dependent, then the excessive tissue needs to be trimmed and repositioned. However, if the attached segment is displaced too far inferiorly either because of prior surgery (the so-called pixie or devil's ear deformity) or by gravitational descent of the lower face, then a V-to-Y advancement is required. Obviously, a combination of pathology mandates selective use of both techniques. If the patient is to undergo a concomitant rhytidectomy, then the attached earlobe position can be set at that time to whatever height deemed aesthetically appropriate by the surgeon, and the fleshy redundancy can be trimmed and recontoured as well.

In order to remove an excessive, unattached, and pendulous lobule, the amount of reduction should be estimated visually. The method by which the lobule is reduced is resection of a vertical wedge or starplasty configuration. A simple wedge whose apex emanates centrally can be used to remove small portions of redundancy, whereas larger areas must be excised with a more generous starplasty technique. The incision is closed with an interrupted 6-0 silk suture. It may be helpful to place the vertical limb of the wedge or star in the slot of the pierced ear to minimize any visible scarring. The reader is referred to the illustration and photographs for proper tissue removal and thereby reduction of the ear lobule (Fig. 5-52A,D–G).

Several techniques are available to correct a pixie ear deformity or to return a long, attached lobule to a more youthful position. For a mild to moderate amount of lobular descent, a V-to-Y advancement may be used to correct this problem (Fig. 5-52B). First, the new, desired position of the lobule should be marked at the lobular–facial interface. A No. 15 blade is used to dissect down through the dermis in a V configuration along the lateral and inferior aspects of the lobule for a distance that matches the desired amount of advancement. However, the lobule maintains its attachment to the deep tissues (subcutaneous fat) directly below. Undermining is undertaken for a short distance around the lobule so that the lobular island pedicle can be easily advanced upward to the desired position in a V-to-Y fashion. The skin is then closed behind the advanced lobule.

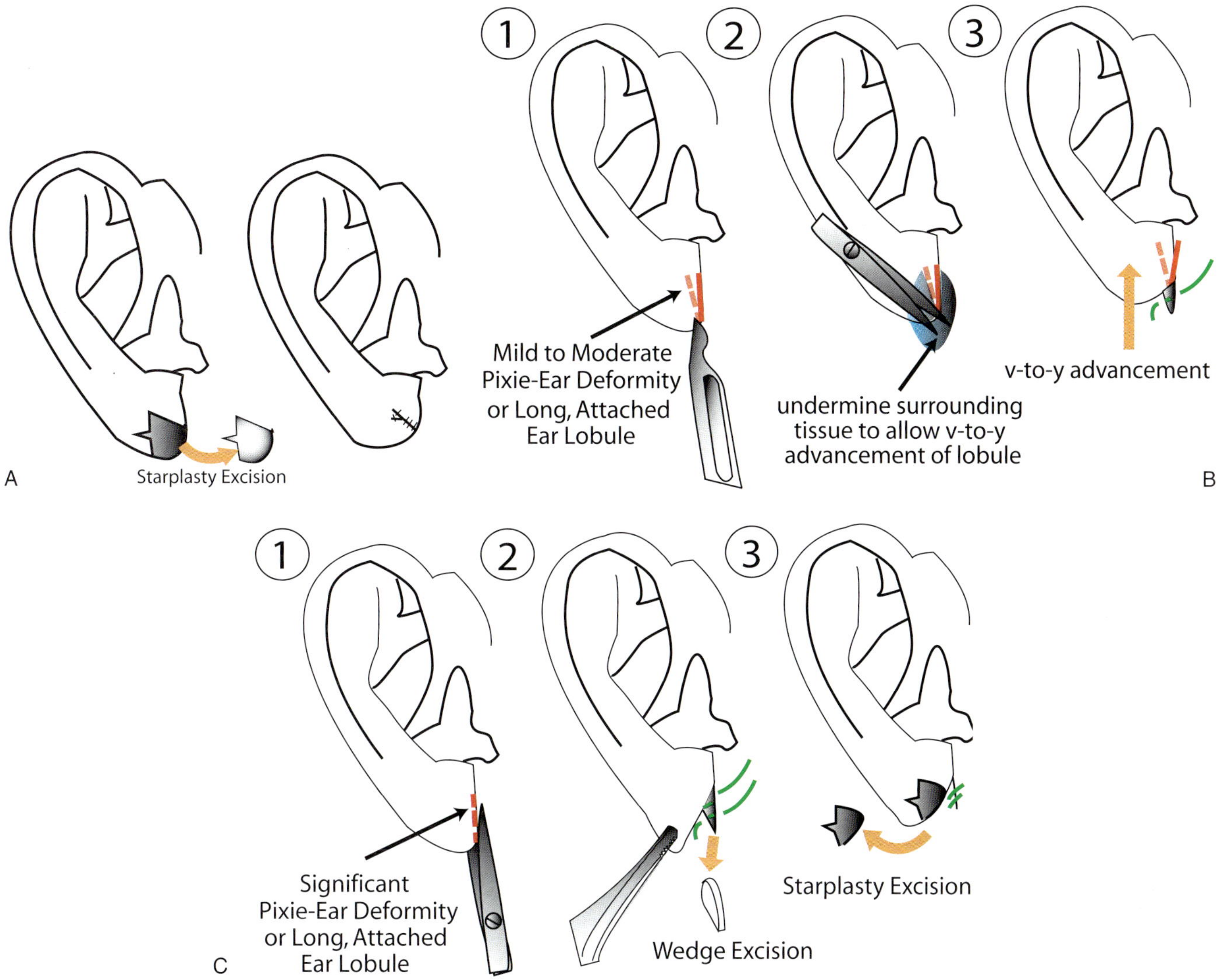

FIGURE 5-52. Lobule Reduction Sequence. A: Illustration showing proper technique for limited lobule reduction using a wedge excision of tissue in which the apex originates centrally and a posterior wedge is incised for larger resections in a "starplasty" technique. For a pixie ear deformity or a long, attached ear lobule, two techniques are available. **B:** For a mild to moderate amount of lobular descent, a V-to-Y advancement may be used to correct this problem. First, the new, desired position of the lobule should be marked at the lobular–facial interface **(1)**. A No. 15 blade is used to dissect down through the dermis in a V configuration along the lateral and inferior aspects of the lobule for a distance that matches the desired amount of advancement. The lobule however maintains its attachment to the deep tissues (subcutaneous fat) directly below. **(2)** Undermining is undertaken for a short distance around the lobule so that **(3)** the lobular island pedicle can be easily advanced upward to the desired position in a V-to-Y fashion. The skin is then closed behind the advanced lobule. **C:** For a significant pixie ear deformity or a very long, attached lobule, the V-to-Y method will not work because the lobule will bunch when advanced superiorly. **(1)** In these more extreme cases, the lobule should be severed from its facial attachment. **(2)** The facial skin can then be reapproximated: A wedge of skin may need to be removed to facilitate easy closure. **(3)** Finally, the excess lobular tissue should be resected and closed in a starplasty fashion. *(continued)*

For a significant pixie ear deformity or a very long, attached lobule, the V-to-Y method will not work because the lobule will bunch when advanced superiorly (Fig. 5-52C). In these more extreme cases, the lobule should be severed from its facial attachment. The facial skin can then be reapproximated: A wedge of skin may need to be removed to facilitate easy closure. Finally, the excess lobular tissue should be resected and closed in a starplasty fashion.

The ear may be repierced 6 weeks later using a very simple technique. After infiltration of local anesthesia, an 18-

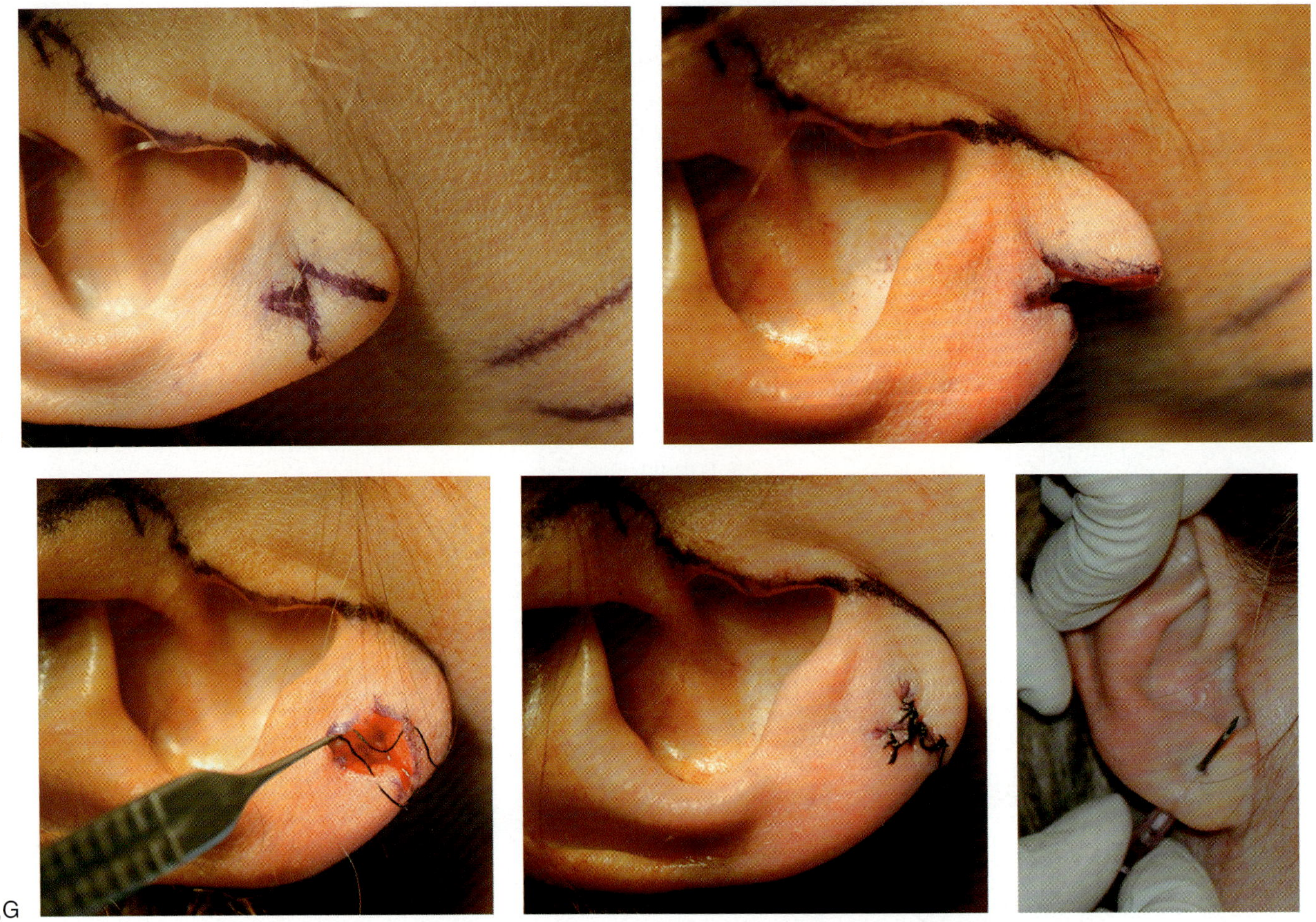

D E F,G H

FIGURE 5-52. *(Continued)* **D:** Photographs showing the planned excision of the excessive lobule in a starplasty design. **E:** After excision of the starplasty wedge. **F:** Trifurcation suture used to close the starplasty incision. **G:** Closure of the ear lobule with 6-0 silk in an interrupted fashion. **H:** The ear is repierced 6 weeks later after lobule reduction using an 18-gauge needle passed posterior to anterior and then the stud should be passed anterior to posterior.

Salient Technical Points

Submentoplasty

1. The submental incision should be placed slightly posterior (approximately 1 mm) to the submental crease to avoid an overly deep crease from developing.
2. Liposuction should be performed only after wide and even undermining with sharp Metzenbaum scissors so that the tunneling, created by the liposuction cannula, will not be observed postoperatively as an irregular skin contour.
3. The aperture of the liposuction cannula always should face downward away from the overlying flap to avoid development of an irregular skin contour.
4. A central lipectomy should be reserved only for patients with limited adipose deposit centrally or used in conjunction with wide liposuction in order to avoid a "cobra" deformity. Platysmal plication also should be carried out after liposuction except in the younger patient, also in order to avoid a cobra deformity.
5. The platysmaplasty should be begun with short back cuts at the level of the cervico-mental angle in order to recreate a more defined appearance of the angle.

Chin Augmentation with Expanded Polytetrafluoroethylene

1. Mersilene mesh is more cost effective than ePTFE but requires greater preparatory effort both preoperatively and intraoperatively and may be associated with slightly more postoperative edema.
2. Chin augmentation can benefit a patient who will undergo a rhytidectomy by augmentation of the

labiomandibular sulci with an extended implant, by providing a point of tension for the overlying skin and SMAS redraping, and by increasing the submental area so that the submental adipose is distributed over a larger area rather than in a discrete bulge.
3. The incision should be placed slightly posterior to the submental crease and even more posteriorly for a larger implant.
4. The implant is placed in a supraperiosteal pocket centrally and a subperiosteal pocket laterally for maximal stability and projection.
5. A buried 4-0 polydioxanone suture is used to close the mentalis muscle and secure the implant prior to skin closure—an unnecessary step for a simple submentoplasty.

Chin Augmentation with Mersilene Mesh

1. The 30- × 30-cm sheet of Mersilene mesh is rolled over a cardboard template (10- × 1-cm in size) nine times to achieve a 10-layered implant.
2. The cardboard template is removed, and the mesh trimmed to the proper size.
3. The rolled implant is held together using a 4-0 polydioxanone suture in an interrupted fashion.
4. The same method is used to fashion the smaller 5- × 1-cm sized implants.
5. Each of these created segments is individually sterilized to be used for insertion at time of surgery.
6. The 10- × 1-cm base segment can be combined with a 5- × 1-cm base segment to achieve a medium-sized augmentation. A smaller amount of augmentation can be obtained with a single 10- × 1-cm implant, whereas large augmentation is accomplished with two 5- × 1-cm segments affixed to a 10- × 1-cm base segment. For the pointed chin, two 10- × 1-cm implants may be used to create a fuller lateral dimension to the chin. The implant segments are sutured together using 4-0 polydioxanone sutures in an interrupted fashion to achieve the desired height and configuration.
7. The lateral edges of the 10- × 1-cm implant are trimmed to a tapered point for ease of insertion.
8. The same technique is used for insertion of the Mersilene mesh implant as for the ePTFE implant (see the preceding).

Primary Rhytidectomy

1. A curvilinear incision that preserves the temporal tuft, follows the posttragal contour, and extends along the entire postauricular sulcus to terminate along the hairline is favored for optimal camouflage and preservation of hair-bearing skin. A small V-notch is placed in the superior aspect of the postauricular sulcus near the junction with the hairline to avoid unfavorable scar contracture.
2. Superficial musculoaponeurotic system sutures are distributed so that the vector of suspension is one half vertical and one half horizontal in direction, except along the jaw line.
3. An imbrication technique (SMAS resection) is favored in order to prevent facial widening with plication and also to harvest the SMAS for reinsertion in the nasolabial or labiomandibular regions. A plication technique may be favored in patients with a very narrow face.
4. The skin is only redraped because tension should be provided by the underlying SMAS. The (preauricular) temporal and the (postauricular) hairline areas should be closed prior to resection of the skin overlying the lobule so that any skin tension is suspended preauricularly and postauricularly and no tension will draw the lobule inferiorly.

Secondary Rhytidectomy

1. Skin resection is at times unnecessary or minimal in extent in a revision rhytidectomy, and the length of the incision can be more abbreviated than in a primary rhytidectomy (e.g., the S-lift incision).
2. An ePTFE sling should be reserved only for the patient who is very fastidious, who will have good follow-up, and who understands that palpability and a constrictive sensation may be present postoperatively. The authors have reserved use of this technique only for those patients who meet the preceding criteria and with whom a long-term relationship already has been established (i.e., in the secondary rhytidectomy setting only).

Lobule Resection

Lobular reduction may be effected either via a V-to-Y advancement, resection of a vertical wedge of tissue, or a starplasty for even greater amounts of tissue removal.

gauge needle is passed through the proposed site to be pierced from the posterior to the anterior side, and the earring post (or stud, the principal part of the earring) is slid onto the 18-gauge needle, which is then withdrawn (Fig. 5-52H). The smaller part of the earring is affixed to the backside of the stud to keep the earring in place, which must remain for a 6-week period to ensure enduring patency of the newly created hole.

POSTOPERATIVE CONSIDERATIONS: CARE, FOLLOW-UP, AND COMPLICATIONS

Postoperative Care and Follow-Up

Postoperative care is relatively straightforward, barring unforeseen complications (see following section). The more sizable dressing, applied at the time of the operation, remains in place overnight. On the following day, the patient returns to have the dressing removed and the wounds inspected. Any evidence of a *minimal* hematoma or seroma can be expressed through the drain site using a rolled 4 × 4 gauze; however, this is a rare necessity. The red rubber catheters are removed from each side, and the incision lines are cleaned of any adherent coagulum with peroxide solution and treated with Bacitracin ointment. A lighter dressing that spans the submental region to the top of the head in a Barton's bandage style is fabricated using several 4 × 4 dressings applied to the exposed incisions and one to two 3-inch conforming bandage (Kling) dressings. The patient may remove this dressing the following day at home (i.e., on second postoperative day).

Every other surgical staple is removed and every other preauricular suture is cut (but not removed) on postoperative day 6. The sutures under the temporal tuft of hair and in the submental region are entirely removed. The remaining sutures and staples are removed on postoperative day 8. The patient is asked to return after 1 month, 6 months, and then yearly. If any concomitant skin resurfacing also was performed, then the more vigilant follow up outlined in Chapter 9 is performed.

After a facelift, men can begin shaving 8 days after surgery when all of the sutures and staples have been removed. An electric razor is preferred for a 30-day period to minimize any trauma to the skin flap. Thereafter, shaving with a straight razor can be resumed. The patient should be counseled to be careful shaving near any incision lines for the first few postoperative weeks.

Complications and Management

Hemorrhage and Hematoma

Hemorrhage and related hematoma account for the most common complication postrhytidectomy. Fortunately, this complication is easily manageable and is often preventable. Certainly, an ounce of prevention is worth a pound (or several pounds) of cure. In the preoperative phase, the patient's blood pressure should be well regulated, both to minimize intraoperative cardiovascular complications and intraoperative and postoperative hemorrhage. All preoperative medications that may compromise effective coagulation must be ceased for a period of 2 weeks prior and 2 weeks postoperatively, including prescription medications (e.g., naproxen, Coumadin, etc.), over-the-counter medications (e.g., aspirin-related products), herbal medications (e.g., St. John's Wort, ginkgo biloba, etc.), vitamin E, and alcohol. The reader is referred to Chapter 3 for a complete list of medications from which the patient should abstain. The patient should also be compliant with a limited physical regimen beginning the morning of surgery until 2 weeks postoperatively at which time he or she can begin brisk ambulation to maintain fitness. However, the patient is always cautioned to be attuned to his or her postoperative energy level and to tailor any physical activity accordingly. In all circumstances, a male patient should always put the surgeon at an increased level of attention given the richer vascularity that the hair-bearing skin of the lower face exhibits and the concomitant risk of hematoma formation.

Despite adherence to the most vigorous prophylactic protocol, a hematoma may still occur. If the hematoma is noted on the first postoperative day and appears to be limited in nature, then a 4 × 4 gauze may be used to roll out the blood through the drain site, and a new pressure dressing is applied. A discrete collection discovered somewhat later may require 7 to 10 days to liquefy before it can be aspirated. However, brisk bleeding, whether arterial or venous, that occurs especially during the initial few hours after surgery is an entirely different matter that requires diligent intervention. The two cardinal signs that indicate the onset or arrival of a disastrous hematoma are *asymmetric pain* and *asymmetric swelling,* which is often accompanied by anxiety and distress. If the patient has already returned home, a phone call to the surgeon that indicates either symptom should alert the surgeon to a possible major hematoma that requires attention. If an expanding or large hematoma is discovered, the patient should return to the operative theater to have the area reexplored, irrigated, and controlled. Persistence of a hematoma predisposes toward flap necrosis and infection. Clearly, flap necrosis is the more devastating of the two complications and should be avoided at all costs. Compounded with other vascular compromising factors such as diabetes mellitus or tobacco usage, the risk of cutaneous necrosis increases exponentially. However, these factors prove to be negligible when compared to the risk that an acute hematoma alone poses on flap vascularity. As mentioned, infection can also arise because of the presence of blood, an excellent culture medium. Therefore, the patient should be on a perioperative antibiotic regimen that counters gram-positive flora.

Infection

As alluded to, infection may arise in the setting of a hematoma. Otherwise, this complication remains quite rare. The authors rely on a perioperative antibiotic course that is commenced the day of surgery and continued for the first postoperative week. However, whether this course of therapy treats the patient or the physician has not been scientifically substantiated. Diabetes and smoking may compromise local vascularity and related wound healing, thereby increasing the risk of infection. However, the authors have found that these predisposing factors prove to be of slight concern given the rich vascularity of the head-and-neck region.

An alloplastic implant (e.g., a chin implant or ePTFE sling) also can prove to be an infectious source. In spite of this, the authors have found that only implants located in an area of great mobility and near the oral cavity (e.g., lip implants) exhibit the greatest tendency toward infection. However, if an abscess develops at the site of implantation, it is almost assured that the implant will require removal. Removal of the implant with reinsertion later when the infection has subsided is the best treatment policy. At the first sign of an infection, a dose of intravenous antibiotics is administered in order to ensure immediate, proper therapeutic levels, followed by a full regimen of broad-spectrum oral antibiotics until the infection clears.

Infection of ear cartilage, or chondritis, should be attentively managed. However, this complication is an infrequent manifestation of postoperative infection. Extensive chondritis can be identified because it extends over the entire ear, except the lobule where no cartilage resides. As gram-negative organisms are likely culprits, an appropriate antibiotic should be selected to thwart these offenders. If oral antibiotics fail to eliminate the infection, broad-spectrum antibiotics and possible hospitalization may be required. At times, a very localized infection at the incision site may be caused by a suture, which acts as the nidus of infection. If this is the case, the suture should be removed, and appropriate gram-positive antibiotic coverage administered.

Protracted Edema

Gentle and expedient surgery is the most reliable method to prevent excessive edema. Additionally, control of blood pressure during the operative case will limit untoward edema. Application of ice directly to the operative site during surgery and for a 24-hour period thereafter is a policy that has proven its value over the years to curb edema. A single dose of intravenous steroids (dexamethasone 8 mg) intraoperatively and oral doses thereafter (8 mg and then 4 mg) during the first day will also hasten resolution of edema. The patient should cooperate with head elevation at all times during the initial week and limit physical exertion, particularly any activity that requires the head to be in a dependent position. A well-configured pressure dressing maintained for the first day and a lighter version applied the following day helps to restrict the amount of edema that can accumulate in the tissues.

If all of these prophylactic measures have been followed, prolonged edema may still arise because an individual's unique physiology or other undetermined factors. Mild to moderate edema that is present for the first two postoperative weeks should be considered within the timeframe of normal healing and not be treated. Patient reassurance is the only recommended intervention. Significant edema over the first two weeks may be treated with a short course of oral steroid medication or a single intravenous dose (e.g., a Medrol dose pack), but further intervention is unwarranted.

If edema persists for greater than 2 weeks, then investigation into the cause may be justified. The surgeon should inquire whether any of the predisposing factors for edema (cited in the preceding) might be culpable. Manual lymphatic massage may also be a helpful adjunctive therapeutic option.

Flap Necrosis

Flap necrosis is a devastating complication that should be avoidable in most circumstances. The reader is referred to the section on hemorrhage/hematoma for a more detailed assessment of prophylactic measures to minimize this adverse occurrence. However, if flap necrosis should arise, then conservative management is the best policy. The wound should be kept moist at all times with Bacitracin, or equivalent, topical antibiotic ointment. As the area becomes more demarcated, limited debridement and wet-to-dry dressings twice daily should be instituted until full epithelialization occurs. An oral antibiotic regimen may also be considered, especially if the etiology is a hematoma given the predilection for infection in this circumstance. The wound should be allowed to heal by secondary intention, and no consideration for flap reconstruction should be entertained during the healing phase. Any skin grafting or rotational flap coverage is contraindicated for a minimum of 9 to 12 months because cutaneous vascularity is already known to be poor.

Facial Nerve Injury

Facial nerve injury is another devastating, but rare, complication. Fortunately, most facial nerve injuries are temporary in nature, although full recovery time may entail 6 months of patience. The buccal area of the face has the most anastomotic redundancy and therefore exhibits the highest chance for full recovery. The fronto-temporal branch is the least likely division to undergo complete recovery. The method of rhytidectomy proposed in which the temporal hair tuft is not violated both spares the sideburn as well as protects against injury to this delicate branch. Obviously, a thorough understanding of facial anatomy is a critical prerequisite for a surgeon who wishes to practice head-and-neck surgery of any kind. A detailed review of facial nerve anatomy and management of facial nerve injury lie beyond the scope of this text, and the reader is referred elsewhere for clarification. However, a basic strategy for facial nerve injury relevant for aesthetic surgery is offered.

If neural transection is not clearly established, then the injury should be regarded as a neurapraxia. Accordingly, patience is the best course of action: Any further surgical exploration only jeopardizes other nerve branches and increases morbidity unnecessarily. Steroid therapy, a single intravenous dose and/or 1 week of oral prednisone, may help to diminish edematous strangulation of the nerve and thereby hasten recovery. If transection is noted during surgery, then reanastomosis of the epineurium with microscopic magnification should be attempted. If the nerve does not recover after 8 to 12 months, then permanent neural damage is likely.

Greater Auricular Neuropathy

The greater auricular nerve can either be severed during surgery or compressed with a nonabsorbable suture. If it is transected, the patient comes to live with the loss of sensation, which improves with time as the patient accommodates to this sensory deficit. If only a single branch is cut, then there should be faster and more complete recovery of sensation. However, compressive neuropathy may be a more difficult problem to manage owing to the acute discomfort that the patient experiences. It usually arises due to suture placement that traps the nerve. Use of 0.5% Marcaine and triamcinolone 10 mg/cc may alleviate the discomfort and expedite resolution of this problem. However, the discomfort may persist in a recalcitrant manner and require unconventional means (e.g., acupuncture) to break the pain cycle.

Scarring

Hypertrophic scarring and keloid formation can arise because of poor surgical technique (excessive skin tension on closure and poor tissue handling) or to a natural predisposition. The reader is referred to the sections on primary and secondary rhytidectomy to review all the surgical techniques that should be followed to avoid this complication. Although keloids may arise in the neck and postauricular regions, the face is relatively immune from true keloid scar formation. Hypertrophic scars, on the other hand, can arise on both the face and neck regions. Individuals of Asian, Latin, and African descent are particularly prone to hypertrophic scarring. Management should include intralesional steroid injection with triamcinolone at 10 mg/mL concentration administered not more frequently than every 3 weeks so that dermal atrophy and hypopigmentation are avoided. Between treatment sessions, topical steroid ointment (e.g., desonide cream; DesOwen, Galderma), or steroid-impregnated tape (e.g., flurandrenolide tape; Cordran tape, Oclassen Pharmaceuticals, Corona, CA) can also be applied to expedite resolution of the scar. Pulsed-dye laser therapy also may serve as a helpful adjunct. If the scar is not localized in an area with very attenuated skin (e.g., the eyelids), then high fluences (12 to 16 J/cm^2) of the pulsed dye laser may be used directly on the scar at frequent intervals (every 2 to 4 weeks) until resolution of the scar. Silicone sheeting also may prove useful in the management scheme, although the authors acknowledge limited experience with this modality. If the scar persists despite these conservative measures, scar revision ultimately may be required.

Asymmetry

Symmetry is a desired objective in every surgical endeavor but is not often achieved. The surgeon may ameliorate a preoperative asymmetry, but flawless symmetry is elusive. The natural physiologic tendency toward asymmetry overcomes the best surgical efforts, and the patient should be counseled about this likely outcome. However, if asymmetry is exacerbated or unrelated to a preoperative state, then this result may be attributed to poor surgical technique. Photographic documentation should be standardized to facilitate proper physician–patient dialog. Asymmetry that arises in the immediate postoperative period is often attributable to uneven edema during the healing phase that should resolve. Facial nerve function should be confirmed to eliminate this possibility, and the wounds carefully inspected for a hematoma or seroma that may be contributing to the asymmetry. Surgical correction of asymmetry is not an easy proposition, especially if it is owing to overzealous excision of skin on one side. The patient should be advised that the safest course of action is expectant observation for a minimum of 6 months before any further surgery should be entertained.

CLINICAL PRESENTATIONS: A SYNTHESIS OF APPROACH

Case #1 (Fig. 5-53A–D)

This patient recently turned 50 and felt that it was time to pursue cosmetic surgery. She was seen 2 years prior in consultation but for various reasons decided against having surgery at that time. She was otherwise healthy and was interested in an opinion as to what would give her the most improvement. On examination, the patient was noted to exhibit both upper and lower facial descent but with a disproportionate amount of lower facial aging. On lateral inspection, she also showed some hypoplasia of her mentum that would benefit from augmentation. The patient was concerned about the puffiness of her lower eyelids and believed that this area also contributed to her overall aged and tired expression.

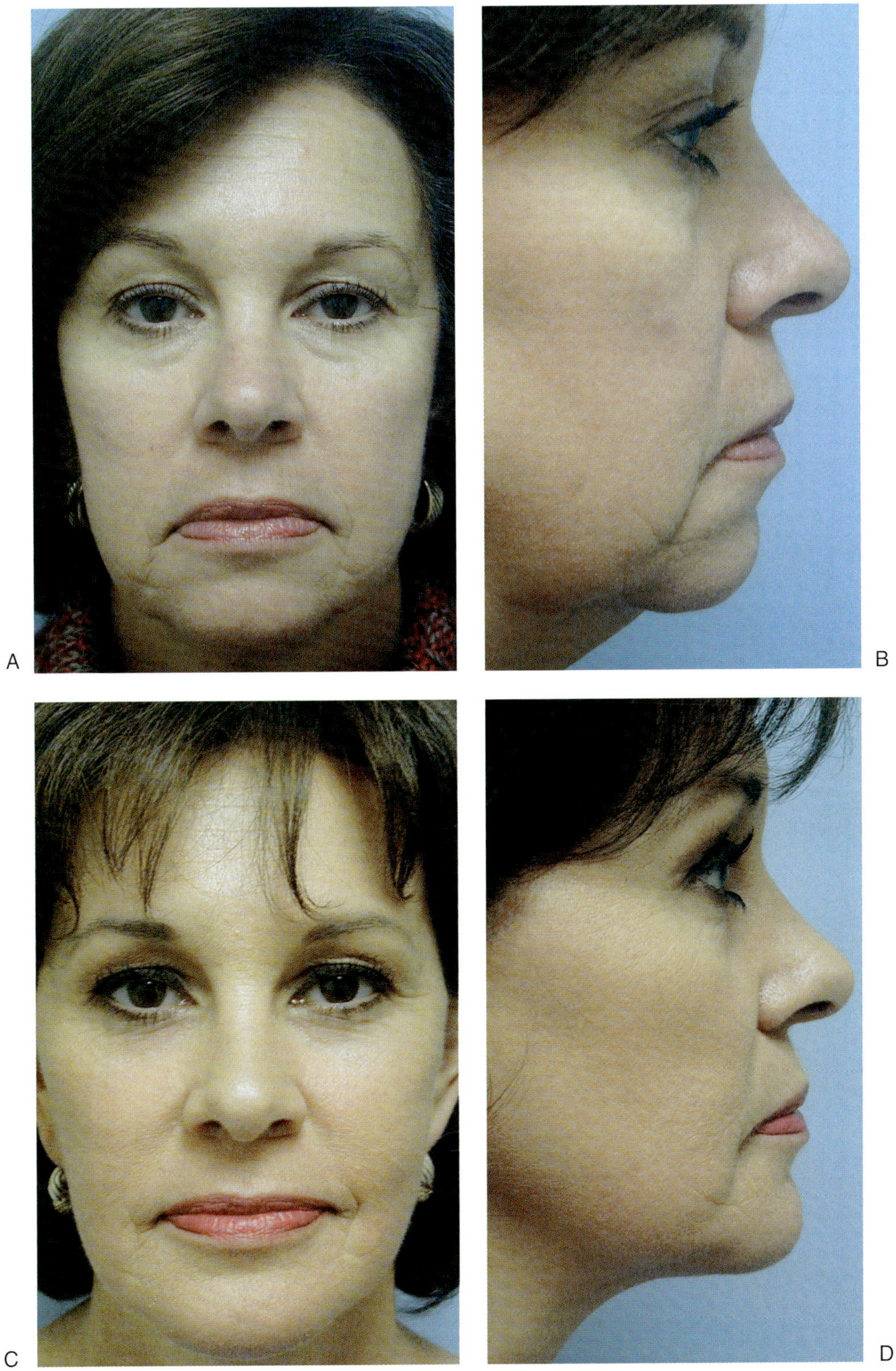

FIGURE 5-53. A–D: This 50-year-old patient exhibits both upper and lower facial aging but with a disproportionate amount in her lower face and neck regions. The patient also shows some hypoplasia of her mentum and relatively deep marionette, or labiomandibular, lines. The patient underwent a lower-eyelid transconjunctival blepharoplasty with lower-eyelid peel with Jessner's/35% trichloroacetic acid, cervical liposuction/submentoplasty, facelift with superficial musculoaponeurotic system (SMAS) plication, and chin augmentation with Mersilene mesh. The chin implant was intended to correct the hypoplastic appearance of her chin and also to address in part the labiomandibular folds. The patient probably would have benefited from a browlift as well as augmentation of her nasolabial and labiomandibular folds with SMAS or comparable soft-tissue filler. She is shown 1 year postoperatively with notable aesthetic improvement in her lower face.

Procedure

The procedure was a transconjunctival lower-eyelid blepharoplasty in conjunction with a Jessner's/35% TCA chemical peel of her lower eyelids, cervical liposuction/submentoplasty, chin augmentation using Mersilene mesh (10- × 1-cm and 5- × 1-cm segments), and extended-dissection SMAS-plication facelift.

Discussion

This patient probably would have benefited from a browlift but was rightfully more concerned about her jaw line and neck. The patient's very deep marionette, or labiomandibular, folds were accentuated by her hypoplastic chin. She showed good dentition and occlusion. It was felt that a moderate chin augmentation would enhance her overall appearance by providing adequate chin projection and also softening her prejowl and jowl mandibular contour. Because of this limitation, the patient was counseled that a facelift alone would be insufficient to eradicate this problem. The patient could have benefited from augmentation of her nasolabial and labiomandibular folds with either SMAS or comparable soft-tissue filler (e.g., acellular dermis or ePTFE).

Case #2 (Fig. 5-54A,B)

This is a 43-year-old businesswoman who presented for an opinion regarding facial rejuvenation. Her concern was mainly directed toward the appearance of her neck and jaw line. The patient stated that her cervical region and jaw line had deteriorated rapidly over the past 6 months and that she had become quite self-conscious about the appearance of her neck. She was particularly sensitive about her aged mien because her line of work involved an aesthetic and beauty practice.

Procedure

The procedure was a cervical liposuction/submentoplasty and extended-flap facelift with SMAS plication.

Discussion

In this age group, patients often present for facial rejuvenation and are interested in an attempt at improving the neckline with liposuction. The early forties are the transition age between those patients who often are treated sufficiently by an isolated liposuction procedure and those in need of lifting as well. Facial, as opposed to cervical, liposuction should be

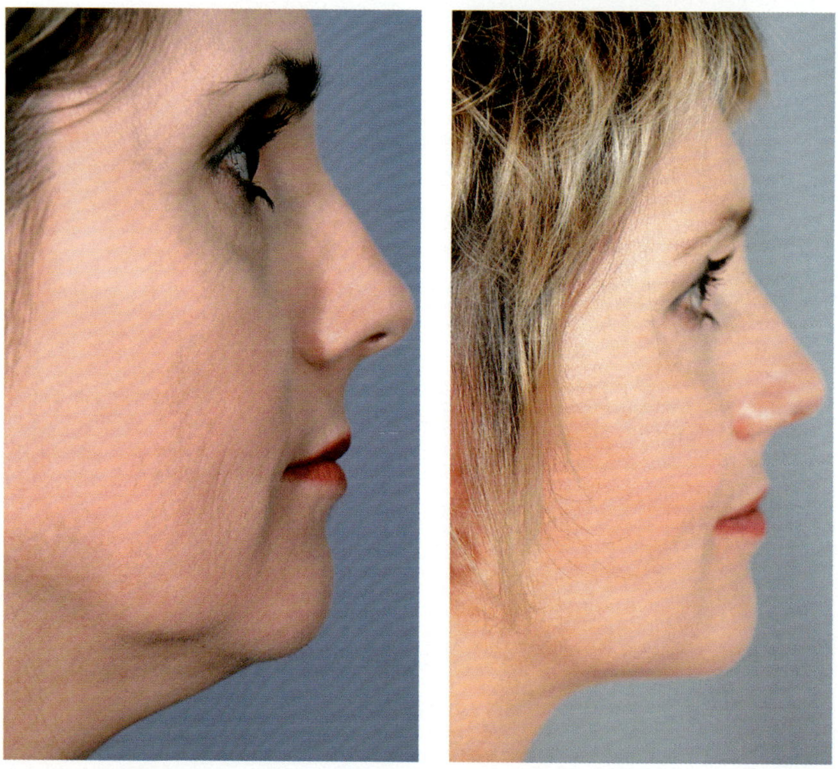

A B

FIGURE 5-54. A,B: This is a 43-year-old businesswoman who exhibited significant lower facial aging over the past 6 months. The patient represents a transition zone in age in which cervical liposuction alone would not suffice because of the jowl formation along the jaw line and the inelastic nature of her skin. The patient underwent a cervical liposuction/submentoplasty and superficial musculoaponeurotic system–plication rhytidectomy. She is shown 1 year postoperatively with notable aesthetic improvement in her lower face.

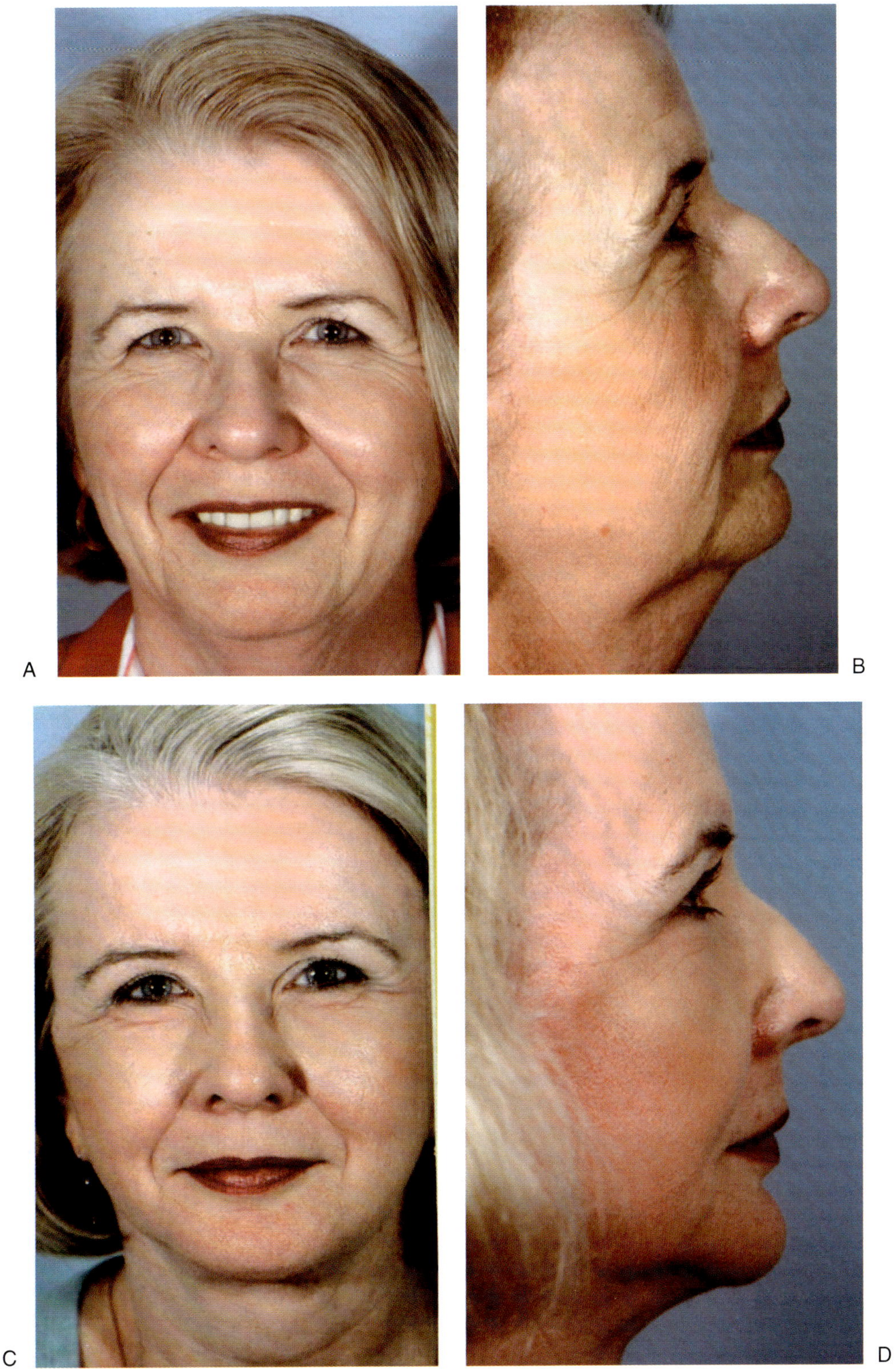

FIGURE 5-55. A–D: This is a 56-year-old woman who expressed concern about her neckline but also the tired expression of her eyes. She was very concerned about having an overdone appearance after surgery. The patient underwent a browlift, subperiosteal midface lift, submentoplasty with cervical liposuction, rhytidectomy, chin augmentation using a medium-sized expanded polytetrafluoroethylene chin implant, transconjunctival lower-eyelid blepharoplasty, CO_2-laser resurfacing of the lower eyelids and periorbital areas, and upper eyelid blepharoplasty. The patient exhibits improvement in her overall facial appearance at 1 year postoperatively.

discouraged or performed in a very conservative fashion as contour problems are much more likely along the jaw line and upper face. If elected, facial liposuction should be undertaken conservatively through an open approach with a patient who exhibits a round face and heavy tissue in the lower face and jaw line. This patient did not undergo facial liposuction. In this particular case, it was felt that there was sufficient loss of elasticity and that cervical liposuction without a facelift would be very limited in its effect. In addition to loss of elasticity, the early jowling that the patient exhibited only could be truly effaced with a combined facelift.

Case #3 (Fig. 5-55A–D)

This is a 56-year-old patient who was concerned about the aged appearance of her neckline and the constantly tired expression of her eyes. She was very interested in facelift surgery but was concerned about having a tight or overdone look. As she exhibited her family trait of a heavy brow, she did not want to look very different from her family members, which she believed would be interpreted as unnatural looking by them. On examination, the patient was found to have a particularly ptotic brow and forehead with significant hooding in the superior lateral orbital area. She was noted to have fair skin, deep periorbital and moderate perioral rhytids that she wished to have addressed at the same time as her facial rejuvenation procedure. There was marked accumulation of submental adipose tissue and a large soft-tissue envelope of the neck and lower face. She also exhibited slight hypoplasia of the chin and parasymphyseal area.

Procedure

The procedure was a minimally invasive browlift, subperiosteal midface lift, submentoplasty with cervical liposuction, rhytidectomy, chin augmentation using a medium-sized ePTFE chin implant, transconjunctival lower-eyelid blepharoplasty, CO_2-laser resurfacing of the lower-eyelids and periorbital areas, and upper-eyelid blepharoplasty.

Discussion

The patient was concerned about overelevation of the forehead because she remarked that she always had a heavy brow. For this reason, care was taken not to over elevate the medial or lateral aspect of the brow. In turn, midfacial suspension was achieved via the standard transbrow approach (Chapter 4). An aggressive submental liposuction and submentoplasty were undertaken with removal of an unusually large amount, approximately 4 to 5 mm, of redundant, medial platysmal muscle on each side prior to plication. Chin and prejowl augmentation were accomplished with a medium-sized ePTFE chin implant. An SMAS plication and intermediately long skin flap were used for the rhytidectomy.

This patient presented with upper, middle, and lower facial descent that each contributed to her overall facial aging. She was particularly concerned with the potential for a "startled" or overpulled look to her brow region. By addressing each particular area of ptotic tissue rather than over treating one area, multiple small contributions in each facial zone assisted in yielding a fairly dramatic yet natural-appearing result.

As mentioned, a medium-sized chin implant was also used in this particular patient, which greatly enhanced the facelift result for several reasons. First, the patient displays some mild hypoplasia of her mentum that detracts from overall facial harmony, especially in light of her larger nose that is particularly evident on the lateral view. Second, the prejowl region can be partially addressed using an extended chin implant that serves to efface the redundancy in this area in part. Finally because a bony, angular face predisposes to a better facelift result, creation of a more prominent mentum permits a focal point around which the neck and jaw line can be redraped. Also, the same incision used for a submentoplasty and cervical liposuction is used for access to insert the chin alloplast.

REFERENCES

1. Duffy MJ, Friedland JA: The superficial-plane rhytidectomy revisited. Plast Reconstr Surg 1994;93:1392–1403.
2. Ivy EJ, Lorenc ZP, Aston SJ: Is there a difference? A prospective study comparing lateral and standard SMAS facelifts with extended SMAS and composite rhytidectomies. Plast Reconstr Surg 1996;98:1135–1143.
3. Becker FF: Deep plane facelift vs. SMAS facelift. A comparative study, lecture given at the 8th International Symposium of Facial Plastic Surgery. New York, May 4, 2002.
4. McCurdy JA Jr, Lam SM: Cosmetic surgery of the Asian face, 2nd ed. New York: Thieme, 2004.
5. Chang EW, Lam SM, Karen M, et al: Sliding genioplasty for correction of chin abnormalities. Arch Facial Plast Surg 2001;3: 8–15.
6. Dedo DD: "How I do it"—plastic surgery. Practical suggestions on facial plastic surgery. A preoperative classification of the neck for cervicofacial rhytidectomy. Laryngoscope 1980;90:1894–1896.
7. Miller TA, Orringer JS: Excision of neck redundancy with single Z-plasty closure. Plast Reconstr Surg 1996;97:219–221.
8. Campbell JP, McCollough EG, Metzinger SE: Posterior cervical rhytidectomy: a valuable adjunct in facial rejuvenation surgery. Otolaryngol Head Neck Surg 1997;116:79–90.
9. Pessa JE, Garza PA, Love VM, et al: The anatomy of the labiomandibular fold. Plast Reconstr Surg 1998;101:482–486.
10. Goin MK, Burgoyne RW, Goin JM: Face-lift operation: the patient's secret motivations and reactions to "informed consent." Plast Reconstr Surg 1976;58:273–278.
11. Webb WF, Slaughter R, Meyer E, et al: Mechanisms of psychological adjustment in patients seeking "face-lift" operation. Psychosomatic Medicine 1965;27:183–199.
12. Edgerton MT Jr, Knorr NJ: Motivational patterns of patients seeking cosmetic (esthetic) surgery. Plast Reconstr Surg 1971;48: 551–557.

13. Kamer FM, Minoli JJ: Postoperative platysmal band deformity. A pitfall of submental liposuction. Arch Otolaryngol Head Neck Surg 1993;119:193–196.
14. Becker DG, Cook TA, Wang TD, et al: A 3-year multi-institutional experience with the liposhaver. Arch Facial Plast Surg 1999; 1:171–176.
15. Gross EJ, Hamilton MM, Ackermann K, et al: Mersilene mesh chin augmentation. A 14-year experience. Arch Facial Plast Surg 1999;1:183–189.
16. Seckel BR: Facial danger zones: avoiding nerve injury in facial plastic surgery. St. Louis, MO: Quality Medical Publishing, 1994:18–23.

6

HAIR RESTORATION

SAMUEL M. LAM
EDWIN F. WILLIAMS III

Cosmetic surgery for men has dramatically increased in popularity over the past decade, spurred in part by mass media images that portray the idealized male form. Aesthetic surgery is a natural extension of the fitness fixation that has captivated the male ego and propelled it on a quixotic quest in pursuit of the Adonis physique. Although many men seek global rejuvenation of the face, societal norms dictate two principal facial regions that receive disproportionate attention: the eyes and the hair. Blepharoplasty offers the male patient who thrives in the competitive workplace a targeted approach toward rejuvenation: Aging eyes often betray fatigue, anger, and sadness that may belie the patient's true emotional state or youthful vigor. Similarly, hair restoration has become a principal concern for the mature, or not quite so mature, man who faces the tragic loss of hair. The ubiquitous media engine often portrays the balding man as a Samson, who stripped of his virile lock, has lost his sexual vitality. Unfortunately, the counterfeit claims of miracle cures that abound on the Internet, on television, and in print do little to provide any meaningful remedy to the bewildered man. Undoubtedly, men fall prey to hormonally incited hair loss to a greater frequency and extent than the opposite sex. Nevertheless, women are susceptible to hair loss, whether androgen-driven or otherwise, and they have sought medical and surgical therapy for their condition as well.

The history of follicular transfer dates back two centuries to Dieffenbach's early experiments.[1] It was not until Orentreich introduced his elegant punch-grafting technique in the 1950s that follicular grafting was more precisely understood and widely implemented.[2] Nevertheless, the original punch graft left an indelible image in the public mind that has been likened to the cornrow appearance of a doll's head. These unsightly "plugs" hindered widespread acceptance of this technique. In the early 1980s, Nordstrom and Marritt pioneered the use of micrografting, or single follicular transfer, that offered a more natural appearance to the grafted scalp.[3,4] Alternatively, scalp reduction with extender placement (see the following) has been useful to correct crown, or vertex,* baldness, because grafting in this area may appear unnatural. Scalp rotation flaps (e.g., the twice-delayed Juri flap) are beneficial for patients who desire rapid, dense coverage to the fronto-temporal region.[5,6] Tissue expansion has also been successfully implemented for hair restoration but has not been exploited in the authors' practices (and accordingly is not discussed herein.) Beyond these varied surgical options, advances in medical treatment have provided sufferers of alopecia a less invasive alternative. The physician who treats alopecia should be acquainted with the diverse treatment methodologies to combat follicular loss and exercise erudition in the selection of the appropriate course of action. This chapter reviews the many surgical and medical treatment strategies that currently exist for hair loss and emphasize a systematic appraisal to guide therapy.

The surgeon whose primary talent is brandishing the scalpel may find the multifaceted approach to hair restoration a daunting ordeal. Accordingly, many disciplines may need to converge, including a medical therapist or physician, an operative technician, and a hairpiece specialist, to provide the balding patient the optimal care that he deserves. Often, a patient may not be ready to undertake surgical hair restoration because of financial constraints, fear, lack of motivation, or insufficient hair loss to justify transplantation. These patients may be better candidates for medical therapy (e.g., minoxidil or finasteride) until surgery becomes a more suitable option. Herbal remedies, albeit often clinically unsubstantiated, may offer an unconventional, yet perhaps beneficial, regimen for alopecia. A physician or a therapist may play a valuable role in dispensing medical or herbal treatments, respectively. Alternatively, the same or another provider can tender services that rely on hairpiece camouflage. Clearly, the field of hair restoration is broad and complex and may require a team working independently or together to achieve the aesthetic objectives of the patient.

*The terms crown and vertex have been used in the literature to denote a region situated either at the most superior aspect of the scalp or the tonsure region posteriorly. This text refers to them as synonymous terms that denote only the tonsure region, that is, where monks or priests of some religious orders bare shaved scalps. The superior aspect of the scalp is referred to as the midscalp.

PREOPERATIVE CONSIDERATIONS: PATIENT SELECTION AND RELEVANT ANATOMY

The first step toward successful surgical hair restoration is proper physician–patient dialog to establish the desire, motivation, and expectation that the patient harbors. Despite what may be glaringly obvious to the transplant surgeon as the most deficient area of alopecia, the patient may hold an altogether different opinion of what troubles him or her. The consultation should aim at unifying patient concerns with the surgeon's objectives in a realistic, achievable fashion. Despite the most talented and extensive grafting efforts, some patients who desire significant density may be left unsatisfied with conventional graft transplantation. Conversely, a patient who expresses trepidation about extensive surgery may not be a suitable candidate for scalp rotation and reduction procedures. Besides the psychological aspects of hair transplantation, the anatomic constraints of a patient's particular hair, scalp, and donor areas should be entered into the equation when selecting the appropriate surgical approach. The following section highlights the salient points regarding proper patient selection given the previously enumerated limitations.[7]

First, a thoughtful and thorough history always should be obtained about a patient's onset, rapidity, and evolution of hair loss. As will be discerned, a mature, stable hairline affords the surgeon a wider range of surgical options than a rapidly progressive hairline of a younger patient. Nevertheless, an apparently very stable hairline may become less so because of both intrinsic or extrinsic factors at any time; and the surgeon should never hold an unwavering conviction that the past is an absolute predictor of the future. Prior medical history that may contribute to the development of alopecia also should be elucidated, including radiation exposure, medication abuse, hormonal imbalances, dietary deficiencies, or other inciting factors. A history of prior medical therapy using approved (finasteride and minoxidil), herbal (saw palmetto and vitamins), experimental (dutasteride), and other medicinal or quasimedicinal compounds should be elicited. The duration of medical therapy may hint at the length of time that the patient has been troubled by his or her hair loss, and to what extremes he or she has pursued various avenues to ameliorate the condition. Prior surgical efforts also should be properly assessed, as well as the patient's satisfaction or displeasure with those interventions.

A focused physical examination should follow of the scalp and hair. Hair color, texture, density, curliness, and distribution should be evaluated along with scalp color, elasticity, and integrity. These attributes determine the overall success of the transplantation, as succeeding portions of this chapter more readily reveal. For instance, dark, thick, straight hair contrasted against a milky white scalp may be the least forgiving combination and may yield a less natural look despite best efforts at follicular unit or micrografting, especially in the region of the vertex. Donor density also must be evaluated: A thick occipital fringe provides ample donor source for grafting transplantation, whereas a robust parietal fringe may contribute more to the success of a scalp flap rotation or reduction. The fronto-temporal recession should be attentively studied, as surgical blunting or effacement of these "character lines" often leads to an unnatural look and may make further camouflage in a rapidly receding hairline difficult. Obviously, the surgeon must plan his or her procedure to provide both immediate benefit but also aim at overall longevity: These twin goals always should be kept in mind.

As alluded to, the psychological dynamics that motivate the patient are central to success of any hair transplantation. The patient's expectations of the transplantation session must be met to ensure surgical triumph. First, the patients' desire for density versus coverage should be determined. Some patients, especially those who have been accustomed to synthetic hairpieces, may not perceive simple coverage in the areas of alopecia to be sufficient and may insist on greater density than can be afforded by grafting sessions. If the photographic results of patients who have undergone "megasession" grafting sessions are nevertheless uninspiring, then scalp rotation and reduction may be entertained to resolve this perceived inadequacy. However, most men are quite satisfied with any coverage they may achieve; therefore, they are usually excellent candidates for transplantation.

In contradistinction, the authors have noted that women, who naturally tend to exhibit less widespread hair loss, often remain discontented with their surgical result despite very extensive transplantation. Unlike discrete areas of androgenic alopecia that preside in the fronto-temporal and crown regions, female-pattern baldness is more evenly distributed across the scalp and less extensive in nature. Accordingly, women tend to be less satisfied with follicular grafting because the amount of hair loss is less perceptible to begin with and surgical enhancement of more dispersed alopecia may be similarly less noticeable. The generalized thinning that occurs in the female sufferer of alopecia has been classified according to the Ludwig scale[8] (Fig. 6-1) as opposed to the Norwood scale for men (Fig. 6-2). As part of an informed preoperative consultation, the surgeon must ensure that the limitations of surgical hair restoration for the female patient are well understood before surgery is contemplated.

Similarly, patients who desire significant density also may express impatience with the 6 months to 1 year required to see the incipient regrowth of the newly transplanted hair. In addition, several transplantation sessions that are necessary to achieve considerable density may further delay noticeable growth and add overall expense if the cumulative number of grafting sessions is tallied. For the minority of patients who are unwilling to wait and who desire rapid, dense growth of hair, a scalp rotation or reduction

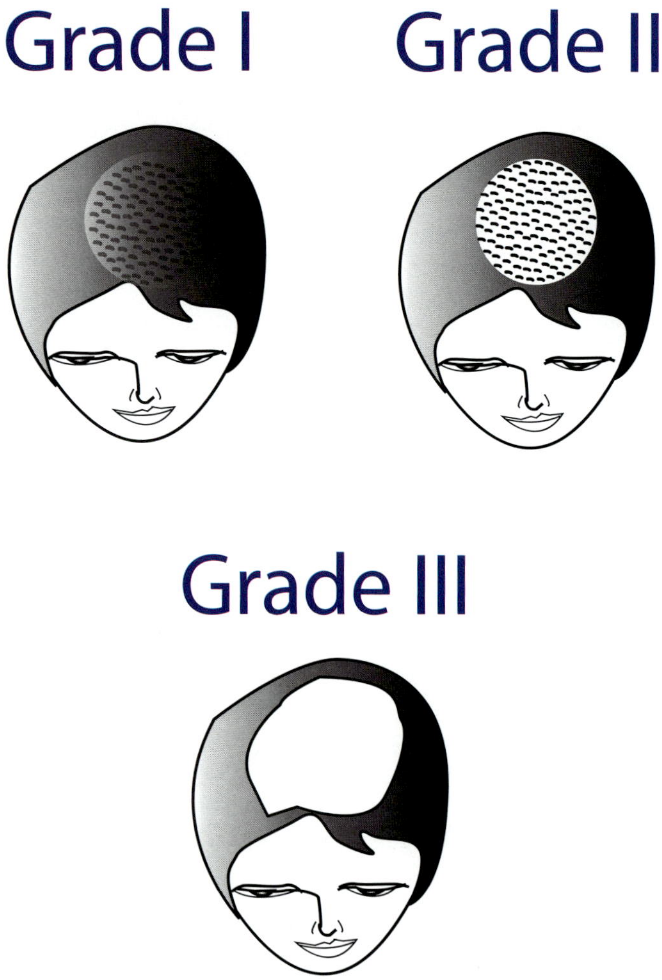

FIGURE 6-1. Illustration showing the classification scheme for female-pattern baldness known as the Ludwig's scale. Thinning tends to be more generalized than in male-pattern baldness, which typically spares the frontal hairline. Instead, the temporoparietal and crown areas are more uniformly affected.

may be the optimal surgical approach for them. All these concerns again must be tempered with the added morbidity of staged flap or reduction procedures that may contribute to an undesirable convalescence.

Patients who may be good candidates for scalp reduction techniques are those who suffer from exclusive crown, or vertex, alopecia and who are of a mature age (more than 40 years old), with stable hair recession. Patients who continue to lose significant hair may expose their suture line and require further sessions of scalp reduction in an already tight and incompletely distensible scalp. In addition, patients should be counseled preoperatively on the likely further loss of some hair near the incision line. As mentioned, preoperative scalp elasticity should be assessed before consideration of scalp reduction. Curiously, scalp distensibility is less of a concern if an extender is used as part of the procedure, because the implanted device tends to overcome some of the unfavorable tensile forces of the inelastic scalp.

Scalp reduction is really only possible as a serious alternative to follicular grafting as a result of Patrick Frechet's brilliant invention, the scalp extender, in 1993.[9] The technique of scalp reduction was first introduced in 1977 by the Blanchards,[10] but has undergone a variable course of success because of two complications: stretchback[11] and slot deformity. Prior to the implementation of an extender, the reduced bald scalp stretches back partially: the surgical equivalent of taking two steps forward and one step back (Fig. 6-3). The Frechet extender consists of a central extensible silastic sheet with titanium hooks attached on both ends: The device is implanted below the reduced scalp so that no stretchback occurs in the reduced bald area (unfavorable stretchback) but only takes place in the hair-bearing periphery (favorable stretchback). Slot deformity refers to the remaining slot-shaped bald area that persists along the incision line after all the scalp-reduction sessions have been completed. The authors have relied on a multiple z-plasty closure to camouflage this potential deformity and occasionally follicular grafting to disguise the defect further if necessary during the last session.

Scalp reduction has proved a reliable method in the authors' hands for select patients with crown baldness. On the other hand, successful follicular grafting of the exposed crown may yield at times a less favorable result. Generally speaking, the crown area may be the most difficult to address because of the so-called "bleacher-stand effect" (i.e., grafts seen from behind and above the patient may appear "pluggy" in appearance). However, if the patient demonstrates a favorable combination of dark-complexioned skin and light-colored hair then follicular grafting to the vertex may be much more forgiving and yield a natural appearance. Intense follicular grafting along follicular unit divisions is the preferred method to graft the exposed crown in order to maximize the likelihood for a natural result. Interestingly, the most labor intensive grafting sessions in the vertex may still be unrewarding, as patients often fail to appreciate an area that is not directly in their daily view unlike the comparatively more ecstatic reviews received for the transplanted fronto-temporal region.

As briefly mentioned, the younger patient (less than 40 years old) or the patient with unstable and rapidly progressive hair loss may not be a suitable candidate for scalp reduction. After closure of the exposed crown, this type of patient may continue to lose significant hair and make incision-line camouflage challenging. Flap design principally involves recruitment of parietal hair into the central defect. Accordingly, donor hair in the parietal fringe should be sufficiently thick to provide density to the exposed crown and to tolerate some degree of stretchback in the donor area. The occipital-fringe donor site is also recruited for closure but tends to be less distensible in tissue advancement owing to the adherence of the occipitalis musculature to the posterior nuchal line.

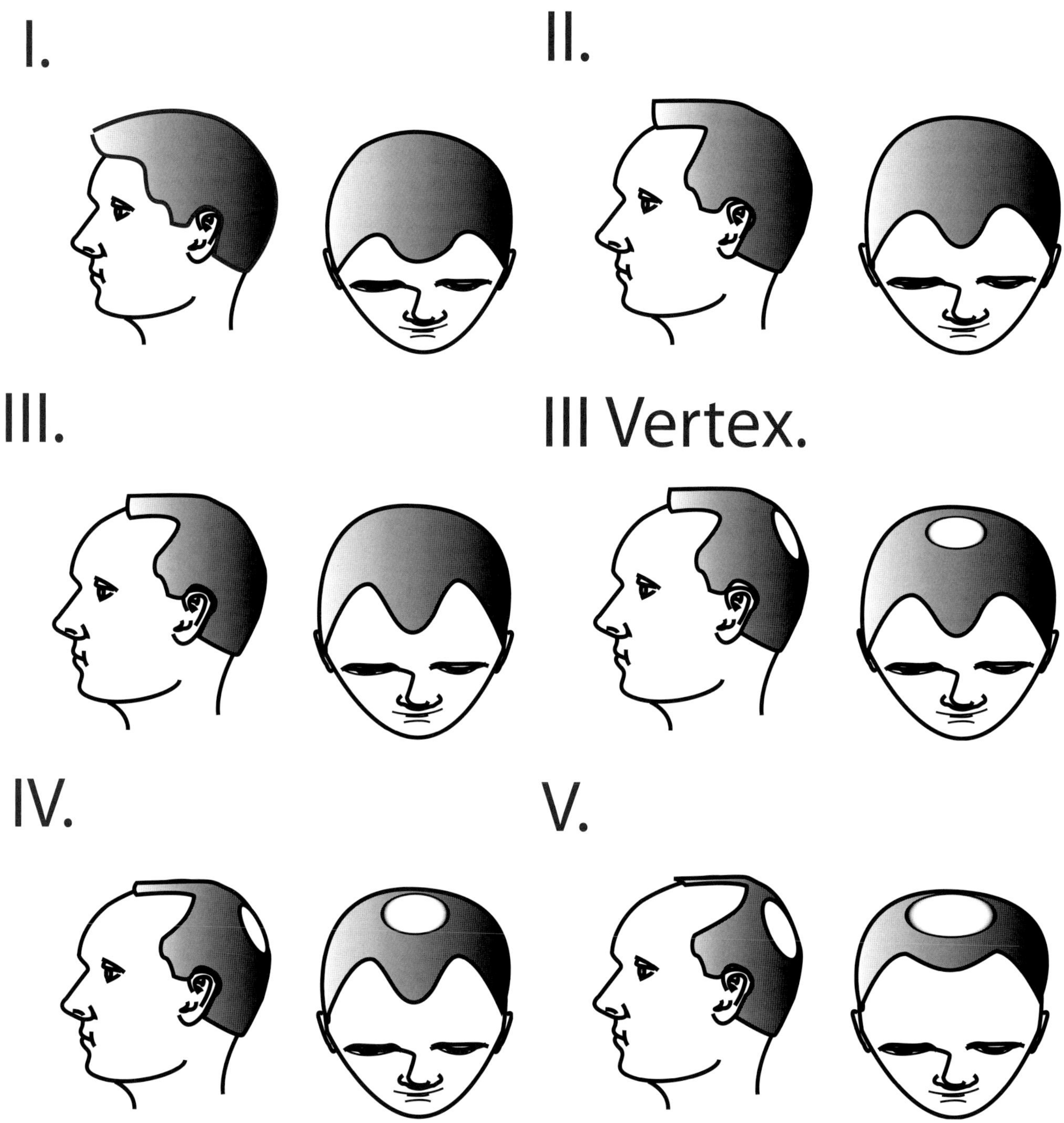

FIGURE 6-2. The Norwood classification for male-pattern baldness is most often used. **Type I** shows minimal to no hair loss along the fronto-temporal expanse. **Type II** exhibits fronto-temporal recession that does not extend further than a line drawn through a coronal plane 2 cm anterior to the external auditory canal. **Type III** hair loss refers to fronto-temporal recession that extends posterior to the coronal plane that lies 2 cm anterior to the external auditory canal. **Type III Vertex** indicates hair loss that primarily affects the vertex (or crown) region with or without accompanying fronto-temporal recession that does not exceed that described in **Type III**. **Type IV** reveals greater fronto-temporal loss than exhibited in **Type III** along with marked hair loss in the crown area but with a moderately dense swath of hair that bridges the intervening expanse between the two areas. **Type V** hair loss shows more extensive hair loss in both the fronto-temporal and vertex areas with only a small bridge of dense hair between the two areas. *(continued)*

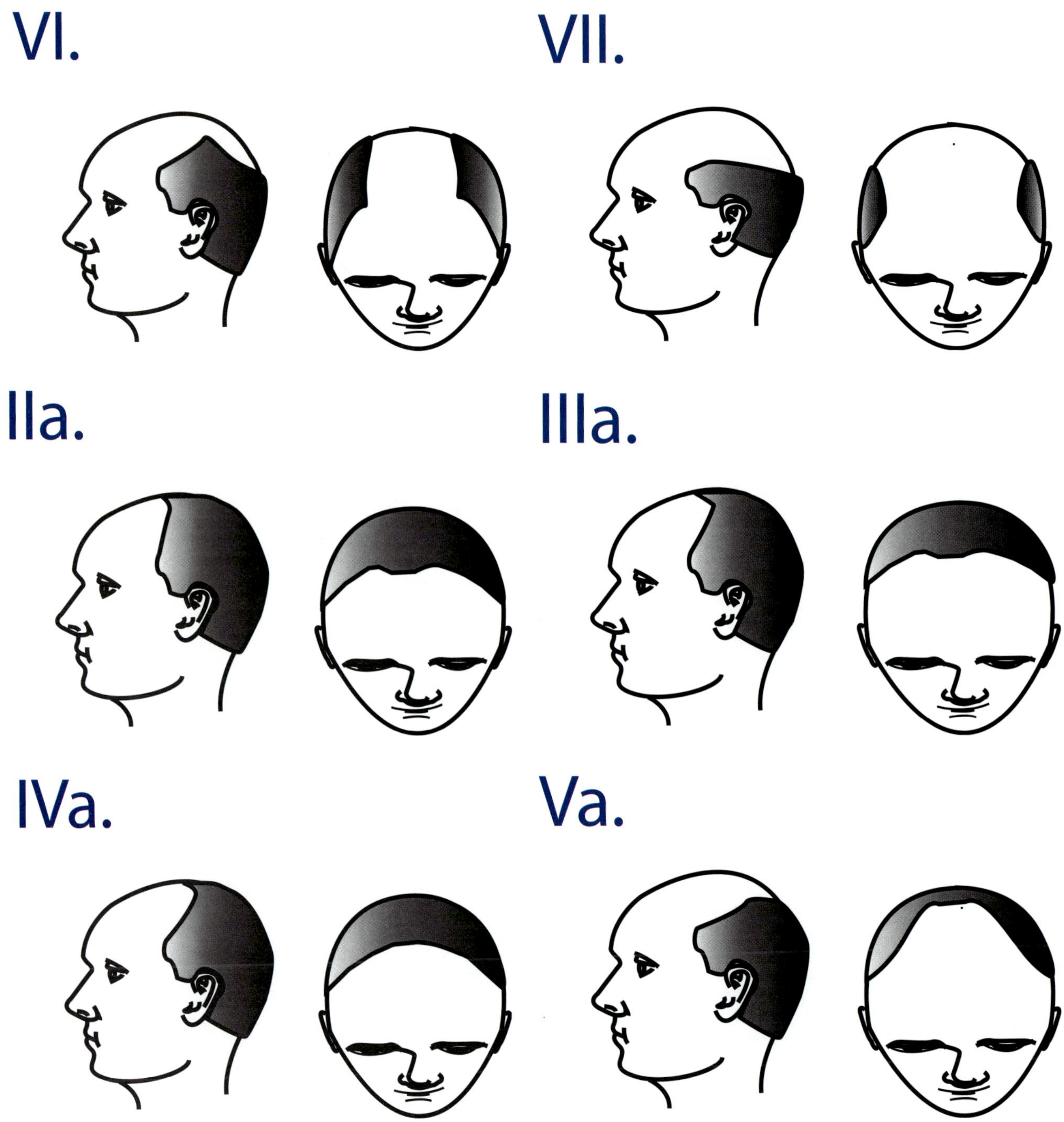

FIGURE 6-2. *(Continued)* **Type VI** hair loss reveals a complete absence of any remaining hair that separates the two now confluent areas of alopecia. In addition, the hair loss is more extensive laterally and posteriorly. **Type VII** represents the most severe expression of male-pattern alopecia with only a narrow-horseshoe configuration that remains along the posterior and lateral border of the hairline. Norwood also classified a variant of hair loss that afflicts approximately 3% of male patients with alopecia in which the fronto-temporal recession marches progressively posteriorly in a uniform fashion without a central, anterior peninsula of hair. **Type IIa** refers to a condition in which the entire anterior hairline is receded uniformly across the forehead but does not extend any further posteriorly than 2 cm anterior to the mid-coronal line. **Type IIIa** reveals alopecia that extends to the mid-coronal line. **Type IVa** signifies alopecia that has extended past this midcoronal line. Finally, **Type Va** indicates significant recession of the hairline into the vertex, and more severe forms of this variant become indistinguishable with **Types V and VI**.

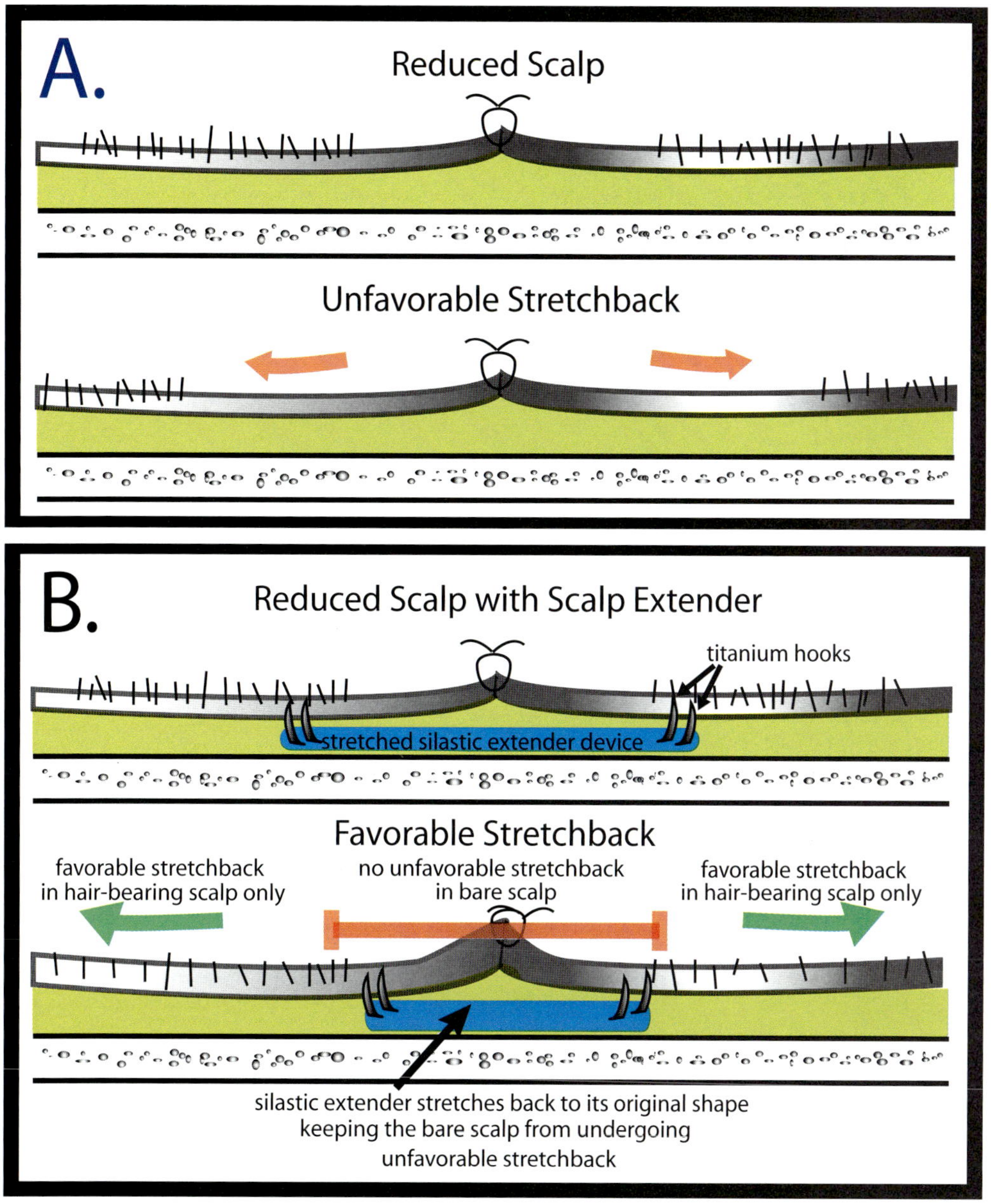

FIGURE 6-3. A: Illustration showing scalp reduction without an extender device leading to unfavorable stretchback in the non–hair-bearing scalp—the surgical equivalent of taking two steps forward and one step back. **B:** Scalp reduction is undertaken with a stretched silastic extender device that retains the non–hair-bearing scalp from undergoing unfavorable stretchback so that all stretchback occurs in the hair-bearing scalp only (favorable stretchback). Note that the extender device actually draws the central non–hair-bearing scalp inward to some degree over the intervening month prior to the next reduction session, which is exhibited by some skin bunching as the extender device loses its stretched configuration.

The patient who desires rapid, dense coverage of the fronto-temporal region and who possesses adequate parietal donor hair may be eligible for scalp rotation with the Juri-designed, twice-delayed, temporo-parietal-occipital flap. In the authors' experience, even patients who have undergone multiple, extensive transplantation sessions are exulted by the unparalleled density that they receive from a single flap rotation procedure. If needed, the contralateral parietal bed may be recruited as a second Juri flap to add density behind the first flap. Unlike scalp reduction, which mandates a more stable pattern of hair recession, fronto-temporal coverage with a flap rotation does not demand this prerequisite. Nevertheless, rapid, ongoing hair loss of the fronto-temporal region may make a scalp rotation less than desirable, be-

Evaluation of the Surgical Candidate

Psychology

What area troubles the patient? (fronto-temporal versus crown)

What are the patient's expectations? (natural hairline, dense coverage)

How long has the patient been concerned about the hair loss and what steps has he or she taken to ameliorate the condition? (hairpieces, sprays, medications, surgery)

History

What are the onset, rapidity, and pattern of hair loss?

What is the patient's general overall health? (diabetes, immunosuppression)

What medications has the patient tried to correct hair loss (including prescribed, herbal, experimental medications)?

Has the patient undergone any surgery or trauma to the scalp or hair?

Has the patient been exposed to any radiation insult to the hair-bearing region?

Any related autoimmune diseases?

Does the patient smoke or use any form of tobacco? Any illicit drug history?

Physical

Hair color, texture, curliness (lighter, thinner, curlier hair is preferred for a natural, less "pluggy" hair transplantation)

Scalp color and elasticity (darker color is preferred for a natural, less "pluggy" hair transplantation)

Donor site: the density, extent, nature, and location of the hair

Recipient site: determine the extent of the area that the patient desires for transplantation

Selection of Surgical Technique

Follicular Grafting

Fronto-temporal region is area of primary concern

Good occipital or temporal donor sites

Scalp Reduction

Crown, or vertex, is area of primary concern

Dark hair and light skin make follicular transfer in crown region more noticeable (the bleacher-stand effect). Therefore, scalp reduction may be preferred.

The area of exposed crown does not exceed 12 cm.

Good scalp distensibility

No significantly progressive hair loss in the crown area

Scalp Rotation

The fronto-temporal region is area of primary concern.

The patient is accustomed to the density provided by a synthetic hairpiece.

The patient desires rapid, dense coverage of the fronto-temporal region.

Good temporo-parietal-occipital donor site(s)

Nonsmoker

Instrumentation and Equipment

Instrumentation/Equipment for Follicular Grafting

Prep/Surgical Stand:**

Nonsterile gloves

Surgical marking pen

Electric razor

Wide paper tape to hold hair away from donor site

Hair comb

10-cc syringe (4), 18-gauge needle with 0.9% normal saline

10-cc syringe (4), 27-gauge needle with lidocaine 1% and 1:100,000 epinephrine

Needle holder

Tori triple-blade handle outfitted with three No. 10 blades

18-gauge NoKor needle (Becton Dickinson & Co., Franklin Lakes, NJ) or SP90 (Micro spear point) blade for graft insertion

Jeweler's forceps (2)

Babcock (or tenaculum)

Adson–Brown forceps

Hand drill with 1.75-mm hollow drill bit (Robbins Instruments, Inc., Chatham, NJ)

**Of note, the preparatory stand is the same as that used during the actual surgical procedure, because a separate sterile stand is not required for hair transplantation. However, a separate table should be prepared for graft dissection and preparation. Also, a dental chair serves as an ideal platform on which to operate, because it permits versatility in patient positioning during the procedure. The patient is in the upright position during donor-site harvesting and placed into a more recumbent position during graft insertion.

2-0 polypropylene C-3 (N/A, CE-2) [C17]† for donor site closure

Graft Dissection/Preparation Table:
- Powder-free gloves (sterile)
- Petri dishes (4)
- Single-edged razor blades
- Magnification visors (loupes or dissecting microscopes)
- Small bowls with normal saline (2), to wash the grafts
- Disposable Plexiglas platforms, for graft dissection
- Illumination view boxes, on which to dissect the grafts
- Adson–Brown forceps (2), to separate the strip grafts
- Jeweler's forceps (4), for individual graft dissection
- Spray bottle with sterile water or normal saline

Instrumentation/Equipment for Scalp Reduction

Prep Stand:
- Nonsterile gloves
- Surgical marking pen
- 10-cc syringe (2), 27-gauge needle with lidocaine 1% and 1:100,000 epinephrine

Surgical Table:
- Bard-Parker No. 10 blade
- Two heavy clamps
- Wide-double hooks
- Large needle holder
- Adson–Brown forceps
- LaRoe undermining forceps (9¾″ and 12¾″, Robbins Instruments, Inc.)
- Frechet-style Scalp Extender‡
- 2-0 polypropylene C-3 (N/A, CE-2) [C17] for wound closure

Instrumentation/Equipment for Scalp Rotation

First Stage:
- Nonsterile gloves
- Surgical marking pen
- 10-cc syringe (2), 27-gauge needle with lidocaine 1% and 1:100,000 epinephrine
- Doppler probe and instrumentation
- Surgical lubricant for Doppler probe
- Basic soft-tissue instrument set (Chapter 4)
- Bipolar cautery
- Skin stapler

Second Stage:
- 10-cc syringe (2), 27-gauge needle with lidocaine 1% and 1:100,000 epinephrine
- Basic soft-tissue instrument set (Chapter 4)
- Bipolar cautery
- Skin stapler

Third Stage:
- Nonsterile gloves
- Surgical marking pen
- 10-cc syringe (2), 27-gauge needle with lidocaine 1% and 1:100,000 epinephrine
- Doppler probe and Instrumentation (optional to confirm patency of vascular pedicle)
- Surgical lubricant for Doppler probe
- Basic soft-tissue instrument set (Chapter 4)
- Bipolar cautery
- Monopolar cautery
- Skin stapler
- 6-0 polypropylene suture, P-3 (P-13, PRE-2) <RE-3> needle
- 3-0 polypropylene suture, PS-2 (P-12, PRE-4) <RE-2> needle (Instead of 3-0 polypropylene, 4-0 polypropylene suture, with a FS-2 (C-13, CE-4) <KTE-6> needle can be used.)
- Jackson-Pratt closed suction drain

---

†The first needle size refers to the Ethicon code. The second parenthetical code refers to the equivalent needle size manufactured by US Surgical/Davis & Geck. Of note, the first code within the parentheses refers to new US Surgical code, and the second number within the parentheses refers to the older Davis & Geck code. The third bracketed code refers to the equivalent needle size made by Look. The fourth code in angle braces refers to the Deknatel needle equivalent.

‡The scalp extender that the authors use is obtained from Advanced Bio-Technologies, Inc. (Silverdale, WA), which can be reached at 1-800-240-8227 (or 360-698-2266), *www.advancedbiotech.com*. The authors stress that they do not have any financial relationship with the company and that the contact information is included only to assist the reader.

cause future follicular grafting sessions are required to camouflage the exposed posterior aspect of the flap. However, a detailed history should also delve into tobacco usage that may unnecessarily jeopardize flap viability. The authors elect to abstain from undertaking any flap procedure in an individual who is actively smoking. Complete cessation of this habit must be ensured 2 weeks before the initial flap elevation and maintained for the duration of all three phases of the procedure; and record of patient compliance must be documented in the medical chart. Once more, it should be emphasized that most patients are more psychologically disposed to hair grafting transplantation, and this technique serves as the primary means by which to address androgenic alopecia and has provided very satisfying results for surgeon and recipient alike.

INTRAOPERATIVE CONSIDERATIONS: TECHNIQUE AND SALIENT TECHNICAL POINTS

DVD Follicular-Grafting Techniques

Although scalp reduction and rotation methods have been used with success in the treatment of alopecia, follicular grafting remains the mainstay of therapy for surgical hair restoration. In the authors' practices, follicular grafting accounts for over 95% of surgical hair restoration; and this technique is the only acceptable method for female-pattern baldness. Over the past decade, the senior author has evolved his technique from minigrafting and micrografting now to incorporate follicular unit grafting as well. These terms are clarified before embarking on the surgical narrative. Other modifications have been made in grafting techniques that stress maximal density, a preeminent concern for the patient with alopecia. The technique outlined herein represents state-of-the-art follicular transfer as the senior author practices today, and the clinical case studies at the end of this chapter reveal some of the important changes that have been implemented over this past decade.

In order to obtain a firm grasp on the particular technique that is advocated in this section, the reader should understand some fundamental terminology only briefly alluded to in the foregoing text. The two principal schools of follicular grafting fall under the rubrics: "follicular unit grafting" and "minigrafting and micrografting." Follicular unit grafting has been a popular method of hair restoration over the past decade.[12] Hair follicles are not evenly distributed across the scalp but grow in discrete clusters of one to four hairs, so-called "follicular units" (Fig. 6-4). Many hair restoration surgeons promote dissection of all follicular grafts along these follicular units in order to achieve the most natural appearance (Fig. 6-5). However, transfer of an entire bald scalp with this technique can be a tedious affair. The terms micrografting (one- to two-hair grafts) and minigrafting (three- to six-hair grafts) represent an alternative method to partition grafts. These terms only describe the number of hairs per single graft, irrespective of how these hairs grow in follicular units. However, during graft dissection, the easiest method to cleave individual grafts is typically along follicular unit divisions. Larger minigrafts that carry five- to six-hair grafts represent more hairs than grow in a follicular unit but may consist instead of two neighboring follicular units. Some surgeons advocate placement of micrografts along the anterior hairline to achieve a natural appearance and then insertion of minigrafts more posteriorly to achieve rapid density in this region. The senior au-

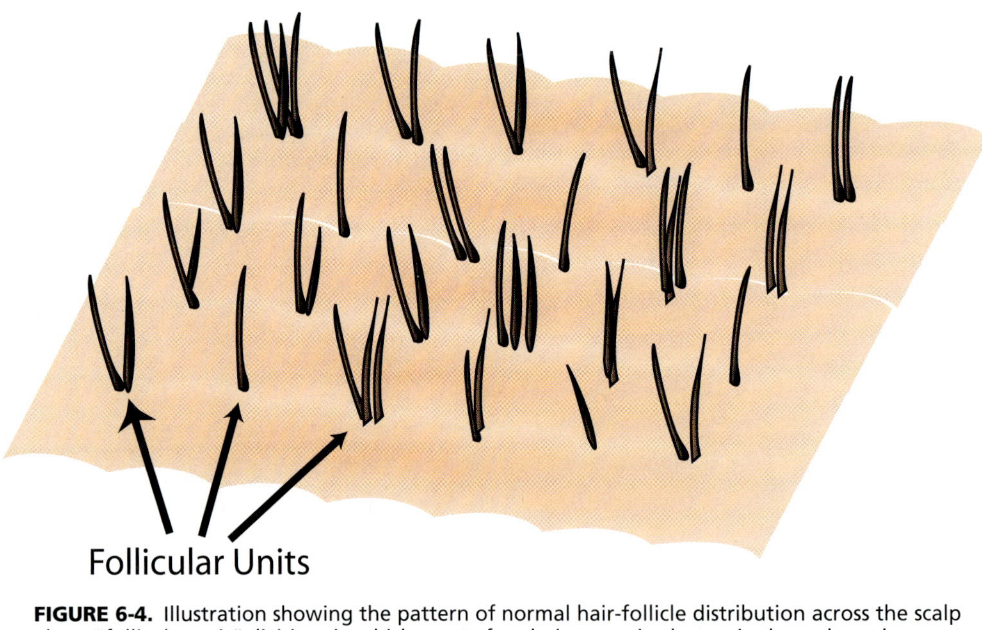

FIGURE 6-4. Illustration showing the pattern of normal hair-follicle distribution across the scalp along "follicular unit" divisions in which one to four hairs grow in clusters in the scalp and are not evenly spaced out as might be erroneously conceived.

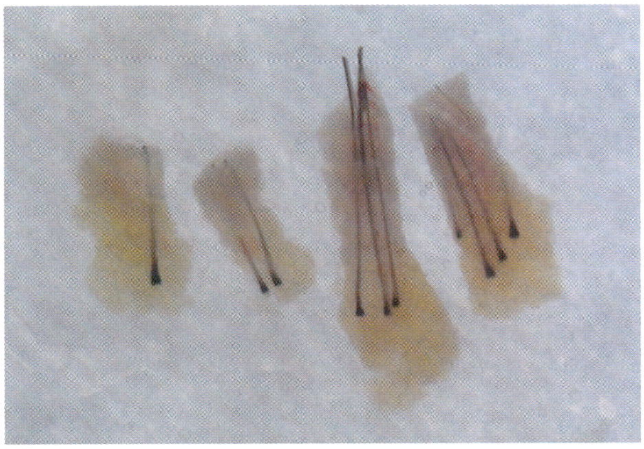

FIGURE 6-5. Close up of four individual follicular unit grafts with (from left to right) one, two, three, and four hairs per graft.

thor relied principally on this technique for many years. Currently, a combination of follicular unit transfer and minigrafting and micrografting is used to achieve a more natural result and optimal density, as explained in the following.

Some of the principles described here are repeated again in detail later in this section but are presented at this point simply as an overview. The anterior hairline may constitute the most important region to address, because the patient and onlookers scrutinize this area most often owing to its high visibility on direct gaze. The remaining scalp posterior to the anterior hairline is relatively camouflaged when viewing the patient directly. Accordingly, the principal concerns when approaching the anterior hairline are creation of a natural appearance and attainment of maximal density. In order to achieve these goals, the senior author relies heavily on densely packed follicular unit grafts along the anterior hairline. To obtain a natural appearance, the finer, vellus hairs located more inferiorly in the posterior occiput are used in the anterior-most rows, and the rows are graduated from one-hair grafts to one- to two-hair grafts to two- to three-hair grafts, with each successive row moving anterior to posterior. In addition, the anterior hairline is designed in an irregularly asymmetrical pattern rather than a straight-line configuration (Fig. 6-6A,B). To gain maximal density, the hairs are placed at different angles to one another, or "cross-hatched," to obscure the naked scalp below (Fig. 6-6C). The central forelock also is more heavily addressed because this area can be viewed from both the left and right sides of the patient; therefore, the grafts are effectively doubled visually in this area (Fig. 6-6D). These concepts are further elaborated later in this section. Creation of the anterior hairline represents the most labor-intensive aspect of follicular grafting but deserves this attention for the stated reasons. The more posteriorly situated scalp extending to the midscalp and crown demand primarily density, which can be more easily achieved with larger "minigrafts" that fall in the five- to six-hairs-per-graft size. A 1.75-mm diameter, round-punch device is used to create the recipient sites for these larger 2-mm grafts. Judicious combination of follicular unit and minigrafting and micrografting techniques permits the most rapid but natural restoration of hair than either technique alone.

Hairline Design

Prior to administration of anesthesia, the surgeon should review with the patient exactly which areas of alopecia concern him.[§§] Accordingly, the surgeon should mark out the proposed hairline and other deficient areas that require surgical attention. The most crucial aspect to achieving a natural result with follicular grafting is recreating a natural-appearing hairline. Two anatomic regions should be kept in mind, the central frontal tuft and the respective fronto-temporal recesses. The new hairline should be recreated using the principle of an irregularly asymmetrical insertion of grafts to mimic a natural hairline. As mentioned, a patient's fronto-temporal recession should be carefully examined and the angle of the fronto-temporal hairline retained to some extent. Advancing the hairline too far forward (usually less than 10 cm from the orbital rim in the central frontal forelock and less than 12 cm from the orbital rim laterally in the fronto-temporal recession) may yield a less natural result and make camouflaging difficult in a younger, rapidly progressive hairline. The textbook paradigm of facial aesthetics dictates that the face ideally should be divided equally into vertical thirds (trichion to glabella, glabella to subnasale, subnasale to menton), but this principle should not apply to hair-restoration surgery. Even if surgery is planned in a younger patient (in his early twenties), the surgeon should consider that this youthful hairline will remain unchanged for the duration of that person's life and begin to appear unnatural as that individual matures. Furthermore, the geographic region of hair loss that occurs behind the transplanted hair will be more sizable (especially in a younger patient who already requires surgical hair restoration) and may demand a considerable effort to camouflage. The isolated island of transplanted hair in an ocean of naked scalp is a dreadful telltale sign of past success and present failure. One always should be cognizant of the long-term outcome that a transplant will exhibit.

When planning the frontal hairline, the surgeon can rely on the Norwood method as a reliable guide to avoid the creation of an unnatural hairline (Fig. 6-7A–D).[13] The construction of the anterior hairline is undertaken by defining three key points: the central, most anterior point of the hairline and the two peaks of the fronto-temporal recession (Fig. 6-7C). The central, anterior point of the hairline should not descend past a level that is situated two finger breadths

[§§]Although women are clearly eligible candidates for hair transplantation, the remainder of this chapter will be devoted in large part to the male patient. Accordingly, for simplicity's sake, pronoun references will be truncated to "him" rather than the use of the more politically correct phrasing of "him or her," and hairline design will refer principally to the male patient. Commentary with regard to female pattern baldness and related therapeutic intervention will be made where deemed appropriate.

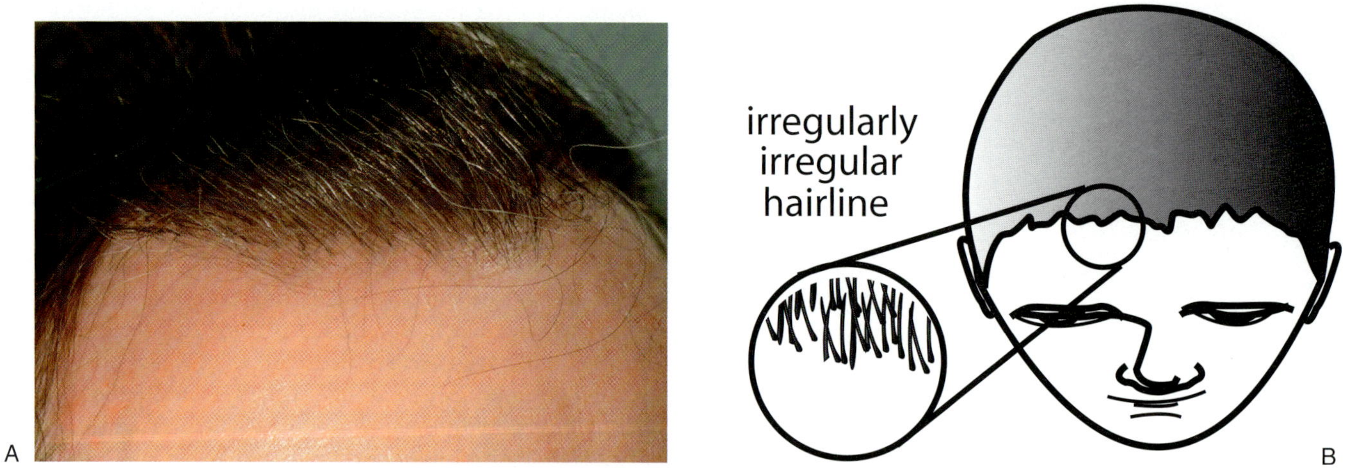

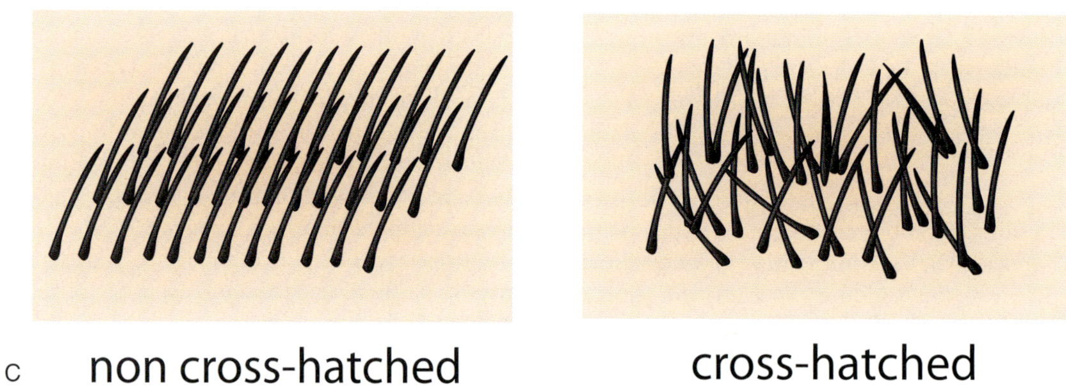

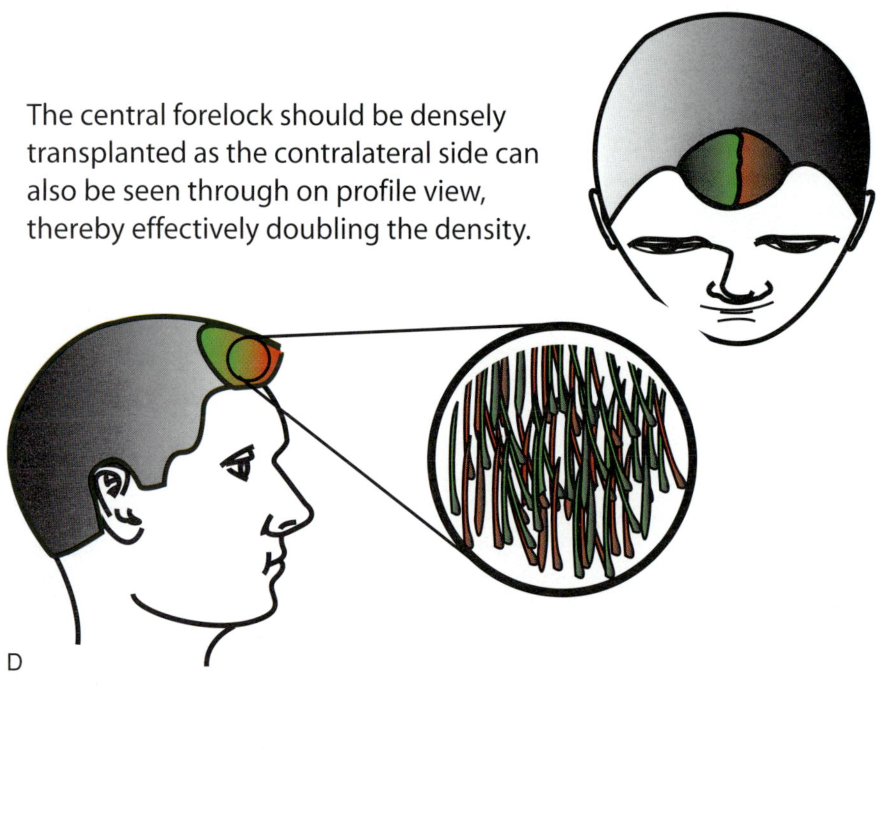

FIGURE 6-6. A: A natural hairline appears to be irregularly asymmetrical in appearance. **B:** The anterior hairline is designed in an irregularly asymmetrical pattern (akin to atrial fibrillation on an electrocardiogram) to mimic a natural hairline and minimize an operated-on appearance. **C:** All hairs are placed at different angles to one another, or "cross-hatched" in order to achieve maximal density and thereby camouflage the underlying bald scalp. **D:** The central forelock along the anterior hairline should receive assiduous attention with concentrated placement of grafts in this area. The central forelock may be viewed from the left and right sides of the patient, which visually doubles the density of the grafts in this region.

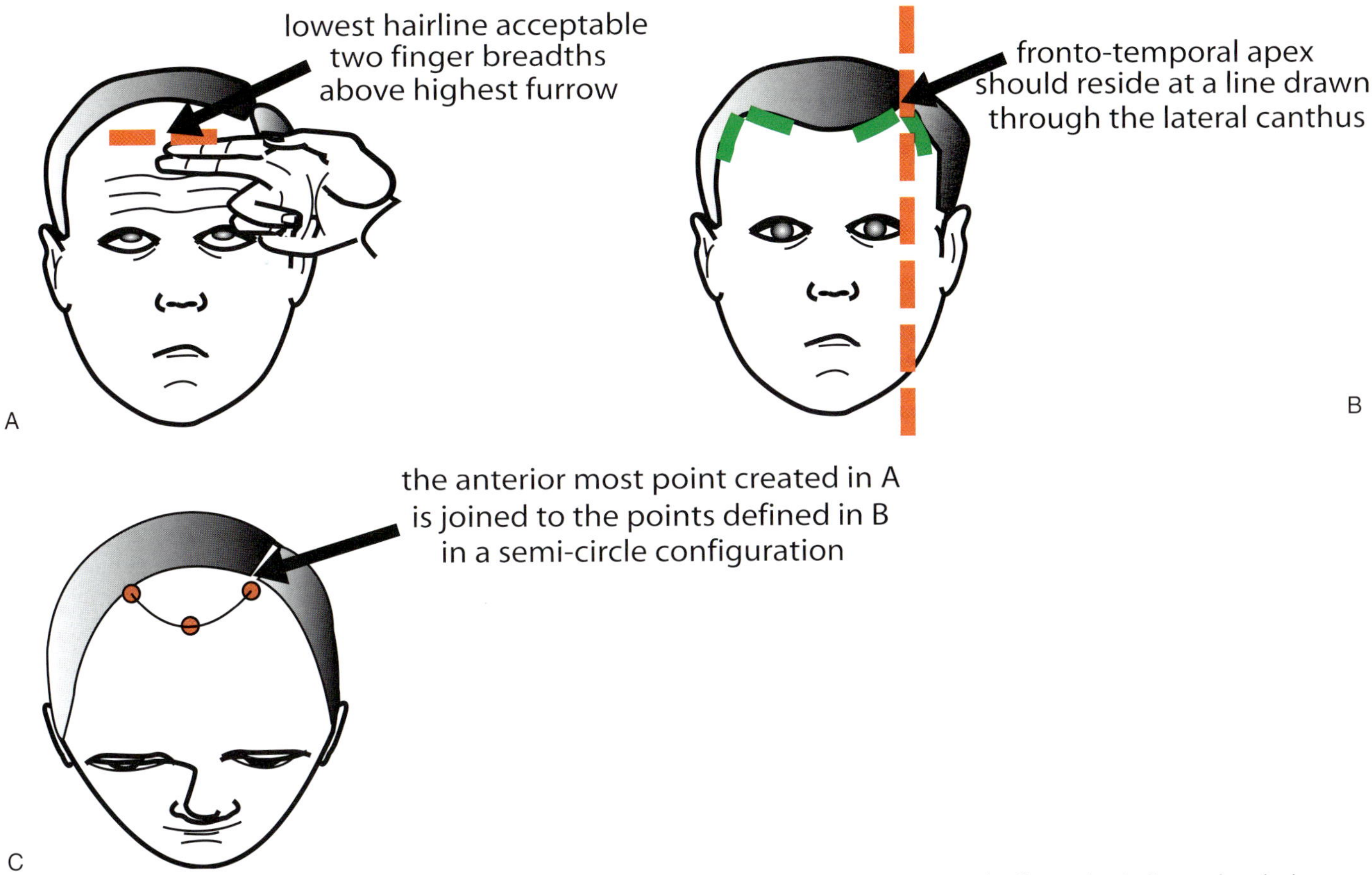

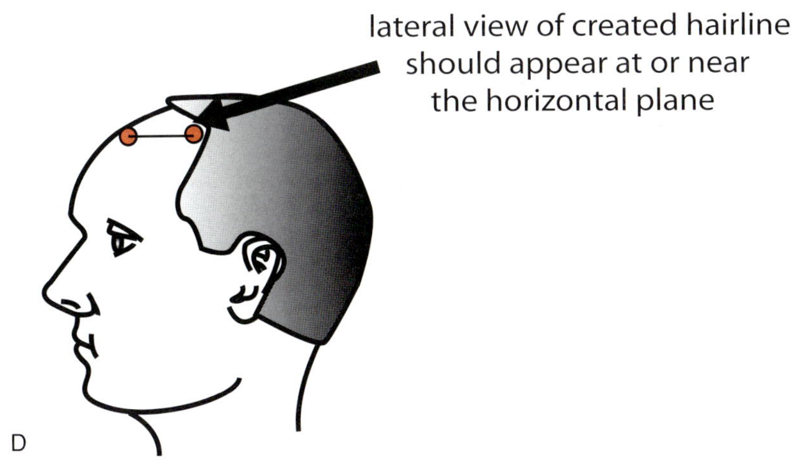

FIGURE 6-7. A: The illustration indicates that the lowest, central hairline should not descend below a point defined at two finger breadths above the highest forehead furrow when the patient gazes upward. This height should be considered only a starting point, because it is often too low for most men. Typically, the created hairline should fall approximately 10 cm above the orbital rim to avoid the risk of an excessively low hairline. **B:** Laterally, two points that define the new peak of the fronto-temporal recession should lie along a vertical axis drawn through the lateral canthus or slightly medial to this line. **C:** The illustration shows the three defining key points: the central, most anterior point of the hairline (**A**) and the two peaks of the fronto-temporal recession (**B**). The three key points should be connected as an open oval shape. **D:** On lateral view, these connected points should appear as a straight line or sloping line angled slightly upward posteriorly (but never downward).

above the highest forehead furrow created when the patient gazes upward (Fig. 6-7A). This line is the absolute lowest that is suitable for position of the hairline and only should be used as a starting, reference point. The surgeon then gauges how much higher the hairline should be positioned based on several factors: the patient's age, fronto-temporal recession, existing hairline, rate of hair loss, and aesthetic opinion. As mentioned, an acceptable starting point for the central forelock is approximately 10 cm from the orbital rim. The lateral two points that define the new peak of the fronto-temporal recession should lie along a vertical axis drawn through the lateral canthus, or slightly medial to this line (Fig. 6-7B). All three points are then connected to form an open oval shape that should appear as a straight line or slightly upward (but never downward) sloping line on lateral view (Fig. 6-7D). Because these guidelines are only meant as a starting point, the hairline should be adjusted to fit the enumerated criteria based on aesthetic judgment.

Anesthesia

Intravenous sedation is the preferred method of anesthesia that should be maintained during the initial portion of the procedure; that is, while the local anesthesia is infiltrated and the donor site harvested (Fig. 6-8). The substantial quantity of local anesthesia required for hair transplantation warrants some sedation to minimize discomfort and achieve amnesia. Patients receive a regimen of intravenous midazolam (Versed) sedation, from 4 to 8 mg. Additional medication, usually at an incremental bolus of 2 mg of midazolam, is administered according to patient requirements. The amount of anesthesia needed for sedation is observed to be directly proportional to the patient's daily or weekly alcohol consumption. Before delivery of intravenous anesthesia, the surgeon may discreetly inquire as to the amount of alcohol that the patient consumes in order to ascertain the necessary amount of anesthetic agent. Generally, this same anesthetic regimen is suitable for all scalp-reduction sessions as well for the first two stages of the Juri-flap procedure. (The reader is referred to the appropriate sections that describe scalp reduction and rotation techniques for detail regarding the proper protocol for anesthesia in those cases.) Further, similar procedures that do not require general anesthesia (e.g., acellular dermis or ePTFE soft-tissue augmentation or chemical peeling) also can employ the same anesthetic technique (Chapters 8 and 9).

Surgical Technique

Preparation of the Donor Site

The initial step in follicular-grafting surgery is selection of appropriate donor hair. The surgeon should evaluate the donor site (typically the occipital region) carefully for density, color, and quality of the hair. Generally speaking, the area immediately below the occipital protuberance but still above the inferior border of the hairline is ideal for donor harvesting (Fig. 6-9A). Removing hair above the occipital protuberance predisposes toward harvesting hair genetically programmed for future hair loss; and doing so at the inferior border of the hairline leaves behind a conspicuous scar. The more inferior-based hair (near the occipital hairline) tends to be well suited for placement along the anterior-most hairline as single- or two-hair grafts, because these grafts are finer in nature than the coarser hair situated more superiorly in the occipital region. The surgeon should attentively evaluate the suitability of the hair for this purpose and direct the technicians accordingly to use this hair to dissect one- and two-follicle–sized grafts. If this area does not appear to be

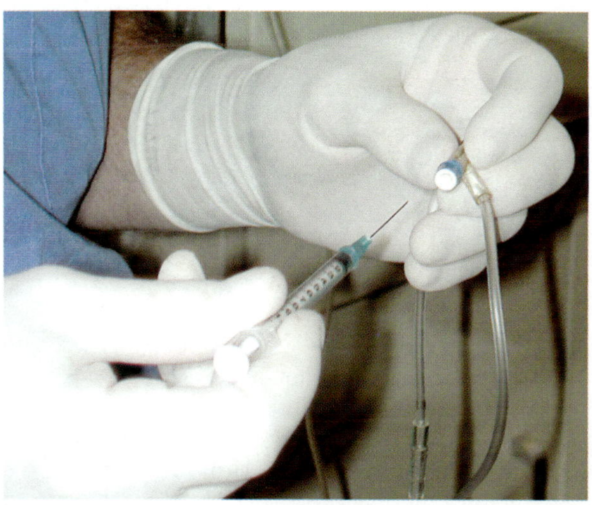

FIGURE 6-8. Intravenous sedation with midazolam provides excellent anesthesia during the most sensitive part of the operation, that is, infiltration of local anesthesia and donor-site harvesting.

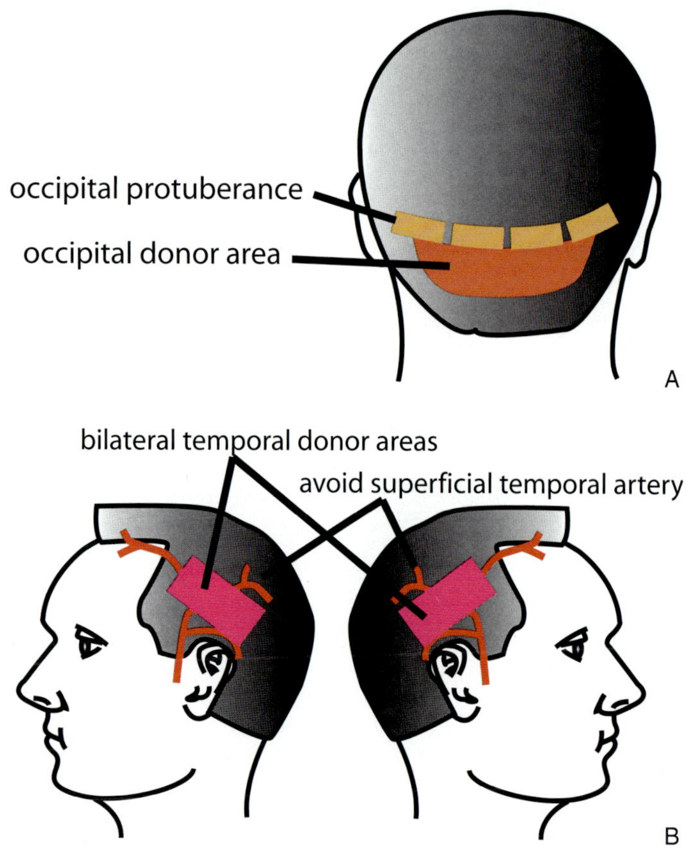

FIGURE 6-9. A: Illustration shows the preferred sites for donor-hair harvesting. The occipital region provides the first choice of donor hair given the large quantity that can be easily harvested. The first time that occipital hair is harvested, the donor hair should be taken from below the occipital protuberance to avoid harvesting hair genetically programmed for hair loss and to yield more vellus hair, which is ideal for anterior-hairline placement. The surgeon should stay above the posterior hairline to camouflage the incision site. **B:** The temporal area can be a suitable alternative for patients who have donor-hair depletion of the occipital region or who lack sufficiently fine hair in the occipital region for anterior-hairline grafting. As advised, smaller segments taken bilaterally from the temporal area are preferable to large excisions in this area to maintain symmetry and to limit tension on closure. Care should be taken to avoid injury to the posterior branch of the superficial temporal artery.

well suited for anterior hairline grafting, the surgeon should entertain the option of harvesting select temporal hair for this purpose (see the following for technique). In addition, the temporal region can serve as an excellent reserve for donor hair when the occipital region has been nearly depleted. When deciding on temporal hair harvesting, the surgeon should be advised to take smaller swaths of hair from targeted areas (e.g., bilateral harvesting of discrete areas) rather than larger passes, which may lead to ultimate asymmetry and tension on closure (Fig. 6-9B).

After the surgeon has decided on which hair will be harvested, the technician or assistant, who is in charge of preparing the surgical instruments (Fig. 6-10A,B), local anesthesia, tumescent solution, and so on, should shave the occipital or temporal region to prepare the donor site. The amount that the occipital region needs to be shaved depends on the extent of the graft session (small, medium, or large). Although these terms are arbitrary in nature, they serve well to communicate to all surgical team members the number of grafts that will be required; therefore, the number of technicians, operative-time allocation, and extent of the donor site that should be shaved. In addition, the surgeon can establish unambiguous dialog with the patient in regard to the intended surgical effort and thereby set a commensurate surgical fee. For convenience, the authors have used the following guidelines: a small session equals approximately 500 to 700 follicular grafts; a medium-size session, 700 to 1,000; a large, 1,000 to 1,500; and a megasession, more than 1,500 grafts.

Based on the size of the grafting session, the technician should shave the occipital region with an electric razor without a guard (Fig. 6-11). An electric razor is preferred over a straight razor because shearing is less traumatic, faster, easier, and more precise. Also, a short amount of follicular height, or stubble, remains after use of an electric razor that facilitates graft orientation. Wide paper tape can be used above and below the shaved area to hold the untrimmed hair out of the surgeon's way. The patient should then have an absorbent chuck underpad secured around the neck to avoid soilage of clothing during the operation. The preferred patient position for most of the procedure is sitting upright except during recipient-site creation, at which time a supine position is favored.

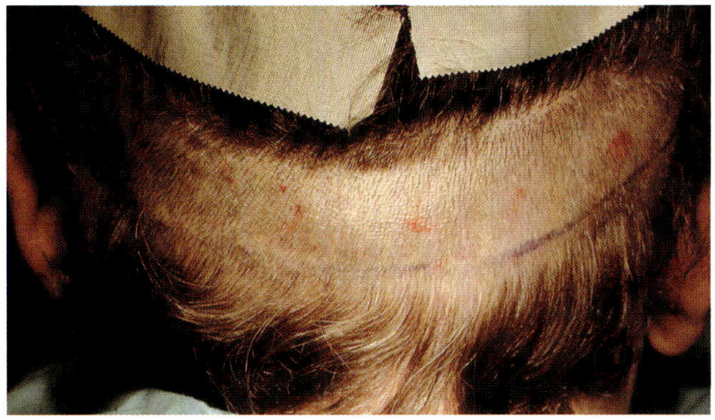

FIGURE 6-11. Follicular Grafting, Step 1. The occipital donor site, which is located below the occipital protuberance but above the posterior hairline, is shaved with an electric razor as a preparatory step. Wide paper tape is used to hold the untrimmed hair away from the donor site during harvesting.

Infiltration of Anesthesia and Harvesting of Donor Site

After the appropriate sedation, 1% lidocaine mixed with 1:100,000 epinephrine is infiltrated into the donor (occipital hair) and the recipient sites (fronto-temporal, midscalp, or vertex). Sterile normal saline then is infiltrated into the

A 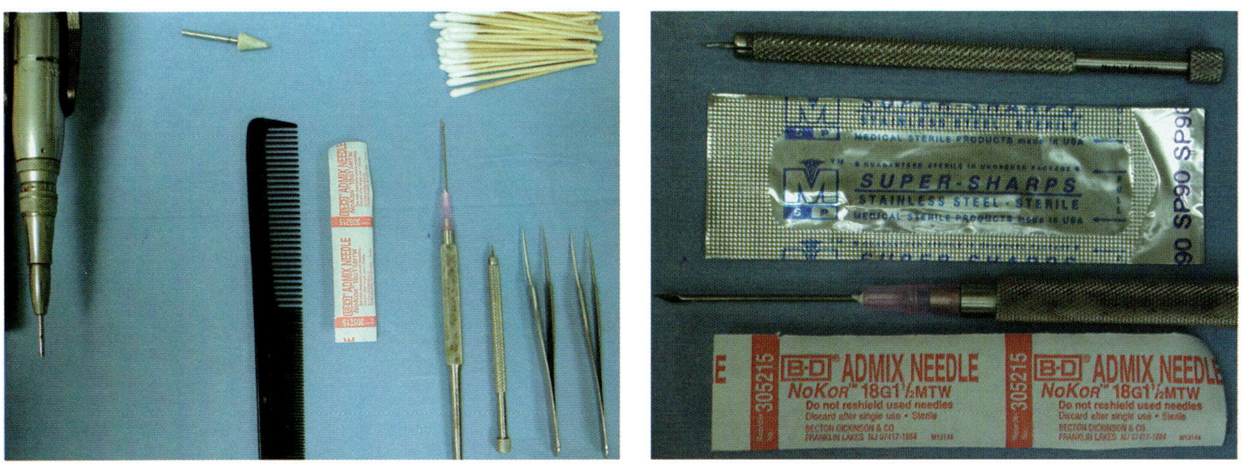 B

FIGURE 6-10. A photograph showing all of the instruments necessary for follicular grafting including the following. **A:** A rotating hand drill with a 1.75-mm round punch for creation of minigraft sites along the midscalp. **B:** An 18-gauge NoKor needle or SP90 blade which can be used interchangeably for creation of follicular unit sites along the anterior hairline.

subcutaneous plane of the donor site using an 18-gauge needle on a 10-cc syringe for tumescent effect and ease of harvest (Fig. 6-12). The end point of saline infiltration should be when the scalp appears tense and blanched and resistance is met when the plunger of the syringe is depressed. Tumescence yields several distinct advantages: (a) the follicles assume a more perpendicular orientation permitting ease of harvest; (b) the increased tension provides a more stable platform for the incision; (c) the proper plane of dissection (i.e., the subcutaneous plane) is more easily maintained because of hydrodissection and increase in overall depth of the subcutaneous plane; and (d) superior hemostasis is achieved by the added pressure of the saline on the vascular bed.

A Tori-style scalpel with 3 No. 10 blades, spaced 2 mm apart, and directed parallel with the hair follicles at 20 to 30 degrees upward is used to harvest two rows of donor hair (Fig. 6-13A,B). Although the tumescent solution tends to straighten the hair follicles somewhat, the overall follicular direction in the occipital region remains downward. During harvesting of the donor site, the surgical assistant should stand in front of the patient to observe for any signs of discomfort (e.g., wincing of the eyes), and should also hold the patient's head steady, because the patient should be quite heavily sedated during this interval. Usually two rows, each 17 cm long, are sufficient to yield approximately 170 grafts that bear three to six hairs ("minigrafts") and about twofold to threefold that number of grafts that bear one to two hairs ("micrografts"). (This estimated total of three- to six-hair minigrafts is simply calculated by multiplying 2-mm width minigrafts over a 1-cm distance, which yields five minigrafts. In turn, five grafts × two rows = 10 grafts/cm × 17 cm = 170 minigrafts in two rows.) Generally, no more than three passes of the Tori scalpel should be undertaken to avoid excessive tension on wound closure.

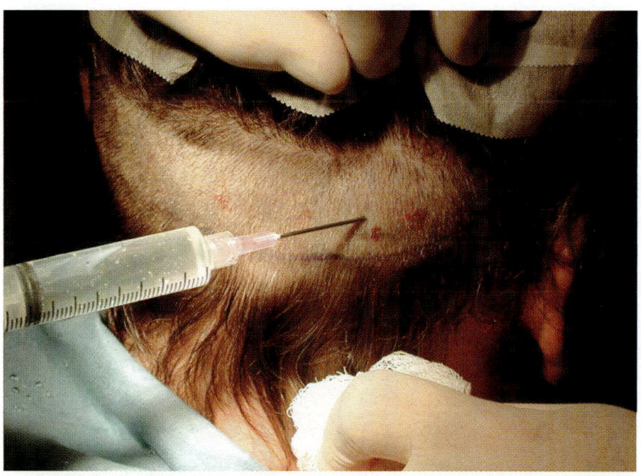

FIGURE 6-12. Follicular Grafting, Step 2. After local anesthesia has been injected into the donor area using 1% lidocaine and 1:100,000 epinephrine, sterile normal saline is then infiltrated into the subcutaneous plane of the donor site using an 18-gauge needle on a 10-cc syringe for tumescent effect and ease of dissection. The end point of saline infiltration should be when the scalp appears tense and blanched and resistance is met when the plunger of the syringe is depressed.

Of note, several key points should be kept in mind if the temporal region is to be harvested. To reiterate, only smaller patches of temporal hair should be removed from any given site to minimize the chance of asymmetry and wound tension on closure. When dissecting the temporal hair bed, the Tori scalpel also should be directed slightly upward at 20 to 30 degrees (just like in the occipital region) to parallel the direction of the hair follicles. The preferred location for temporal harvesting is several centimeters above the auricle running in an anterior-to-posterior direction. Unlike occipital-based harvesting, the depth of the incision cannot be as indiscriminate because the posterior branch of the superficial temporal artery resides immediately below the hair follicles and may be transected during harvesting (Fig. 6-9B). Therefore, care should be taken to harvest the graft as superficially as possible without violating the base of the hair shaft. Transection of the superficial temporal artery does not have any adverse effect on wound healing but only makes the task of hemostasis an avoidable nuisance.

After all the parallel rows have been dissected with the Tori scalpel, they can then be harvested from the scalp. First, a No. 10 blade is used to taper each collective end of the rows into a fusiform point: The back of the head should resemble the outline of a long football after dissection of all the rows. A tenaculum is affixed to one fusiform end to grasp all the collective rows in its tines, and a No. 10 blade is used to cleave all the rows in the midsubcutaneous plane (Fig. 6-14). The surgeon should carefully observe that the follicular shaft is not being transected during harvesting and that only a small cuff of adipose tissue (about 1 to 2 mm) remains below the hair follicle, because excessive fat below the hair bulb requires additional trimming at the time of graft preparation. The harvested strip grafts then are deposited into a bowl of saline for individual graft dissection and preparation. The donor site is closed with a running, locking 2-0 polypropylene suture that will be removed 2 weeks postoperatively (Fig. 6-15A,B). In the past, surgical staples were used; however, they irritated patients and provided less hemostasis than a locking suture. Of note, any bleeding that appears before wound closure should not be cauterized, because the locking suture will preclude any hematoma or seroma from arising.

Graft Preparation

After the donor site has been harvested, the team of technicians should begin to dissect the individual grafts (Fig. 6-16). Typically, three to four technicians are needed to expedite the dissection process, which can be the most arduous aspect of hair transplantation, followed only by graft insertion for level of technical labor. Graft preparation should be carried out on a large flat surface with good illumination and proper loupe or microscope magnification.

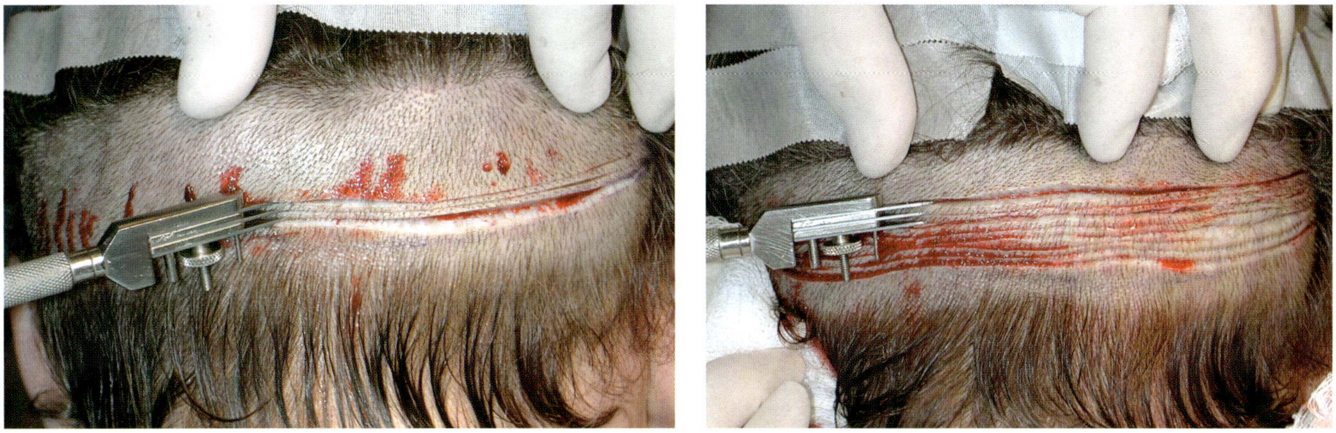

A B

FIGURE 6-13. Follicular Grafting, Step 3. A,B: Donor hair is harvested using a Tori-scalpel that holds three No. 10 blades that permit dissection of two parallel rows of hair simultaneously. Additional rows can be harvested above these rows as necessary. In accordance with good surgical principles, harvesting from an inferior to superior direction avoids blood from dripping downward that would obscure dissection.

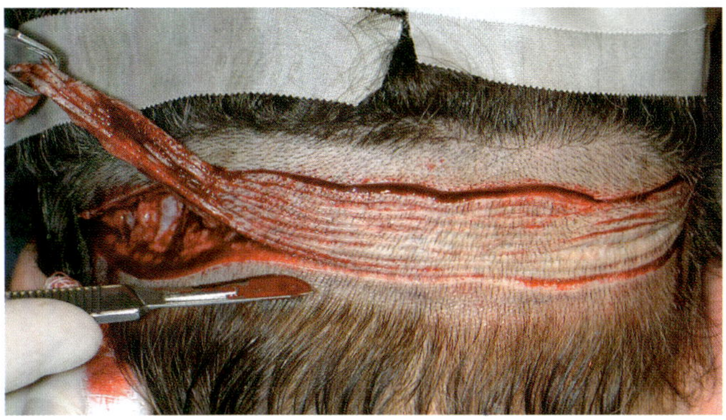

FIGURE 6-14. Follicular Grafting, Step 4. After the ends of the donor site are tapered to a fusiform point with a No. 10 blade, a tenaculum is affixed to one fusiform end to grasp all the collective rows in its tines, and a No. 10 blade is used to cleave all the rows in the midsubcutaneous plane. The surgeon should carefully observe that the follicular shaft is not being transected during harvesting and that only a small cuff of adipose tissue (about 1 to 2 mm) remains below the hair follicle.

Magnification visors are recommended because they are inexpensive and induce less eyestrain than use of a dissecting microscope. Generally, 2½ times magnification is sufficient for proper inspection of the grafts and reduction of eye fatigue. Flat, tabletop view boxes provide transillumination of the tissue, which facilitates ease of graft dissection. Disposable, Plexiglas sheets should be placed on top of the view box as a cutting board on which the grafts may be dissected without injury to the underlying view box screen. In order to reduce the glare of excessive light from the view box, a surgical drape should cover most of the view box except for the immediate field of dissection.

All the collected strip grafts should be bathed in a bowl of sterile saline until time for graft preparation. The saline removes any excess blood that may cling to the grafts and prevent desiccation. *Gentle handling of graft material and constant moisture are critical for graft viability.* A spray bottle with saline should be kept nearby that can be used to

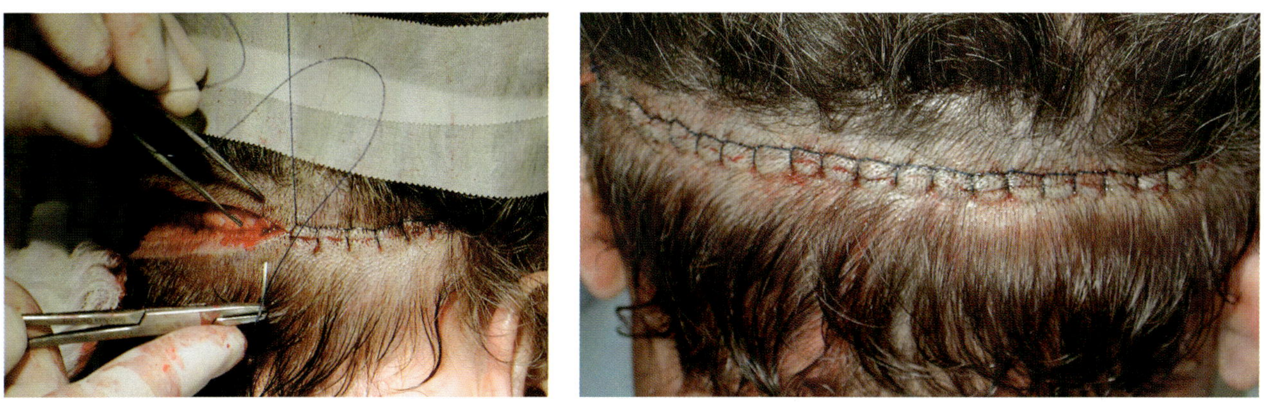

A B

FIGURE 6-15. Follicular Grafting, Step 5. A,B: The donor site is closed with a running, locking 2-0 polypropylene suture that will be removed 2 weeks postoperatively. Of note, undermining of the wound edges is both unnecessary and traumatic to future donor hair. Any bleeding that appears before wound closure should not be cauterized, because the locking suture limits the risk of a hematoma or seroma.

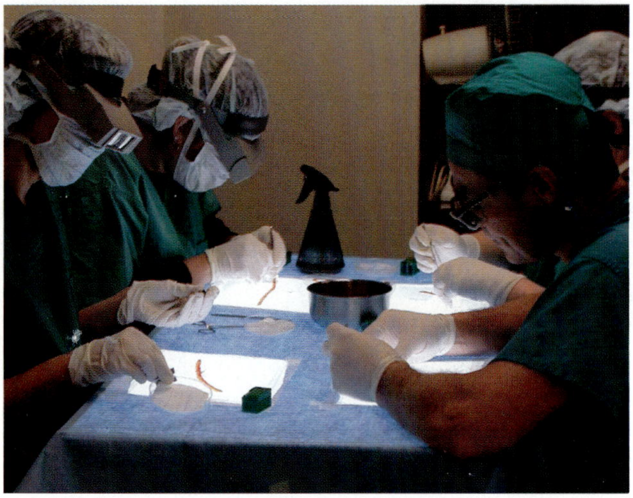

FIGURE 6-16. Follicular Grafting, Step 6A. A team of three to four technicians should dissect the grafts on a large flat table with illuminated view boxes and proper loupe or visor illumination. Protective, disposable Plexiglas sheets should be placed atop the view box for cutting to avoid injury to the view box.

moisten the grafts periodically during the period of preparation and insertion. After the strip grafts have been properly cleansed, they should be separated from one another at both ends with a No. 10 blade (Fig. 6-17). (The reader is reminded that all of the individual strip grafts are still joined together at both ends after strip graft harvesting.) Any excess adipose tissue (greater than 1 mm) that remains below the base of the hair shafts should be trimmed before further graft dissection.

At this point, the strip grafts are dissected into discrete follicular grafts for transplantation using a straight razor. The amount of epidermal, dermal, and adipose tissue that should remain on each graft is negligible, with only about a 1-millimeter cuff surrounding the graft on all sides (Fig. 6-5). In order to achieve the density of grafts in a particular area, the follicular graft must be relatively devoid of excessive tissue. To obtain this degree of accuracy, the technician must rely on magnification and illumination, as previously discussed. In contradistinction, the larger grafts that are distributed across the midscalp (i.e., behind the 3-cm anterior hairline) are larger and can have a 2-mm adipose cuff surrounding the hair shaft. Precise insertion techniques and placement of different sized grafts is discussed in the following section. During graft preparation, the surgeon and two assistants can begin graft insertion with the grafts that have already been dissected. The grafts should be dissected mainly along follicular units for ease of graft harvesting and to achieve an optimal aesthetic result. However, the principle of follicular unit transfer is not strictly adhered to, because larger grafts (four to six hairs per graft) also are dissected. Furthermore, the finer-caliber hair grafts that are harvested more inferiorly along the occipital or temporal fringe should be cleaved into one- or two-hair grafts (despite follicular unit divisions) so that they can be destined for anterior hairline placement. After dissecting each graft, the technician should position the grafts on a Petri dish according to graft size. A line of demarcation should be drawn on each Petri dish that separates one-, two-, three-, three- to four-, and five- to six-hair grafts (Fig. 6-18). Alternatively, a Petri dish can be assigned to each of the graft sizes.

Graft Insertion

Follicular grafting of the balding scalp may be divided into two principal areas of concern: the frontal hairline and the more posteriorly situated midscalp (Fig. 6-19). The area that is most noticeable to the patient and casual observer alike is the frontal hairline, which deserves commensurate attention and labor by the surgical team. The technique to address the anterior hairline differs markedly from that used to recreate the density required for the remaining scalp. Accordingly, this section is subdivided into management of the frontal hairline and that of the posterior scalp.

Anterior Hairline

The creation of a natural hairline in both height and configuration already has been addressed. This section focuses on the technique of graft insertion into the anterior hairline that ensures maximal density yet retains a nonsurgical appearance. Three key surgical aspects of frontal hairline creation are explained: (a) the concept of cross-hatching; (b) the importance of the frontal forelock; and (c) the technique of graduated follicular grafting.

A 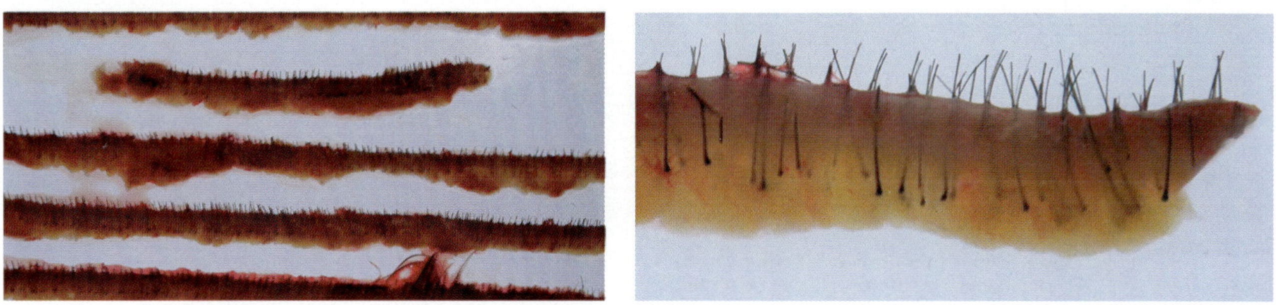 B

FIGURE 6-17. Follicular Grafting, Step 6B. A: Multiple strip grafts shown atop a view box. **B:** A single, close-up view of a strip graft, which will be dissected in turn into individual follicular grafts.

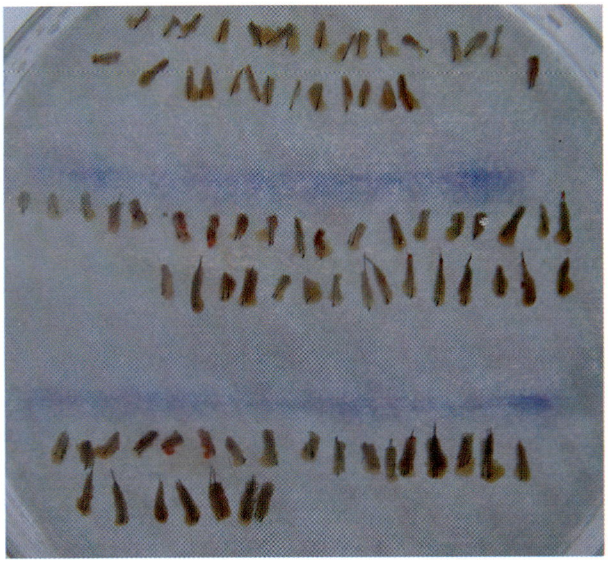

FIGURE 6-18. Follicular Grafting, Step 6C. Petri dish with lines of demarcation showing one-,two-, and three-hair grafts from top to bottom.

Placement of individual follicular grafts at different angles to one another permits maximal camouflage of the bald scalp. This technique is known as cross-hatching. If grafts are all placed in the same alignment, the bare scalp will be more visible to the naked eye than if they are placed in varying orientation to one another. Therefore, cross-hatching increases the perceived density of the hair. Similarly, the frontal forelock should be targeted for placement of a greater concentration of grafts because this central area can be observed from both sides of the head. Accordingly, every graft that is placed in this region is seen when the observer is viewing the patient from either the right or left side. Conversely, grafts placed along the right side of the hairline are only visible when the observer is situated to the right of the patient. The same limited view that the observer has on the left side of the patient is applicable to the left side of the hairline. The grafts placed along the central forelock have double the exposure time than laterally placed grafts. Further, because the central tuft of hair can be seen from either vantage point, the hair in this area appears to gain twice the perceived density, because twice the number of grafts are being viewed concurrently.

Besides overall height and configuration of a hairline, several other key factors contribute to its natural appearance. The hairline should assume an irregularly asymmetrical pattern (i.e., the hairs should not be situated in a straight-line configuration across the proposed hairline). When creating the hairline, the surgeon should attempt to stagger each graft a bit anterior or posterior to the previously placed graft without any consistent pattern. This haphazard arrangement mimics a natural hairline. The aforementioned principle of cross-hatching further enhances the irregular design of the hairline. The anterior most row of the hairline should consist of fine, single-hair strands as opposed to coarse, three- to four-hair follicular grafts. By placing finer-caliber and single-hair grafts along the anterior-most hairline, the surgeon emulates a natural hairline and thereby prevents a "pluggy" appearance to the surgical result. Each

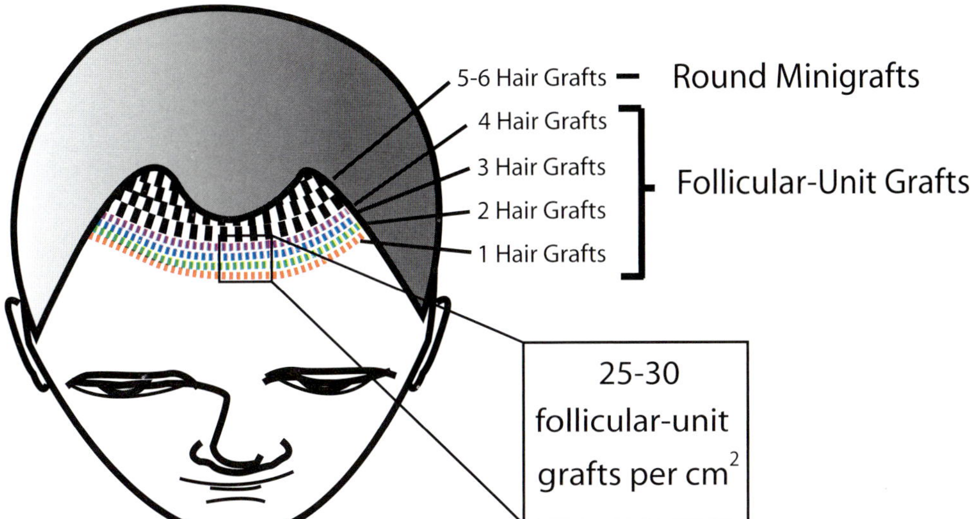

FIGURE 6-19. The illustration shows the two principal regions for follicular grafting: the anterior hairline and posteriorly situated midscalp. The frontal hairline should be addressed with graduated follicular unit grafts (from the anterior row with only one-hair grafts with an increase in number in each successive row posterior to the front row). The midscalp is addressed with larger minigrafts. If the area of alopecia extends to the crown, then the area posterior to the minigrafts should be gradually feathered with additional smaller follicular unit grafts toward the bald scalp if that remaining area is not intended for operative camouflage.

successive row posterior to the most anterior row should show an increase in the number of hairs per graft and thickness of the hair-shaft caliber. The surgeon ensures optimal density and a natural result by following all of these tenets.

As mentioned, local anesthesia in the recipient site should be administered at the inception of the case when the midazolam is delivered. During graft insertion, the patient may be fully awake and express anxiety over his lucid state. However, the surgeon should resist the temptation to grant additional intravenous sedation, because the more protracted recovery period that ensues typically does not justify another bolus of medication at this point.

The anterior hairline to be constructed constitutes on average a 10-cm distance along its length and a 3-cm distance from anterior to posterior extent. Therefore, the total scalp void that typically must be transplanted is approximately 30 cm^2. Per square centimeter, approximately 20 to 25 follicular grafts should be inserted to achieve maximal density. Accordingly, 600 to 750 grafts should be placed to occupy a 3-cm recession of the anterior hairline. Additional grafts may be placed posterior to this 3-cm deep hairline if required for additional camouflage. However, generally speaking, larger 2-mm, three- to six-hair "minigrafts" may be used behind this anterior hairline to achieve more rapid density. (See the following section on the midscalp.)

The surgeon and two assistants should be in charge of graft insertion. The technique involves the surgeon creating a recipient site, the first assistant then filling that recipient site with an appropriate graft, and the second assistant handing the first assistant another graft for insertion (Figs. 6-20 and 6-21A–C). More precisely, the surgeon uses an 18-gauge NoKor needle or SP90 blade (according to preference) to create the recipient site using the principles of cross-hatching and irregularly asymmetrical placement (as explained). The second assistant hands the first assistant the appropriate size and caliber graft with a pair of jeweler's forceps; the first assistant then places the graft into the recipient site according to the direction that the surgeon created. The first assistant must maintain his or her line of vision constantly on the surgeon's hand in order to recognize in what direction the recipient site was created so that placement of the graft matches that same direction. Therefore, the role of the second assistant is critical so that the first assistant need not look away from the hairline to obtain the appropriate graft for insertion. Graft insertion proceeds across the entire hairline row by row. As the surgeon returns to fill in the next row, which should be one to two hairs per graft larger than the row immediately anterior, some of the previously placed grafts may be noted to have fallen out of the recipient site. Unfortunately, this problem is frequently encountered, as edema increases and the crowding of densely packed grafts force neighboring grafts out of their nestled position. Care must be taken to return these displaced grafts back into the recipient site. Dislodgement of the graft is less likely after a fibrin clot has formed in the recipient site.

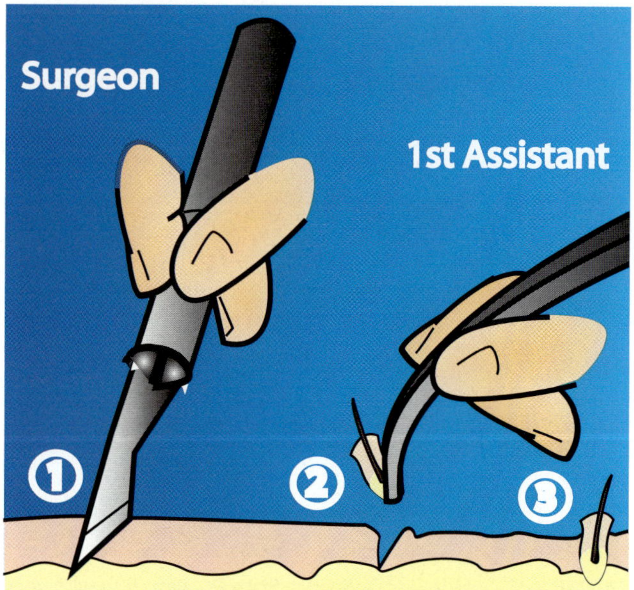

FIGURE 6-20. The illustration shows proper graft insertion technique in which the chief surgeon creates a recipient site. Paying careful attention to the angle in which the surgeon created the recipient site, the first assistant places the graft into the site at the same prescribed angle. The second assistant then hands the first assistant the appropriate sized graft for the next graft placement (not shown).

The Midscalp

Behind the hairline and extending over the midscalp, the surgeon should create larger recipient sites that can accommodate five- to six-hair grafts. These larger sites are created with a rotating hand drill that carves out 1.75-mm circular defects into which these 2-mm sized grafts may be inserted (Fig. 6-22A,B). It is important that the same principle of cross-hatching be applied to achieve maximal density. It is very easy for the rotating drill to ensnare the neighboring hair and thereby temporarily depopulate more hair than will actually be grafted. This unnecessary hair removal can be quite distressing to the patient, who will already undergo additional hair loss in several weeks to months—a condition known as telogenic effluvium that typically occurs 2 to 4 weeks posttransplantation because of the trauma caused by surgical manipulation. The inadvertent entanglement of adjacent hair by the rotating instrument can be reduced by the following techniques: (a) wet the hair and hold the hair out of the way with the nondominant hand; and (b) limit the time that the hand drill is in rotation (i.e., start the drill rotating when the instrument is in contact with the scalp and stop the drill rotating before removing the instrument from the scalp). If a foot pedal is used to control the hand drill, the foot should only briefly tap the foot pedal rather than depress it for any sustained duration. After each graft is created, the tissue core within each site should be removed with a Brown–Adson forceps so that the larger grafts can be placed into the resulting divot.

At the end of the session, a commercial hair dryer that uses radiating heat rather than a dynamic air stream can be

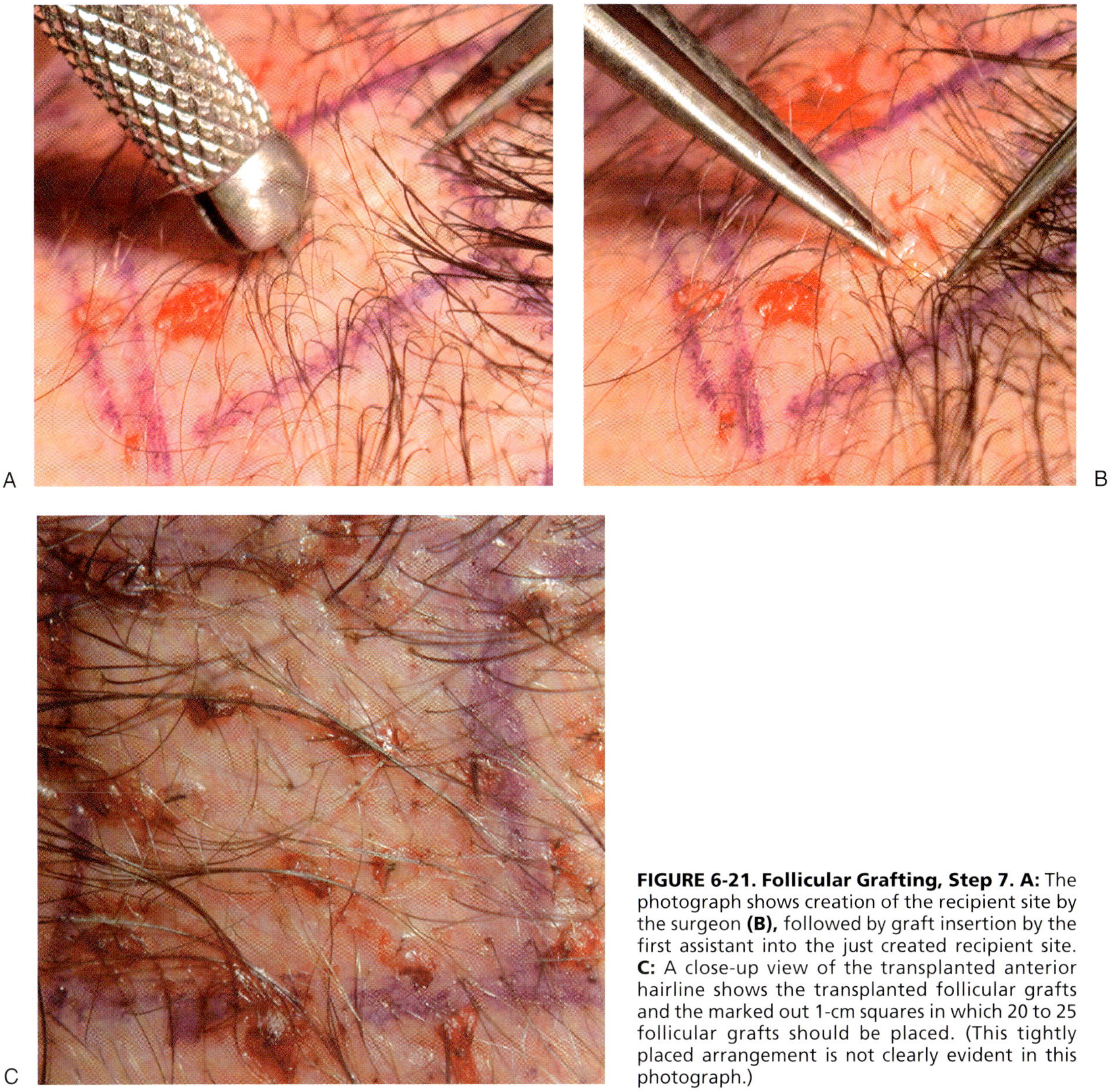

FIGURE 6-21. Follicular Grafting, Step 7. A: The photograph shows creation of the recipient site by the surgeon (B), followed by graft insertion by the first assistant into the just created recipient site. C: A close-up view of the transplanted anterior hairline shows the transplanted follicular grafts and the marked out 1-cm squares in which 20 to 25 follicular grafts should be placed. (This tightly placed arrangement is not clearly evident in this photograph.)

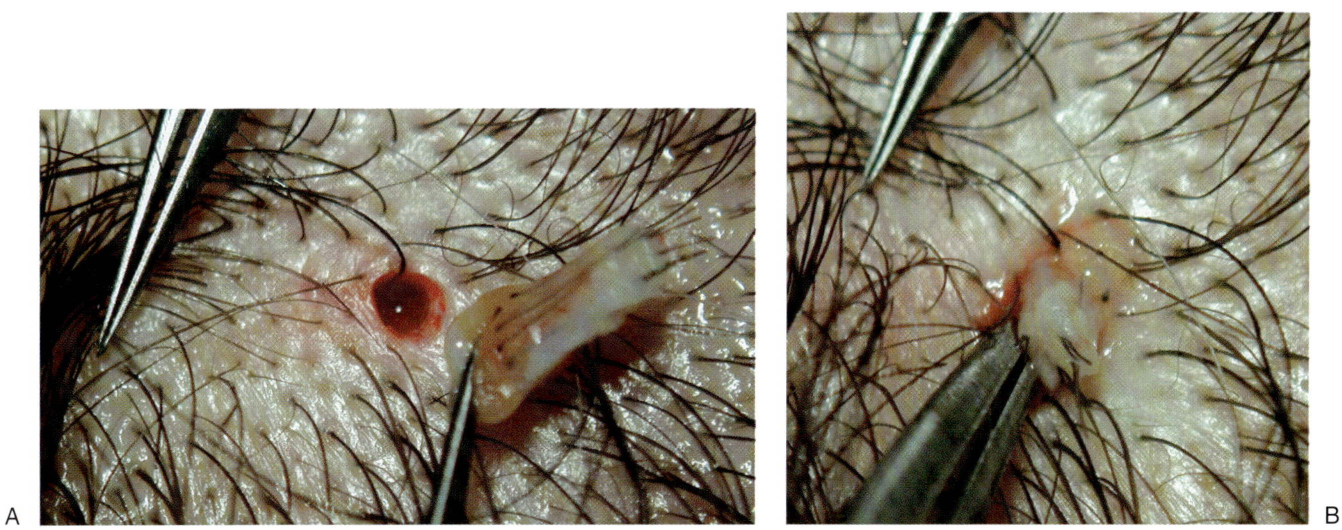

FIGURE 6-22. Follicular Grafting, Step 8. A,B: A larger recipient site is created for minigraft placement in the midscalp region using a rotating hand drill that carves out 1.75-mm circular defects. The resulting divot should be removed with Brown–Adson forceps so that the larger minigraft (with five to six hairs) can be placed into the defect.

used to dry the hair before placement of a bandage. Several layers of 4 × 4 gauze are applied directly on top of the transplanted hair and kept in place with a baseball cap. Because the hair has been air dried, the 4 × 4 gauze does not tend to adhere to the scalp or the inserted grafts.

DVD Scalp Reduction Techniques (Scalp Reduction with Extender)

General Considerations

As a quick review, the ideal candidate for scalp reduction is a more mature patient (more than 40 years old) with a relatively stable pattern of hair recession who desires camouflage of his exposed crown, or vertex, area. *The diameter of the bald vertex cannot exceed 13 cm for successful closure of the area.* The patient also must be psychologically prepared for multiple sessions of scalp reduction to achieve complete closure. Four sessions are anticipated for complete closure of 10 to 12 cm of exposure. Similarly, three sessions should be sufficient for closure of 8 to 9 cm. As mentioned, greater than 13 cm of baldness proves to be difficult to close entirely, despite numerous sessions.

Typically, the first session permits approximately 4 cm of tissue mobilization from the parietal fringe (2 cm from each side) and about 1 to 2 cm from the occipital fringe (Fig. 6-23). Subsequent sessions permit less tissue advancement with about 3 cm of total tissue recruitment laterally and less than 1 cm posteriorly. Remaining scalp exposure may be addressed with minigrafts and micrografts to the central slot deformity after appropriate multiple z-plasty closures are performed (Fig. 6-24A,B). If the patient exhibits fronto-temporal recession and is motivated, then concurrent minigrafting and micrografting may be undertaken in that region even if significant undermining is planned in the area of proposed grafting. Although graft viability tends to be good despite undermining, the authors are inclined to discourage combined approaches (grafting and scalp reduction) to minimize risk of graft loss and the potential morbidity of protracted and extensive surgical manipulation.

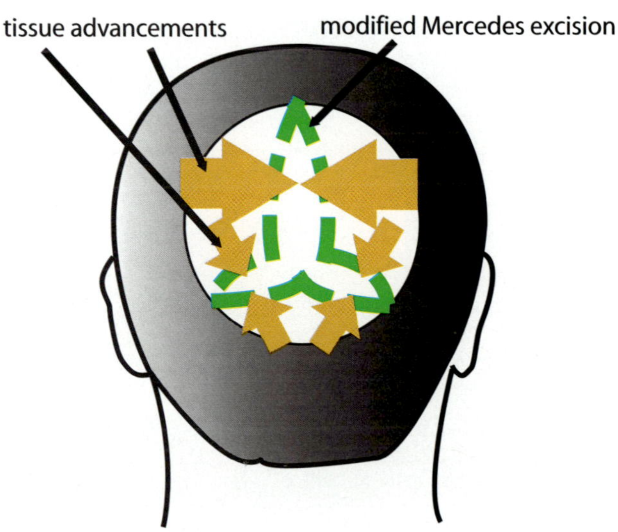

FIGURE 6-23. The illustration shows the modified Mercedes configuration that permits greater parietal reduction with the larger limb and two smaller occipital-based limbs.

Anesthesia

Generally, intravenous sedation using the protocol described in the preceding for follicular grafting is sufficient for all scalp-reduction sessions. In addition, local anesthesia of 1% lidocaine with 1:100,000 epinephrine is infiltrated as a ring-block around the perimeter of the area to be dissected and undermined.

Surgical Technique

A modified Mercedes configuration is designed over the exposed crown with the longer limb in the midsagittal plane and the shorter limbs extending postero-laterally. This inverted-Y incision has yielded the largest area of scalp recruitment by drawing more mobile parietal scalp centrally and advancing less of the adherent occipital scalp. The rich occipital vasculature also makes surgical manipulation in this area less than desirable. The size of each limb of the Mercedes should follow the guidelines described earlier for recommended tissue advancement; e.g., a 4-cm width of the vertical limb to recruit 2 cm of parietal donor hair from each side and a 1- to 2-cm width of the horizontal limb to advance a respective 1 to 2 cm of occipital hair during the first session. In subsequent sessions, narrower limbs (e.g., a 3-cm wide vertical limb and a 1-cm, horizontal limb) should be used, because the scalp becomes less elastic.

The initial incision can be undertaken after appropriate intravenous and local anesthesia are administered. The dissection is taken down through the galea aponeurotica and carried out in a subgaleal plane all the way down to just above the ears laterally and over the occipital protuberance posteriorly (i.e., to the nuchal line). As mentioned, use of an extender is mandatory to achieve maximal reduction, and minimal unfavorable stretchback (Fig. 6-3), and to shorten the interval between sessions.[¶] Before the use of an extender, concomitant stretchback could prolong total reduction time to upward of 18 months, including all reduction sessions. Now, not only is unfavorable stretchback eliminated, but also the biomechanical advantage imparted by the extender permits a markedly reduced interval between sessions, with an average of 30 days.

¶The reader is referred to the instrumentation and equipment section of this chapter for contact information regarding where a scalp extender device can be obtained.

A 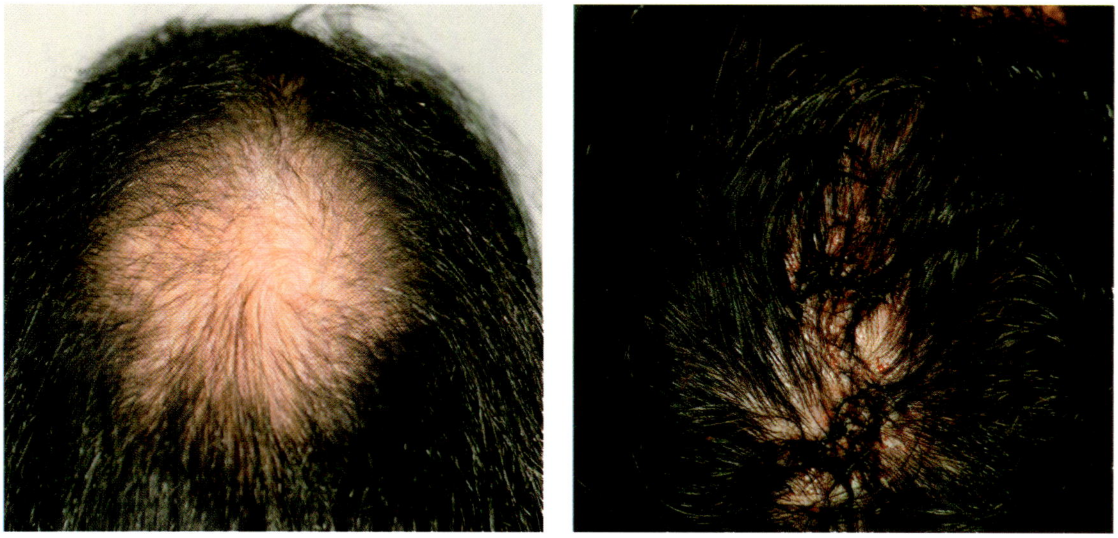 B

FIGURE 6-24. A: Posterior view of the scalp before scalp reduction, and **(B)** after three reduction sessions with final z-plasty closure.

After the bald scalp is excised in the aforementioned modified Mercedes configuration, appropriate undermining is accomplished in the subgaleal plane with a LaRoe undermining forceps (Fig. 6-25A). The extender can then be positioned prior to scalp closure (Fig. 6-25B). The titanium hooks of the extender should be secured under one parietal wound edge first. As one assistant holds the scalp down in position, the surgeon advances the other free edge of the extender toward the contralateral parietal wound edge, grasping the device with a pair of clamps and placing the distensible silastic under tension. The second assistant maintains the free parietal wound edge in an elevated position with a wide, double-pronged retractor as the surgeon positions the unsecured titanium hooks under the described free parietal edge. The cutaneous closure of the wound then can be properly undertaken after the extender device is securely fashioned to the underlying galea: A 2-0 polypropylene is used to close the wound in a running, locking fashion. The sutures are removed 2 weeks postoperatively. As mentioned, reduction sessions can be spaced 1 month apart if an extender is used.

The number of reduction sessions is predicated on the initial size of baldness and scalp elasticity that will permit complete closure. At the time of the final reduction session, a concurrent, multiple z-plasty closure is planned for several reasons. This type of closure visually disrupts the scar and

A 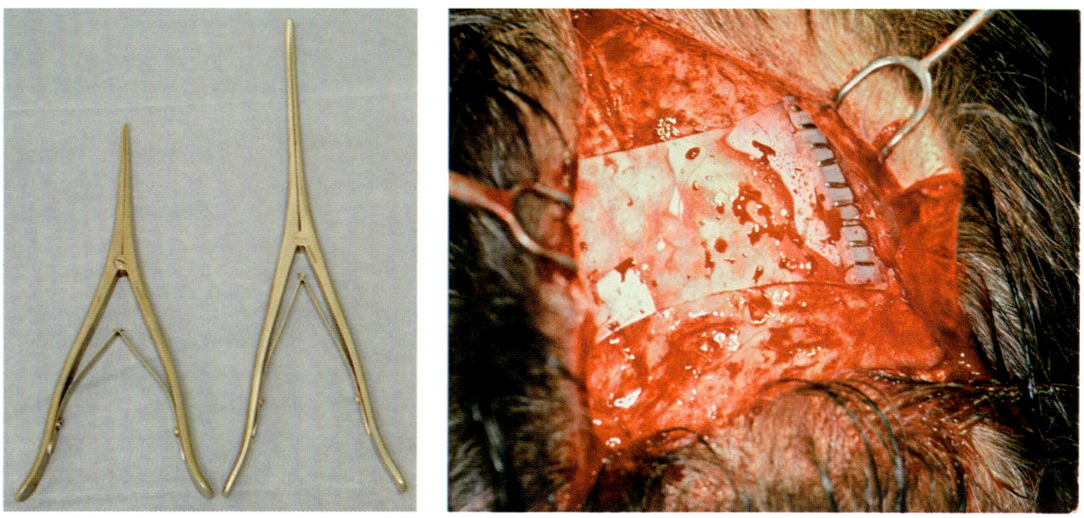 B

FIGURE 6-25. Scalp Reduction. A: Undermining is undertaken with a specialized pair of forceps LaRoe undermining forceps ($9\frac{3}{4}$" and $12\frac{1}{4}$", Robbins Instruments, Inc.). **B:** The intraoperative photograph that shows the extender device placed during scalp reduction, as viewed through the surgical defect.

reduces the risk of unfavorable scar contracture. With ensuing mild alopecia in the area of the z-plasty closure, the complex arrangement of transposition flaps camouflages any minor hair loss. In the authors' practices, no revision cases have been needed over the past 10 years, and satisfaction has been uniformly high.

Scalp Rotation Techniques (The Juri Twice-Delayed Temporo-Parietal-Occipital Flap)

General Considerations

In brief review, scalp-rotation procedures should be reserved for those patients who desire rapid, dense coverage to the fronto-temporal region and who tolerate more invasive, multistage surgery (Fig. 6-26). The density provided by this surgical method is unparalleled when compared with traditional grafting techniques. The rate of fronto-temporal recession usually does not pose a problem. However, the area immediately behind the flap may become exposed over time if excessive hair loss continues. A contralateral flap or micrografting and minigrafting will disguise this problem if it should arise. The temporo-parieto-occipital region should exhibit dense, undisturbed donor hair for rotation, and the patient's vascular integrity must be ascertained (i.e., no recent smoking history or other vascular compromise). The patient also should understand that the frontal hairline might appear excessively thick and the fronto-temporal regions blunted. For these reasons, the prospective patient should anticipate the potential for additional micrografting sessions to achieve the desired aesthetic result. Further, revision of a standing-cone deformity may be required in a few instances if this problem does not resolve after several months.

Although several variations of scalp rotational procedures exist in the literature,[14–16] the authors have found consistently excellent results with the twice-delayed flap originally proposed by Jose Juri. Unlike the single-delayed temporo-parietal flap, the Juri flap yields twice the length and breadth of the aforementioned flap. The more abbreviated temporo-parietal flap is too short to traverse the entire frontal hairline and a contralateral flap usually is required to bridge the gap. Unfortunately, this more diminutive flap often appears unnatural, especially if further recession of hair arises behind the flap, leaving an isolated, narrow strip of hair that serves as the manufactured frontal hairline. Conversely, the Juri flap provides a longer flap that usually spans the entire arc of the frontal hairline and gives adequate width (typically 4-cm versus the temporo-parietal's paltry 2-cm girth, for a comparative fourfold increase in surface area). Again, a second Juri flap can be planned as a staged procedure after a 6-month minimum but preferably at 1-year postfinal flap inset.

Anesthesia

For the first two stages of the Juri flap (in which the flap is prepared for transposition), the protocol for intravenous sedation as outlined in the previous section on follicular-grafting techniques may be appropriate. However, the extensive undermining and surgical mobilization that is required for the third and final stage of the Juri flap usually require deeper sedation or general anesthesia under the care of an anesthesiologist or trained anesthetist. As far as local anesthesia is concerned, 1% lidocaine with 1:100,000 epinephrine is injected circumferentially around the Juri flap, taking care to avoid infusion of anesthetic agent directly into or near the nutrient arteries to the flap. At the time of the first stage of the Juri flap, the surgeon should carefully delineate the vascular pedicle with a Doppler device prior to infiltration of local anesthesia so that the safe perimeter for injection may be determined.

Surgical Technique

First Stage

The initial task that must be addressed is determination of a suitable hairline on which the surgeon and patient can agree. The desired new frontal hairline should be constructed both in terms of configuration (peaked versus straighter with less fronto-temporal recession) and height (from the orbital rim). Clearly, the proposed hairline cannot extend 4 cm below the existing hairline, because the 4-cm width of the T-P-O flap must bridge this gap. If the patient and surgeon believe that the hairline should descend much more than 4 cm from the existing hairline position, then a contralateral flap will be required to bring the hairline down further. However, if the patient exhibits significant hair recession so that even two T-P-O flaps will not bridge the gap between the original and proposed hairline, then a Juri flap may not be the ideal solution to the patient's particular condition of alopecia. Alternatively, for the very bald patient, bilateral T-P-O flaps may be rotated into position to create a dense new hairline and micrografting and minigrafting used to soften the transition with the naked scalp posterior to the flap.

The T-P-O flap is based axially on the posterior branch of the superficial temporal artery (STA) and distally on the postauricular and occipital arteries in a random fashion (Fig. 6-27A). As part of the first stage of the operation, the proximal flap should be mapped out according to Doppler analysis of the posterior branch of the STA (Fig. 6-28A–C). Because the distal aspect of the flap is random, a doppler reading is unwarranted. The proximal third of the flap lies behind the new hairline, whereas the distal two thirds of the flap serves to recreate the new hairline. Therefore, the peak of the flap should be designed at the junction of the middle and distal thirds. The base of the flap should commence 4 cm above the helical crus and span a distance of 4-cm width at an angle of 30 to 40 degrees with the horizontal (Fig. 6-

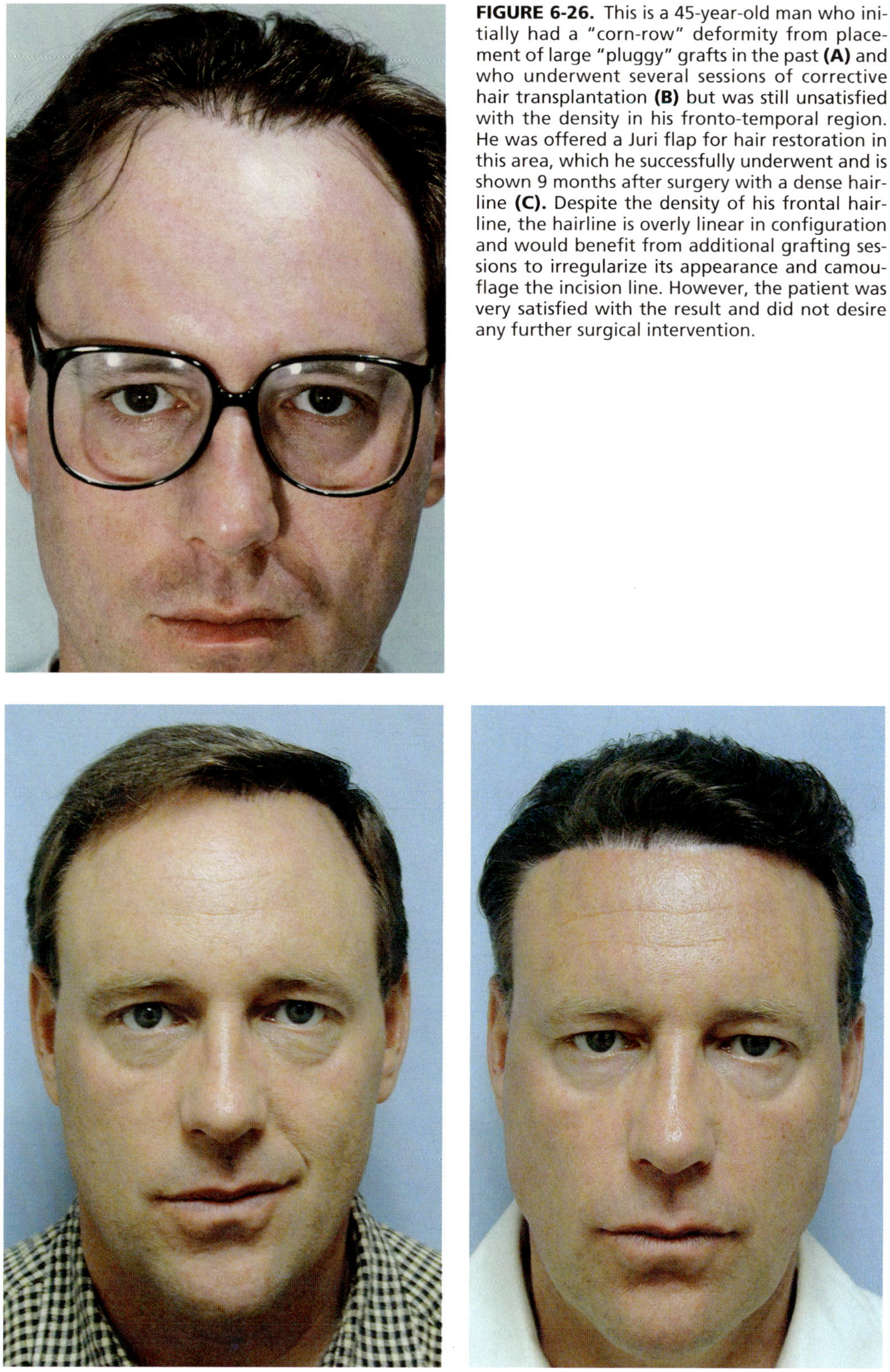

A

B

C

FIGURE 6-26. This is a 45-year-old man who initially had a "corn-row" deformity from placement of large "pluggy" grafts in the past **(A)** and who underwent several sessions of corrective hair transplantation **(B)** but was still unsatisfied with the density in his fronto-temporal region. He was offered a Juri flap for hair restoration in this area, which he successfully underwent and is shown 9 months after surgery with a dense hairline **(C).** Despite the density of his frontal hairline, the hairline is overly linear in configuration and would benefit from additional grafting sessions to irregularize its appearance and camouflage the incision line. However, the patient was very satisfied with the result and did not desire any further surgical intervention.

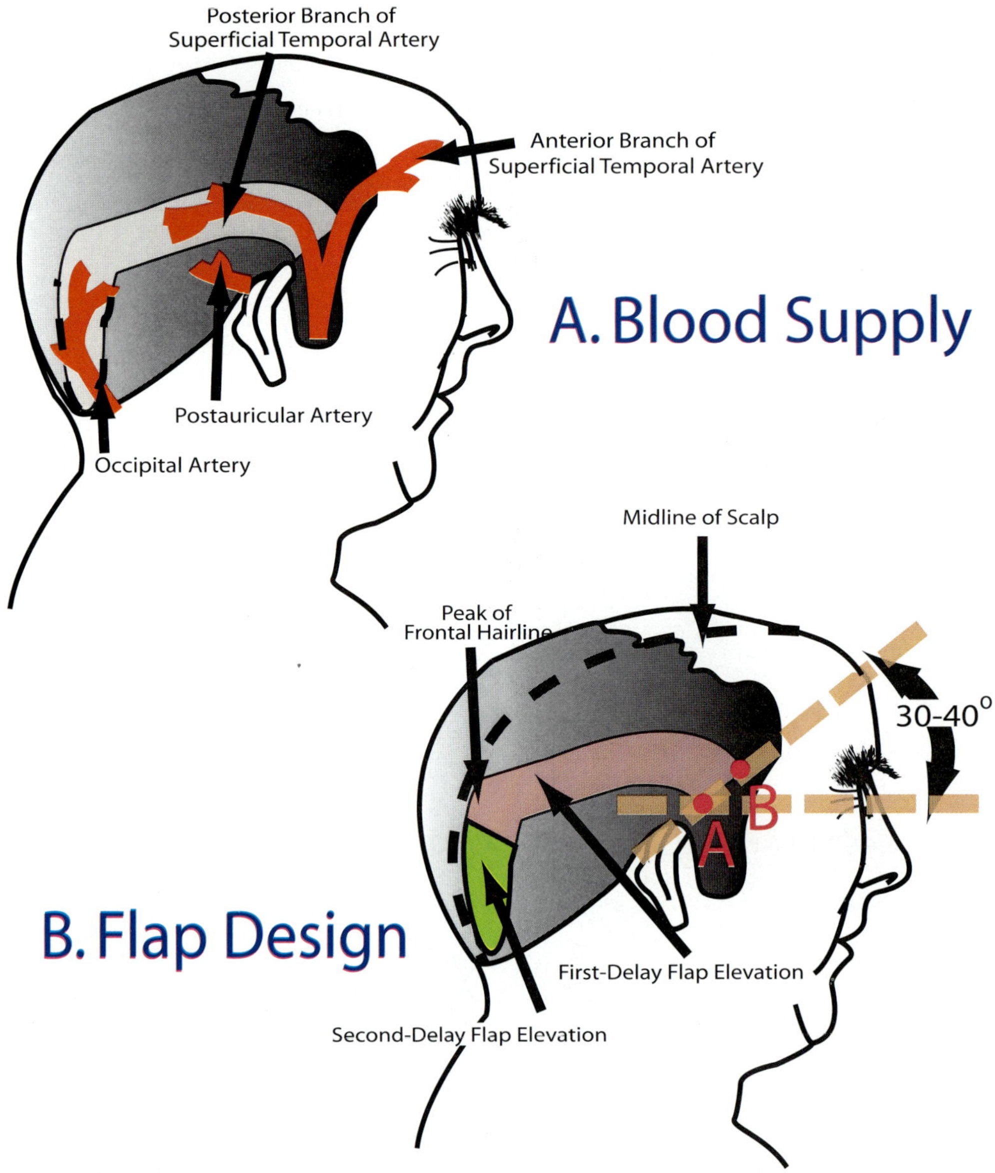

FIGURE 6-27. A: The temporo-parieto-occipital (Juri) flap is based on the posterior branch of the superficial temporal artery (STA) in an axial fashion and distally on the postauricular and occipital arteries in a random fashion. **B:** The flap should originate 4 cm above the helical crus (*point A*) and span a distance of 4 cm angled 30 to 40 degrees upward (*point B*). The flap then extends ipsilaterally in a posterior direction along the Doppler reading of the STA. The proximal flap (*in pink*) should be elevated and reset into its native position for the first phase of surgery. After 1 week, the distal flap (*in green*) should be elevated and reset into its native position. *(continued)*

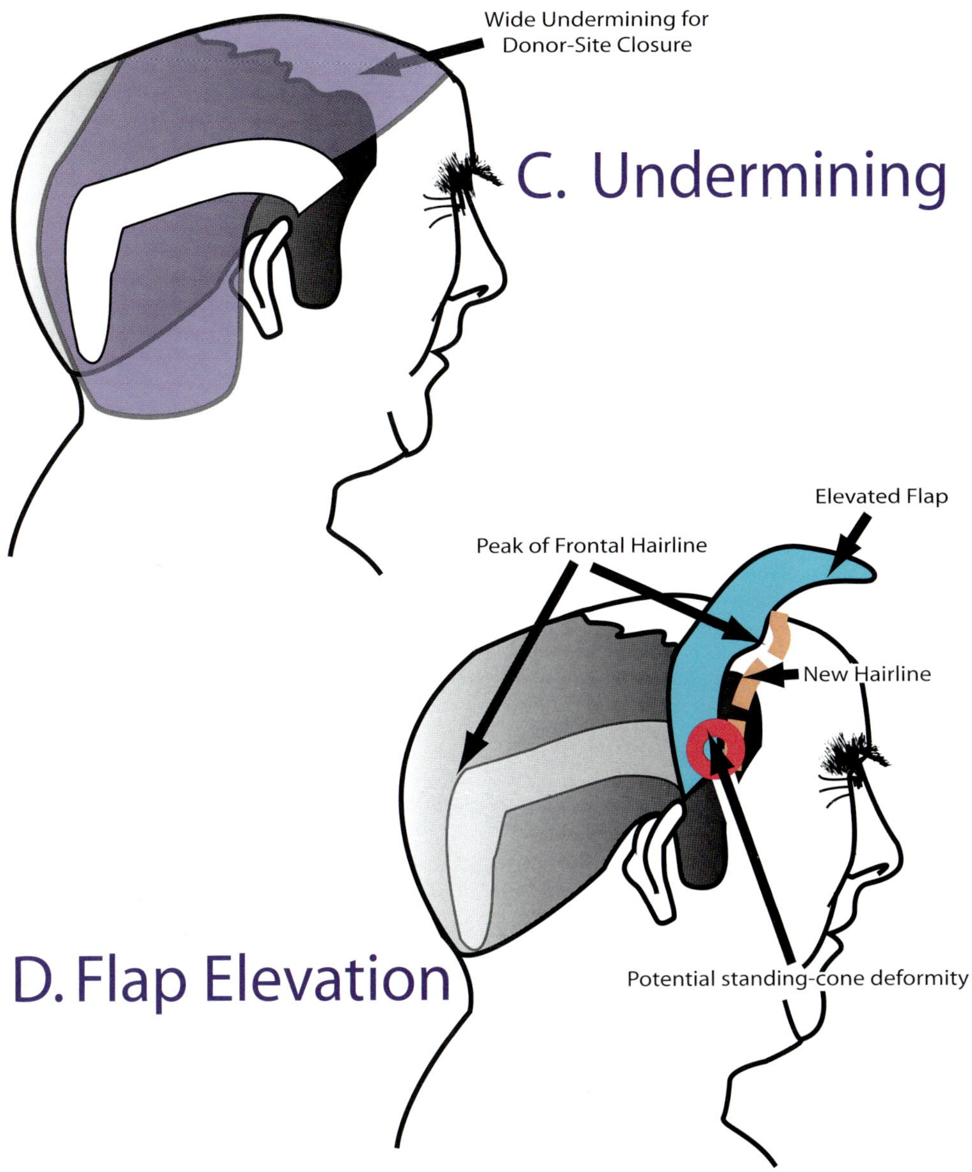

FIGURE 6-27. *(Continued)* **C,D:** After another week, the flap should be elevated and transposed. The area of undermining (in the subgaleal plane) must be broad (*in purple*) in order to ensure closure of the donor area. The flap is then transposed to the new hairline (*in orange*). A standing-cone deformity, or "dog ear" (*red circle*) may develop at the medial base of the flap after it has been inset. Typically, this deformity resolves over time but may require some trimming after a few months.

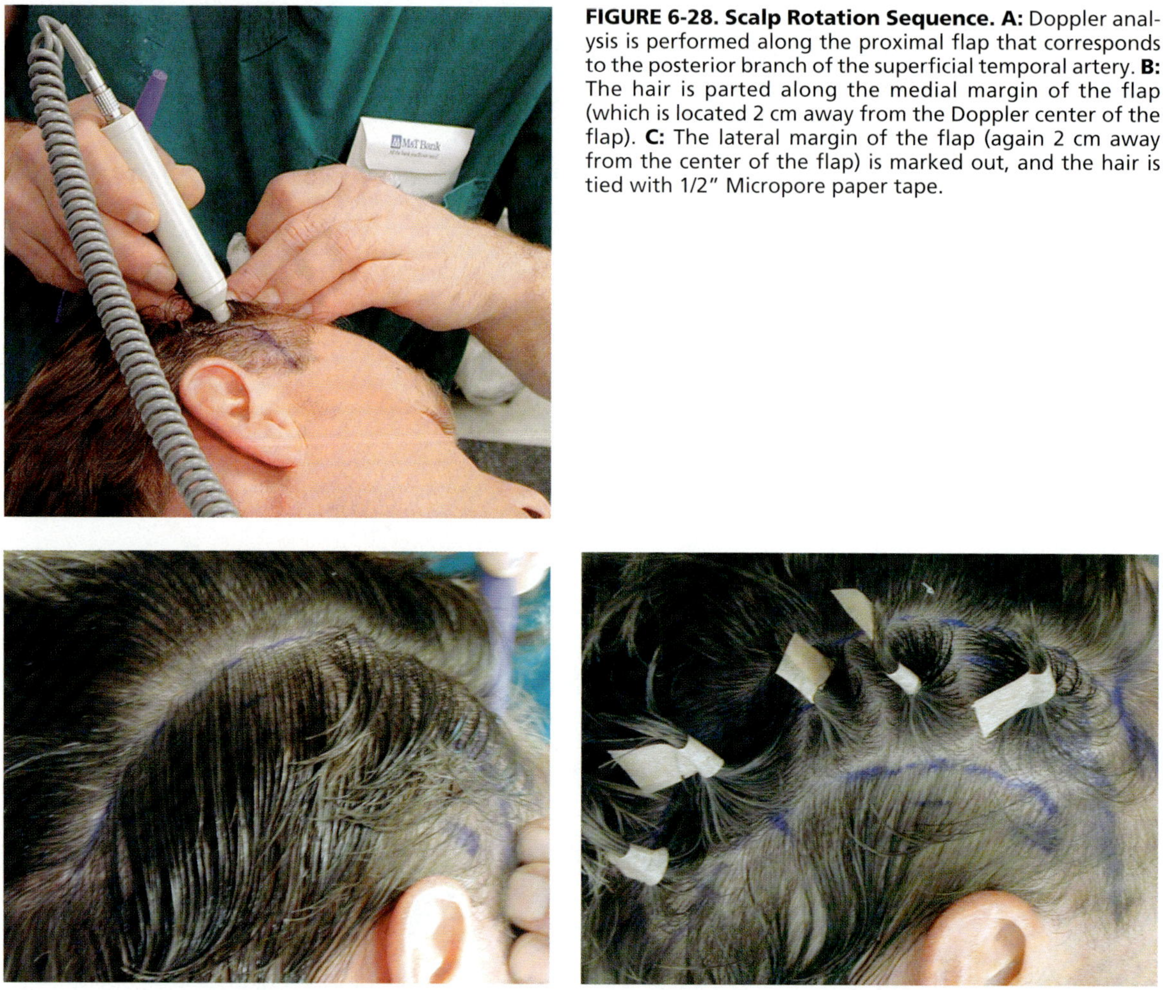

A B C

FIGURE 6-28. Scalp Rotation Sequence. A: Doppler analysis is performed along the proximal flap that corresponds to the posterior branch of the superficial temporal artery. **B:** The hair is parted along the medial margin of the flap (which is located 2 cm away from the Doppler center of the flap). **C:** The lateral margin of the flap (again 2 cm away from the center of the flap) is marked out, and the hair is tied with 1/2" Micropore paper tape.

27B). The distal extent of the flap should remain on the ipsilateral side of the head and not reach the midline if possible, unless greater flap length is mandatory.[17]

Proper flap and hairline design are imperative for a successful operation. Therefore, the surgeon must accord considerable deliberation and patience to this task rather than hasten forward to actual surgery. The flap length that is marked out should be confirmed to be adequate for hairline creation (Fig. 6-29A,B). An unraveled 4 × 4 gauze can be held at the base of the proposed flap and stretched across the constructed hairline, so that the gauze pivots to cover two thirds the length of the flap. After the flap design has been established and corroborated with the patient, the proximal two-thirds of the flap are raised from its bed and returned to its native position. A No. 10 blade can be used for the incision and flap elevation. The level of dissection is subgaleal, which is a natural and bloodless cleavage plane. Hemostasis along the cut edges of the flap may be attained with bipolar cautery (Fig. 6-30). Monopolar cautery should be avoided to minimize injury to the neighboring vascular pedicle. Placement of a closed suction drain is helpful along with light compressive dressings that remain in place until the first postoperative day, both of which serve to eliminate the risk of hematoma or seroma. Surgical staples are the most efficient way to close the scalp, and they also should be placed along the proposed outline for the distal flap so that the second stage flap elevation may be carried out easily.

Second Stage

The second stage of the Juri flap is the least demanding step of all three stages, lacking the deliberative effort required for the first stage and the technical labor for the third stage. Accordingly, the actual time expenditure for surgery is more cursory, and anesthesia requirements should be tailored to the limited nature of the surgical endeavor. Generally, short-acting intravenous sedation complements the infiltration of local anesthesia but may not be needed for the more stoic patient.

The second stage is undertaken 1 week after the first stage. However, delay of any stage of the procedure may be warranted if signs of impending flap compromise are evi-

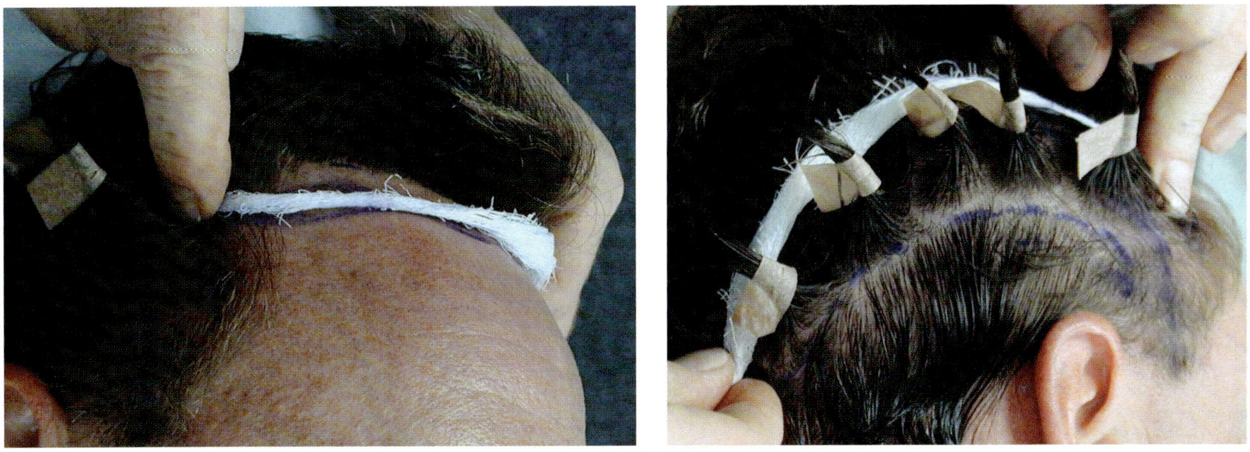

FIGURE 6-29. Scalp Rotation Sequence. A: After the desired hairline is marked out, an unraveled 4 × 4 gauze is used to measure the distance of the proposed, new hairline. **B:** Then, the length of the flap is verified to be sufficient to traverse the constructed hairline using the same 4 × 4 gauze.

dent. Using the staples from the first stage of surgery as a guide, the distal portion of the flap (i.e., the remaining one-third of the flap that has not already been elevated) is then temporarily raised out of its native position and set back into position. The surgeon should be very careful not to raise inadvertently the proximal two-thirds of the flap while elevating the proximal portion. This problem can be averted by removing the staples that hold the proximal two-thirds of the flap only *after* elevation and inset of the distal third of the flap. The dissection of the distal flap should follow the subgaleal plane, as outlined for the first stage of the procedure. In order to avoid injury to the vascular pedicle, the flap should be elevated gently with blunt scissors in a spreading fashion. After the distal third of the flap has been elevated, the flap is returned to its original position and secured in place with staples. Of note, the previous staples placed along the proximal extent of the flap can be removed at this time. No compressive dressing or drains are applied after the second stage.

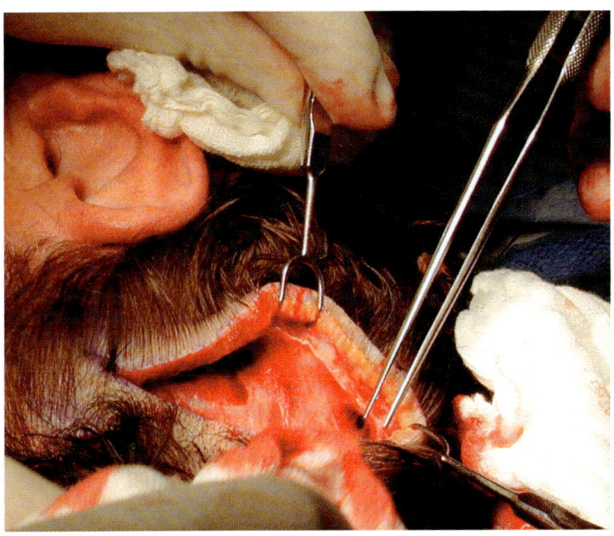

FIGURE 6-30. Scalp Rotation Sequence. Dissection is carried out in subgaleal plane. All cautery must be undertaken with a bipolar device, as monopolar cautery may jeopardize the flap integrity.

Third Stage

After an additional 1-week delay, the entire flap may be elevated, mobilized, and rotated into position (Fig. 6-27C,D). Because flap viability is critical for this stage of surgery, any evidence of vascular congestion or arterial insufficiency should be sufficient reason to delay the stage another week or two. Doppler analysis may help render appropriate judgment if the surgeon is uncertain as to the integrity of the flap. The proposed hairline should be redrawn with a surgical marking pen and confirmed with the patient before any incision is carried out along this line. In addition, flap length should be assessed to determine adequacy for hairline coverage, using a stretched-out 4 × 4 gauze, as previously described. (The reader should review the salient points of hairline design as described in the first stage of flap surgery before embarking on the third stage.) This stage of surgery is the most labor intensive. Protracted surgery, extensive dissection, and significant blood loss justify general endotracheal anesthesia or deep intravenous sedation for patient comfort and compliance. Infiltration of local anesthesia with the standard 1% lidocaine and 1:100,000 epinephrine should be carried out along the constructed hairline where the flap will be received and around the entire periphery of the planned area of dissection; i.e., ipsilateral to the flap laterally down to the superior helical crus, posteriorly down to the nuchal ridge but not past the midline, for the sake of flap viability. This extensive area of infiltration corresponds to the area that needs to be undermined for donor-site closure. However, the surgeon should be careful to avoid infiltration of the vasoconstrictive anesthetic directly into the flap or immediately adjacent to it.

Salient Technical Points

Follicular Grafting

1. The Norwood method is a reliable starting point for hairline design. The lowest extent of the central frontal forelock should be two finger breadths above the highest furrow created on upward gaze. Laterally, the fronto-temporal recess should lie at or slightly medial to a vertical line drawn through the lateral canthus. The half-open oval that is created by connecting these three points should be viewed as a straight line or slight upward sloping line, when the patient is viewed on profile. Further adjustments in hairline design are dictated by aesthetic judgment and in collaboration with the patient.
2. Intravenous midazolam sedation is preferable for patient comfort during infiltration of local anesthesia and donor-site harvesting.
3. The tumescent technique is favored for donor-site harvesting in order to increase ease of dissection, improve hemostasis, and minimize injury to the hair follicles.
4. The more inferiorly situated occipital hair tends to be finer, more vellus in character than the superiorly positioned hair: It is ideal for the anterior-most row of the hairline. If the occipital donor site has been depleted or if velluslike hair cannot be found in this region, then temporal hair may need to be harvested. Temporal hair should be taken in smaller swaths bilaterally to avoid asymmetry and tension on closure. Depth of dissection should be carefully observed to avoid inadvertent transection of the posterior branch of the superficial temporal artery, which leads to unnecessary bleeding.
5. Generally, no more than three passes of the Tori scalpel should be undertaken in the occipital region to avoid difficulty closing the donor site. 2-0 polypropylene is preferred to close the donor area in a running, locking fashion.
6. Graft preparation should be carried out with three to four technicians who should divide the grafts in individual Petri dishes according to graft size: one-hair grafts, two-hair grafts, three-hair grafts, three- to four-hair grafts, and five- to six-hair grafts. Dissection should be undertaken with a straight razor over a transilluminated view box protected by a disposable Plexiglas sheet. Magnification visors facilitate precise dissection and reduce eye fatigue.
7. The most attention should be paid to creation of a natural and dense anterior hairline using the principle of follicular unit transfer. Twenty to 25 follicular unit grafts should be placed per square centimeter to achieve this density. Three principles should be followed to achieve maximal density and a natural hairline:
   a. Cross-hatching. The grafts should be placed in varying orientations to one another to obscure the exposed scalp.
   b. Central-forelock coverage. The density of grafts should be focused in the central aspect of the hairline, because the density in this area is visually doubled by virtue of it being seen from both the left and right side of the patient.
   c. Graduated graft placement. The anterior most row of the hairline should be recreated with one-hair grafts, followed by one- to two-hair grafts, three-hair grafts, and three- to four-hair grafts for each successive row moving anterior to posterior.
8. The area posterior to the anterior hairline and the midscalp region should be addressed through use of larger five- to six-hair minigrafts, which can provide rapid density. A 1.75-mm round punch is used to create the recipient sites that will accommodate the 2-mm sized grafts.
9. The technique of graft insertion involves the surgeon creating a recipient site, the first assistant then filling that recipient site with an appropriate graft, and the second assistant handing the first assistant another graft for insertion. The surgeon uses an 18-gauge NoKor needle or SP90 blade to create the recipient site using the principles of cross-hatching and irregularly asymmetrical placement. The second assistant hands the first assistant the appropriate size and caliber graft with a pair of jeweler's forceps, who then in turn places the graft into the recipient site according to the direction that the surgeon created the site. The first assistant must maintain his or her line of vision constantly on the surgeon's hand in order to recognize in what direction the recipient site was created so that placement of the graft will match that same direction.
10. The patient's scalp is subjected to a hair dryer before a layered 4×4 gauze dressing is applied over the graft sites, which in turn is covered with a baseball cap.
11. The donor site sutures are removed 2 weeks postoperatively.

Scalp Reduction

1. The ideal candidate for scalp reduction is a more mature patient (more than 40 years old) with a relatively stable pattern of hair recession who desires camouflage of his exposed crown, or vertex, area.
2. The diameter of the bald vertex cannot exceed 13 cm in diameter for successful closure.
3. For 10 to 12 cm of exposure, four sessions are antici-

pated for complete closure. Similarly, three sessions should be sufficient for closure of 8 to 9 cm.

4. Typically, the first session permits approximately 4 cm of tissue mobilization from the parietal fringe (2 cm from each side) and about 1 to 2 cm from the occipital fringe. Subsequent sessions permit less tissue advancement with about 3 cm of total tissue recruitment laterally and less than 1 cm posteriorly.
5. A modified Mercedes configuration is designed over the exposed crown with the longer limb in the midsagittal plane and the shorter limbs extending posterolaterally.
6. A scalp extender minimizes unfavorable stretchback and reduces the interval between sessions to 1 month.
7. A z-plasty closure is recommended to disguise a potential slot deformity, and minigrafting and micrografting may be further needed for additional camouflage.

Scalp Rotation

1. Scalp rotation procedures should be reserved for those patients who desire rapid, dense coverage to the fronto-temporal region and who tolerate more invasive, multistage surgery. The density provided by this surgical method is unparalleled when compared with traditional grafting techniques.
2. The proposed hairline cannot extend 4 cm below the existing hairline, because the 4-cm width of the T-P-O flap must bridge this gap. If the patient and surgeon believe that the hairline should descend much more than 4 cm from the existing hairline position, then a contralateral flap will be required to bring the hairline down further.
3. As part of the first stage of the operation, the proximal flap should be mapped out according to Doppler analysis of the posterior branch of the STA. Because the distal aspect of the flap is random, a Doppler reading is unwarranted.
4. The proximal third of the flap lies behind the new hairline, whereas the distal two thirds of the flap serves to recreate the new hairline. Therefore, the peak of the flap should be designed at the junction of the middle and distal thirds. The base of the flap should commence 4 cm above the helical crus and span a distance of 4 cm width at an angle of 30 to 40 degrees with the horizontal. The distal extent of the flap should remain on the ipsilateral side of the head and not reach the midline if possible, unless greater flap length is mandatory.
5. In the first stage of the procedure, the proximal two-thirds of the flap are elevated and returned to its position. The remaining distal third of the flap should be outlined with staples in order to facilitate easy identification for the second stage of the operation.
6. The second stage of the operation is undertaken 1 week after the first stage but should be delayed if there is any evidence of vascular compromise to the flap. The second stage involves elevating and returning the distal one-third of the flap back to its original position without inadvertently raising the proximal two-thirds of the flap. This problem can be averted by removing the staples that hold the proximal flap only *after* elevation and inset of the distal flap.
7. Protracted surgery, extensive dissection, and significant blood loss justify general endotracheal anesthesia or deep intravenous sedation for patient comfort and compliance during the third stage of the Juri flap.
8. The proposed hairline should be incised so that the knife blade is beveled anteriorly. This angulation permits growth of hair from the flap through the scar for increased camouflage. The intervening bald scalp between the original and proposed hairline should be excised in the subgaleal plane to accommodate flap inset.
9. Closure of the donor site usually requires considerable undermining both laterally and posteriorly down past the nuchal line and toward the contralateral side as well as anteriorly toward the forehead in the subgaleal plane.
10. Given the marked hemorrhage during the procedure and the need for absolute hemostasis to assure flap viability, placement of a closed-suctions drain should be placed only after diligent hemostasis has been obtained.

The two critical aspects that define success of this surgical stage are proper rotation and inset of the T-P-O flap and closure of the donor site. The proposed hairline should be incised so that the knife blade is beveled anteriorly. This angulation permits growth of hair from the flap through the scar for increased camouflage. The intervening bald scalp between the original and proposed hairline should be excised in the subgaleal plane to accommodate flap inset. The flap is then carefully elevated in the subgaleal plane, and initial undermining is performed in the surrounding tissues to permit tension-free flap elevation and rotation. No undermining should be carried out anterior to the new hairline in order to avoid translocation of the hairline level. If the flap does not exactly fit the recipient site, then it can be conservatively trimmed until it is closer in dimension and shape. The newly created anterior hairline may be sutured into place using 6-0 polypropylene and the posterior aspect of the flap may be secured with 3-0 or 4-0 polypropylene.

Closure of the donor site usually requires considerable undermining both laterally and posteriorly down past the nuchal line and toward the contralateral side as well as anteriorly toward the forehead in the subgaleal plane (Fig. 6-27C). Blunt scissor dissection along this natural cleavage plane facilitates atraumatic, expeditious surgery. Considerable blood loss usually accompanies this part of the procedure, which should not alarm the surgeon. The standing-cone deformity that arises at the proximal base of the flap usually resolves partially within a few weeks and often entirely so after several months. Patients should be counseled preoperatively as to this inevitable unnatural protuberance whose size is proportionate to the dimensions of the flap raised and the arc of rotation undertaken. Given the marked hemorrhage during the procedure and the need for absolute hemostasis to assure flap viability, placement of a closed-suction drain should be placed only after diligent hemostasis has been obtained. The drain can be removed on the first postoperative day. The donor site can be closed with surgical staples, which should remain for a 2-week period.

POSTOPERATIVE CONSIDERATIONS: CARE, FOLLOW-UP, AND COMPLICATIONS

Postoperative Care and Follow-Up

Follicular Grafting

For the first two postoperative weeks, a baseball cap permits a convenient method to camouflage the surgery site until most swelling has dissipated and crusting has fallen away. The patient can begin cleaning his hair with a gentle, nonirritating baby shampoo the following morning on a daily basis. Shampoos without sodium lauryl sulfate should be selected to minimize scalp and graft irritation, especially during the healing period. Vigorous scalp and hair cleaning should be avoided so as not to disrupt the graft sites. Dexpanthenol (see medial therapies) also may be applied locally to the graft sites with a cotton-tipped applicator to reduce crust buildup and can be used to clean the donor site as well. Donor-site sutures are removed after a 2-week period. Donor site incisions heal inconspicuously without unfavorable cicatricial formation. Traumatic telogenic loss of existing nontransplanted hair is temporary, and shed follicles eventually return. Patients should be properly reassured about the transient nature of this hair loss, so that undue anxiety need not be experienced.

Further grafting sessions can be planned as early as 1 month postoperatively, but this early intervention generally is ill advised because the transplanted grafts need several months to begin to manifest. Accordingly, a minimum of 3 months should be expected before the next grafting session is planned. However, a longer period of 6 to 12 months is preferred to permit maximal hair growth before embarking on another surgical venture.

Scalp Reduction

Between scalp reduction sessions, very little care is required. The sutures used to close the incision are removed 2 weeks postoperatively (i.e., 2 weeks before the next session). After all the sessions have been completed, the patient should be followed closely for any signs of alopecia or unfavorable stretch-back. If this problem should arise, then an additional session of micrografting to the exposed area can be performed after all incisions have healed (i.e., after a minimum of 3 weeks).

Scalp Rotation

Minimal postoperative care is necessary after each of the first two surgical stages, because the next session follows only a week later. No drains are placed after the first two stages. Bandages are removed on the first postoperative day, and the patient is instructed to refrain from hair washing for 2 days. Thereafter, he can begin a gentle cleaning regimen with a nonirritating formula such as baby shampoo. The surgeon should keep an observant eye on flap viability so that the following stage can be appropriately delayed if any signs of flap compromise are evident. If the patient has no adverse reaction, topical antibiotic ointment, such as Bacitracin, can be sparingly applied to the flap edges to keep them moist between stages, but this is not compulsory.

After the third stage, the surgeon should pay close attention to the health of the flap. The surgeon should not be unduly alarmed if the flap appears dusky or pale because this coloration is typical immediately postoperatively. However, if the flap color appears to worsen after the first day, then a few sutures may have to be loosened or removed to increase flap vascularity. Beyond these conservative measures, the surgeon has a paucity of tactics in his or her arsenal to combat flap necrosis. Fortunately, this devastating complication is quite rare beyond mild distal flap loss. The surgical drains should remain in place until the drainage output has begun to taper or remains below 30 cc over a 24-hour period. Typically, the drains should remain between 1 to 3 days until the preceding criteria are met, because flap compromise may arise from excessive fluid accumulation under the flap. After 1 week, the 6-0 polypropylene sutures along the new frontal hairline can be removed; and after 2 weeks, the remaining sutures and staples can be safely removed. The patient should be followed on a daily basis for the initial 2 to 3 days until flap viability does not appear to be at risk. Only the most conservative debridement of an eschar should be undertaken, because aggressive tissue resection may jeopardize the potential for future hair growth in the flap.

Complications and Management

Follicular Grafting

Fortunately, complications after follicular transfer remain quite rare. The donor and recipient sites heal very well, and the transplanted grafts take root tenaciously. As mentioned, the traumatic hair loss that arises several weeks to months following hair transplantation, known as telogenic effluvium, is a temporary condition, for which the patient should receive reassurance. However, a few uncommon complications will be mentioned that may be attributed largely to technical error and therefore should be avoided.

Divoting and Cobblestoning

Placement of hair grafts that lie above or below the level of the surrounding tissue may result in this complication. Fortunately, minor discrepancies rarely translate into an appreciable defect. The best policy in the immediate postoperative period is expectant. However, if the surface irregularities persist after several months and should disturb the patient, then correction is warranted. A raised graft area can be simply amputated flush with the surrounding tissue with a No. 15 blade. The underlying transplanted follicle should grow if the hair bulb is retained. If the graft site appears depressed, then it should be excised or punched out; and the wound edges approximated with an absorbable suture. Despite these theoretical risks, the authors have not experienced any of these complications to date.

Compression and Donuting

These complications have been elaborated on in the section describing operative technique for follicular grafting. In review, compression occurs when a graft contains numerous follicles (more than six hairs per graft) or is relatively large in size; and the surrounding tissue compresses all the grafts into a central core area to resemble a single thick stalk. The result is an unnatural "pluggy" look that can be corrected by simple punch excision of the graft site and closure. Donuting occurs when a large graft is inserted into a recipient site, and the vascular supply to the center of the graft is insufficient to maintain its viability. Therefore, the follicles that usually reside in the central aspect of the graft do not survive. If the result appears unnatural, then the graft can be eliminated by punch removal and closed. However, this result rarely causes a cosmetic deformity.

Cyst Formation

If a follicular graft is accidentally placed upside down into the recipient site, the trapped epithelial surface may be expressed as a cyst. However, they may simply represent a small ledge of trapped epithelium of the graft under the neighboring skin and not an inverted graft. These cysts may be unroofed and the contents expressed. If they persist, then the graft site may need to be removed with a punch instrument. Cysts are a relatively common occurrence after a follicular transplantation and most often resolve spontaneously.

Hair Loss

As mentioned, telogenic effluvium is a common postoperative event and should not be strictly classified as a complication. The traumatized hair follicles undergo a return to telogen phase at 8 to 10 weeks postoperatively, which manifests as hair loss that should return by 3 to 4 months. No treatment is necessary except calm reassurance. The midscalp is an area that is hypovascular relative to the neighboring regions of the scalp and prone to less graft viability. However, this difference in vascular supply only poses a negligible risk and rarely causes a cosmetic concern.

Cornrow Deformity

The unnatural appearance, caused by placing large punch grafts, can be avoided simply by using no graft larger than six hairs. However, if the surgeon should encounter this unsightly complication owing to his or her colleague's handiwork or one's own surgical misadventure, then surgical revision is justifiable. Three routes of revision surgery are available. The surgeon can camouflage the cornrow sites by placing minigrafts and micrografts anterior to and around the existing grafts. However, if the donor hair is scarce or a large region needs be covered with additional grafting, the surgeon can partially correct the situation in the following manner: The large graft sites can be partly removed with a small 2-mm punch instrument and transplanted elsewhere. Although this approach appears ideal, the amount of usable graft material from the excised cornrow sites is far less than 100%. Alternatively, the entire cornrow graft site can be excised and closed. Obviously, a combination of all three techniques may be required to achieve an optimal result.

Folliculitis

This condition presents as focal (or less commonly global) scalp erythema with associated pustule formation around the base of a hair shaft(s). Folliculitis typically occurs 2 weeks to 3 months postoperatively. Local hydrogen peroxide to the infected hair follicles with a cotton-tipped applicator and systemic oral antistaphylococcal antibiotics should eradicate this problem.

Unfavorable Scarring

This is a rare complication in the fairer-complexioned patient but may occur in darker-skinned individuals, particularly those who are prone to keloid or hypertrophic scarring. If this problem occurs along the donor site, then intralesional steroid injection or pulsed-dye laser treatment can ameliorate the condition. For further details, the reader is referred to the complications section of Chapter 5.

Scalp Reduction

Fortunately, complications with scalp reduction are infrequent so long as proper patient selection is carried out and realistic expectations are delineated.

Unfavorable Scarring

Scarring may occur along the incision site and should be addressed conservatively, as outlined in the complications section of Chapter 5. However, if the incision line fails to improve after less aggressive intervention, then scar revision may be needed. Direct scar excision with intralesional steroid injection at the time of revision surgery is a good first attempt before more elaborate scar-revision techniques are employed. Additional micrografting along the incision line may camouflage this deformity.

Slot Deformity

This complication usually arises because of continued hair loss in the vertex region. This problem may be circumvented if the patient is properly selected for stable recession. However, prediction of future hair loss is never absolutely accurate. Therefore, if this complication should manifest, then correction can entail another scalp reduction session if the scalp is distensible enough or camouflaged with micrografting and minigrafting.

Scalp Rotation

Although luckily frank flap necrosis is rare, imperfect surgical results may be frequent, especially for the surgical tyro. Revision surgery usually entails minor flap adjustments and micrograft camouflaging.

Standing-Cone Deformity

Postoperative anxiety should be allayed that the raised contour at the proximal bend of the flap should most likely settle down but may rarely require minor surgical correction with a Burrows-type triangle reduction if several months of patience have not been rewarded with improvement in the contour.

Flap Necrosis

Clearly, the most ominous complication that plagues regional flap rotation is complete flap loss. Although no significant flap demise has arisen, the authors have remarked a few cases of minimal flap loss at the distal tip, which heals completely with secondary intention. If these areas become unaesthetic after healing, then excision or grafting may remove this unattractive stigma. For basic care after flap necrosis, the reader is referred to the complications section in Chapter 5.

An Unnatural, Blunted Frontal Hairline

The extreme density of the grafted hair often may need to be softened with micrografting, and occasionally minigrafting, anterior to the incision line. Micrografts can effectively irregularize the hairline and increase the transition zone to fully dense hair. A blunted appearance to the hairline can be prevented by configuring the flap to have a peaked shape. However, if the hairline still appears too linear, then central minigrafting and micrografting may restore the appearance of the fronto-temporal gullies by building up the frontal forelock.

MEDICAL MANAGEMENT OF HAIR LOSS

The sophisticated patient today often desires the full gamut of restorative techniques available for alopecia, including medical, surgical, and synthetic coverage options. Although a discussion of hairpieces lies beyond the scope of expertise and interest of the authors, a review of current medical solutions is given herein. The introduction of finasteride has reawakened interest in medical treatment for hair loss. With the advent of the Internet, innumerable treatments that lack any scientific foundation have been touted as panaceas for alopecia. The following section highlights the many proven and unproven methods that exist, with dutiful circumspection for the more dubious remedies. Although medical management has been scientifically validated for minoxidil and finasteride, long-term treatment can be expensive and equal that of surgical restoration over time; but, unlike surgery, it is only temporary after cessation of usage. Nevertheless, the physician should be well versed with at least the fundamental medical options available to respond to patients' queries intelligently. Furthermore, adjunctive use of medical therapy before, during, and after a hair transplantation may contribute favorably to the longevity of the transplant result.[18] However, patients may be reluctant to remain on a maintenance regimen for life because of the added expense and labor involved.

Byzantine methods of medical hair treatment abound today and offer the physician and patient a dizzying array of options. Some are founded on controlled clinical trials and others are merely products of hype. Two established medical therapies for androgenic alopecia (AGA), approved by the Food and Drug Administration (FDA), are topical minoxidil and oral finasteride. In addition, systemic antiandrogen receptor antagonists, such as spironolactone and cyproterone acetate, may be beneficial for female patients exhibiting AGA. Newer pharmaceutical agents that have shown initial promising results are under rigorous scientific investigation, such as dutasteride, a combined Type I and II, 5 alpha-reductase inhibitor, and vascular endothelial growth factor (VEGF). Also, minoxidil and finasteride are subjects of recent studies in which these medications have been applied in higher-percentage formulations (15% minoxidil and 1.25-mg finasteride [under current investigation at the senior author's institution]) and via unconventional routes of administration (topical finasteride [also being investigated at the senior author's institution and seen previously to be beneficial in a mouse model]).[19] In addition to all the pharmaceutical-grade therapies, a host of natural, herbal medications have been introduced, with less definitive scientific bases. Adjunctive measures that aim to improve scalp and hair hygiene (e.g., shampooing products) and that attempt to enrich the local vascularity of the scalp (e.g., laser therapy) also have been marketed to sufferers of alopecia. This chapter reviews the traditional and newer methods of medical hair therapy to provide the reader with a more comprehensive understanding of what is available and the scientific underpinnings that support various treatment options. Discussion of hair physiology, patient selection, and coverage options lies beyond the scope of this chapter.

Established Medical Therapies

Pharmaceutical therapies that have proven efficacy in AGA may be classified into two categories: biologic-response modifiers and androgen-blocking agents. Biologic-response modifiers exert their control over follicular growth via regulation of cellular differentiation as well as a host of mechanisms, including mitogenic, immunosuppressive, vasodilatory, angiogenic, and growth-factor–related. Androgenic blockade may be then further divided into 5-alpha reductase inhibitors (finasteride) and androgen receptor antagonists (spironolactone and cyproterone acetate).[20]

Biologic Response Modifiers

Many biologic response modifiers are under current investigation, but the most well known example of this category is minoxidil.

Minoxidil

Minoxidil is a piperidinopyrimidine derivative that was originally devised as an antihypertensive medication but was found to have hypertrichosis as a side effect and consequently introduced as the first FDA-approved medical therapy for AGA. Although the mechanism of action is not completely apparent, minoxidil may exert its effect via positive modulation of potassium channels, mitogenic growth of epidermal keratinocytes, or increasing local vascularity.[21–24] These proposed mechanisms may not fully explain all the beneficial effects on follicular growth that minoxidil yields.

Many large-scale, multicenter, double-blind trials have confirmed the efficacy of 2% and 3% minoxidil in the treatment of AGA, with greater benefit seen in the 5% strength.[25–29] Although many studies have shown that overall minoxidil effectively treats AGA, only 10% of men demonstrate noticeable regrowth of hair and 30% experience stabilization.[30–32] Maximal effects may be evident at 1 year and diminishes somewhat thereafter. Minoxidil also has been proved beneficial in female patients with a 50% stabilization and 13% regrowth rate.[33] However, discontinuation of medication usually results in loss of regrowth over a period of 6 months. As evident, minoxidil may be more effective in preservation of hair than significant regrowth. Further, minoxidil works by converting miniaturized, telogenic hairs into more active, anagenic shafts but is less successful in a totally exposed pate. Combination with topical tretinoin in minimal concentrations (0.025%) appears to enhance absorption of minoxidil and may increase efficacy.[34] Side effects exhibited by minoxidil are more local (usually an irritative dermatitis in 7.5% of patients) than systemic. Facial hypertrichosis may be evident in 5% of female patients but is usually transitory and rarely requires any intervention.

As mentioned before, use of minoxidil or finasteride has been recently advocated as an adjunctive measure to hair transplantation by many leading experts in the field of hair transplantation.[18] Uncontrolled studies have found that perioperative minoxidil usage led to hair regrowth without the typical telogen effluvium that occurs 2 to 4 weeks after surgery in some cases and earlier regrowth of hair approximately 4 weeks after telogen effluvium rather than the normal 3 to 5 months afterward in other cases.[35] It has been recommended that minoxidil or finasteride be instituted at the initial consultation with the understanding that it may require 2 to 4 months for the medication to begin to exhibit any effect. Minoxidil should be stopped 2 to 3 days prior to surgery to reduce the theoretical risk of increased intraoperative bleeding that may ensue owing to the vasodilatory effects of the medication and recommenced 2 to 14 days after surgery so as to minimize the theoretical risk of damage to the transplanted hair follicles by the propylene-glycol base. Finasteride, on the other hand, is continued without interruption.[18]

Androgen-Blocking Agents

Finasteride (5 Alpha-Reductase Inhibitor)

Finasteride, a relative newcomer, was the second FDA-approved medication to treat AGA and arrived on the market in December 1997. Finasteride, a steroidal derivative, inhibits Type II 5 alpha-reductase, which converts testosterone to the more potent androgen, dihydrotestosterone (DHT). Type II 5 alpha-reductase is found primarily in scalp follicles and the urogenital system, whereas Type I is more ubiquitously present in sebaceous glands, keratinocytes, apocrine glands, and dermal papillae. This selective inhibition of the Type II enzyme prevents the deleterious action of DHT on hair follicles without any significant effect on circulating testosterone levels. Fortunately, DHT possesses little benefit to the adult male, contributing only to prostatic hypertrophy, hirsutism, and acne.

Large-scale, controlled multicenter studies have proven the objective (standardized photographic analysis and hair counts) and the subjective (patient reports) benefits that finasteride has on hair restoration. Eighty-three percent of finasteride-treated hair counts revealed stabilization at 1 year compared with 72% of controls who showed advancing hair loss. Further, 66% of the finasteride-treated group showed some regrowth of hair by year 2.[36,37] However, the patients who terminated use of finasteride exhibited loss of regrown hair. An extended study at 5 years demonstrated durable improvement in the treated group compared with progressive loss in controls.[38] A smaller study of nine pairs of monozygotic twins also corroborated the objective and subjective benefit to the treated versus the placebo group.[39] A dose-finding study determined that a 1-mg oral dose was optimal for hair growth. Interestingly, another study found no benefit in postmenopausal women after a 12-month period.[40]

Sexual dysfunction may arise with a frequency just above that of the placebo group (4.2% versus 2.2%) and resolves with discontinuation of the drug and even in 58% who continue with therapy.[41] Finasteride should be withheld from women of childbearing age because crushed tablets may expose a male fetus to genital abnormalities.

Spironolactone

Like cyproterone acetate, spironolactone acts as an androgen receptor blocker; therefore, these types of medications that bear systemic antiandrogen effects are contraindicated in men. Oral spironolactone, an aldosterone antagonist, competitively inhibits the androgenic receptor and weakly interferes with adrenal androgen biosynthesis. A few clinical trials have supported the use of spironolactone in AGA, but further work is necessary to confirm these initial findings.[42,43] Oral spironolactone has demonstrated a greater role in the treatment of hirsutism than in AGA. Topical spironolactone also has been evaluated for use in male patients with AGA but is now only in a preliminary phase of investigation. Side effects of spironolactone principally concern menstrual difficulties but also may give rise to precipitous hyperkalemia. Like finasteride and cyproterone, a very real threat to the male fetal genitalia exists, and all women of childbearing age must be maintained on an oral contraceptive regimen.

Cyproterone Acetate

Cyproterone acetate, an androgen receptor antagonist and progestin, should only be used in women, given the aforementioned risk of systemic feminization. Albeit of proven benefit in hirsutism and acne, controlled clinical trials on AGA have yet to be performed. Again, the woman of childbearing age should be admonished as to the potential risk to a developing male fetus and accordingly placed on contraceptive medication during use of cyproterone. Other side effects that have been manifested include menstrual irregularities, weight gain, breast tenderness, depression, nausea, and diminution of libido.

Experimental Medical Therapies

The following medical therapies are currently under investigation and have yet to enter the market to treat AGA. However, preliminary experiments and trials have demonstrated favorable results that have sparked interest in these agents.

Dutasteride

Like finasteride, dutasteride (GI198745) is a potent inhibitor of 5 alpha-reductase; but, unlike finasteride, it targets both Type I and II enzymes. This dual action has been proposed as one mechanism by which dutasteride may be more efficacious in treatment of AGA. Although Type II 5 alpha-reductase is the principal enzyme localized to the scalp, Type I 5 alpha-reductase may still have an effect on the development of AGA. Men born with only the Type I 5-alpha reductase enzyme experienced hair loss when administered testosterone (Ertel J. Phase-II FDA study results for dutasteride [GI198745]). In a pharmacokinetic model, dutasteride was evaluated against finasteride in 48 healthy male subjects. The study found that dutasteride was threefold more potent in inhibition of Type II 5 alpha-reductase.[44] Animal models (rat and dog) have shown the greater reduction of DHT levels by dutasteride over that by finasteride.[45] Currently, dutasteride has received FDA approval for treatment of benign prostatic hyperplasia and should be available on the market for that indication shortly. Preliminary clinical results have shown favorable results with dutasteride in treatment of AGA, but Phase-III trials are on hold at this time.

Vascular Endothelial Growth Factor

Vascular endothelial growth factor is a cytokine that stimulates angiogenesis in vascular endothelial cells. Vascular endothelial growth factor was originally identified in neoplasia, wound healing, and psoriasis, as well as in normal physiologic processes. Studies have documented the role of VEGF in normal hair growth, in which anagenic hair follicles express VEGF.[46] Angiogenesis is stimulated as the hair cycle enters anagen. A recent study examined the role of VEGF in hair-follicle control using a mouse model and found that VEGF-expressed transgenic mice exhibited more robust and numerous anagenic follicles, whereas VEGF-deprived mice showed delayed conversion from telogen to anagen and smaller anagenic follicles.[47] Culture studies showed that the presence of VEGF did not directly stimulate growth but the increased vascularity derived by VEGF was responsible for follicular stimulation. A prior study determined that minoxidil may promote hair growth via upregulation of VEGF.[48] At this time, VEGF has yet to undergo any definitive clinical investigation.

Nitroxide, TEMPOL

The nitroxide radical TEMPOL (4-hydroxy-2,2,6,6-tetramethylpiperidine-1-oxyl) acts to protect against superoxide, hydrogen peroxide, and x-ray–mediated cytotoxicity. Topical application of TEMPOL to the guinea pig scalp with radiation-induced alopecia showed protective effects on hair loss and increased rate of hair recovery.[49,50]

Although approved for use in cancer patients with alopecia, TEMPOL is awaiting further clinical trials for AGA before it becomes available.

Natural Herbal Therapies

Occidental medicine justifiably has a long tradition of skepticism toward nontraditional, herbal, or Eastern remedies that lack rigorous scientific validity. Unapproved concoctions abound that entice the desperate and unwitting patient who suffers from AGA to subscribe to any therapy that offers hope. The following section is not meant to substantiate the divers herbal extracts and preparations available on the market but rather to offer a brief introduction to some of the common therapies that exist in order to provide the physician with some educated thought on the subject.

Saw Palmetto (Serenoa Repens)

The extract taken from the red saw palmetto berries of the small plant called Serenoa Repens is thought to inhibit 5-alpha reductase and the binding of DHT to androgen receptors. A few double-blind, placebo-controlled studies conducted in Europe have determined its efficacy in treatment of BPH.[51,52] However, the 5 alpha-reductase inhibiting capacity is known to be significantly less than finasteride. The results of 5 alpha-reductase inhibitory activity have been equivocal.[53,54] A preliminary study in hair regrowth has shown some favorable results with combined oral and topical application (Ortiz R and Carlisi DJ, unpublished data). Saw palmetto apparently exerts its effects without significant systemic alteration of circulating hormone levels.[55]

Vitamins

Vitamin deficiency has been implicated in hair loss, but definitive benefit as to their efficacy has yet to be proved. Biotin is a water-soluble vitamin that most often is absent in patients sustained on exclusive parenteral nutrition. These individuals demonstrate symptoms that include alopecia and a scaly dermatitis and that respond to biotin supplementation. A few congenital disorders of biotin metabolism, biotinidase and holocarboxylase deficiency also cause alopecia, and addition of dietary biotin tends to ameliorate the degree of hair loss.[56,57] However, extrapolating from these facts that biotin supplementation may be beneficial to combat AGA may be flawed, and no valid clinical trials have been undertaken to date. Another vitamin that often has been cited as a critical cofactor in hair metabolism is vitamin D. Total-body alopecia may be exhibited in the congenital condition, vitamin D-dependent rickets type II.[58,59] Topical vitamin D has also been used to correct chemotherapy-induced alopecia in an animal model.[60] Many oral and topical formulations of various substances are promoted as panaceas for hair loss, including zinc, amino acids, numerous vitamins, hormones, jojoba oil, urea, wheat germ oil, and exotic herbs.[61] Despite claims that these products benefit AGA, stringent scientific evidence is lacking.

Adjunctive Therapies

Scalp and Hair Hygiene Products

Numerous products that address scalp and hair hygiene have been advocated as vital adjuncts in the treatment of AGA. These products claim to enhance absorption of pharmaceutical products, such as minoxidil, by creating a favorable scalp environment. Alternatively, these lotions and cleansers attempt to rid the hair–scalp complex of excessive sebum that may choke local vascularity to the follicle. Unfortunately, shampoos and conditioners that make these claims have not undergone any substantive clinical trials and are yet of unproved benefit.

Dexpanthenol

Dexpanthenol has been a constituent used in some hair care products designed to treat AGA. Controlled studies have looked at the favorable effect that this topical ingredient has imparted on hydration of the stratum corneum via prevention of transepidermal water loss.[62] It has been proposed that this effect on the scalp allows for improved permeability to the hair shaft, but direct evidence of this is unavailable. Further, occasional contact dermatitis arising from use of this product also has been reported.[63]

Copper Peptide

Copper-containing products have been marketed widely to facilitate wound healing and stimulate hair growth. Copper peptide complexes may be found in both topical treatment products as well as in shampoos. The exact mechanism of action is unknown. An animal study showed follicular enlargement on a rat's dorsum when exposed to a topical copper-binding peptide (PC1031).[64] A Phase-II, single-center, double-blind study revealed the subjective improvement in patients compared with placebo controls as well as objective increase in hair count using the higher-strength 2.5% concentration of PC1358 that was statistically significant, but no difference in hair weight was found between the groups.

Laser Therapy

Although laser therapy for temporary hair removal has shown efficacy, laser therapy for hair growth is still largely unproved. One study showed an increase in blood flow with the diode laser compared with a decrease in blood flow with noncoherent, monochromatic light using Doppler analysis.[65] Obviously, increase in local blood flow does not necessarily translate into short- or long-term hair growth. Clinical trials currently are underway to investigate the utility of this new modality.

The Future of Medical Therapy

Newer generation systemic antiandrogens and various other medical therapies offer hope that androgenic alopecia will be more effectively managed in the coming years. Scientific inquiry also has been directed at methods that target the genetic basis for hair loss. Currently, animal studies are underway to investigate the efficacy of topical administration of liposomes bearing entrapped DNA that could restrict local androgen receptor expression.[66] These studies are in the preliminary stages and may prove to be the mainstay of therapy in the future.

CLINICAL PRESENTATIONS: A SYNTHESIS OF APPROACH

Case #1 (Fig. 6-31A,B)

This patient is a 38-year-old medical technologist who had experienced significant hair loss over the past decade. He had tried various hair replacement schemes in the past but abandoned this modality because of the labor-intensive maintenance and incompatibility with his lifestyle. On examination, this man exhibited coarse, black hair and a fair complexion. The caliber of his donor hair was moderately dense with over 24 hair follicles/cm^2. After a thorough consultation, the patient expressed realistic objectives for surgical restoration; namely, that more than one grafting session might be required to attain the ultimate result and subsequent sessions might be needed to maintain his look in the face of ongoing hair loss.

Procedure

Four separate grafting sessions were undertaken, spaced at 6- to 8-month intervals. Each transplantation session involved 400 minigrafts (three- to six-hair grafts) distributed across the midscalp to achieve density; and 75 to 125 follicular unit grafts of various sizes were transplanted along the anterior hairline according to the method described in the text. Black hair and a fair complexion placed the patient in a less than desirable category for ideal refinement, and for that reason particular emphasis was placed on harvesting the follicular unit grafts from the more inferior aspect of the donor site that corresponded to a softer, more vellus and more terminal type hair.

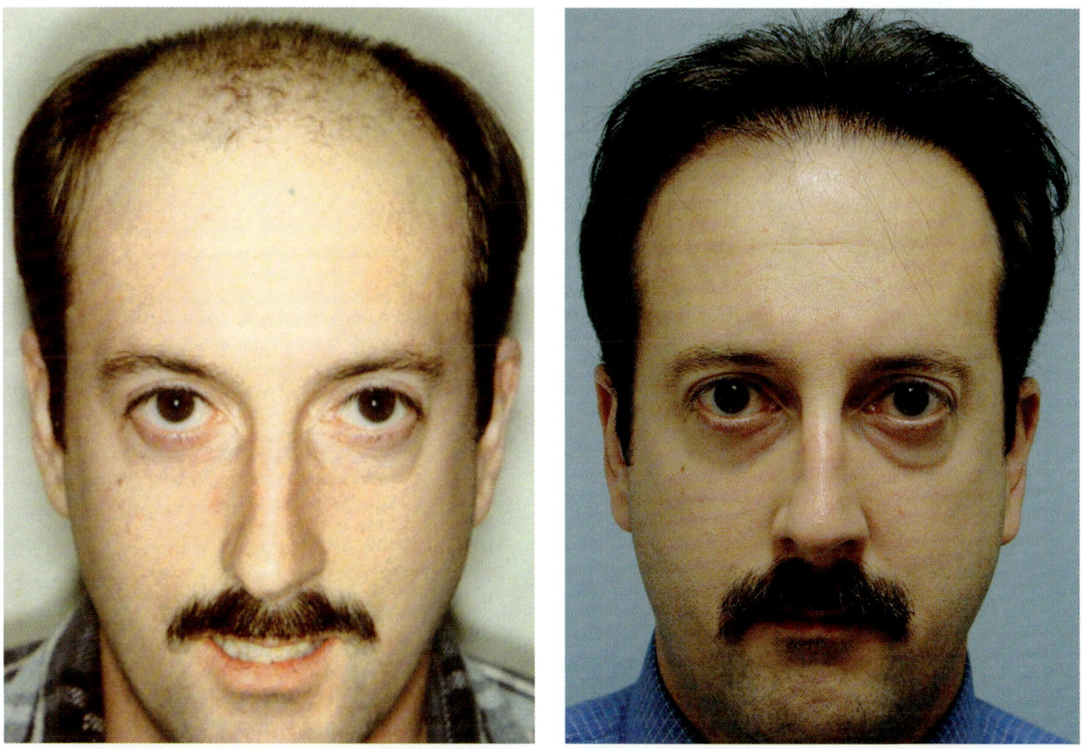

A B

FIGURE 6-31. A,B: This is a 38-year-old man who had tried various hair-replacement schemes (including hairpieces) but was unsatisfied with these labor-intensive regimens. He demonstrates an unfavorable combination for follicular transfer (i.e., straight, coarse, black hair and a milky-white scalp). Nevertheless, understanding the limitations of transplantation given these anatomic constraints, he elected to proceed with follicular grafting. He underwent four sessions spaced 6 to 8 months apart using 400 minigrafts and 75 to 125 follicular unit grafts per session. The patient is shown 1½ years after his last grafting session with notable improvement.

Discussion

As with any cosmetic endeavor, the surgeon should attempt to assess the patient's expectations and ensure that the surgical objectives can be met to the patient's satisfaction. The combination of coarse, straight black hair and milky white skin, as this patient exhibited, made natural, nonpluggy, looking grafting a difficult task. Straight, black hair that arises atop a white scalp looks like a transplanted shaft. Intentional harvesting of softer, more vellus hair that arises near the posterior hairline is preferred for anterior hairline transplantation, especially in a patient with very dark, straight hair. In addition, the shiny, white, exposed scalp can be visually reduced by densely packing follicular units along the anterior hairline and by cross-hatching the hairs at various angles. Reduction of the visible, white scalp minimizes the contrast between the hair shaft and the scalp and thereby ameliorates the unnatural graft appearance. Although these surgical techniques are particularly well suited in the patient with dark hair and light scalp, it is advocated for all patients undergoing follicular transplantation in order to attain maximal density. Nevertheless, the patient with this color combination must be fully cognizant of the limitations of his anatomy prior to electing to proceed with surgery.

Case #2 (Fig. 6-32A–D)

This is a 32-year-old entertainer who began losing his hair in his early twenties. Having had a significant amount of hair loss during the intervening years, he felt that his balding had somewhat stabilized over the past several years and presented for evaluation for surgical hair restoration. The patient wore a hat while on stage to camouflage his receding hairline. The patient desired to have fuller density to his hair so that he could appear on stage without a hat and not bear the stigma of obvious premature alopecia. His expectations and goals were realistic: He did not desire a prepubescently low hairline or effacement of his fronto-temporal recession but rather wanted a hairline that would be suitable for his age and still look natural over the coming years. The patient underwent two transplantation sessions separated by approximately 6 months and is shown approximately 2 years after the second session.

Procedure

Two hair-transplantation sessions were performed at a 6-month interval with approximately 350 minigrafts with 200 micrografts for each session.

Discussion

As evident, this patient exhibited a deep fronto-temporal recession. With such an anterior hairline configuration, the surgeon must exercise restraint when deciding on the anterior limit of the proposed hairline. Drawing the hairline very far forward requires significant effort to camouflage the increased fronto-temporal distance after density to the frontal, central hairline has been established. In addition, the age of the patient was taken into consideration, given the likelihood that at this younger age additional thinning and loss would increase the need for numerous sessions to chase the temporal recession. Also, creation of a "30-year-old" hairline would look preposterous when the patient became more mature. For these reasons, a very conservative hairline was drawn approximately 9.5 cm from the glabella with a gentle curvature back along the fronto-temporal recession. Of note, the patient was a relatively good candidate for hair restoration surgery because he had a fair complexion and sandy brown hair.

Case #3 (Fig. 6-33A–E)

This is a 40-year-old man who had been contemplating hair restoration surgery for several years but was not satisfied with the density that follicular transfer could offer. He had not tried any medical treatments or hairpieces in the past, nor had he undergone any previous grafting sessions. He was interested in maximal density in as short a period as possible. On physical examination, he showed fronto-temporal recession without overt loss of crown hair. His hair was relatively dark and straight and his skin tone was also darker (Fitzpatrick III to IV) given his Middle Eastern descent. He was a nonsmoker and was not diabetic. He appeared to be a good candidate for a Juri flap and was offered the risks, benefits, and limitations for both follicular transfer and Juri flap surgery. He chose the latter.

Procedure

The procedure was a twice-delayed, temporo-parieto-occipital (Juri) flap from the right side.

Discussion

As emphasized throughout the text, a twice-delayed, temporo-parieto-occipital flap is only suitable for a very small minority of patients. The ideal candidate desires significant density in the fronto-temporal region and is willing to accept the morbidity of a multistaged operative procedure. The patient should not show significant fronto-temporal recession that exceeds approximately 4 cm (the width of the flap). However, two flaps (bilateral) can be positioned in a staged fashion for greater recession (obviously, up to 8 cm). If a bilateral Juri flap is entertained, the first flap should be placed to create the new hairline and the second flap positioned behind the first flap. If the patient shows recession that extends into the crown, or vertex, additional follicular grafts behind the flap should be placed to camouflage the

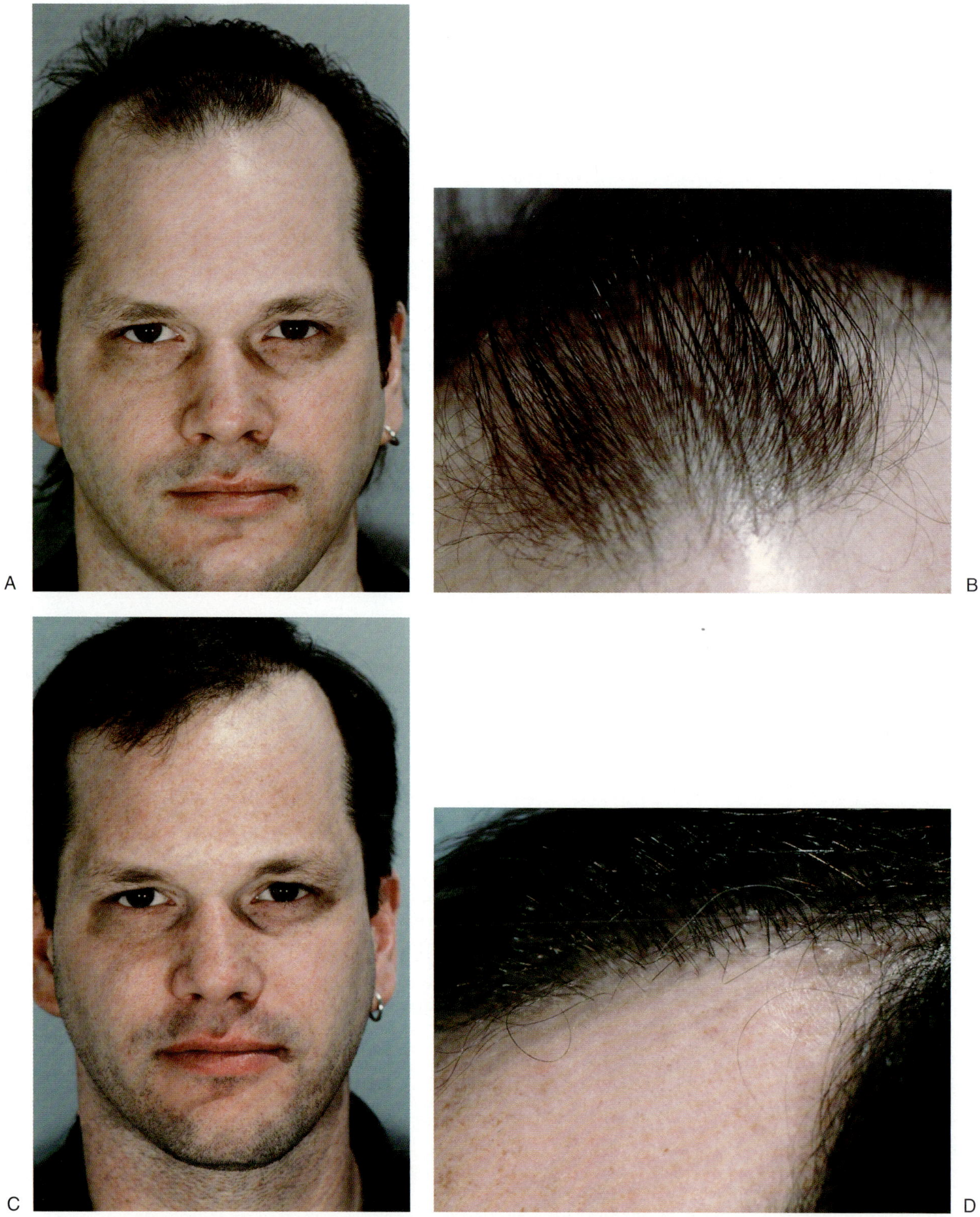

FIGURE 6-32. A–D: This is a 32-year-old entertainer who sported a cap on stage in order to camouflage his receding hairline. He had realistic expectations about surgical hair restoration and wanted a natural appearing hairline. He underwent two grafting sessions consisting of 350 minigrafts and 200 micrografts done with a 6-month interval and is shown 2 years after the second session with good improvement. Given the patient's young age, the height of the hairline must be designed with further hair loss in mind as well as what would be considered a natural-appearing hairline when he is more mature.

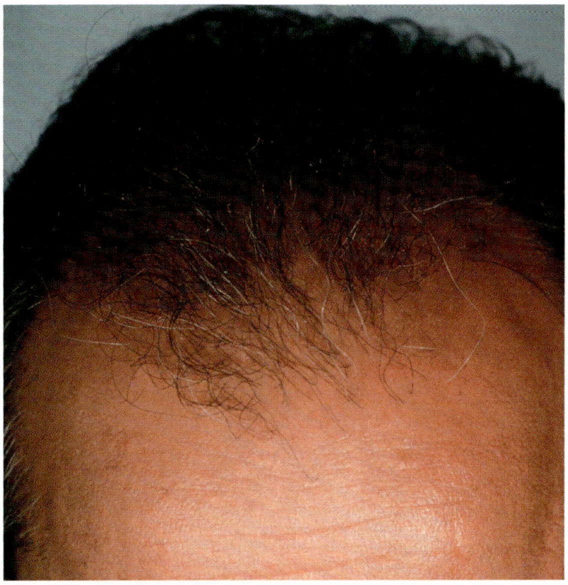

A

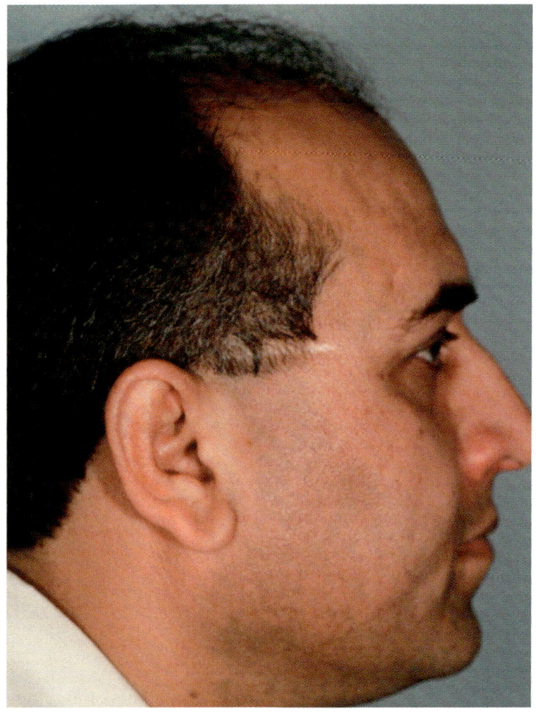

B

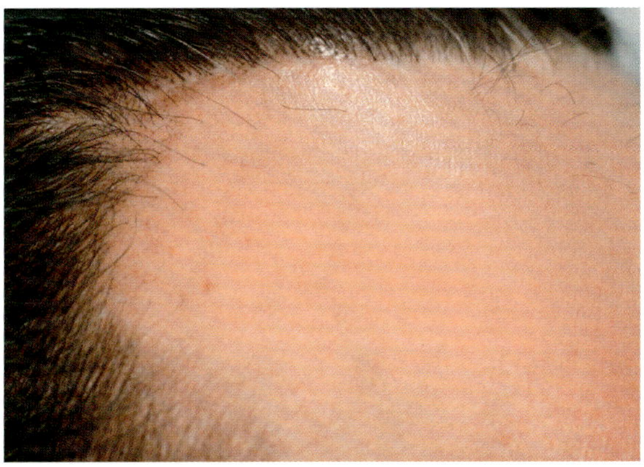

C

FIGURE 6-33. A–E: This is a 40-year-old man who desires rapid hair restoration and is willing to undergo a multistaged operation to achieve this aesthetic objective. He is Middle Eastern by descent and exhibits dark hair and dark skin. He exhibits principally frontotemporal recession with adequate coverage more posteriorly. He underwent a twice-delayed temporoparieto-occipital (Juri) flap with notable aesthetic improvement. Given his dark complexion, a fine, white incision line is perceptible, but the patient refused any additional follicular sessions to camouflage this area and improve the appearance of his hairline because he was very satisfied already with the surgical outcome. **A:** Preoperative, close-up, bird's-eye view; **B:** preoperative, lateral view; **C:** postoperative, close-up view; **D:** postoperative, bird's eye view; **E:** postoperative lateral view.

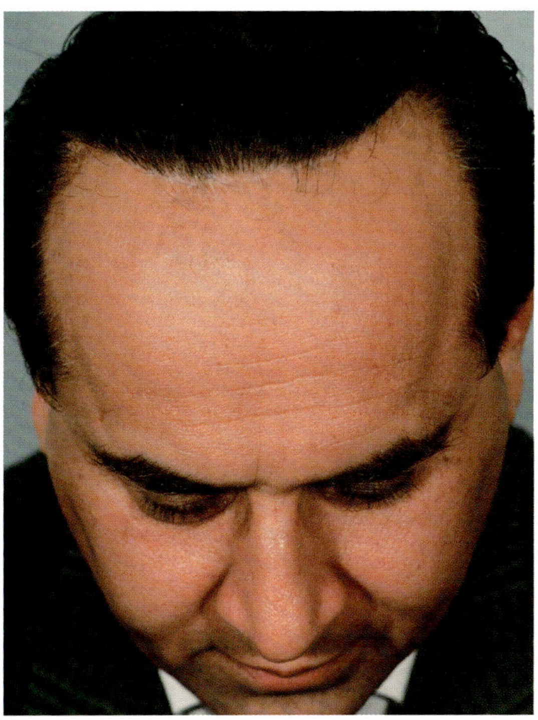

D

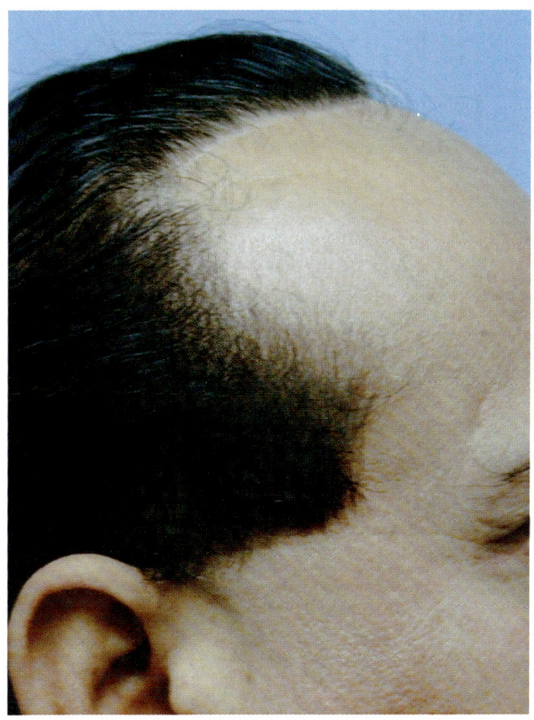

E

abrupt transition to non–hair-bearing skin. Additionally, patients should understand in the preoperative setting that follicular grafting should be placed anterior to the flap several months after flap transfer to soften the linear configuration of the flap and create a more natural-appearing hairline. However, many patients have expressed satisfaction with the appearance and refused to undergo this added surgical endeavor (as in this particular case). If the patient shows significant recession along the fronto-temporal valleys, the flap will have to extend over a greater arc and distance, making the potential for a persistent standing cone deformity ("dog ear") at the point of rotation (i.e., at the base of the flap) much higher and the likelihood that the flap will extend the entire, intended distance less probable. This patient exhibited very deep fronto-temporal alleys that engendered a protracted standing-cone deformity requiring months to resolve. No revision surgery for this protuberance ultimately was needed. Unlike follicular-transfer surgery, light hair and dark skin are not an ideal combination. This patient who had darker-complexioned skin developed a fine, visible white, incision line that would have benefited from follicular camouflage. On the other hand, lighter skin would have served to mask this fine incision line considerably better. Light hair color is preferred, but for a different reason than given for follicular transfer. Because individual grafts are not used, the risk of a "pluggy" look does not constitute an aesthetic problem. Instead, the linear configuration of the anterior hairline is less noticeable by virtue of the lighter hair color. Further, subsequent follicular transfer anterior to the flap benefits from the camouflaging effect of the lighter hair color. One important contraindication that has been mentioned before deserves reiteration here: Patients who risk flap loss are smokers or diabetics, and these patients are ineligible for a Juri flap.

Case #4 (Fig. 6-34A,B)

This is a 47-year-old man who suffers from crown balding with some fronto-temporal thinning as well. He was principally concerned with his crown baldness and wanted this area addressed. He had not tried any medical or surgical options in the past for his hair loss. He was otherwise healthy and had a stable pattern of hair loss over the past 5 years. On physical examination, he was noted to have a Fitzpatrick-II skin color with curly hair and a total of 11 cm diameter of crown baldness. He elected to undergo scalp reduction to achieve his aesthetic objectives.

Procedure

The procedure consisted of three sessions of scalp reduction using a silastic extender with each session spaced at a 1-month interval. Scalp reduction was accomplished with 4.5 cm advancement during the first reduction session, 3.5 cm

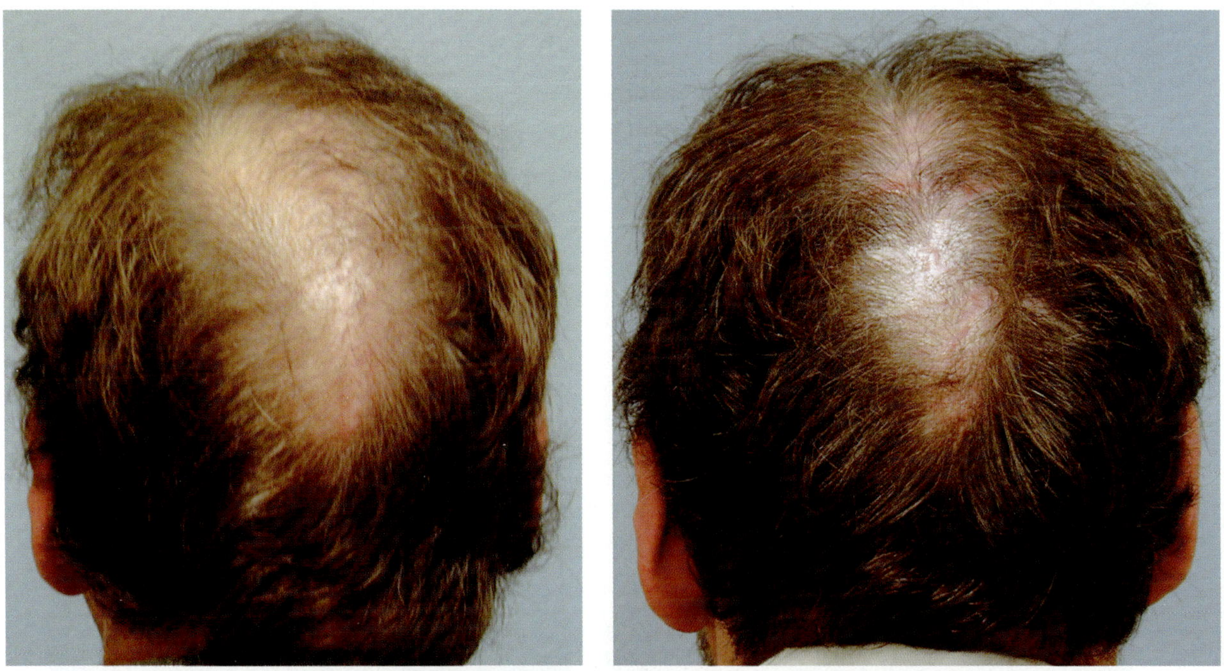

A B

FIGURE 6-34. A,B: This is a 47-year-old man who is principally concerned about his crown baldness and who elected to undergo scalp reduction to correct this aesthetic concern. The patient exhibited a total of 11 cm of bald crown scalp. He underwent three scalp reduction sessions with the assistance of an extender device and with each session spaced 1 month apart. During the last session, the patient had his extender removed and the wound closed in a z-plasty configuration.

for the following session, and 3 cm for the final session. The scalp extender was removed at the last session and the wound closed in a z-plasty configuration.

Discussion

Generally, crown baldness is a less satisfying area to manage because the patient and onlooker do not readily view this area on a regular basis. Nevertheless, patients who suffer from this area may be quite self-conscious about their naked pate and desire intervention. The appropriate candidate for this procedure is one who is over 40 years of age and who has a relatively stable pattern of hair loss in the crown region that extends no greater than 12 cm in total diameter. Use of an extender device has greatly reduced the number of sessions required and accelerated the process so that only 1-month intervals are required to achieve reduction. A z-plasty closure minimizes unfavorable scar contracture and also avoids the appearance of a slot deformity despite some further hair loss. If the incision site becomes exposed over time, then follicular grafting should be offered to the patient to camouflage this area.

REFERENCES

1. Dieffenbach JF: Nonnulla de regeneratione et transplantatione. Dissertation inauguralis 1822.
2. Orentreich N: Autografts in alopecia and other selected dermatological conditions. Ann NY Acad Sci 1959;83:463.
3. Nordström R: "Micrografts" for improvement of the frontal hairline after hair transplantation. Aesthetic Plast Surg 1981;5:97.
4. Marritt E: Single-hair transplantation for hairline refinement: a practical solution. J Dermatol Surg Oncol 1984;10:962–963.
5. Juri J: Use of parieto-occipital flaps in the surgical treatment of baldness. Plast Reconstr Surg 1975;55:456–460.
6. Juri J, Juri C: Temporo-parieto-occipital flap for the treatment of baldness. Clin Plast Surg 1982;9:255–261.
7. Lam SM, Hempstead BR, Williams EF: A philosophy and strategy for surgical hair restoration: a ten-year experience. Dermatol Surg 2002;28:1035–1042.
8. Ludwig E: Classification of the types of androgenetic alopecia (common baldness) occurring in the female sex. Br J Dermatol 1977;97:247–254.
9. Frechet P: Scalp extension. J Dermatol Surg Oncol 1993;10: 616–622.
10. Blanchard G, Blanchard B: Obliteration of alopecia by hair lifting. J Natl Med Assoc 1977;69:639–641.
11. Nordström RE: "Stretch-back" in scalp reductions for male-pattern baldness. Plast Reconstr Surg 1984;73:422–426.
12. Bernstein RM, Rassman WR, Stough D: In support of follicular unit transplantation. Dermatol Surg 2000;26:160–162.
13. Norwood OT, Taylor BJ: Hairline design and placement. J Dermatol Surg Oncol 1991;17:510–518.
14. Ezaki, Kasori Y: The occipito-parietal flap method in the treatment of male baldness. Aesthetic Plast Surg 1995;19:469–472.
15. Nordstrom RE: One variety of a long, delayed temporo-parieto-occipital flap. J Dermatol Surg Oncol 1988;14:755–761.
16. Elliott RA Jr: The lateral scalp flap for anterior hairline reconstruction. Clin Plast Surg 1982;9:179–196.
17. Kabaker SS: Juri flap procedure for the treatment of baldness: two-year experience. Arch Otolaryngol 1979;105:509–514.
18. Avram MR, Cole JP, Gandelman M, et al: The potential role of minoxidil in the hair transplantation setting. Dermatol Surg 2002;28:894–900.
19. Sintov A, Serafimovich S, Gilhar A: New topical antiandrogenic formulations can stimulate hair growth in human bald scalp grafted onto mice. Int J Pharm 2000;20:125–134.
20. Wiseman M, Shapiro J: Therapeutic approach to androgenetic alopecia. J Cutan Med Surg 1999;3 Suppl:S21–S27.
21. Buhl AE: Minoxidil's action in hair follicles. J Invest Dermatol 1991;96:73S–74S.
22. Buhl AE, Waldon DJ, Conrad SJ, et al: Potassium channel conductance: a mechanism affecting hair growth both in vitro and in vivo. J Invest Dermatol 1992:98:315–319.
23. Kurata S, Uno H, Allen-Hoffmann BL: Effects of hypertrichotic agents on follicular and nonfollicular cells in vitro. Skin Pharmacol 1996;9:3–8.
24. Wester RC, Maibach HI, Guy RH, et al: Minoxidil stimulates cutaneous blood flow in human balding scalps. J Invest Dermatol 1984;82:90–93.
25. Civatte J, Laux B, Simpson NB, et al: Two percent topical minoxidil solution in male-pattern baldness: preliminary European results. Dermatologica 1987;175(Suppl 2):42–49.
26. Connors TJ, Cooke DE, De Launey WE, et al: Australian trial of topical minoxidil and placebo in early male-pattern baldness. Australas J Dermatol 1990;31:17–25.
27. Koperski JA, Orenberg EK, Wilkonson DI: Topical minoxidil therapy for androgenetic alopecia. A 30-month study. Arch Dermatol 1987;123:1483–1487.
28. Rietschel RL, Duncan SH: Safety and efficacy of topical minoxidil in the management of androgenetic alopecia. J Am Acad Dermatol 1987;16:677–685.
29. Savin RC: Use of topical minoxidil in the treatment of male-pattern baldness. J Am Acad Dermatol 1987;16:696–704.
30. Price V, Menefee E: Quantitative estimation of hair growth: comparative changes in weight and hair count with 5% and 2% minoxidil, placebo and no treatment. In: Van Neste D, Randall V, eds. Hair research for the next millennium. Amsterdam: Elsevier Science, 1996:67–68.
31. Olsen EA: Treatment of androgenetic alopecia with topical minoxidil in early male-pattern baldness. J Am Acad Dermatol 1985;113:185–192.
32. DeVillez RL: Topical minoxidil for androgenetic alopecia: optimizing the chance for success by appropriate patient selection. Dermatologica 1987;175(Suppl 2):50–53.
33. DeVillez RL, Jacobs JP, Szpunar CA, et al: Adrogenetic alopecia in the female: treatment with 2% minoxidil solution. Arch Dermatol 1994;130:303–307.
34. Bazzano GS, Terezakis N, Galen W: Topical tretinoin for hair growth promotion. J Am Acad Dermatol 1986;15: 880–883,890–893.
35. Kassimir JJ: Use of topical minoxidil as a possible adjunct to hair transplant surgery. J Am Acad Dermatol 1987;16:685–687.
36. Kaufman K, Olsen EA, Whiting D, et al: Finasteride in the treatment of men with androgenetic alopecia. Finasteride male pattern hair loss study group. J Am Acad Dermatol 1998;39: 578–589.
37. Leyden J, Dunlap F, Miller B, et al: Finasteride in the treatment of men with frontal male pattern hair loss. J Am Acad Dermatol 1999;40:930–937.
38. Kaufman KD: Long-term (5-year) multinational experience with finasteride 1 mg in the treatment of men with androgenetic alopecia. Eur J Dermatol 2002;12:38–49.
39. Stough DB, Rao NA, Kaufman KD, et al: Finasteride improves male pattern hair loss in a randomized study in identical twins. Eur J Dermatol 2002;12:32–37.

40. Whiting DA, Waldstreicher J, Sanchez M, et al: Measuring reversal of hair miniaturization in androgenetic alopecia by follicular counts in horizontal sections of serial scalp biopsies: results of finasteride 1 mg treatment of men and post menopausal women. J Invest Dermatol Symposium Proceedings 1999;4:282–284.
41. Whiting DA: Advances in the treatment of male androgenetic alopecia: A brief review of finasteride studies. Eur J Dermatol 2001;11:332–324.
42. Burke B, Cunliffe W: Oral spironolactone therapy for female patients with acne, hirsutism or androgenic alopecia. Br J Dermatol 1985;112:124–125.
43. Rushton DH: Quantitative assessment of spironolactone treatment in women with diffuse androgen-dependent alopecia. J Soc Cosmet Chemists 1991;42:317–325.
44. Giseleskog PO, Hermann D, Hammarlund-Udenaes M, et al: A model for the turnover of dihydrotestosterone in the presence of the irreversible 5 alpha-reductase inhibitors GI198745 and finasteride. Clin Pharmacol Ther 1998;64:636–647.
45. Bramson HN, Hermann D, Batchelor KW, et al: Unique preclinical characteristics of GG745, a potent dual inhibitor of 5AR. J Pharmacol Exp Ther 1997;282:1496–1502.
46. Goldman CK, Tsai JC, Soroceanu L, et al: Loss of vascular endothelial growth factor in human alopecia hair follicles. J Invest Dermatol 1995;104:18S–20S.
47. Yano K, Brown LF, Detmar M: Control of hair growth and follicle size by VEGF-mediated angiogenesis. J Clin Invest 2001; 107:409–417.
48. Lachgar S, Charveron M, Gail Y, et al: Minoxidil upregulates the expression of vascular endothelial growth factor in human hair dermal papilla cells. Br J Dermatol 1998;138:407–411.
49. Goffman T, Cuscela D, Glass J, et al: Topical application of nitroxide protects radiation-induced alopecia in guinea pigs. Int J Radiat Oncol Biol Phys 1992;22:803–806.
50. Cuscela D, Coffin D, Lupton GP, et al: Protection from radiation-induced alopecia with topical application of nitroxides: fractionated studies. Cancer J Sci Am 1996;2:273.
51. DiSilverio F, D'Eramo G, Lubramo C, et al: Evidence that Serenoa repens extract displays an antiestrogenic activity in prostatic tissue of benign prostatic hypertrophy patients. Eur Urol 1992;21:309–314.
52. Champauli G, Patel JC, Bonnard AM: A double-blind trial of an extract of the plant Serenoa repens in benign prostatic hyperplasia. Br J Clin Pharmacol 1984;18:461–462.
53. el-Sheikh MM, Dakkkak MR, Saddique A: The effect of Permixon on androgen receptors. Acta Obstet Gynecol Scand 1988;67:397–399.
54. Rhodes L, Primka RL, Berman C, et al: Comparison of finasteride (Proscar), a 5 alpha reductase inhibitor, and various commercial plant extracts in in vitro and in vivo alpha reductase inhibition. Prostate 1993;22:43–51.
55. Casarosa C, Cosci di Coscio M, Fratta M: Lack of effects of a lyposterolic extract of Serenoa repens on plasma levels of testosterone, follicle-stimulating hormone, and luteinizing hormone. Clin Ther 1988;10:585–588.
56. Baumgartner ER, Suormala T: Multiple carboxylase deficiency: inherited and acquired disorders of biotin metabolism. Int J Vitam Nutr Res 1997;57:377–384.
57. Wolf B, Heard GS, Weissbecker KA, et al: Biotinidase deficiency: initial clinical features and rapid diagnosis. Ann Neurol 1985; 18:614–617.
58. Gupta PC, Patwari AK, Mullick DN: Alopecia with rickets: an end organ unresponsiveness to 1,25-dihydroxyvitamin D-a case report. Indian J Med Sci 1990;44:239–243.
59. Höchberg Z, Benderli A, Levy J, et al: 1,25-Dihydroxyvitamin D resistance, rickets, and alopecia. Am J Med 1984;77:805–811.
60. Paus R, Schilli MB, Handjiski B, et al: Topical calcitriol enhances normal hair regrowth but does not prevent chemotherapy-induced alopecia in mice. Cancer Res 1996;56:4438–4443.
61. Wolfe H, Kunte C: Current management of androgenetic alopecia in men. Eur J Dermatol 1999;9:606–609.
62. Gehring W, Gloor M: Effect of topically applied Dexpanthenol on epidermal barrier function and stratum corneum hydration. Results of a human in vivo study. Arzneimittenlforschung 2000; 50:659–663 (in German).
63. Hahn C, Roseler S, Fritzsche R, et al: Allergic contact reaction to dexpanthenol: lymphocyte transformation test and evidence for microsomal-dependent metabolism of the allergen. Contact Dermatitis 1993;28:81–83.
64. Uno H, Kurata S: Chemical agents and peptides affect hair growth. J Invest Dermatol 1993;101 (1 Suppl):143S–147S.
65. Pontinen PJ, Aaltokallio T, Kolari PJ: Comparative effects of exposure to different light sources (He-Ne laser, InGaA1 diode laser, a specific type of noncoherent LED) on skin blood flow for the head. Acupunct Electrother Res 1996;21:105–118.
66. Li L, Hoffman RM: The feasibility of target selective gene therapy of the hair follicle. Nature Med 1995;1:705–706.

7

REJUVENATION OF THE AGING NOSE

SAMUEL M. LAM
EDWIN F. WILLIAMS III

At first glance, a chapter dedicated to rhinoplasty in a book devoted to rejuvenation of the aging face appears misguided. However, the nose undergoes unmistakable signs of aging that should not be ignored by the aesthetic surgeon. Whereas the eye and brow complex draws attention on direct gaze, the neck and chin complex is more acutely noted on lateral view. However, the central position and projection of the nose make it a feature that attracts scrutiny from both the frontal and profile perspectives. The elongated, crooked appearance that the aged nose assumes is particularly remarkable on lateral view and can undermine the surgically rejuvenated appearance of the remainder of the face. The protuberant, irregular proboscis that is the hallmark for rhinophyma may be disfiguring to the individual and, worse yet, may harbor occult carcinoma. With these general aesthetic considerations in mind, the facial plastic surgeon can determine judiciously when rhinoplasty may be warranted for the patient who displays the classic signs of the aging nose.

Besides aesthetic concerns, the aging nose may prove to cripple the patient functionally as well. The inelastic, descended, mature nose exhibits less structural integrity than its younger counterpart and can obstruct nasal airflow substantially. Both the internal and external valves may be compromised by the weakened architecture. Further, the heavy soft-tissue envelope of the rhinophymatous nose may add considerable weight to the nose to compress both nasal valves further. The male patient often suffers from the ravages of nasal aging more so than the female because of the heavier, less angulated attitude that characterizes even the younger masculine nose. Also, rhinophyma appears to be a disease that afflicts the male patient almost exclusively. Therefore, the mature male patient may present more frequently to the physician for corrective surgery than the female because of these preponderant functional concerns. Along with ameliorating the functional deficits of the ptotic, unsupported nose, the surgeon, per force, concurrently addresses some, or most, of the aesthetic attributes. Therefore, the aesthetic and functional dimensions are often inseparable entities; and this chapter elucidates the surgical role for both conditions.

Although this chapter dwells on the peculiar characteristics that define the aging nose, the authors outline a rhinoplasty treatment strategy that may be more broadly applied to all situations. A ptotic tip is not exclusive to the aging nose, and many aesthetic flaws that mar a mature nose detract from the beauty of a more youthful nose. This proviso applies to the functional deficits that characterize the aging nose as well. The diligent rhinoplasty surgeon should tailor his or her surgical strategy to fit a particular patient's nose but should approach all noses with a systematic policy. This philosophy that embraces simplicity, flexibility, and planning is further detailed in the forthcoming section.

PREOPERATIVE CONSIDERATIONS: PATIENT SELECTION AND RELEVANT ANATOMY

Relevant Anatomy of the Aging Nose

Although the nose plays a central role in facial aesthetics, it remains chiefly a respiratory organ that warms, humidifies, and cleanses the ambient air on inspiration. The primacy of nasal function should not escape the surgeon's consideration when operating on this vital appendage: The responsibility to maintain nasal patency should inform even strictly aesthetic endeavors. Hence, the anatomy is reviewed in terms of both the external aesthetic attributes and the internal functional underpinnings.[1]

The nose is divided into three constituent elements: the lower flexible third (alar cartilages), middle semiflexible third (upper lateral cartilages), and rigid upper third (the nasal bones) (Fig. 7-1). The flared lower lateral, or alar, cartilages are winged, tapered structures that define the external nares and thereby the external nasal valve. More precisely, the external valve consists of the curved alar cartilage and the nasal floor to complete the circular, valvular ring (Fig. 7-2). The integrity of the external nasal valve is commonly compromised by aggressive rhinoplasty but may be affected by numerous other factors, including congenital weakness, trauma, thermal injury, tumor, and aging. After rhinoplasty, the external valve may collapse either owing to cartilaginous weakening (cephalic resection, domal division,

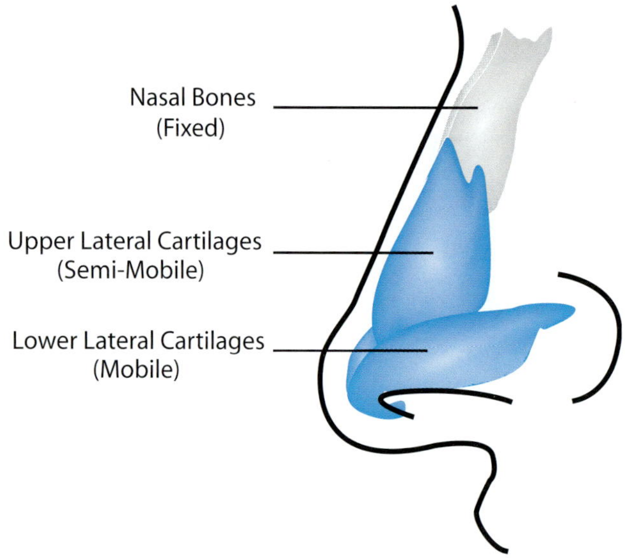

FIGURE 7-1. The illustration shows the three constituent components of the nose: the lower, flexible third (alar cartilages); the middle, semiflexible third (upper lateral cartilages); and the rigid, upper third (the nasal bones).

and various incisions that weaken tip support) or soft-tissue retraction and scarring. Similarly, cartilaginous or soft-tissue weakness predispose toward valvular collapse in the aging nose. During the aging process, the soft tissue loses elasticity and the tissues become attenuated, both of which contribute to the inability to overcome gravitational force and eventual tip ptosis. In addition, the cartilaginous structures of the nose lose some of their tensile strength and the ligamentous structures that bind the cartilages together (scroll, interdomal ligament, etc.) and fasten the cartilage to the surrounding soft tissue (the minor tip-supporting mechanisms) experience some erosion to their strength. The increased sebaceous quality of the nasal tip, known in extreme as rhinophyma, adds weight to the nasal tip and actually may occlude the external naris. All of these factors lead to compromise of the external valve in the aging nose that may require surgical intervention to correct.

The internal nasal valve, also known as the limen vestibuli, is the major regulator of nasal airflow in the White nose. Mesorrhine and platyrrhine noses that typify the Asian and African noses, respectively, have a much broader cross-section in the region of the internal valve; therefore, they rarely suffer from internal nasal valve collapse. The nasal structures that comprise the internal valve include the caudal border of the upper lateral cartilage, the nasal septum, and the anterior head of the inferior turbinate. The angle formed by the union of the nasal septum and upper lateral cartilages should be a minimum of 10 to 15 degrees in order to ensure patency (Fig. 7-3). A high septal deflection can impinge the upper lateral cartilage and thereby narrow the described angle. The weakening of the cartilaginous support that marks the aging nose can contribute to internal valve collapse. Prior rhinoplasty can detrimentally affect the internal valve (e.g., dorsal reduction severs the upper lateral cartilage–septal union and may predispose toward valvular compromise). A bulbous anterior head of the inferior turbinate, which may arise from allergy, infection, or tumor, or may be a congenital structural anomaly, also can lead to diminished airflow and increased turbulence. All of these structures should be carefully examined during the preoperative consultation (*vide infra*).

Rhinophyma represents a distinct clinical entity that can cause significant cosmetic and functional disturbance in the aging nose (Case #1). Older men, in particular, are the primary victims of this deforming disease. The comic actor, W.C. Fields, sported perhaps the most notorious example of this elephantine nose. The increased sebaceous activity in the lower third of the nose occurs because of an idiopathic rise in sebaceous gland hypertrophy. Part of the mechanism by which this process may be triggered is attributed to

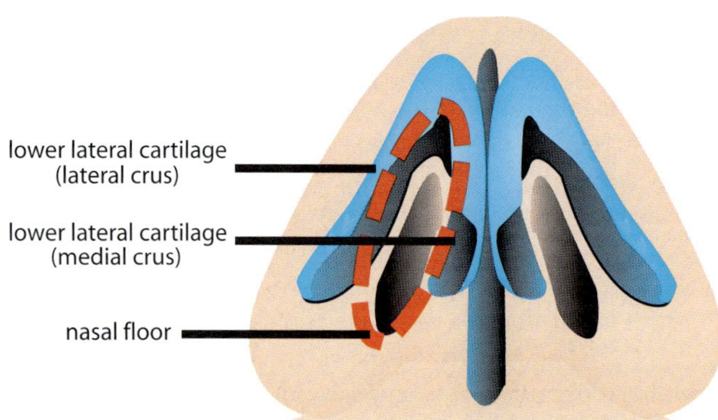

FIGURE 7-2. The flared lower lateral, or alar, cartilages are winged, tapered structures that define the external nares and thereby the external nasal valve. More precisely, the external valve consists of the curved alar cartilage and the nasal floor to complete the circular, valvular ring.

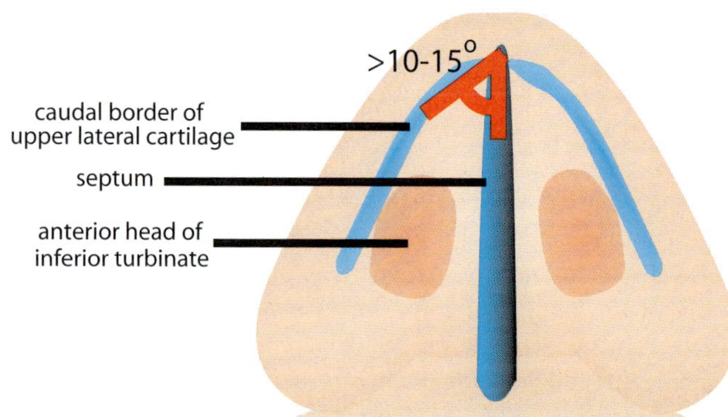

FIGURE 7-3. The nasal structures that comprise the internal valve include the caudal border of the upper lateral cartilage, the nasal septum, and the anterior head of the inferior turbinate. The angle that is formed by the union of the nasal septum and the upper lateral cartilages should be a minimum of 10 to 15 degrees in order to ensure patency.

proliferation of the bacterium, *Demodex follicularis*. Rhinophyma has been viewed as the end stage of acne rosacea, a dermatologic condition that afflicts the central oilier regions of the face. Topical tetracycline applied regularly during the incipient phase of this disease may control the spread and possibly reverse it. However, once the malady is in full bloom, medical management does little to efface this now-impregnable entity. Of note, the often-cited belief that rhinophyma originates from alcoholic intemperance is a fallacy that should not be propagated. As mentioned, correction of rhinophyma should address both the aesthetic and functional problems, which include the potential insidious presence of basal cell carcinoma. The most suspicious areas should be sent for pathologic review in the preoperative phase (or intraoperatively at least) if highly suspicious to obtain insurance coverage.

A Systematic Approach to Rhinoplasty

Although this chapter is devoted to the surgical management of the aging nose, the reader is encouraged to approach every rhinoplasty in a systematic fashion. This section elucidates the authors' philosophical approach to all rhinoplasty, which the reader can adapt to fit the circumstance at hand. The three cornerstones that define successful rhinoplasty surgery are simplicity, planning, and flexibility.[2] Although these principles appear to be broadly conceived and ill defined, the reader is urged to review this section carefully and contemplate the guiding tenets outlined. After diligent study, the reader will hopefully come to realize the importance that these dictates exemplify.

Simplicity

The guiding principle of simplicity always should be recalled during the preparatory and execution phases of rhinoplasty. Simplicity entails undertaking rhinoplasty with the fewest steps necessary to achieve the aesthetic or functional goals. For instance, a patient who exhibits cephalic fullness to the lower lateral cartilages without notable bifidus should be an eligible candidate for a closed, nondelivery, transcartilaginous technique. The nondelivery technique affords the most expedient and targeted approach to the aesthetic deficit without undue, protracted operative dissection. In contrast, rhinoplasty surgery that entails major architectural destruction followed by extensive structural reconstitution should be condemned if conducted in an indiscriminate fashion. Not every nose justifies aggressive resection: Prolonged surgical manipulation increases variability because of scar contracture over time that may transform a beautiful immediate result into a disaster down the road. The effect of skin "shrink wrapping" over time may reveal any minor flaws in surgical technique or even expose the outline of structural grafts that have been perfectly executed.

Categorically, plastic surgeons are perfectionists by inclination; for that reason, the targeted goal is consistently 100% in every rhinoplasty endeavor. However, if achievement of 100% entails 5 hours of surgery, then the ultimate result may fall far short of the intended mark because of the aforesaid variability that arises from radical surgery. The law of diminishing returns takes hold, because edema distorts anatomy and the hemostatic effects of the local anesthetic dissipate after an hour and a half of operative time.

Instead, the surgeon should think systematically how he or she could arrive at the maximal aesthetic achievement with the minimal of surgical maneuvers. Accordingly, a realistic goal for surgery may be 90% rather than 100%. This is not to concede that 100% is not achievable but rather that it may not be preferable because by doing so the result may approach 80%. These percentages are only presented to help instruct the rhinoplasty surgeon understand the principle of simplicity more precisely and clearly do not represent actual conceived numerical values.

Planning

Planning goes hand in hand with simplicity. In order to achieve the most straightforward, simplest strategy to every rhinoplasty endeavor, proper planning should begin from the first patient encounter. At the conclusion of the initial consultation, the surgeon should outline a plan for surgery that may involve as basic as a few marginal notes jotted down to a more elaborate and complete dictation. Either method of documentation is acceptable so long as the surgeon can readily refer to the proposed plan at the time of surgery and recall what should be done at that later date. With a hectic schedule, it is a wasteful and troubling exercise to begin afresh with surgical planning moments before the actual procedure. Using simplicity as a guide, the surgeon should deliberate seriously whether an external, transcolumellar incision is justifiable. The authors believe that open structure rhinoplasty is a worthwhile venture in select cases but should not be undertaken in every circumstance. The external approach adds increased surgical dissection and operative time that may not be required. Conversely, difficult revision cases may not be suitable to an endonasal approach because of the needs for better visualization and greater structural reconstitution. Letting the punishment fit the crime should dictate how much surgical dissection is necessary. The forthcoming section on operative considerations presents treatment strategies that are based on these guiding tenets of planning and simplicity.

Flexibility

Flexibility constitutes the final consideration that should inform every rhinoplasty effort. Although this principle really refers to intraoperative decision making, it is mentioned in the preoperative section so that the reader can understand the three guiding tenets of simplicity, planning, and flexibility together. Despite the best efforts at planning an effective strategy, the vicissitudes that may arise during surgery occasionally justify a change in the course of action. This decision to undertake a different surgical tactic defines flexibility. The surgeon should not rigidly adhere to a preconceived plan if that plan begins to appear ill suited to the current situation. For instance, placement of a columellar strut and a transdomal suture may be all that are required to correct a ptotic tip during intraoperative analysis, and the plan for a lateral crural overlay may be justifiably abandoned given the perceived situation. With all three cornerstones in mind, the surgeon should be able to formulate a reliable, systematic strategy for every rhinoplasty and adapt that strategy according to individual constraints. Diligent study of long-term postoperative results confirm or alter future surgical endeavors; and the successful rhinoplasty surgeon should remain a pupil for life.

Preoperative Evaluation

The three elements of a proper preoperative evaluation include assessment of the psychological motivations and expectations, the history of the patient's problem, and physical assessment of the aesthetic and functional features of the patient's nose.

Psychological Evaluation

The psychological inquiry that is mandatory for every cosmetic consultation has been well outlined in Chapter 3. Nevertheless, rhinoplasty often carries with it more psychological overtones than routine, aging-face surgery and deserves special mention herein. Although rhinoplasty of the aging nose is primarily restorative, aesthetic enhancement beyond one's former, youthful nasal shape may be requested. For example, a mild dorsal hump that is present at youth may become accentuated over time because of nasal tip ptosis. The patient may desire not only correction of nasal ptosis but also removal of the hump altogether. Alternatively, the patient may request aesthetic tip refinement along with improvement of nasal function. As the nose is prominently situated in the center of the face, changing the aesthetic features of the nose may have significant psychological repercussions. Accordingly, the surgeon should decipher the exact aesthetic and functional goals that the patient desires and work to match those objectives after careful investigation of the underlying motivations and expectations.

As mentioned, the male patient often suffers the effects of nasal aging (ptosis or rhinophyma) more acutely than his female counterpart. Unfortunately, men may exhibit a more profound psychological dilemma when electing aesthetic or functional rhinoplasty. Studies have revealed that men are less tolerant of change to their physical facial features. This fact is particularly true for the more mature male patient who already has developed a rather static self-image, as opposed to the more mutable self-perception of the adolescent male.[3,4] Although women can adapt easily to their newly shaped visage, men gaze into their reflected image and see an altogether foreign expression. Furthermore, the altered nose proves to be most troublesome aspect of the face for men to accept. Freudian connotations have been made of the nasal appendage mimicking a phallus and surgical correction of which is commensurate with castration. This analogy may strike the reader as grossly absurd; however, significant nasal reduction may be viewed as a form of emasculation, because the strong nasal profile is a hallmark of masculinity. Besides the aesthetic patient, the functional male rhinoplasty patient may prove equally frustrating. The classic, "engineer"-minded individual approaches the physician, often clutching in tow elaborate, self-executed diagrams that attempt to instruct the physician how best to alleviate the nasal impairment. Typically, these illustrations serve to impart little substantive information but only to underscore the fixated frame of mind that the patient is exhibiting. Most often, this type of patient has already journeyed tirelessly to find the elusive surgeon who will address his or her every complaint. The plastic surgeon always should be attentive during the preoperative phase to determine not only which patient should be operated on but more important, which one should not.

Historical Evaluation

A thorough and complete history should be taken to ascertain the patient's aesthetic and functional concerns. The details of good history taking already should be well understood by the physician. Nevertheless, a few salient points that are particular to rhinoplasty are mentioned here. The psychological motivation for aesthetic improvement has been addressed in the previous section. Apart from psychological issues, the surgeon must endeavor to determine exactly what aesthetic flaws concern the patient. The consultation process should reflect the progressive union of the patient's desires with the educated opinion of the surgeon. Aesthetic goals that may compromise nasal function should be tempered appropriately. For instance, overly narrowing the nose may not be achievable given poor elasticity or already impaired nasal airflow. A crooked nose is a very difficult entity to correct fully, and the surgeon should declare the limitations of surgical intervention to establish realistic expectations. History that should be elucidated includes prior trauma, nasal and sinus surgery (both aesthetic and functional), allergy and sinus disease, and other related systemic illnesses. The precise nature and extent of prior surgery should be delineated so that planning for the current endeavor can be maximized. Previous operative dictation can be helpful but often is misleading or vague. Therefore, an in-depth history and attentive physical examination may serve as a next best proxy for this lack of knowledge.

For functional complaints, the surgeon should probe the exact circumstances when the nasal impairment occurs or is exacerbated. If the nasal obstruction arises only temporarily, then surgical intervention may not be justified and medical therapy may be warranted instead. If allergy or other medical conditions can be ruled out, then precise localization of the nasal impairment often is uncovered during the physical examination.

Physical Examination

Nasal aesthetic and functional flaws may be most clearly ascertained with a thorough physical examination. Most of the physical examination may be completed during the initial portion of the consultation in which the patient reports the aesthetic problems that trouble him or her. Therefore, the physical examination may be integrated into the dialog with the patient and any remaining aspects of the examination that were not formally covered early on are evaluated at this point. First, the nose is inspected for symmetry and compliance with aesthetic guidelines.

Ideal nasal and facial aesthetic proportions have been reported widely. However, a brief review is included herein. The nasal length (from glabella to nasal tip) should occupy approximately one third of the total vertical height of the face. The upper one third of the face should extend from the hairline to the glabella, and the lower one third should cover the distance from the bottom of the nose to the lower aspect of the chin, or menton (Fig. 7-4A). As the patient matures, the nose elongates because of gravity and loss of elasticity so the nose comes to occupy more than one third of the vertical facial height. Similarly, the lower third of the face shortens because of the encroachment of the longer nose over the upper lip. As the male patient matures, the loss of frontal hair translates into a longer upper one third of the face. However, as the chapter on hair restoration details, the upper third of the face should not be shortened to the golden one-third distance to avoid a prepubescent appearance of the hairline. Horizontally, the nasal width should equal that of an eye, forming one fifth of the total distance across the face. The distance from the lateral canthus to the lateral aspect of the flared ear should occupy the remaining one fifth of the face (Fig. 7-4B). Aging does little to impact on the proportion of the horizontally divided face.

On profile view, nasal projection has been defined by many formulae. A simple method that has proved clinically reliable is the one described by Goode: The distance from the alar–facial groove to the nasal tip should equal to 0.55 to 0.60 of the distance from the nasion to the alar–facial groove (Fig. 7-5). Generally speaking, the male nose can tolerate a

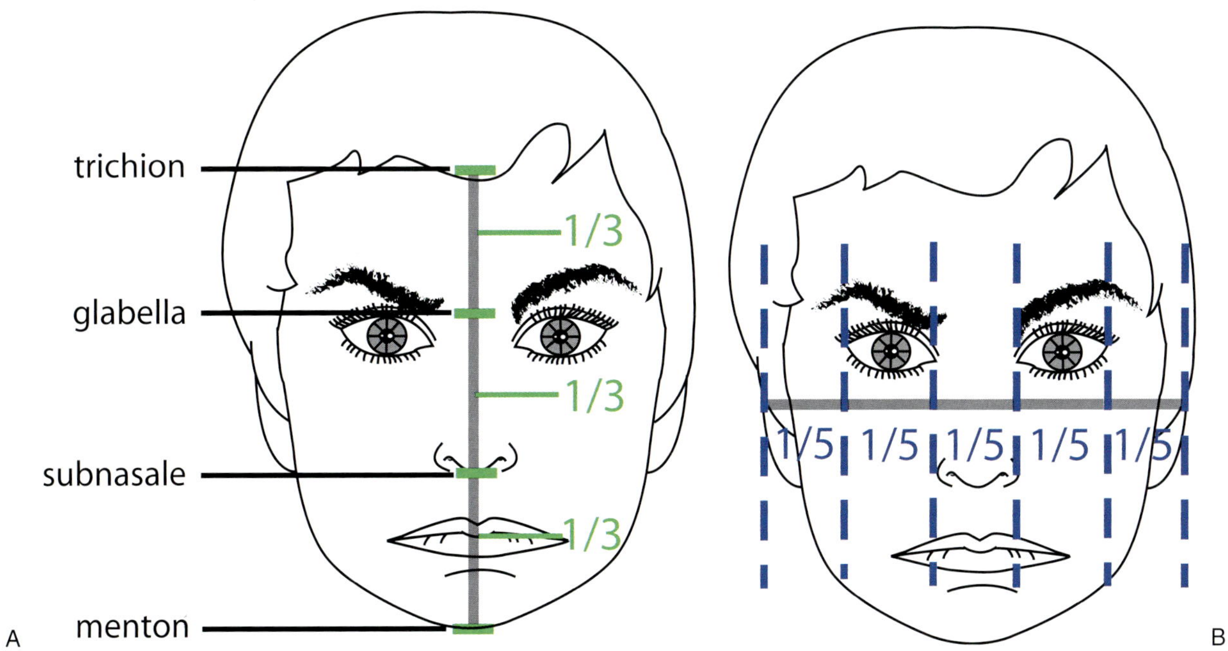

FIGURE 7-4. A: The nasal length (from glabella to nasal tip) should occupy approximately one third of the total vertical height of the face. The upper one third of the face should extend from the hairline to the glabella, and the lower one third should cover the distance from the bottom of the nose to the lower aspect of the chin, or menton. As the patient matures, the nose elongates because of gravity and loss of elasticity so that the nose comes to occupy more than one third of the vertical facial height. Similarly, the lower third of the face shortens due to the encroachment of the longer nose over the upper lip. As the male patient matures, the loss of frontal hair translates into a longer upper one third of the face. **B:** Horizontally, the nasal width should equal that of the eye, forming one fifth of the total distance across the face. The distance from the lateral canthus to the lateral aspect of the ear should occupy the remaining fifth of the face.

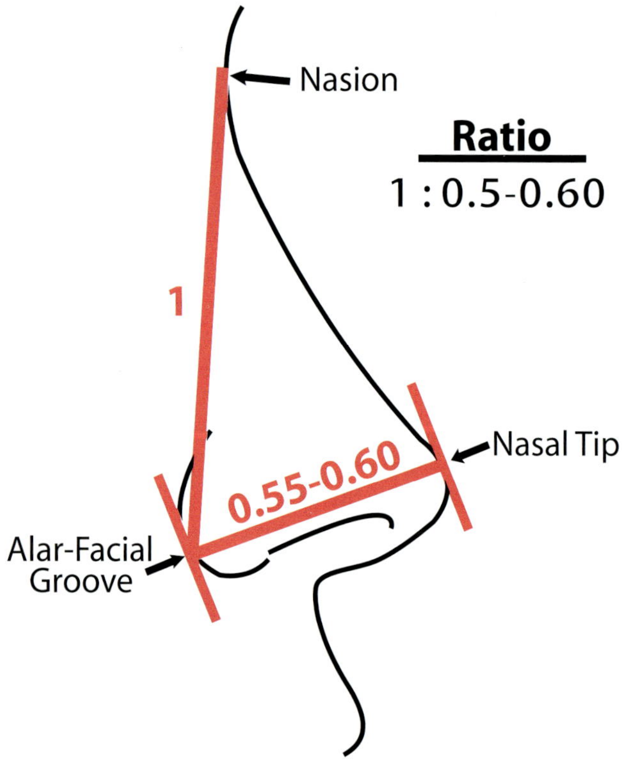

FIGURE 7-5. Nasal projection can be measured by many different formulae. The Goode method describes a simple technique to determine ideal nasal projection: The distance from the alar–facial groove to the nasal tip should equal 0.55 to 0.60 of the distance from the nasion to the alar–facial groove.

greater degree of projection than that of the female nose. The rotation of the nose defined by the columellar–labial angle should be more perpendicular for the male, approximately at 90 to 95 degrees, whereas the ideal female rotation rests between 95 to 105 degrees (Fig. 7-6A,B). As the patient matures, this angle becomes more acute, and restorative surgery should aim to return the nose to the ideal attitude. The nasofrontal angle is narrower for the male, ranging ideally between 115 to 120 degrees owing to the heavier male brow and is more open for the female, situated between 120 to 130 degrees (Fig. 7-6A,B). On profile, the male nose can tolerate a slight dorsal convexity, or hump, whereas the female nose should be relatively straight in contour. A slight supratip break, or depression, is a favorable aesthetic attribute for the female but is not so for the male. A double-break contour of the columella-lobule region is a natural and pleasing configuration that should be maintained or improved with surgery. Finally, the alar–columellar relationship should be such that a perfect oval shape of the nostril is viewed laterally with the distance from the ala to the columella approximating 1 to 2 mm (Fig. 7-7). An entire book can be dedicated to the description of ideal aesthetic values, but this brief review should serve as a basic framework with which the rhinoplasty surgeon can assess the patient's nasal features.

After the nasal anatomy has been studied visually, the surgeon should evaluate the nasal soft tissues by palpation. The nasal tip should be depressed with a finger and released to determine tip recoil (Fig. 7-8A). If the lower lateral cartilages splay easily under pressure and do not spring back to their normal configuration after release, then surgery should be tailored to reflect the weaker condition of the cartilages. For instance, significant trimming of the lower lateral cartilages should be avoided in these circumstances. The skin thickness also should be appreciated, because thin skin may expose any surgical imperfections over time and thick skin may camouflage the surgical result (Fig. 7-8B). Therefore, medium–thick skin is ideal for rhinoplasty. The length of the nasal bones should be palpated because short bones predispose toward an inverted-V deformity. This complication appears as a cutaneous, inverted-V depression between the nasal bones and upper lateral cartilages, because the middle vault collapses owing to lack of bony support after surgical manipulation. In these cases, osteotomies may need to be avoided or spreader grafts placed to buttress the upper lateral cartilages (the middle vault) against inward collapse. Any bony irregularities also should be studiously palpated and recorded.

After all of these external landmarks and structures have been adequately assessed, the surgeon should then turn his or her attention to the internal aspect of the nose. If the patient reports nasal obstruction, the surgeon should begin the nasal examination by observing the patency of the external nasal valve. Without touching the patient's nose or inserting a nasal speculum, the surgeon observes the nares in repose and in dynamic contraction during quiet respiration. At rest, the external valve already may appear to be compromised by virtue of a narrowed nostril aperture. Alternatively, the external valve may appear to collapse only with inspiration owing to weak lateral alar support. If either condition is noted, then a cotton-tipped applicator can be used to stent the nostril open to determine if this action alleviates the nasal obstruction. A finger that is positioned just lateral to the ala on the cheek skin can be used to distract the cheek laterally and thereby open the nostril. If these techniques improve symptomatic nasal airflow, then external nasal valve collapse is present. For the aging nose, the external valve may be reduced by nasal tip ptosis. Therefore, lifting the nasal tip back to a more upright position may eliminate nasal congestion that corroborates external valvular compromise. The following section describes methods to address external valvular problems.

Next, the internal nasal cavity should be inspected for signs of septal, turbinate, or internal valvular compromise. A nasal speculum can be placed to widen the nasal aperture for better visualization of the internal anatomy, and a headlight provides proper illumination. The septum should be checked for deviation, and a comparative view of both nasal cavities may render a more accurate assessment as to the presence of a septal deflection. A high septal deflection lo-

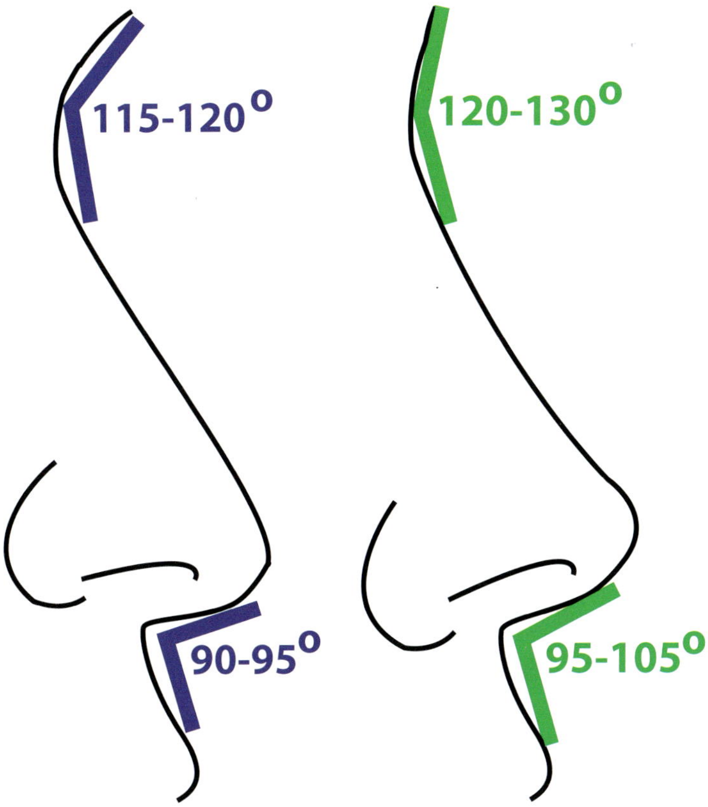

A,B

FIGURE 7-6. A: For the male, the ideal nasolabial (or columellar-labial) angle should be approximately 90 to 95 degrees; and the nasofrontal angle, 115 to 120 degrees. **B:** For the female, the ideal nasolabial (or columellar-labial) angle should be approximately 95 to 105 degrees; and the nasofrontal angle, 120 to 130 degrees.

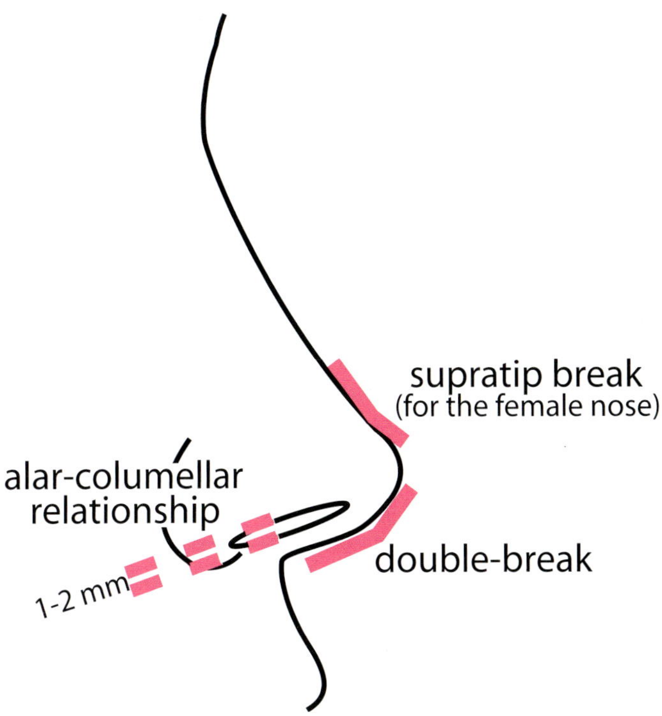

FIGURE 7-7. A slight supratip break, or depression, is a favorable aesthetic attribute for the female nose. For both sexes, a double-break contour of the columella-lobule region is a natural and pleasing configuration that should be maintained or improved with surgery. The alar–columellar relationship should be such that a perfect oval shape of the nostril is viewed laterally with the distance from the ala to the columella approximately 1 to 2 mm.

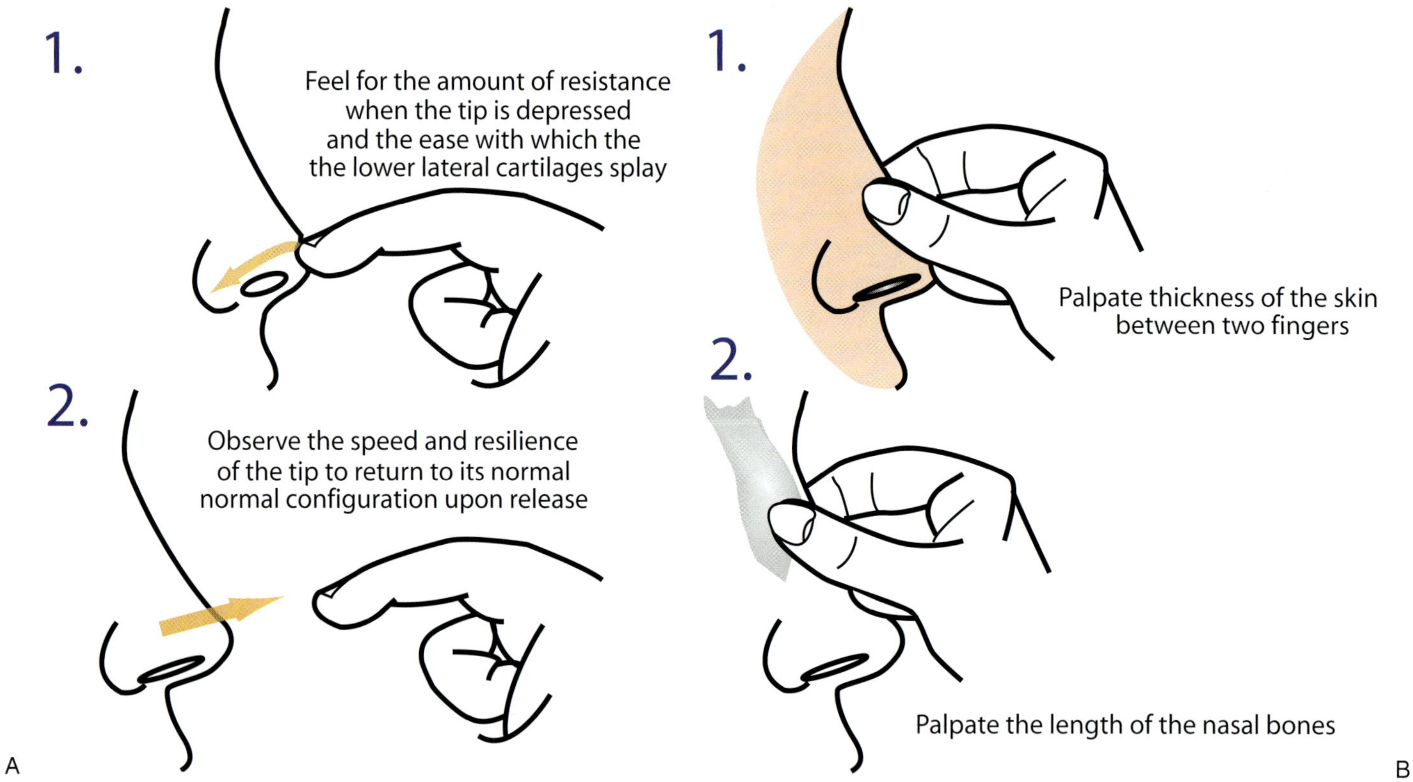

FIGURE 7-8. A: As part of the preoperative examination for aesthetic rhinoplasty, the nasal tip should be depressed and tip recoil should be assessed. **B:** The skin thickness also should be appreciated, because thin skin may expose any surgical imperfections over time and thick skin may camouflage the surgical result. Medium–thick skin remains ideal for rhinoplasty. The length of the nasal bones also should be palpated, because short bones predispose toward an inverted-V deformity.

cated at the junction of the upper lateral cartilage and septum should be carefully studied, because this narrowed passage may be related to internal valve restriction. As mentioned, the anterior head of the inferior turbinate is also a constituent element of the internal nasal valve, and enlargement of this tissue may restrict nasal airflow. Erythematous, purulent turbinates suggest a bacterial etiology for the inflammation, whereas pale to violaceous and edematous mucosa may indicate an allergic source. After anterior rhinoscopy has been concluded, the nasal speculum should be removed. Then, if internal valve collapse is entertained, a cotton-tipped applicator should be gently inserted into the nose to stent the upper lateral cartilage away from the septum. The applicator tip should be applied against the upper lateral cartilage near the septal-upper lateral cartilage junction (Fig. 7-9A). If the patient is equivocal about the improvement, then the contralateral side should be tested in a similar fashion to offer the patient a comparative perspective. Finally, the cheek should be distracted immediately lateral to the upper lateral cartilage very gently to determine if there is any improvement with this technique (Cottle maneuver) (Fig. 7-9B). This method carries value only if the finger distracts the upper lateral cartilage (at the internal nasal valve) and not the nostril (i.e., the external nasal valve.) Similarly, the external valve can be stented open with a cotton-tipped applicator, nasal speculum, or finger distraction against the cheek. The following section on surgical technique elaborates on correction of internal valvular collapse.

INTRAOPERATIVE CONSIDERATIONS: TECHNIQUE AND SALIENT TECHNICAL POINTS

Aesthetic and Functional Rhinoplasty of the Aging Nose

General Remarks

Rhinoplasty is a vast and complicated subject that would require several volumes of writing to do it justice. Although the previous section outlined a general approach to rhinoplasty, this section on intraoperative management only details the surgical maneuvers relevant to correction of the aging nose (both functional and aesthetic). The preoperative section presented broader themes in order provide the reader with a framework with which to approach rhinoplasty according to the authors' philosophy. This section remains true to the objective of this book (i.e., surgery for facial rejuvenation). If the reader requires more in-depth knowledge about rhinoplasty, he or she is referred to Eugene Tardy's masterpiece, *Rhinoplasty: The Art and the Science,*[5] or Jack Sheen's illustrious text, *Aesthetic Rhinoplasty,*[6] for

Instrumentation and Equipment

Instrumentation/Equipment for Rhinoplasty

Prep Stand:
- Nonsterile gloves
- 10-cc syringe, 27-gauge (1¼ inch long) needle with 1% lidocaine and 1:50,000 epinephrine
- Bowl with four long nasal pledgets soaked in equal parts of oxymetazoline and Pontocaine
- Nasal speculum
- Bayonet forceps
- Surgical marking pen

Instruments:
- Nasal tray that includes:
  - Takahashi forceps
  - Large Rubin elevators
  - Medium Rubin elevator
  - Unguarded 2-mm osteotome
  - Unguarded 3-mm osteotome
  - Dissection block (for graft carving)
  - Mallet
  - Medium DeBakey forceps
  - Fine, toothed forceps
  - Double-ended rasp
  - Freer elevator
  - Cottle elevator
  - Frazier suction

Sutures:
- 4-0 chromic suture, PS-4 (P-24, PR-4) <RE-4>* needle
- 5-0 chromic suture, P-3 (P-13, PRE-2) <RE-3> needle
- 7-0 polypropylene or nylon, P-1 (P-10, PRE-1) [C1] <EDR-1> (for skin closure or external incision)
- 4-0 polydioxanone, PS-3 (P-11, PRE-3) [PC-34] needle (suture for graft fixation and for suturing cartilage)

*The first needle size refers to the Ethicon code. The second parenthetical code refers to the equivalent needle size manufactured by US Surgical/Davis & Geck. Of note, the first code within the parentheses refers to newer US Surgical code, and the second number within the parentheses refers to the older Davis & Geck code. The third bracketed code refers to the equivalent needle size made by Look. The fourth code in angle braces refers to the Deknatel needle equivalent.

Other Supplies:
- 10-cc syringe, 27-gauge (1¼ inch long) needle with 1% lidocaine and 1:50,000 epinephrine
- Cotton-tipped applicators
- 4 × 4 gauze
- Bowl of saline
- Bowl of hydrogen peroxide
- No. 15c blades (3)
- Bipolar cautery
- Suction tubing

Dressing:
- Telfa (cut into two strips ¾ inch long)
- Eye pad cut into half (as a nasal tip dressing)
- ½ inch Brown Micropore tape for the dorsum
- Bacitracin ointment in 5-cc syringe
- Mayo scissors
- 4 × 4 gauze
- Benzoin adhesive
- Denver splint

Instrumentation/Equipment for Rhinophyma Resection

Prep Stand:
- Nonsterile gloves
- 27-gauge (1¼ inch long) needle with 1% lidocaine and 1:50,000 epinephrine
- Surgical marking pen
- 4 × 4 gauze

Instruments:
- No. 10 blade (3)
- Wire brush dermabrader

Other Supplies:
- CO_2 laser (or thrombin spray and monopolar electrocautery)
- 27-gauge (1¼ inch long) needle with 1% lidocaine and 1:50,000 epinephrine
- 4 × 4 gauze

Dressing:
- Bacitracin
- Xeroform gauze
- Eye pad cut into half or a 2 × 2 gauze (for nasal tip dressing)

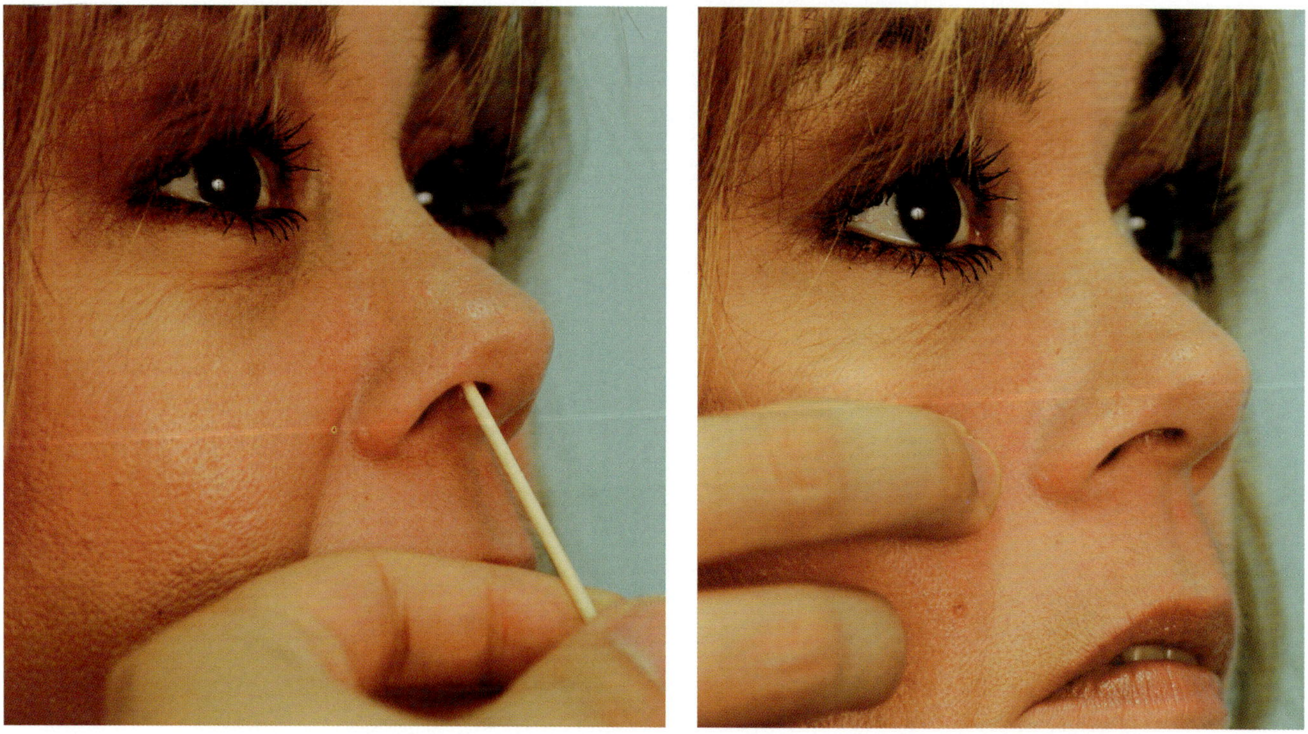

A B

FIGURE 7-9. A: To evaluate internal valve compromise, a cotton-tipped applicator should be gently inserted to distract the upper lateral cartilage away from the septum to determine whether this maneuver alleviates internal valvular collapse. **B:** Alternatively, a Cottle maneuver can be tried in which the cheek is distracted laterally to stent open the internal valve. It is important to place the finger only adjacent to the upper lateral cartilage, where the internal valve resides, and not along the nostril, where the external valve is located. (This photograph really depicts stenting the external valve.) In addition, only gentle pressure should be applied in order to avoid stenting both valves open.

greater detail. Interestingly, even texts that are dedicated to rhinoplasty often fail to include a chapter that specifically outlines a treatment strategy for the aging nose. Certainly, rhinophyma resection is considered too outré for inclusion within the subject of most rhinoplasty textbooks. This chapter hopefully adds a rational treatment strategy for the aging nose to the existing body of literature.

Surgical Maneuvers: Correction of the Ptotic Nose

Septal Angle Resection

Resection of the septal angle, or antero-inferior margin of the septum, is an effective method of elevation of an underrotated nose in the younger patient. However, this simple strategy may not work as well for the aging nose. This maneuver is predicated on the elasticity of the nose, which allows the soft tissue to retract over the resected angle—a state that may not exist in the mature nose. Septal-angle resection still may constitute a viable technique in the following two conditions. If sufficient elasticity still is noted in the nose, then septal-angle resection can be attempted *in conjunction with* other restorative maneuvers. Because the nose is ptotic usually owing to loss of elasticity, this technique often does not work alone or at all. If the septum appears to be very long and the tip resists upward transposition with digital pressure, then appropriate angle resection may be indicated in this circumstance to permit freedom of the nasal tip to ride upward.

Septal-angle resection may be undertaken through an external or endonasal approach, with the latter preferred for its simplicity and direct access. A *near* complete transfixion incision is undertaken to expose the caudal margin of the septum.** As a technical point, it is easier to incise the mucosa directly over the septal cartilage (about 1 mm cephalad to its caudal border) so that the plane of dissection can be established easily for septoplasty. Then, in order to expose the septal angle, fine curved scissors are used to retrodissect the mucosa off of the caudal border of the septum to expose the antero-inferior margin, or angle. A No. 15 blade can then be

**As clarification, a hemitransfixion incision only transects halfway or less through the mucosa caudal to the septum to expose one side of the septum. A transfixion incision is a through-and-through transection of the mucosa at the caudal border of the septum; and a near complete transfixion passes 80% to 90% through the mucosal distance to expose the entire caudal end of the septum without passing through the other side of the mucosa.

used to transect a triangular wedge off of the caudal septum with its base along the anterior border so that the nasal tip will then be transposed superiorly (Fig. 7-10A,B).

Columellar Strut

According to Anderson's tripod theory, lengthening of the central leg (the medial crura) or shortening of the lateral legs (the lateral crura) rotates the nose upward (Fig. 7-11). As the nose ages, the central tripod limb (i.e., the medial crura) loses support, and the nose rotates downward. To counterbalance the force of gravity, a columellar strut should be placed in most, if not all, cases of nasal tip ptosis, especially considering that the rhinoplasty surgery alone causes loss of tip support. Even in standard rhinoplasty cases in which nasal ptosis does not exist, the columellar strut can serve a useful function to prevent future tip ptosis. A good rule to follow is that if one thinks that a columellar strut may be beneficial, it should be placed. The ease of surgical placement justifies its role in the majority of rhinoplasty cases, and it represents the minimum surgical maneuver for the ptotic nose. A columellar strut may be used alone only if very mild tip ptosis is present (i.e., the columellar–labial angle does not exceed 20 degrees downward from the desired position and tissue integrity is not excessively flaccid). After placing and securing the columellar strut, the new columellar–labial angle should be verified and tip resilience palpated to determine whether additional steps should be carried out to raise the tip further. The nose descends approximately 10 degrees over time because of a mild loss of structural support, and slight overcorrection is warranted.

In accordance with simplicity, the endonasal approach is favored if the nose does not need to be opened for any another reason. Septal cartilage serves as a better donor material, because it is more rigid and straighter than auricular cartilage and thereby acts as a more effective buttress. However, if septal cartilage is deficient, then auricular cartilage may be used instead. In order to increase the tensile strength of conchal cartilage, the portion of cartilage should be harvested with twice the width (approximately 4 mm) and transected along its length through the entire thickness while retaining one perichondrial surface intact. The strut is then folded onto itself pedicled on the perichondrium in order to increase the rigidity of the cartilage. Prior to insertion, the folded cartilage should be secured with 5-0 chromic suture in a mattress configuration to prevent the cartilage segments from unfolding (Fig. 7-12).

A

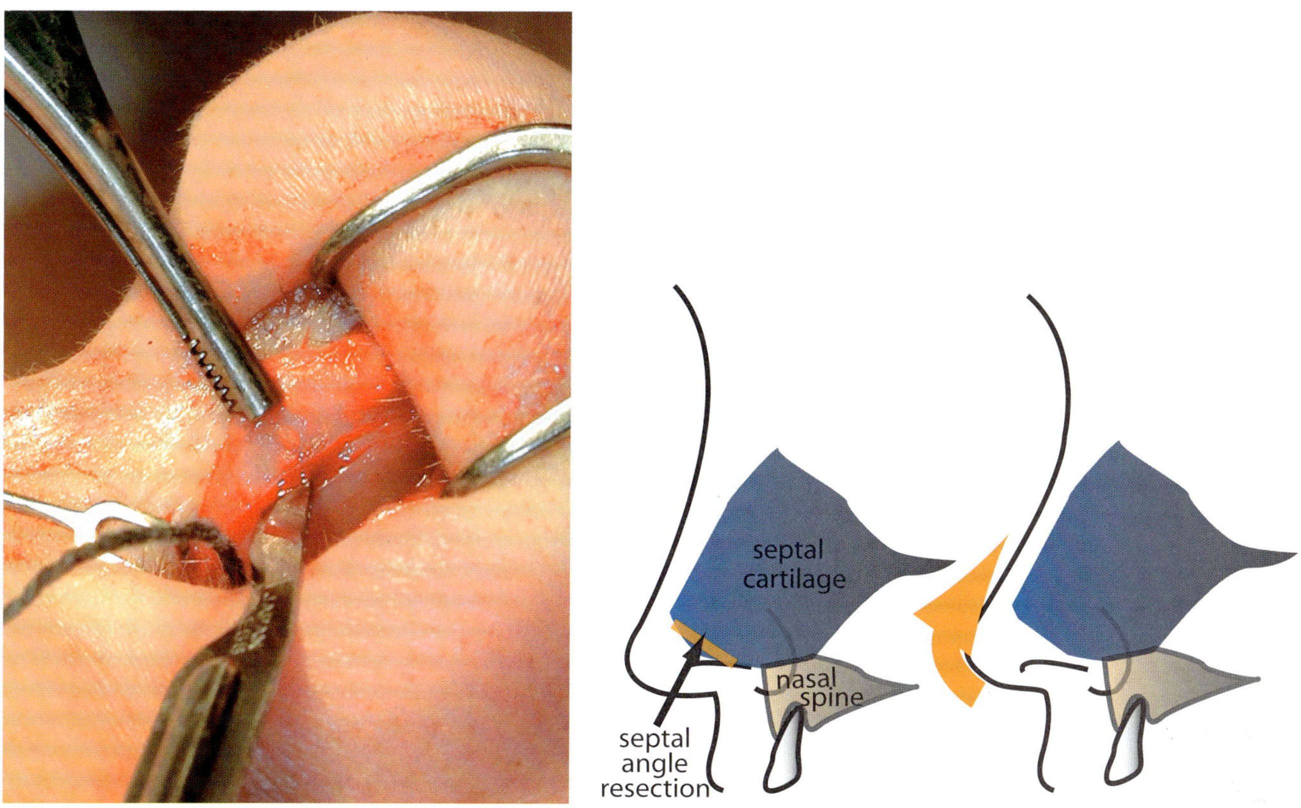

B

FIGURE 7-10. A: Septal-angle resection is generally a more ideal technique for underrotated, younger noses than for similar older noses because this maneuver is predicated on nasal tissue resilience to rotate the nose upward. (Please see text for the precise indications when this technique is suitable for the mature nose.) The photograph shows septal-angle resection through an endonasal approach in the left naris. **B:** Illustration shows the location and extent of septal angle resection with resulting tip rotation.

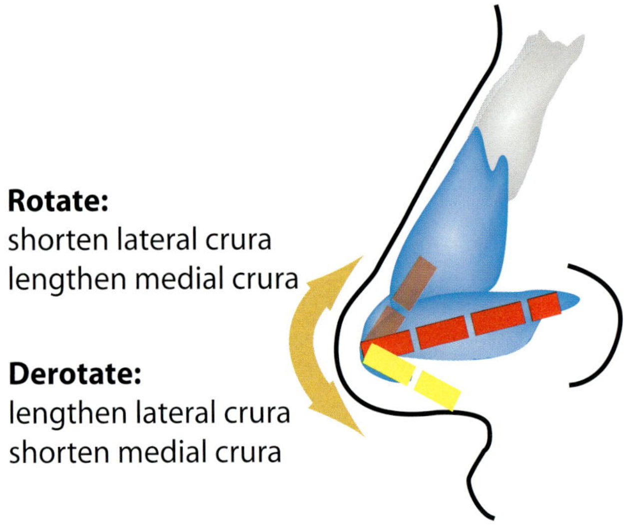

FIGURE 7-11. Anderson's tripod theory states that lengthening of the central limb (the medial crura) or shortening of the lateral limbs (the lateral crura) rotates the nose upward. The converse is also true (i.e., shortening the medial crura or lengthening the lateral crura derotates the nasal tip downward).

Via the endonasal approach, the columella should be accessed via a separate incision contralateral to that used to access the septum during septoplasty. A 3-mm vertical (i.e., running perpendicular to the orientation of a transfixion-style incision) incision is made just caudal to the caudal septal border midway between the septal angle and nasal spine. Fine curved scissors are used to dissect a pocket between the medial crura up toward the nasal tip and down toward the nasal spine. The pocket stops short of the actual nasal spine in order to avoid the strut from clicking on the bony prominence during animated expression. The columellar strut is then inserted into this pocket through the aforementioned 3-mm stab incision and secured into place via the pocket principle, because suture fixation is unnecessary (Fig. 7-13). Of note, the strut theoretically should be ensconced between the limbs of the medial crura but in actuality is typically situated slightly higher bordered by the caudal septum superiorly and the medial crura inferiorly. In the external approach, the columellar strut is placed by dissecting a pocket starting from the anterior aspect of the medial crura between the domes down toward the spine. After securing the graft in position, any excess that remains beyond the domes should be transected. As mentioned, tip position and support should be confirmed before completion of the operation.

Lateral–Crural Overlay

The lateral–crural overlay technique represents a more radical solution to nasal tip ptosis and is indicated in cases in which the nasal tip is moderately to severely ptotic. This technique relies on the principle of shortening the lateral limbs of the tripod to effect rotation of the nasal tip upward (Fig. 7-14). Although this technique can be carried out via the endonasal approach, it is not recommended, because proper visualization, ease of surgery, and accurate assessment of symmetry and height all mandate use of the external approach. The lateral–crural overlay technique can correct even the most significant downturn of the nose. Furthermore, the degree of rotation can be adjusted by overlapping the cartilaginous segments to the desired extent. This technique readily addresses the lateral limbs of the tri-

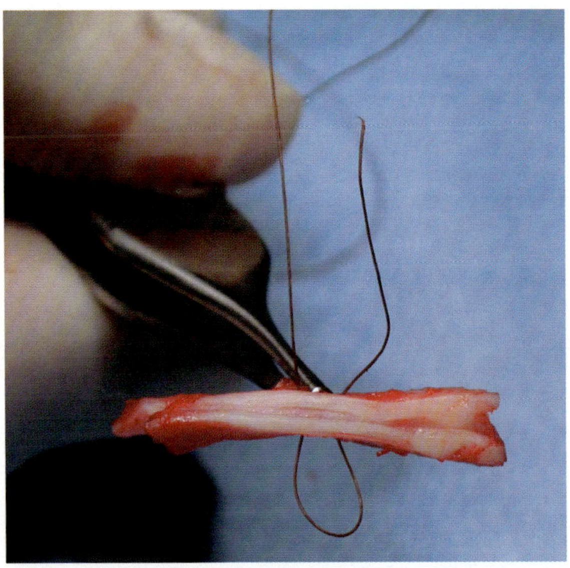

FIGURE 7-12. If auricular cartilage is used as a columellar strut, it must be folded on itself in order to increase its tensile strength before insertion (see text). A 5-0 chromic suture is used to hold the two segments together in the desired configuration.

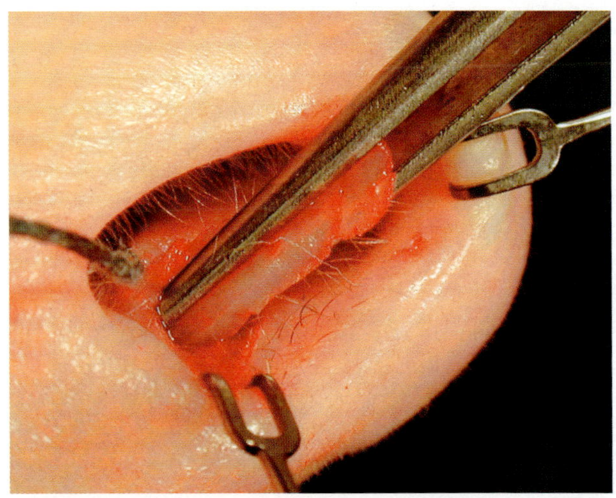

FIGURE 7-13. After dissection of a separate pocket on the contralateral side to the hemitransfixion incision, the columellar strut is inserted through the 3-mm stab incision and secured via the pocket principle. The photograph shows insertion of the columellar strut with fine-toothed forceps through the right naris.

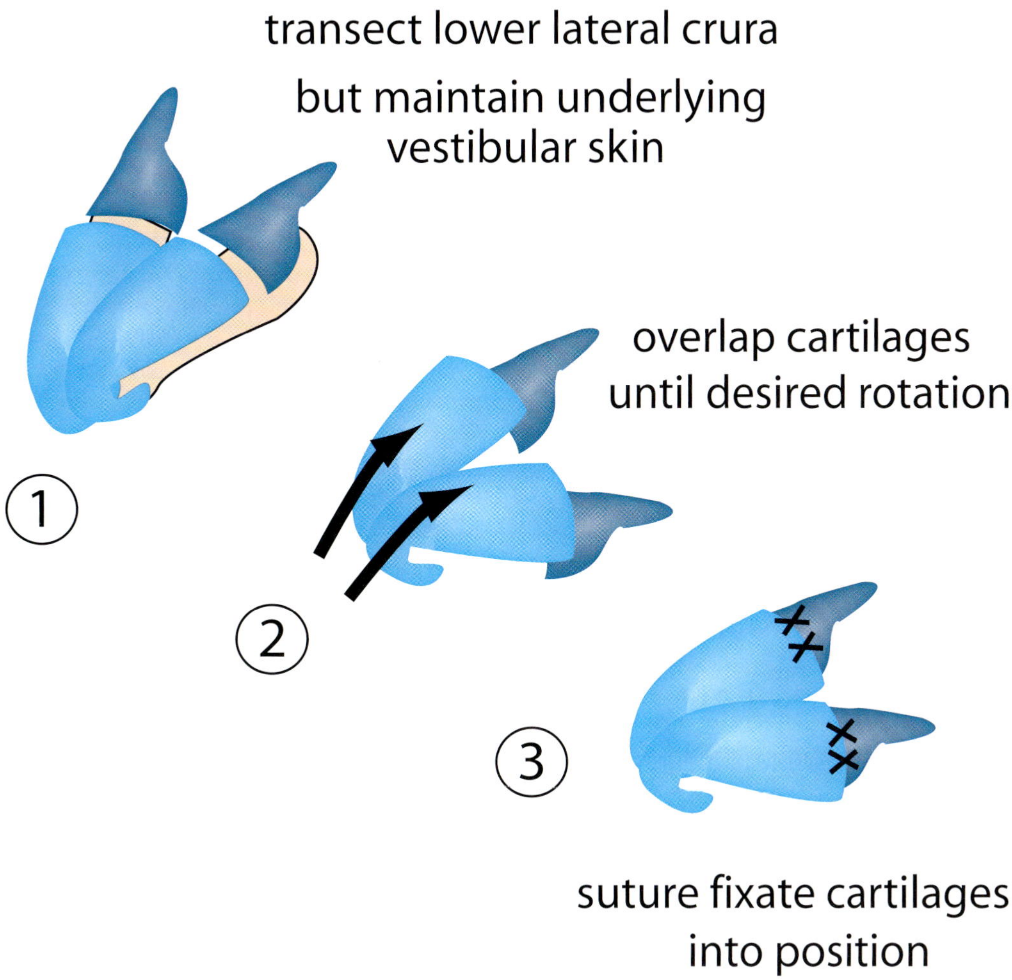

FIGURE 7-14. The lateral–crural overlay technique provides significant nasal tip rotation by shortening the lateral limbs of the tripod. The external-rhinoplasty approach is favored for technical ease and more precise visualization and adjustment. The illustration shows the overlap and suturing of the cartilaginous segments of the lateral crura: (**1**) After the lower lateral cartilages are exposed through an external-rhinoplasty incision, the cartilages are transected vertically with a No. 15 blade without disturbing the integrity of the underlying vestibular skin. To avoid injury to the vestibular skin, a pair of fine, dissecting scissors should first be used to undermine the cartilage from the vestibular skin (Fig. 7-15) and left in place as a cutting board until the cartilage has been completely transected. The cartilage should be cut closer to the pyriform aperture, but enough cartilage should be present laterally to permit overlap of the segments. (**2**) The cartilage segments should be overlapped until the desired tip rotation is evident. (**3**) Finally, the overlapped cartilage segments are sutured in place with a 5-0 polydioxanone suture. Slight overcorrection should be attempted.

pod (i.e., the lateral crura) and works effectively when combined with other ancillary surgical maneuvers that help buttress the medial, central limb (e.g., a columellar strut).

First, an inverted-V incision is marked at the midcolumellar aspect. After local anesthesia is administered, the skin and soft-tissue envelope is opened along the supraperichondrial, sub–superficial musculoaponeurotic system (SMAS) plane until the nasal tip is fully exposed.[7] Dissection should be carried out toward the pyriform aperture, because the full length of the lateral crura should be in view for lateral–crural overlay. The extent of dissection laterally may be slightly more than what is required for simple nasal tip surgery. A columellar strut may be placed at this time via the external approach and secured in place. By strengthening the central limb (the columella) and shortening the lateral limbs (the lateral crura), the nose can be rotated and maintained in that position for the greatest duration.

Sharp, angled Converse scissors should then be used to undermine several millimeters of vestibular skin away from the overlying lateral crus at approximately one third the distance from the pyriform aperture to the dome (i.e., nearer the pyriform aperture) (Fig. 7-15).† A No. 15 blade then should be used to transect the lateral crus completely in a vertical fashion without injuring the underlying vestibular skin. The medial edge of the transected lateral crus then can be brought to lie over the lateral edge and secured in place with a buried, horizontal mattress suture of 5-0 polydioxanone. As mentioned, the amount of nasal elevation desired dictates the degree of overlap. The contralateral side is approached in the same fashion. Even with marked tip ptosis, the amount of cartilage overlap should be approximately 1 to 2 mm at a maximum during the initial attempt because of the significant degree of rotation that this surgical maneuver offers.

Transcutaneous Nasal Elevation

The preceding surgical techniques serve as reliable methods to address nasal tip ptosis in the overwhelming majority of cases. However, in the recalcitrant case, a more radical option may be elected. The nose can be lifted upward via excision of a wedge of skin at the nasal root and suspended upward to the new level (Fig. 7-16). Clearly, this technique should be reserved for the patient who is more advanced in age and who desires to undergo an expedient method to correct his or her nasal ptosis. Although the blood supply to the nose emanates principally from vessels that reside lateral to the pyriform aperture, a transcolumellar incision may be safely combined with this extensive incision superiorly without jeopardy to the vascularity of the skin flap.

†The distance of one third toward the pyriform aperture is chosen for several reasons. If the point is too far lateral, there will be insufficient cartilage laterally to which the medial edge may be sutured. Also, a far lateral point does not allow enough distance for the medial edge to travel over the lateral segment. A point chosen too far medially may show the cut edges of cartilage along the midpoint of the lateral crus after translocation.

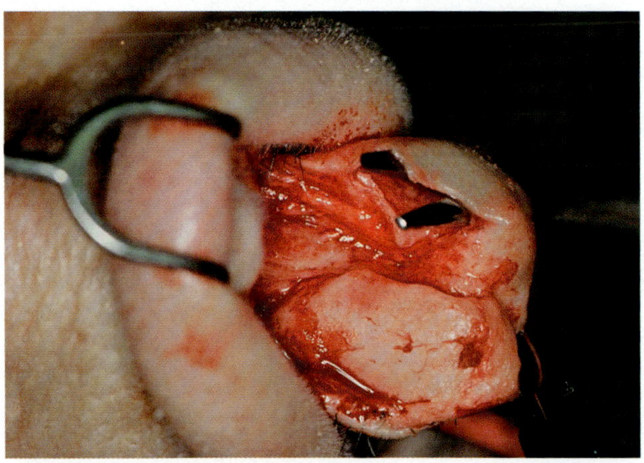

FIGURE 7-15. Photograph showing a bird's eye view of the nose with the skin envelope retracted in the standard external-rhinoplasty approach and the left lower lateral cartilage separated from the underlying vestibular skin using fine, sharp scissors as part of the lateral–crural overlay technique for nasal rotation (Fig. 7-14).

The patient should be asked to depress the brow and raise the nose in a snarl so that the deeper rhytids can be ascertained. A fusiform line that extends across the nasal root, or nasion, should be drawn that is centered over the midline and that extends just lateral to the nasal width. Forceps should be used to grasp the skin and soft tissue to determine how wide the fusiform incision should be in order to effect nasal tip elevation. Dissection is taken down to the periosteum, and the skin island is removed and discarded. Undermining should be undertaken only below the inferior wound edge to mobilize the tissues for elevation. Generally speaking, dissection is usually taken down in a sub–SMAS plane until sufficient tissue mobilization becomes apparent: Wide undermining is typically necessary to achieve this goal. 4-0 Polydioxanone is used to suspend the inferior flap through the periosteum and soft tissue of the upper flap until the desired nasal height is achieved. After the desired nasal tip position is attained, the skin is closed with a running 6-0 nylon suture. If the patient has concomitant nasal obstruction, the procedure should be carried out with minimal sedation so that the patient can report whether elevation of the tip has provided subjective nasal airflow improvement. Although a cutaneous incision in a highly conspicuous location such as the nasal dorsum may seem a rather poor decision, this incision has healed uniformly well in patients who have undergone this procedure in the authors' practices.

Surgical Maneuvers: Correction of Valvular Collapse

If the patient presents with a ptotic nasal tip, he or she may have external and possibly even internal nasal valve collapse. Accordingly, correction of the ptotic nasal tip may ameliorate or eliminate the associated nasal obstruction. If not, then the following maneuvers may need to be undertaken to address internal and external valvular collapse, respectively. Assuming knowledge of fundamental nasal surgery, basic septoplasty and turbinoplasty techniques are not reviewed. Further, scarred or deficient anatomy that results from prior trauma or surgery and that leads to valvular compromise fall outside the scope of this chapter.

Spreader Graft

A spreader graft may be placed through an external or endonasal approach (Fig. 7-17); however, the internal valve can be stented more effectively through the internal approach. As Toriumi reported, the cantilever effect on the internal valve is only achievable via an endonasal approach; therefore, this method is preferred (Fig. 7-18). The endonasal approach for spreader graft placement is easy to perform and can be done in 10 to 15 minutes with the patient under minimal sedation. By doing so, the patient can report subjective improvement immediately after graft insertion and thereby confirm success of the operation.

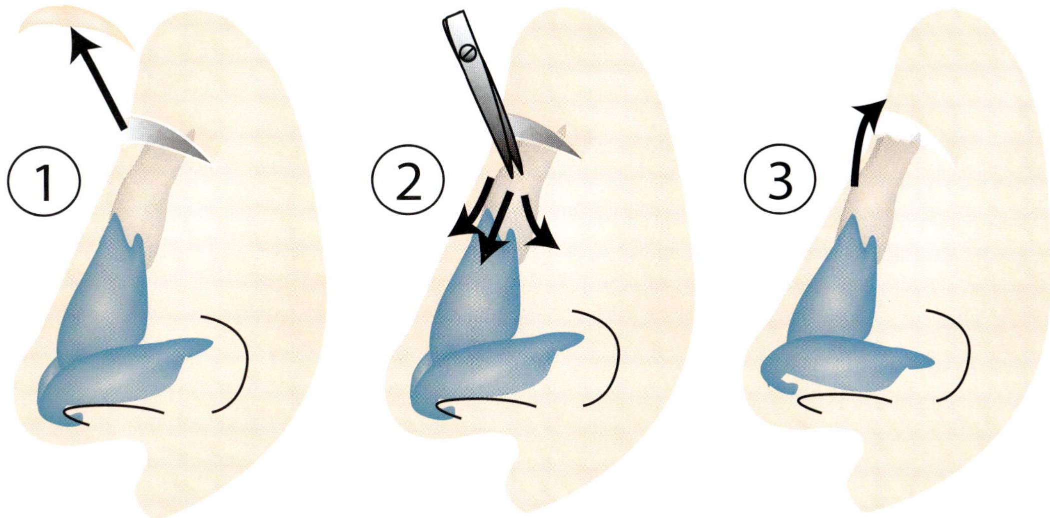

FIGURE 7-16. Illustration showing the transcutaneous nasal wedge excision for more radical nasal rotation. The lines of the fusiform excision are hidden in horizontal rhytids, and dissection is carried out in a sub–SMAS plane only under the inferior flap until sufficient tissue mobilization is achieved.

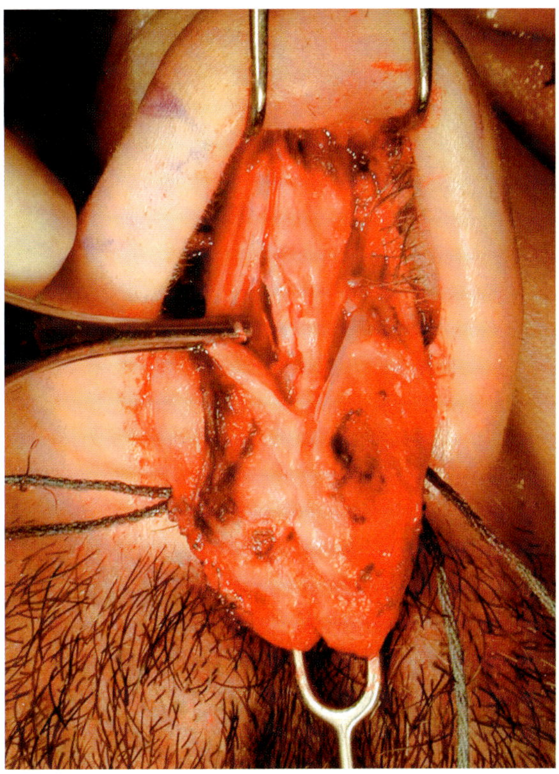

FIGURE 7-17. A photograph showing the external approach to spreader graft placement in which a septal cartilage spreader graft has been inserted between the separated upper lateral cartilage and septum. After contralateral placement of the same graft, the grafts are fixated into position using a mattress-style suture of 5-0 polydioxanone.

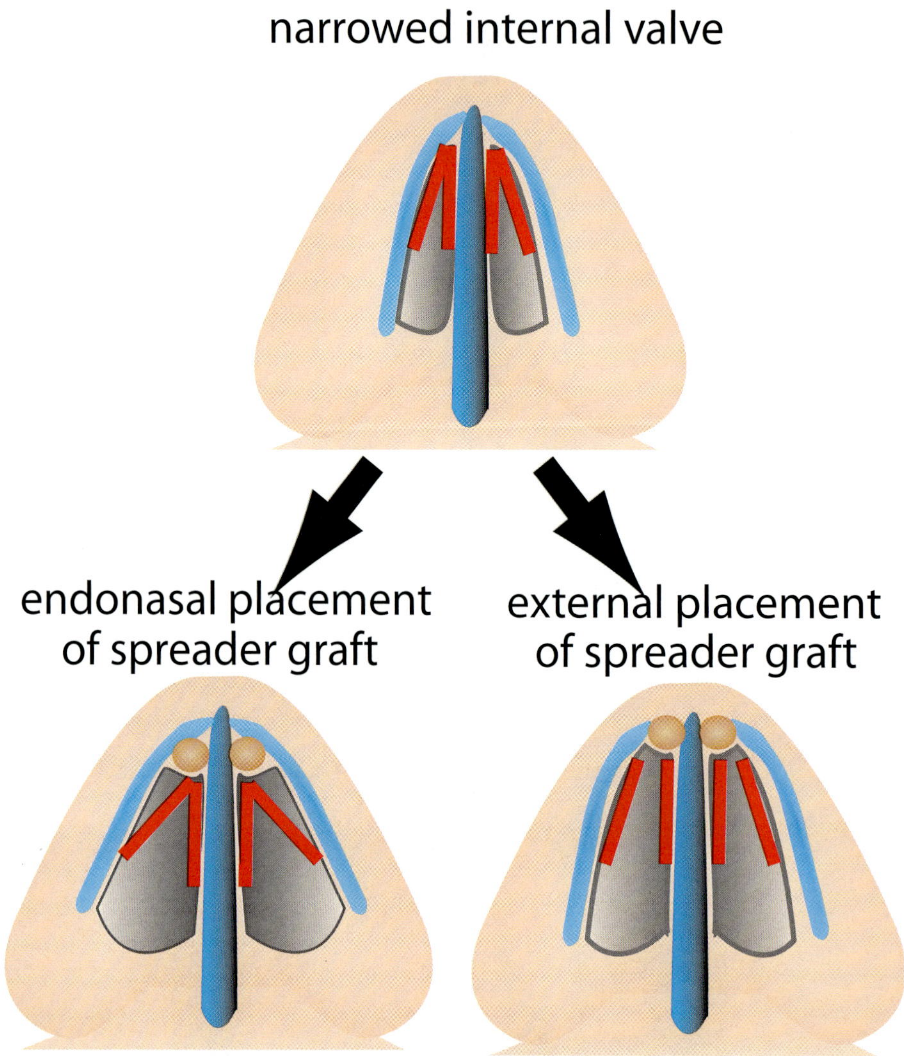

FIGURE 7-18. Illustration showing the cantilever effect on the upper lateral cartilage when a spreader graft is placed via the endonasal approach versus the simple displacement of the upper lateral cartilage when an external approach is undertaken.

After the septum has been anesthetized, a No. 15 blade is used to make a 2- to 3-mm incision along the dorsal aspect of the septum approximately 2 to 3 mm cephalad to the caudal septal border. A Freer or Cottle elevator is used to dissect a narrow subperichondrial pocket as wide as the elevator tip until the midportion of the upper lateral cartilage is reached (Fig. 7-19A). Because the pocket remains narrow and high along the septum, the elevator should be nudged forward slowly rather than swept up and down in a broad path. When the pocket has been completed, the elevator tip is pressed against the upper lateral cartilage–septal junction and pulled back forcibly along this junction to ensure that the graft will be placed as high as possible at the upper lateral cartilage–septal interface. However, the surgeon should be careful not to sever the connection between the septum and upper lateral cartilage, otherwise no cantilever effect can be obtained. By placing the graft tightly within this recess, the upper lateral cartilage can be properly cantilevered outward to open the internal valve (Fig. 7-19B). The contralateral side is carried out in the exact same method before harvesting the graft material. By creating the recipient site first, the dissected pocket will have achieved complete hemostasis by the time the graft is ready to be inserted.

If the grafting material is to be derived from the septum, then septoplasty should be performed at this time. It is imperative that the septoplasty be conducted in a separate, discrete pocket that does not communicate with the higher graft pocket described in the preceding. If the two pockets are joined by accident, then a mattress suture can be placed to fixate the graft in place. However, this is far from ideal, because the graft is less securely positioned and the task of placing a suture very high cephalically is not an easy propo-

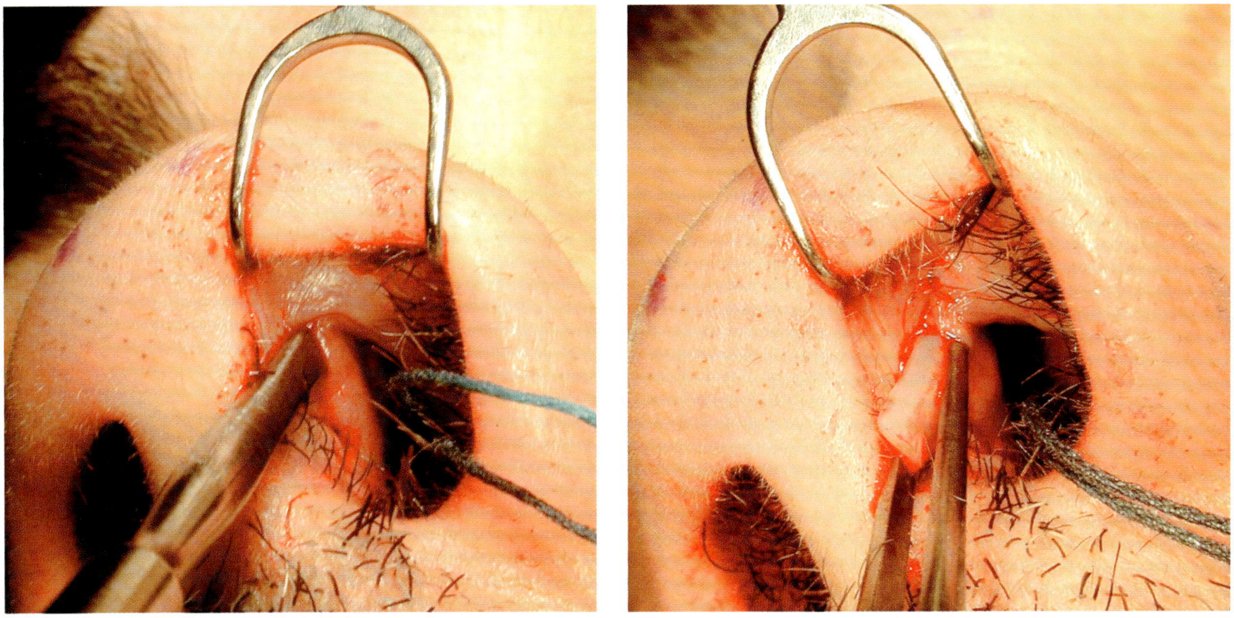

A B

FIGURE 7-19. A: The endonasal approach for spreader-graft placement is preferred due to technical ease and desired functional effect (Fig. 7-18). After a No. 15 blade is used to make a 2- to 3-mm incision along the dorsal aspect of the septum, approximately 2 to 3 mm cephalad to the caudal septal border, a Freer or Cottle elevator is used to dissect a narrow, subperichondrial pocket as wide as the elevator tip until the midportion of the upper lateral cartilage is reached. As the pocket remains narrow and high along the septum, the elevator should be nudged forward slowly rather than swept up and down in a broad path. When the pocket has been completed, the elevator tip is pressed against the upper lateral cartilage–septal junction and pulled back forcibly along this junction to ensure that the graft will be placed as high as possible at the upper lateral cartilage–septal interface. **B:** The graft is then inserted into this high, narrow pocket in order to cantilever the upper lateral cartilage outward. (Of note, if a septoplasty is undertaken for graft harvest or for functional reasons, the septoplasty pocket should not communicate with the dissected spreader graft pocket.)

sition. If the graft cannot be adequately sutured into position, then the nose may be opened to permit increased visualization and external suture fixation.

After the graft is harvested, two rectangular pieces of cartilage (one for each side of the nose) should be created that measure approximately 2 to 2.5 mm × 20 to 25 mm in size. The spreader grafts should be taken from the thickest portion of septal cartilage, which is typically situated along the posterior bony–cartilaginous junction. The thicker cartilage can more effectively stent the nasal valve open. A fine, toothed forceps can be used to insert the graft into the narrow pocket under direct visualization. Often, if the graft is placed correctly, the upper lateral cartilage can be observed to move laterally under the pressure of the spreader graft. If the patient is under lighter sedation, then he or she should be asked to comment on the nasal improvement to ascertain whether a thicker graft is needed. At times, a double layer of septal cartilage may be required if the patient still presents with nasal obstruction after graft insertion. However, it is more difficult to place a double-layered graft into the tight, cephalic pocket. After the graft is inserted, the incision can be closed with a simple mucosal suture or a through-and-through mattress to close both incisions at the same time.

Alar–Batten Graft

Like the spreader graft, the alar–batten graft can be placed via the endonasal approach, which affords the simplest and fastest method to improve external valve collapse. Also similar to internal spreader graft placement, the pocket should be created first to permit maximal hemostasis before graft insertion. An abbreviated, 4-mm incision should be made along the caudal aspect of the lower crus just lateral to the vestibular dome (Fig. 7-20). A fine pair of sharp scissors should be used to dissect a pocket over (i.e., superficial to) the lateral crus toward the pyriform aperture. The tendency is to dissect a pocket angled too superiorly. Therefore, the surgeon should make a conscientious effort to turn the wrist laterally toward the pyriform aperture. The pocket is created so that the graft will be situated partly over the lateral crus and partly over the soft tissue that lies inferiorly and that is devoid of cartilage. Further, the pocket should be dissected all the way to the pyriform aperture.

Septal or auricular cartilage should be harvested as grafting material. Although auricular cartilage reproduces the natural curvature of the lateral crus, it lacks the tensile strength needed to stent the external valve sufficiently. Therefore, septal cartilage is much preferred as an

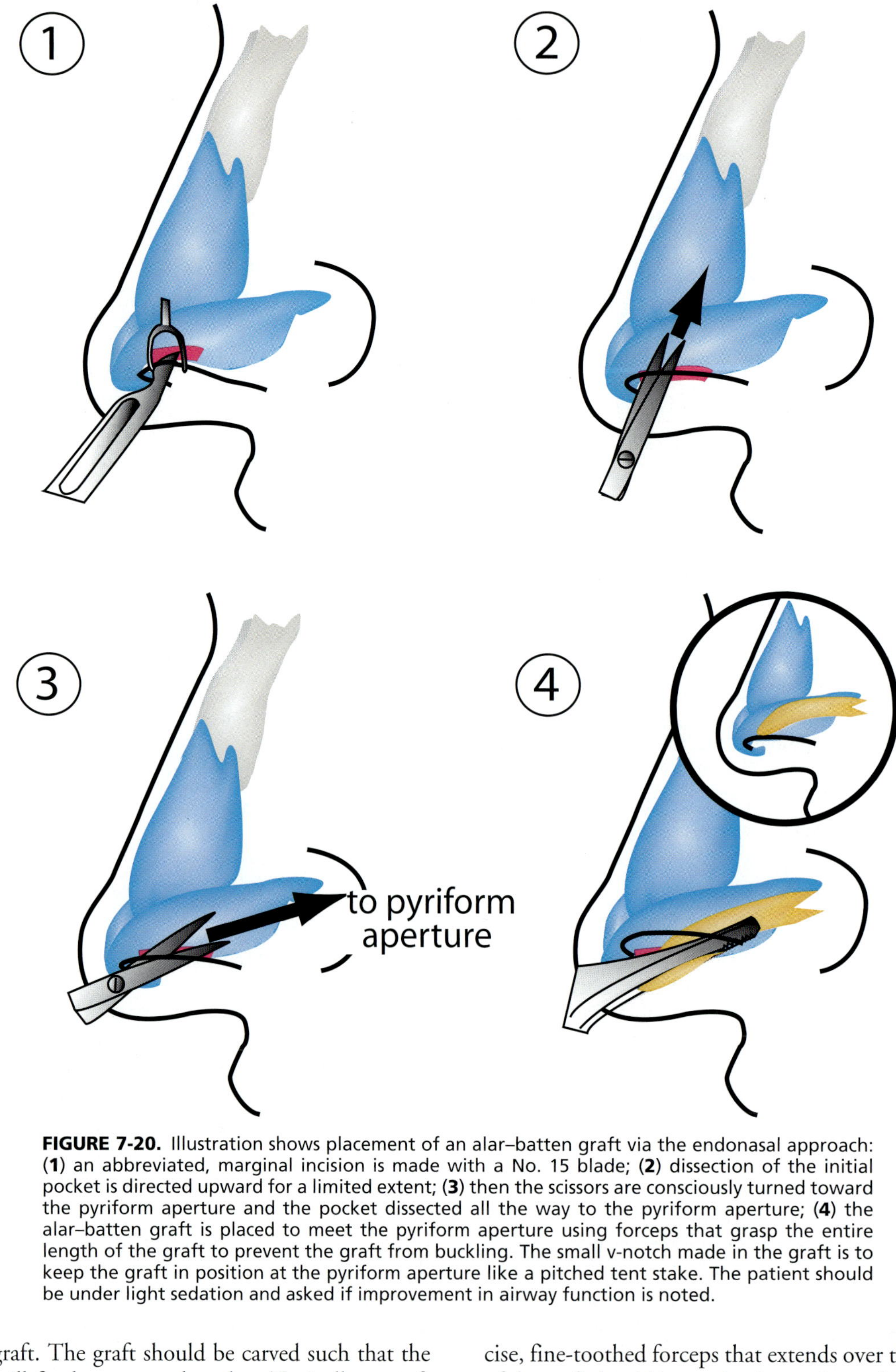

FIGURE 7-20. Illustration shows placement of an alar–batten graft via the endonasal approach: (**1**) an abbreviated, marginal incision is made with a No. 15 blade; (**2**) dissection of the initial pocket is directed upward for a limited extent; (**3**) then the scissors are consciously turned toward the pyriform aperture and the pocket dissected all the way to the pyriform aperture; (**4**) the alar–batten graft is placed to meet the pyriform aperture using forceps that grasp the entire length of the graft to prevent the graft from buckling. The small v-notch made in the graft is to keep the graft in position at the pyriform aperture like a pitched tent stake. The patient should be under light sedation and asked if improvement in airway function is noted.

alar–batten graft. The graft should be carved such that the dimensions will fit the proposed pocket. Typically, a graft size of 3 to 4 × 15 to 20 mm is acceptable. The lateral end of the graft should have a small-V wedge removed, such that the graft is firmly anchored into the soft tissue near the pyriform aperture like a tent pole. The most technically difficult aspect of this procedure is graft insertion and may require several attempts even in the most experienced hands. A precise, fine-toothed forceps that extends over the entire length of the graft should be used to insert the graft into the pocket: The forceps held in this fashion protects the graft from buckling or tearing and guides the graft properly into the pocket. It is imperative that the graft extends all the way to the pyriform aperture. If the graft falls short of this distance, it will merely contribute to the weight of the ala and exacerbate external valve collapse rather than relieve it. A graft that reaches the pyriform aperture acts like a Romanesque buttress to add rigidity and lend support to the external valve. The endonasal approach is preferred so that the patient can remain under minimal sedation and can report the improvement in nasal obstruction immediately after graft placement. The entire procedure should be relatively quick, like internal spreader graft insertion. The incision then can be closed with a single absorbable 5-0 chromic suture.

Correction of Rhinophyma

Rhinophyma is a disfiguring disease, and treatment can be a very rewarding experience for the surgeon and patient alike (Fig. 7-21). Success can be ensured if the surgeon follows a few basic guidelines. Although rhinophyma afflicts the nose, correction of this disease is more a task of dermatologic surgery than rhinoplasty. The philosophical approach in which a combination of resurfacing techniques is used is highlighted in Chapter 9. However, this chapter deals more in depth with the precise method of treatment and explains how to avert disaster if the reader subscribes to the conservative strategy outlined.

General endotracheal anesthesia is preferred for patient comfort, compliance, and airway control because this surgery can be quite hemorrhagic. However, intravenous sedation can be used without undue concern. After the patient has been properly anesthetized, 1% lidocaine with 1:50,000 epinephrine should be infiltrated endonasally along the nasal bones, nasal tip, and alae. Minimization of local anesthetic in the superficial tissue planes can obscure the intended area of resection. Therefore, transmucosal infiltration of the anesthetic prevents cutaneous tissue distortion but promote adequate hemostasis. After 10 minutes are allowed to elapse, actual surgery can safely commence.

First, a Bard-Parker No. 10 blade is used to trim the excessive tissue off the nose (Fig. 7-22). Usually, significant hemorrhage is encountered at this point. It is very important that the blade be angled parallel with the skin surface, as tangential dissection may leave large divots that may be difficult to camouflage (Fig. 7-23). In order to aid resection near the alae, a moistened 4 × 4 gauze can be opened and inserted into each nostril to absorb excessive blood and to serve as a platform for dissection. Dissection should proceed in an orderly, systematic sequence following the nasal subunits:

A 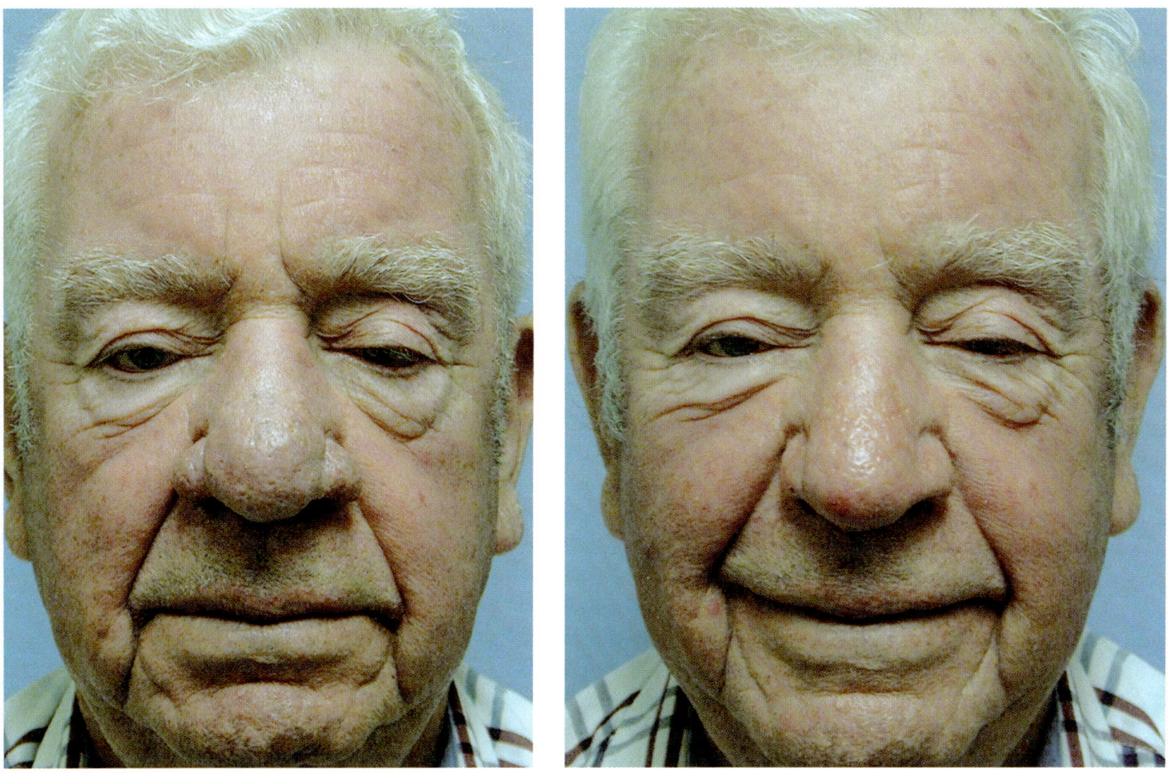 B

FIGURE 7-21. A,B: These photographs show a 76-year-old man with a moderate amount of rhinophymatous changes to his external nose. He did not complain of any symptomatic nasal obstruction from the weight or encroachment of his rhinophymatous tissue. Of note, he had failed multiple topical treatments, including topical metronidazole ointment, that were very irritating to his sensitive skin and provided little aesthetic benefit. He underwent a combined resurfacing technique using cold knife dermaplaning with a No. 10 blade for gross tissue resection followed by wire-brush dermabrasion for contour refinement, and finally CO_2 laser for hemostasis and further tissue contraction. He is shown 8 months after the surgery and is very satisfied with the cosmetic outcome.

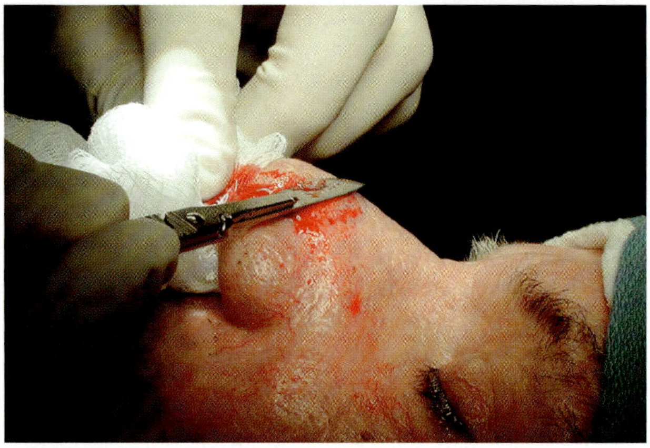

FIGURE 7-22. Rhinophyma, Step 1A. After anesthesia has been infiltrated endonasally for increased hemostasis, a No. 10 blade is used to trim the excessive tissue off of the nose. Using a No. 10 blade permits rapid debulking of tissue.

nasal dorsum, sidewalls, alae, tip, and columella. It is important that the surgeon continue symmetrically as well, so that each nasal sidewall and ala is completed in a successive fashion, verifying accurate symmetry by both visual assessment and palpation. For instance, alar thickness can be assessed by removing the gauze and pinching the ala between two fingers to determine the remaining thickness. Compared with other regions of the nose, it is imperative that the surgeon not overthin the nasal alae. The tendency toward scar contracture is much higher in the alae, as no cartilaginous support exists in their inferior aspect. The authors have corrected several cases of subsequent external valve collapse in patients who had their surgery performed elsewhere by less experienced hands. *At this point, it is worth stating a very important point about the rationale for surgical technique: The use of a cold knife technique should be the principal method by which rhinophymatous resection is undertaken. Laser or cautery techniques cause excessive thermal injury and may leave the nasal tissue atrophied, attenuated, and uneven.* Thermal injury is particularly problematic for the nasal alae, as the risk of scarification and contracture are amplified. Several No. 10 blades should be kept ready for use, because repeated tissue transection quickly dulls the edge. The end point for tissue removal can be determined by examining the nose on profile when the normal contour and height are reestablished. Clearly, some underlying dermis must be retained to provide a source for epidermal regeneration. Typically, the novice surgeon mistakes the transected sebaceous tissue as adipose and fear that he or she has gone too deep. However, sebaceous glands are more compact and whiter than adipose, and the two can be easily distinguished after some scrutiny.

Cold knife dissection offers a rapid method of reducing tissue bulk down to a favorable height and general contour. However, the remaining tissue does not appear even in nature because the tissue left in the wake of the knife blade is still crudely carved, despite the most rigorous attention. Therefore, a dermabrader must be used to refine the contour and ensure a smooth and even terrain (Fig. 7-24). However, the use of a dermabrader alone for the entire procedure without initial cold knife excision is a tedious, time-consuming, and inefficient enterprise. The reader is reminded that a portion of the nasal tissue removed with the knife should be sent for pathological review if it appears excessively irregular or exuberant in nature, because basal cell carcinoma may be present within the tissue. The preferred type of dermabrader is a wire brush rather than a diamond fraise.[‡] Fortunately, dermabrasion for rhinophyma is much

[‡]The details of dermabrasion have been elaborated in Chapter 9. However, some salient points that are particular for rhinophyma resection are reiterated herein.

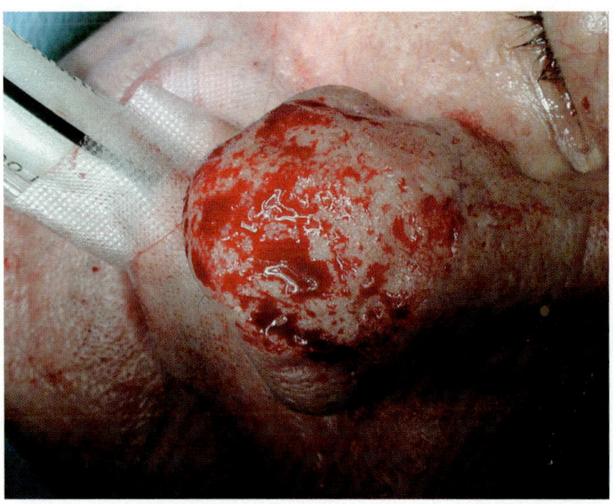

FIGURE 7-23. Rhinophyma, Step 1B. It is very important that the blade be angled parallel with the skin surface because tangential dissection may leave large divots that, in turn, may be difficult to camouflage.

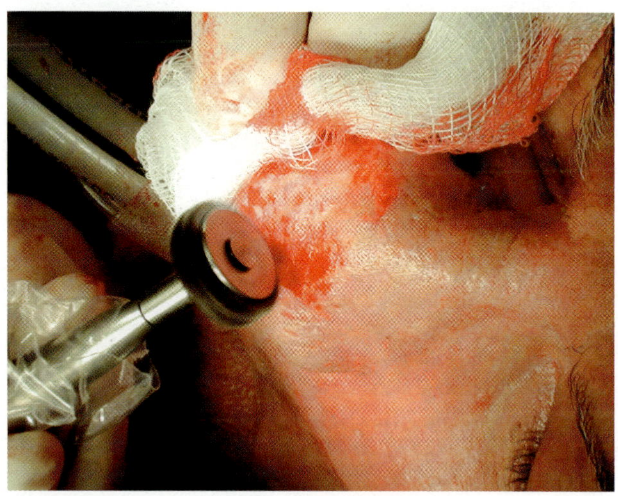

FIGURE 7-24. Rhinophyma, Step 2. After overall debulking has been achieved with the No. 10 blade, the contour is refined and made even using a wire brush dermabrader. Visual inspection and palpation will ensure that the terrain has achieved optimal smoothness.

Salient Technical Points

Correction of the Ptotic Nose

1. Septal angle resection provides limited benefit to nasal elevation in the aging nose. An incision should be made 1 to 2 mm cephalad to the caudal septal border rather than on the mucosa inferior to the septal border because determination of the septal dissection plane (for septoplasty) is much more difficult if the incision is made in the standard transfixion position. A fine pair of sharp scissors should be used to retrodissect the cartilaginous septal angle from the surrounding tissue.
2. A columellar strut should represent the minimum necessary to correct a ptotic nose and can be effectively combined with other techniques to achieve maximal nasal elevation and maintain longevity of the result. An endonasal technique is preferred for simplicity and direct access.
3. Lateral–crural overlay represents the workhorse technique to correct moderate to severe nasal tip ptosis. An external approach is advocated in order to enhance visualization and assessment and to facilitate ease of surgical dissection and suture fixation. The lateral crus should be transected approximately one third the distance from the pyriform aperture to the nasal tip, nearer to the pyriform aperture; and only 1 to 2 mm of cartilage should be overlapped for the initial attempt because significant tissue rotation occurs even with minimal tissue overlap.
4. Transcutaneous nasal elevation should be reserved for the more mature patient who desires an expedient but effective method for severe nasal tip ptosis. Although this technique may appear to stand contrary to aesthetic principles, the scar tends to heal exceptionally well and has not been a conspicuous entity in the patients who have undergone this procedure. The fusiform excision should be centered over the midnasion and dissection should be carried out only under the inferior wound edge until the nasal tip is adequately mobilized for elevation. Periosteal fixation sutures retain the nose in the desired height.

Correction of Nasal Valve Collapse

1. The spreader graft alleviates internal valve collapse and achieves the most dynamic expansion of the valvular region via the endonasal approach. The closed technique also permits a rapid and simple method for graft insertion in which the patient can report symptoms of nasal improvement when light sedation is used. The pocket should be made first before graft harvesting in order to permit time for hemostasis to be achieved. The pocket also should be created high along the dorsal aspect of the septum approximately the width of the elevator tip by nudging the elevator forward rather than a sweeping motion. And the pocket should be made as high as possible by pulling the elevator back along the upper lateral cartilage–septal junction. The thickest portion of septal cartilage located at the posterior bony–cartilaginous junction facilitates the most cantilever action of the upper lateral cartilage.
2. The alar–batten graft is intended for correction of external valve collapse. An endonasal approach is preferable for the ease and rapidity of the surgery. Septal cartilage should be used if possible in order to achieve the requisite rigidity to maintain valvular patency. Also, the cartilage must be inserted all the way to the pyriform aperture so that the cartilage provides a buttress effect rather than contributing to additional weight of the ala if it is too short. The pocket should be created in a supraperichondrial sub–SMAS plane superficial to the lateral crus, aiming the scissors laterally toward the pyriform aperture.

Correction of Rhinophyma

1. A No. 10 blade should be used to remove the large majority of the bulbous excess before wire brush dermabrasion is used to refine the nasal contour. Thermal injury is avoided by using this combined cold technique.
2. The affected nasal regions should be approached in a systematic sequence advancing from subunit to subunit and working in a symmetrical fashion. The ala should be cautiously approached so that adequate tissue is preserved to avoid unfavorable scar contracture and external valve compromise. The dermabrader always should be directed toward the alar margin to avoid ensnarement of the alar edge.
3. Careful palpation of any irregular contour should guide dermabrasion. CO_2 laser or selective cautery can be used to achieve more complete hemostasis before completion of the procedure.
4. Liberal Bacitracin ointment should be applied and continued to maintain a moist environment, and Xeroform gauze should be left in place for a 2-week period until complete reepithelialization has occurred.

more forgiving and technically less demanding than for standard cutaneous resurfacing.

A finger should be passed over the nose to determine where the irregularities reside and thereby guide dermabrasion. Often, irregularities are only palpated rather than seen because the subtle contour differences may not be appreciated by the naked eye. Again, the ala should be gently handled. As the ala represents the most freely mobile tissue, the dermabrader should be delicately used near or on the ala. The direction of the dermabrader should always be directed toward the free alar margin (i.e., superiorly to inferiorly) to avoid inadvertent ensnarement of the edge by the dermabrader wheel.

After the entire surface has been adequately dermabraded, any remaining hemorrhagic points can be effectively cauterized with a CO_2 laser. The CO_2 laser should be used sparingly to seal any major bleeding and passed lightly over the entire nasal surface to increase hemostasis and effect some mild tissue tightening. The caveat that thermal injury is an unfavorable factor for tissue healing is emphasized, and laser technology should be used only at the conclusion of the case for the stated reasons rather than as an instrument for tissue ablation. Alternatively, if a laser is unavailable, then selective cautery can be used for any major sites of bleeding (Fig. 7-25A) and thrombin adhesive can be applied liberally to enhance hemostasis further (Fig. 7-25B).

At the conclusion of the procedure, liberal application of Bacitracin ointment should be applied and continued for 2 weeks until complete epithelialization has occurred in order to maintain a moist environment that expedites epithelial regeneration. Of note, the abnormal rhinophymatous tissue requires a longer time to complete epithelialization than after skin resurfacing of normal skin areas. Therefore, the antibiotic ointment is maintained for the longer 2-week period required for completed epithelialization. Light Xeroform gauze is applied to the resurfaced areas of the nose and left intact for the first two postoperative weeks as a biologic dressing (Fig. 7-26). This covering serves to minimize bleeding and camouflage the unsightly appearance of the resurfaced nose.

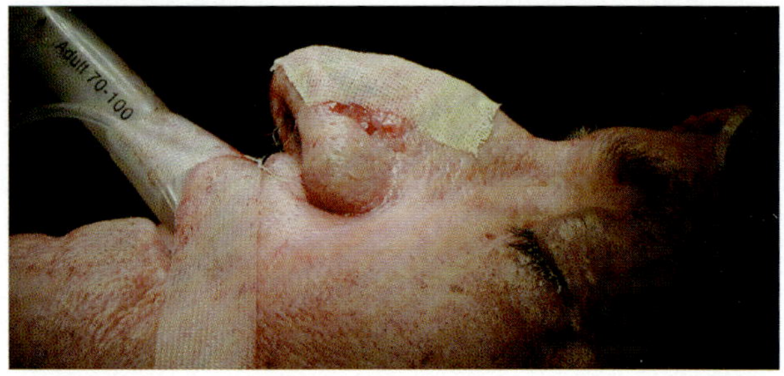

FIGURE 7-26. Rhinophyma, Step 5. Light Xeroform gauze is placed over the resurfaced areas of the nose and left intact for the first two postoperative weeks as a biologic dressing, and Bacitracin is liberally applied over the dressing during this same period. Two full weeks often are needed for complete epithelialization because the tissue is abnormal and requires a longer period of time for healing.

POSTOPERATIVE CONSIDERATIONS: CARE, FOLLOW-UP, AND COMPLICATIONS

Postoperative Care and Follow-Up

Postoperative Care for Rhinoplasty

Nasal postoperative care is straightforward, but certain subtleties should be underscored so that the most favorable result is ensured. The patient should refrain from any vigorous activity and should not bend over or place undue pressure with Valsalva maneuvers or other stressors. Unlike other surgery, ice is not applied to the nose if a nasal splint

A 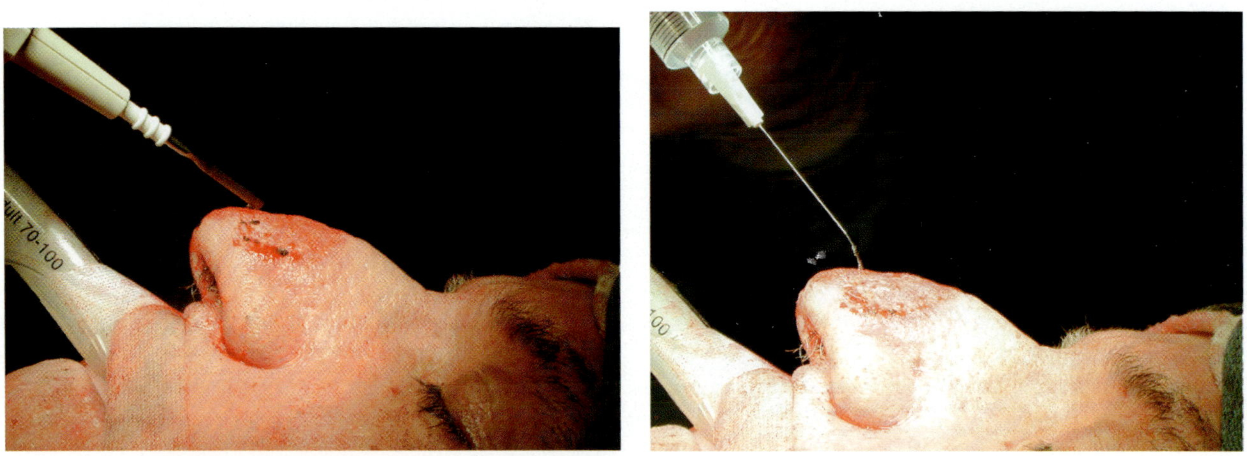 B

FIGURE 7-25. Rhinophyma, Step 3 and 4. A,B: In lieu of CO_2-laser cauterization, monopolar cautery and thrombin may be applied to achieve hemostasis at the conclusion of the case. It should be recalled that only selective application of the CO_2 laser or cautery should be used, especially along the nasal alae, because of risk of thermal injury and subsequent scarring and functional impairment.

is in place so that the precipitation from the ice pack will not loosen the nasal splint. As with all facial surgery, the patient should prop his or her head up and sleep in an inclined position to minimize collected edema. On the morning of the first postoperative day, the patient is instructed to remove the nasal Telfa tampons but to continue with nasal tip dressings until all sero-sanguinous discharge has abated. If a nasal splint or adhesive is present, then the patient should also not shower or immerse the head, otherwise both are liable to come unfastened. On the morning of the seventh postoperative day, the patient should take a steam shower to loosen or remove the nasal splint or adhesive. When the patient arrives at the surgeon's office, the nasal splint and adhesive should be easy to remove or have already fallen off. Use of 100% Acetone on a cotton-tipped applicator facilitates easy removal of the nasal dressing as well as of the colored adhesive that remains on the skin after dressing removal. Any remaining purple marks left by the surgical marking pen can be removed effectively with 100% alcohol. External incisional sutures should be removed at this time, and gentle cleaning of internal debris and clot should be performed with a cotton-tipped applicator soaked in peroxide solution.

Photographic documentation (only lateral and frontal views) should be obtained at the 1-week visit for medico-legal purposes: If the patient sustains injury to the nose thereafter, a record will be present to attest to its state in the immediate postoperative period. Photographs are taken at 1 month, 6 months, and 1 year postoperatively, and yearly thereafter. Patients should never be discharged but encouraged to return for visits. As mentioned, the surgeon should always be a diligent student of his or her work in a formal manner. Rather than a casual glance at the patient's nose, the surgeon should study the comparative preoperative and postoperative views critically on a yearly basis at a very minimum. A surgeon improves his or her skills only after careful scrutiny of all previous work. The rational, systematic approach that has been advocated in the preceding has been culled from meticulous and repeated study of postoperative results. The authors contend that indiscriminate external rhinoplasty with major structural grafting leads to unpredictable results 5 to 10 years later. Conservative rhinoplasty always should be the guiding tenet.

Postoperative Care for Rhinophyma

Unlike rhinoplasty, rhinophyma care may be less involved. Because no nasal splint is present, an ice pack may be applied to the face during the first 24 to 48 hours. As stated, the patient should maintain a diligent regimen of Bacitracin application over the Xeroform gauze to facilitate epidermal regeneration. The Xeroform gauze is retained in place for a full 2-week period unless epidermal regeneration appears to be complete and the patient is intolerant of the presence of the nasal dressing. A folded 4 × 4 gauze can be used to absorb any excessive exudate and can be particularly helpful at night to maintain the dressing in place and minimize soiling of the bed linens. After epidermal regeneration is complete, the patient should be followed for both functional and cosmetic complications. If a conservative resection of the nasal ala was performed, then the chance for cosmetic or functional deformity of the external valve is minimal. Repeated evaluation is important because acne rosacea and rhinophyma are ongoing disease processes that may worsen over time.

Complications and Management

Rhinoplasty

Perhaps a golden rule to follow is patience above all else. The unsatisfied patient is quick to temper, and the object of that frustration is the surgeon. However, the surgeon should decline revision surgery in the first 6 to 12 months after the initial procedure for several reasons. First, the surgical result that is perceived immediately afterward is camouflaged by edema and does not represent a more final outcome. Second, the patient's emotion may reflect an inner turmoil over the altered look that is disproportionate to reality. Third, surgical manipulation in the proximal postoperative period is impaired by increased edema and hemorrhage. However, with judicious discretion, the surgeon should determine select cases that meet criteria for early intervention (e.g., a grossly displaced graft or misaligned nasal bone).

Asymmetry

Preexisting asymmetry is a very difficult entity to correct completely. Asymmetric nasal bones can be straightened but may still reveal slight deviation because of a high septal deflection or inherent tissue recoil. The patient always should be informed of this likely postoperative reality so that expectations are properly adjusted. If asymmetry exists postoperatively, patience may be rewarded by resolution of the matter as edema subsides. However, intervention is warranted if asymmetry exists past the 6- to 12-month mark and the patient is still unsatisfied. Accordingly, osteotomies should be undertaken if the upper third of the nose is crooked. A spreader or onlay graft may be necessary if the middle third of the nose is askew. Onlay grafts or direct cartilage reorientation may be needed to correct the problem if the lower third is deviated. The three cornerstones—planning, simplicity, and flexibility—should be recalled even in revision surgery.

Nasal Hump

The reemergence of nasal convexity may be caused by return of nasal tip ptosis. Alternatively, dorsal convexity may have arisen because of imperfect nasal osteotomies. In this case, small imperfections can be corrected with a nasal rasp technique via a unilateral intercartilaginous incision in the office setting. Nasal adhesive and a splint should be applied for 1 week to control postoperative edema.

Nasal Ptosis

Nasal ptosis may arise postsurgically because of surgical violation of tip-supporting mechanisms or natural loss of tissue turgor that follows further aging. A small degree of ptosis (less than 10 degrees) is expected as a postsurgical sequela. As mentioned, a columellar strut should be placed as a minimum step to prevent postoperative ptosis. If significant dissection was undertaken, the strut often only counteracts the destructive surgical maneuvers rather than increase preoperative nasal tip support. At the conclusion of the procedure, the surgeon should ensure that all incisions are properly closed, even mucosal, so that nasal integrity is restored and thereby tip support strengthened.

If nasal tip ptosis returns, then the surgeon faces the same strategy that was encountered prior to the first surgery. The nasal tip integrity should be assessed through assiduous inspection and palpation, and the angle of underrotation should be determined. Based on the same criteria, the surgeon can proceed to address the ptotic nose in a systematic, graduated fashion.

Nasal Obstruction

After ruling out medical conditions that may be causing obstruction (e.g., rhinitis, sinusitis, nasal polyposis, etc.), the surgeon can investigate any mechanical aspect that may be affecting nasal airflow. If nasal ptosis has returned, then nasal obstruction may be attributed to this condition and alleviated by lifting the nasal tip to a more perpendicular attitude. Internal and external valvular collapse should be carefully examined in the prescribed method outlined in the preceding. Valvular compromise may result from a weakened postsurgical architecture. Septal deflection should have been addressed during the primary rhinoplasty procedure and is a difficult task in the secondary setting. As mentioned, high deflections may be more safely addressed with internal spreader grafts. Lower nasal vault obstruction may be exacerbated by turbinate hypertrophy, and a targeted resection of the anterior head of the inferior turbinate may be undertaken to ameliorate this problem. Synechiae or frank strictures may be the most dreaded complication that leads to airflow obstruction, and treatment of this condition may not be a straightforward matter. Lysis of synechiae, adjuvant steroid injection, and Silastic splinting may be effective and may require repeated intervention. Further details regarding reconstructive options lie beyond the scope of this text.

Rhinophyma

Aesthetic Compromise

Generally speaking, any improvement of the deformed nasal exterior that accompanies rhinophyma is welcome. Underresection can be more easily corrected than overresec-

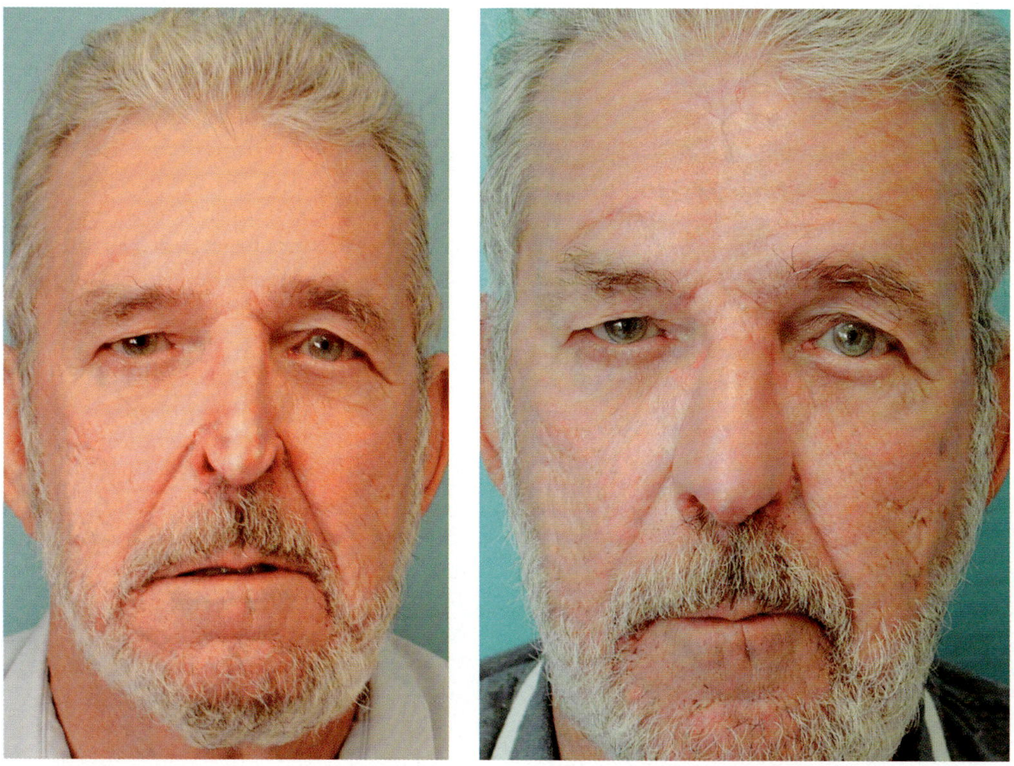

A B

FIGURE 7-27. A,B: This patient presented to the clinic after having undergone overaggressive thermal cauterization for his rhinophyma at another institution, leaving him nasally crippled, both functionally and aesthetically. Staged reconstruction of his nose using a paramedian forehead flap and auricular composite grafts provided limited improvement of his aesthetic and functional condition.

tion, the former requiring only an additional surgical procedure. Unfortunately, overresection may be a difficult condition to correct, especially if significant thermal injury has been imparted to the nasal tissue. Scarring, atrophy, and alar retraction are the hallmarks of overaggressive resection (Fig. 7-27). The authors have even undertaken a paramedian forehead flap and auricular composite grafts to restore the nasal appearance after radical surgery that was done elsewhere left a patient nasally crippled. The results were only of limited success because of the patient's poor vascular status.

Functional Compromise

The most common type of functional compromise that occurs after rhinophyma resection is external valve collapse. As stated, a weakened ala is the principal culprit that can lead to valvular problems. If conservative alar resection is undertaken, then this complication should not arise. The endonasal approach has served as an expedient method to correct external valve compromise after rhinophyma resection in several cases. The authors have not required more aggressive treatment for this complication. Internal valve compromise has not been encountered following rhinophyma resection. These functional impairments have only been witnessed in patients who have undergone overzealous resection by less experienced hands.

CLINICAL PRESENTATIONS: A SYNTHESIS OF APPROACH

Case #1 (Fig. 7-28A,B)

This is a 75-year-old affable restaurant worker who was dissatisfied with the way that his nose appeared and also complained of nasal obstruction. Over the past 10 years, he has noted progressive nasal tip ptosis to the point where his nose has almost reached his upper lip. He also stated that over this same period, he experienced difficulty breathing easily through his nose. On physical examination, the patient was noted to have significant nasal tip ptosis and thick, sebaceous skin. When the patient's nasal tip was manually elevated, he stated that he could breathe more freely through his nose. With the nose tip held up to normal elevation, the nostril rim

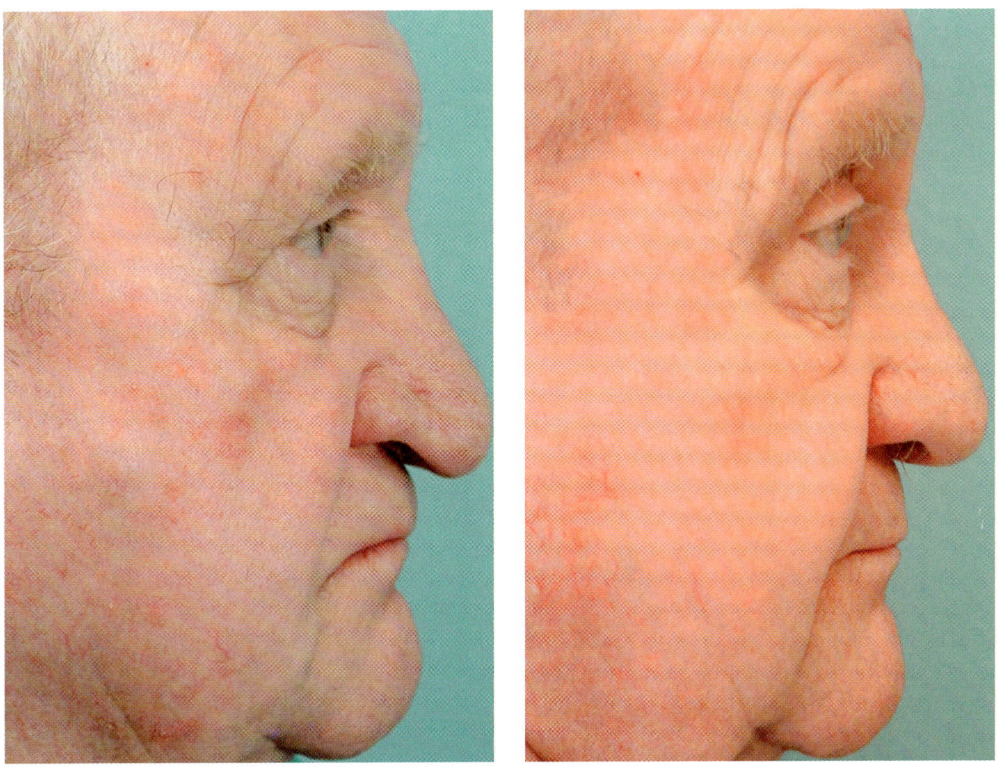

FIGURE 7-28. A,B: These photographs show a 75-year-old man who exhibits both functional and aesthetic nasal compromise because of descent of his aging nasal tip to the point that it almost rests on his upper lip. The patient's nasal airway improved with manual elevation of his nasal tip to a normal position and was further improved by stenting open his right internal nasal valve owing to a high, right-sided, septal deflection. The patient underwent a right-sided spreader graft via an endonasal approach, and a columellar strut and lateral–crural overlay via the external approach. The patient is shown 6 months after surgery with favorable return of his nasal tip to a more youthful position. He also was very satisfied by the improved nasal airflow after surgery.

was evaluated for any evidence of dynamic collapse, which was not evident. On intranasal speculum examination, the patient was noted to have a high septal deflection to the right side but normal caliber inferior turbinates and normal mucosa. With a cotton-tipped applicator inserted into the nose to distract the caudal border of the upper lateral cartilage laterally, the patient noted improved air passage only on the right side. The patient was informed that surgical intervention would be directed toward both aesthetic improvement as well as functional restoration using various surgical maneuvers that are elaborated in the following.

Procedure

The procedure is a bilateral lateral–crural overlay through an external-rhinoplasty technique, columellar strut, and right-sided unilateral endonasally placed spreader graft.

The patient had a septoplasty performed under general anesthesia in order to harvest appropriate grafting material. The septum appeared to be relatively straight other than the high septal deflection. Of note, the septoplasty was not undertaken to correct any deviation, as a high deflection could not be corrected simply by removing septum, which would risk dorsal collapse. Although an external approach to the nose was used to facilitate accurate and easy execution of the lateral–crural overlay, the patient still underwent an endonasal spreader-graft placement in order to maximize functional airway improvement. During septoplasty, attention was paid to maintain a high pocket for the spreader graft that would be separate from that of the principal septal dissection pocket. The spreader graft fashioned from the harvested septum was inserted endonasally while observing displacement of the upper lateral cartilage. Of note, patients who only require an internal spreader graft (or alar–batten graft for that matter) should be under light sedation so that they can report nasal airway improvement at the time of the operation to ensure that the procedure is successful. Next, a transcolumellar incision was made to elevate the soft-tissue envelope in the standard sub–SMAS plane of dissection until the lower lateral cartilages were fully exposed. After the vestibular skin was separated from the overlying lower lateral cartilage, the lateral crus was divided bilaterally, and the amount of overlap estimated by the observed nasal tip rotation. In order to achieve the desired rotation, only 3 mm of lateral–crural overlap was required. After suture fixation, a columellar strut was fashioned and inserted into a pocket through the standard external approach.

Discussion

As patients mature, both functional and aesthetic nasal compromise can arise simultaneously. This patient was concerned as much about his appearance as he was about the functional airway impairment. He exhibited both external and internal valve collapse that contributed to his overall nasal airway obstruction. The high septal deflection that caused his internal valve collapse was most likely present all of his life. However, symptomatic nasal obstruction did not arise until the nasal tip ptosis brought about collapse of his external valve, or nares. The patient underwent a combination of endonasal and external approaches to rectify his breathing problem and external appearance in order to achieve a maximal result. For significant nasal tip ptosis, the lateral–crural overlay technique serves as a workhorse to return the nose to a normal attitude even in the most extreme cases. Excision of dorsal skin is a radical solution that generally is unnecessary, albeit well camouflaged. Finally, a columellar strut is an important and simple adjunct to many rhinoplasty endeavors, as most operative steps undermine integrity of the nasal support. The general rule that if one thinks of placing a columellar strut that one should do so is always advisable.

Case #2 (Fig. 7-29A–D)

This is a 78-year-old retired man who sought aesthetic improvement of his nose. He had never undertaken or even considered other cosmetic surgical intervention in the past but has led a relatively cloistered life over the past decade because of the embarrassment that his nasal appearance has caused him. He stated that whenever he went out in public people inevitably gawked at his deformed, irregular, and prominent nose, which had been ravaged by rhinophymatous changes. He denied any related symptomatic nasal obstruction. Of note, the patient exhibited severe photo damage with numerous actinic–keratotic lesions scattered across his face, but denied any prior history of skin cancer. He also denied any recent changes to the appearance of his nose or other skin lesions, particularly evidence of bleeding, increase in diameter, or change in color.

Procedure

The procedure used was combined resurfacing technique of his external nose using cold knife excision, wire-brush dermabrasion, and thrombin mixture application for hemostasis. Tissue specimens were sent for pathologic review, with one section that returned confirmatory for basal cell carcinoma.

Discussion

Rhinophyma can be a disfiguring disease, and this unsightly entity may cross the boundary between cosmetic and reconstructive surgery. Many different techniques have been advocated for rhinophyma resection, including laser or cautery excision. These particular modalities have won popularity because of their expediency and excellent hemostasis. Nevertheless, hot knife dissection of any kind risks thermal

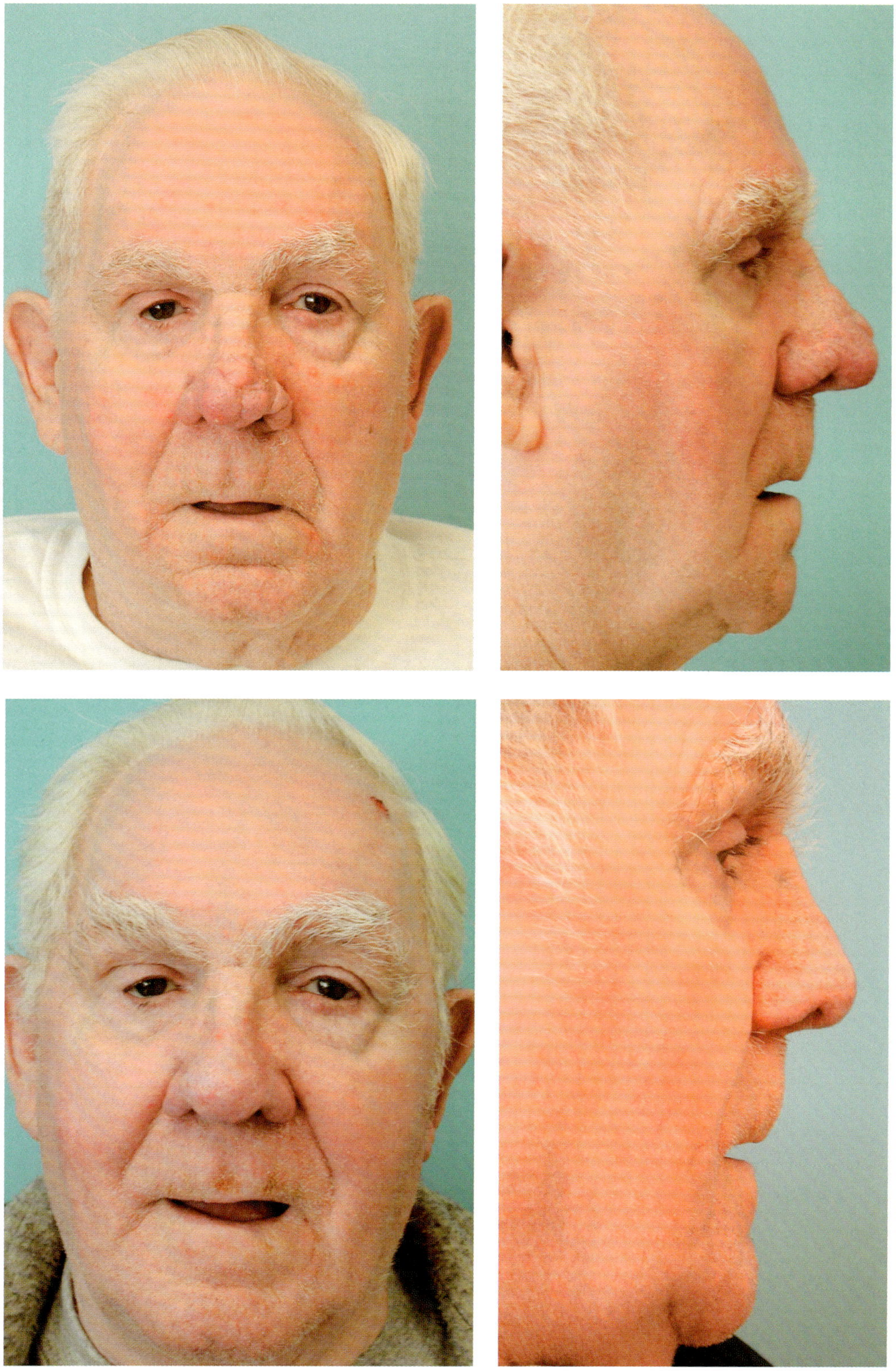

A B C D

FIGURE 7-29. A–D: These photographs show a 78-year-old retired man who presents with disfiguring rhinophyma that has worsened over the past decade, leaving him socially crippled. He underwent a combined resurfacing technique that involved gross resection of abnormal nasal tissue using a No. 10 blade, followed by wire-brush dermabrasion for contour refinement, and conservative cauterization with monopolar cautery and thrombin spray for maximal hemostasis. Abnormal tissue sent for pathological review revealed the presence of basal cell carcinoma in one specimen. The patient is shown 10 months following surgery with notable aesthetic improvement.

injury that can lead to uncontrolled scarring. Because significant hemorrhage accompanies cold knife dissection, the surgeon may be dissuaded easily from this technique but should remain steadfast because of the ultimate benefit that this modality affords the patient. Details of the technique can be reviewed in the appropriate section of this chapter. However, it is worth reiterating that only conservative tissue resection should be undertaken in the alar subunits to avoid subsequent alar retraction and external valve collapse even when only cold knife dissection is used. Finally, the presence of occult skin cancer may be masked by the surrounding exuberant tissue but should be suspected in areas that have grown disproportionately large relative to other portions of the nose. All suspicious areas should be sent for routine pathologic review to ensure that a cutaneous malignancy is not overlooked.

REFERENCES

1. Lam SM, Williams EF: Anatomic considerations in aesthetic rhinoplasty. Facial Plast Surg 2002;18:209–214.
2. Williams EF, Lam SM: A systematic, graduated approach to rhinoplasty. Facial Plast Surg 2002;18:215–222.
3. McGrath MH, Mukerji S: Plastic surgery and the teenage patient. J Pediatr Adolesc Gynecol 2000;13:105–118.
4. Tardy ME Jr: Rhinoplasty in midlife. Otolaryngol Clin North Am 1980;13:289–303.
5. Tardy ME Jr: Rhinoplasty: the art and the science. Philadelphia: WB Saunders, 1997.
6. Sheen JH, Sheen AP: Aesthetic rhinoplasty, 2nd ed. St. Louis: Quality Medical Publishing, 1997.
7. Toriumi DM, Mueller RA, Grosch T, et al: Vascular anatomy of the nose and the external-rhinoplasty approach. Arch Otolaryngol Head Neck Surg 1996;122:24–34.

8

ADJUNCTIVE PROCEDURES FOR REJUVENATION

SAMUEL M. LAM
EDWIN F. WILLIAMS III

Rejuvenative surgery for the face has undergone nothing short of a revolution this past decade, from minimally invasive brow techniques to diverse approaches to the midface. The trend in surgical technique has been toward less invasive strategies that facilitate faster recovery. As part of this Zeitgeist, adjunctive procedures have risen to the forefront in the rejuvenative armamentarium to respond to the demand for quick fixes. Younger patients, who do not require extensive surgical intervention, are seeking prophylactic treatments (e.g., botulinum toxin) and minor improvements with soft-tissue injectables and solid fillers. Adjunctive therapies work equally well in more mature patients as part of a global strategy for rejuvenation. Technological triumphs have kept pace with public demand, and a myriad array of soft-tissue replacement products are under investigation or have entered the market.

Unfortunately, no ideal treatment material or method exists today; that is, biocompatible, natural, permanent, and yet removable. This quandary is the crux of the problem. An alloplast must be stable and well integrated for perpetuity, yet be pliable and natural to palpation and examination, and be easily removable in the event of rejection or infection. Solid fillers may have a firm texture that is intolerable to some patients and may have a higher extrusion or infection rate. Injectable agents may achieve a more natural feel but should be temporary in nature so that they will disappear should infection or other deleterious outcome manifest. Permanent injectables (e.g., Artecoll, Bioplastique, and Dermalive) not currently approved in the United States, have been reported to engender granulomatous reaction several years after implantation and may be only partially extracted with mutilating surgical excision.[1–3] Appropriately chosen materials and properly performed procedures ensure patient satisfaction and optimal aesthetic benefit.

PREOPERATIVE CONSIDERATIONS: PATIENT SELECTION AND RELEVANT ANATOMY

Perhaps the first order of business for any patient who presents to the facial plastic surgeon for consultation is what that patient desires corrected. Besides the aesthetic deficit that the patient perceives, the surgeon usually should promptly establish whether the patient intends to undergo larger flap-type surgery or envisions only a more limited "adjunctive" procedure with less recovery time. Astute attention to the patient's inclination toward less or more surgery facilitates good rapport and ensures a mutual strategy for success. A patient's demeanor and comments may serve as invaluable clues to the surgeon as to the patient's true intentions and objectives. Furthermore, the patient may express hesitation as to whether a certain "look" would be ultimately attractive for him or her and request a temporary measure that can approximate a permanent solution. For instance, botulinum toxin (BTX) may act as a useful agent to demonstrate to the patient the benefit of a potential browlift in the future. Alternatively, collagen may act as a reliable indicator as to how the nasolabial fold would appear with a permanent solid filler (e.g., expanded polytetrafluoroethylene [ePTFE] or acellular dermis). The age of the patient also guides the surgeon as to what recommendations to make: A younger patient may not require or desire invasive surgical intervention, making a limited surgical or dermatological procedure more appropriate.

This section on preoperative considerations is divided according to particular zones of the face that would benefit from an adjunctive-type procedure (e.g., the glabellar frown lines; the lateral–canthal crow's feet; the nasolabial smile lines and marionette labiomandibular lines; thin, hypoplastic lips; and perioral rhagades). By classifying anatomic deficiencies in this manner, the surgeon can evaluate a particular patient complaint and work through the exercise of the modality that is most applicable in a certain situation. The following section on intraoperative considerations elaborates on each method of rejuvenation in a detailed and stepwise fashion.

Generally, a reasonable treatment strategy for adjunctive procedures divides the face into two vertical portions with an imaginary horizontal line drawn through the bottom of the nose (Fig. 8-1). Botulinum toxin therapy is particularly well suited for early wrinkles present in animation above this line, but may be less appropriate for wrinkles below this line.

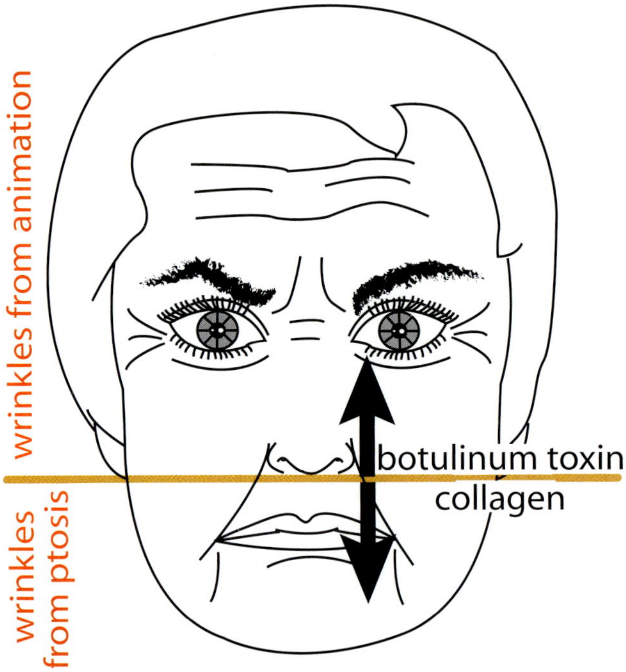

FIGURE 8-1. Illustration shows the benefit of adjunctive procedures based on an imaginary line drawn through the nasal base. Wrinkles above this line are typically attributed to animation, whereas below this line, wrinkles develop principally because of tissue descent. Accordingly, botulinum toxin (BTX) is well suited to address incipient or early wrinkles above this horizontal line; and collagen is preferable to augment the ptotic tissues. Although BTX has been successfully used below this line, and collagen above this line, the authors believe that the risk outweighs the benefits. (Refer to the text for further details.)

Perioral BTX therapy for an overactive depressor offers limited benefit with the attendant risk of oral incompetence. However, soft-tissue augmentation is effective below this horizontal line but less so above it. A fundamental difference in wrinkle quality above versus below this line explains the authors' rationale for this strategy. Wrinkle lines that form above this line are generally etched-in lines from repeated motion and benefit from either BTX therapy early (incipient lines) or resurfacing later (mature lines). Deeper glabellar lines also may be appropriately excised if very advanced. Solid or liquid soft-tissue augmentation in the periocular region cannot readily and evenly efface the fine etched-in lines in this region. Although the glabella tolerates this type of augmentation, liquid fillers are contraindicated because of skin necrosis and retrograde thrombosis and blindness;[4] and solid augmentation may not be the best modality to treat this area. (Consider either resurfacing or excision as better alternatives.) Nevertheless, solid soft-tissue augmentation has been successful for those patients willing to tolerate some palpability in this area.

Below this horizontal axis, the lines that develop usually do so because of gravitational ptosis (e.g., the nasolabial and labiomandibular folds). These folds, rather than wrinkles, are more amenable to soft-tissue augmentation with either liquid or solid fillers rather than BTX therapy. The one exception to this rule is the perioral rhagades, or smoker's lines. These fine crevices around the mouth are more akin to the fine lines that circumscribe the eye. Therefore, solid or liquid augmentation of these lines is not very effective. Unlike the periocular rhytids, however, the perioral rhagades are not as amenable to BTX (which may be an apparent caveat) but should be treated with laser ablation or dermabrasion. Hypoplastic lips, on the other hand, may be appropriately treated with soft-tissue augmentation materials like the other areas described below this horizontal axis.

Glabellar Frown Lines

As a review of basic anatomy, the vertical rhytidosis that forms in the glabellar region may be attributed to the overactivity of the horizontally aligned corrugator supercilii musculature. The horizontal rhytids, usually situated somewhat lower, arise from repeated motion of the procerus muscle. These furrows that form may either be present at rest and in motion or only in motion: This consideration largely determines which intervention is most suitable for a particular patient. The deep glabellar lines engender two aesthetically unattractive features: (a) glabellar creases themselves connote to the observer a sign of aging; and (b) deeper furrows may impart the impression of an angry, worried, or tired visage that may belie the patient's true emotional disposition.

The medial–brow complex is a recalcitrant area to brow-suspension surgery (Chapter 4). Meticulous dissection of the medial–brow complex during brow surgery can lead to many undesirable complications (e.g., uneven contour deformity, return of function, inability to reduce established glabellar rhytidosis, and worse yet frank cutaneous necrosis). For all these reasons, the medial–brow region is more amenable to localized adjunctive therapy.

Younger patients with rhytidosis limited only to animation or those who have incipient rhytidosis are best treated with BTX. Unfortunately, this procedure is only temporary and can be expensive with repeated treatment sessions. However, BTX injection is the best and only therapy that is recommended for early rhytidosis.

With glabellar rhytidosis that is present both at rest and in motion, more aggressive therapy may be warranted. Early, incipient rhytids may be treated with BTX as a first step to see whether the formed line will soften over time owing to muscle inactivity. Alternatively, if the patient has other dyschromias or signs of photodamage, a Jessner's/35% trichloroacetic acid (TCA) peel may efface limited rhytidosis (Chapter 9).

More severe rhytidosis requires carbon dioxide laser ablation in this area. As discussed in Chapter 9, full-face laser therapy may be followed by a protracted recovery time that is insufferable to many patients. Therefore, a chemical peel may be done elsewhere on the face with a targeted laser ablation of the glabella to achieve a more uniform resurfacing if more global photodamage would cause treatment with laser alone in the glabella to appear discontinuous with the adjacent unresurfaced skin. Other temporary soft-tissue augmentation materials (e.g., collagen) have been associated with skin necrosis and retrograde retinal thrombosis and consequent blindness and are contraindicated in the glabella.

Besides laser ablation for deeper wrinkles, solid soft-tissue fillers (e.g., ePTFE or acellular dermis) may provide benefit for the patient and be well tolerated in the thicker glabellar skin. However, as with all solid fillers, the patient must understand the limitations of such augmentation (e.g., palpability, possible mobility and migration, potential visibility, and some risk of extrusion and infection). Given these limitations, a well-established and proven method of rejuvenation of the glabella is direct excision of the rhytid, attenuation of the underlying muscle, reconstruction with a geometric broken-line repair, and possible delayed dermabrasion. (See the following section for a detailed description.) Surgical excision of the rhytid should be reserved only for corrugator-derived vertical rhytids and not the procerus-related horizontal rhytids. The latter rhytids tend to be shallower in depth and do not tolerate this type of surgical technique. Albeit ostensibly aggressive, this technique has stood the test of time and proved valuable in the surgical armamentarium. However, this modality is not necessarily appropriate in other facial areas; for example, excision of the nasolabial fold appears uniformly poor and is not recommended, as the scar ineluctably widens with repeated movement.

Lateral–Canthal Crow's Feet

Similar to glabellar frown lines, the presence of lateral–canthal crow's feet should be classified as lines present at rest and motion versus motion only. The latter condition is amenable to BTX therapy to abort the development of the former problem (i.e., so that the animated lines do not become permanently etched-in lines). Botulinum toxin must be continued indefinitely to ensure that the development of more permanent rhytids do not arise. The notion that the muscles become progressively more attenuated and eventually do not require BTX is a fallacy that has been proved with histological evidence. Nevertheless, patients often report that they "unlearn" certain behaviors that caused the wrinkles in the first place after many months and years of muscular inactivity, thus perpetuating the longevity of BTX.

Another preventative measure that can abort incipient lines and minimize the development of further rhytidosis is the newer technique of nonablative therapy (Chapter 9). Various laser and light devices have been used for nonablative therapy, including the pulsed-dye laser, the Q-switched 1064-nm Nd:YAG laser, 980-nm diode laser, 1320-nm Nd:YAG laser, Erbium:Glass laser, Erbium:YAG laser, and intense pulsed light. Nonablative therapy, which has no discernible downtime (no ecchymosis, erythema, or edema if the parameters are properly adjusted), works by stimulating the underlying dermal collagen that can in turn even out the overlying epidermis. However, nonablative therapy only effectively treats fine and early periocular wrinkles and has limited benefit for deeper, perioral rhagades. The patient in his or her thirties who is a good candidate for BTX therapy may be equally well suited for nonablative laser therapy, which can be combined with BTX treatment. The results after a 3- to 6-month period can be outstanding if a patient understands the limitations of this technology.

More established, etched-in lines should be treated instead with an ablative resurfacing modality. Other than actual redundant skin that requires a blepharoplasty, the surgeon should be attentive to fine lower and lateral eyelid wrinkles that should be addressed with a chosen resurfacing technique. Excising skin when only rhytidosis is present can lead to vertical shortening of the lower lid and malpositioning. Fine wrinkles can be treated quite effectively with a Jessner's/35% TCA peel, whereas deeper wrinkles may benefit from CO_2-laser ablation (if the patient is willing to accept the longer recovery period).

The Nasolabial Smile Lines and the Labiomandibular Marionette Lines

As mentioned, the nasolabial and labiomandibular folds are poorly treated with BTX therapy, because these lines represent actual ptosis of tissue rather than wrinkles in animation. Instead, these lines can be augmented with a soft-tissue filler, whether a temporary liquid injectable or a more permanent solid material, to soften these ptotic folds. The patient should be fully cognizant of the limitations in completely effacing these lines and understand that limited improvement is the goal and not the exception. In addition, the patient should realize that a liquid filler (e.g., collagen) is only temporary and that a permanent filler (e.g., ePTFE) may at times be both palpable and visible and may risk extrusion and infection. Furthermore, if this anatomic area is the primary focus of grievance, then the patient should understand that a facelift, whether deep plane or superficial musculoaponeurotic system (SMAS), will do little to improve this line and may actually worsen it on occasion.

If the patient is willing to accept these limitations, then the surgeon can reasonably discuss the possible types of favorable treatment options. Although hyaluronic acid (Restylane) has shown promising aesthetic benefit and longevity abroad, this liquid injectable material has not yet been approved for use in the United States. Although hyaluronic acid should be free of antigenicity (i.e., no skin test is required), the major adverse reaction that has been reported worldwide, albeit on a small scale, is hypersensitivity (0.06% to 0.15%).[5–7] At this time, bovine collagen remains a mainstay of temporary liquid augmentation. The authors have the greatest experience with Zyplast, which has greater longevity than Zyderm, and is favored by the authors as the only type of collagen for lower facial rejuvenation. As mentioned, the authors do not support the use of collagen, or equivalent augmentation material, in the upper face or periorbital region. Therefore, Zyplast has served well as the only type of collagen needed. Other liquid implants (e.g., Cymetra, Dermalogen, Isologen) can be expensive or temporary and have not been reliably used in the authors' experience. As a practical matter, stocking only one liquid injectable eases the burden of inventory and reduces confusion for the patient and surgeon alike.

If the patient elects to have a permanent soft-tissue filler, then ePTFE may be the most suitable option. Expanded polytetrafluoroethylene comes in many brands, each touting a theoretic advantage based on porosity and pliability. However, in the authors' experience with these different implants, these considerations remain squarely within the realm of theory and carry very little practical import. As mentioned, the limitations that concern this type of implant are palpability (particularly when smiling or during extreme animation of the lower face), and possible visibility, migration, extrusion, and infection. These latter three complications are relatively rare and can be managed by simple excision and removal of the implant if need be. Women tend to tolerate the issue of palpability much better than men, as is generally true for most cosmetic endeavors.

Alternatively, acellular dermis may prove to be a favorable compromise between a permanent substance such as ePTFE and a temporary liquid injectable such as collagen. Although touted as permanent, the authors have found that acellular dermis is semipermanent to permanent, depending on the patient's biophysiologic ability to degrade the foreign material. The benefit of acellular dermis is that usually the substance lasts considerably longer than collagen and is not as palpable (if at all) compared with Gore-Tex (W.L. Gore and Associates, Inc., Flagstaff, AZ) or another type of ePTFE. However, the degree of augmentation may be somewhat less than what may be achievable with ePTFE. The patient should be educated as to the derivation of acellular dermis (e.g., processed cadaveric dermis) and should understand the rigorous screening and mechanical process through which the materials have been subjected. Based on these advantages and drawbacks, the surgeon and patient can then arrive at a mutually agreed on, suitable modality.

Although not truly applicable in this chapter dedicated to "adjunctive" therapies, the nasolabial and labiomandibular folds also may be softened with SMAS excised during an SMAS-imbrication rhytidectomy. If the patient consents for this treatment option, he or she may have the best of all possibilities: an autogenous, pliable material that should not be readily palpable and have an enduring quality. In addition, the risk of extrusion and infection is almost unheard of given the autogenous nature of the implant. The implant also does not cost any extra in terms of harvesting time, donor-site morbidity, or purchase cost. Therefore, the perfect candidate for this procedure is the individual who is undergoing a concurrent rhytidectomy and who exhibits notable marionette, or labiomandibular, folds.

Perioral Rhagades or Smoker's Lines

Perioral rhagades, or smoker's lines, are best treated with a resurfacing modality (Chapter 9). However, treatment of this pathology is mentioned again in this chapter for sake of completeness and to caution the reader about the use of soft-tissue augmentation or BTX to address this entity. These deeply etched lines can be effectively treated only with laser therapy or dermabrasion and attain limited improvement with a TCA peel. Phenol, which is not covered in this book, is a viable alternative. Soft-tissue augmentation with collagen, equivalent filler, or solid implant does very little to address these wrinkles and is not advisable.

Thin, Hypoplastic Lips

Full, pouty lips are an emblem of sensuality, and thin, attenuated lips signify aging and reduced sexual allure. Many young women who are born with congenitally thin lips seek to amplify their lip volume even at a relatively tender age. More mature women suffer from a longer white lip, reduced vermilion height, and less pronounced Cupid's bow. Treatment of hypoplastic lips may be divided into two principal strategies: soft-tissue augmentation and advancement cheiloplasty.

As described, soft-tissue augmentation may be effected with either temporary liquid injectables (e.g., collagen) or more permanent materials (e.g., acellular dermis or ePTFE). The patient must weigh the benefits and drawbacks (already explained) to decide what is most appropriate for that individual. However, the authors emphasize that Gore-Tex, or any kind of ePTFE, may not be the most suitable choice for lip augmentation. Unlike the nasolabial fold, the lip is subjected to much more movement and is more proximal to the contaminated oral cavity. For these two reasons, the incidence of infection with lip augmentation tends to be much higher than with nasolabial-fold augmentation, especially with ePTFE. However, acellular dermis has been noted to be much less prone to extrusion and infection and less palpable than ePTFE. Therefore, acellular dermis may be a reasonable alternative for semipermanent to permanent lip augmentation. These conclusions have been arrived at after many years of trial and error and represent empiric observation rather than a controlled study protocol.

Advancement cheiloplasty, or lip advancement, should be discouraged, because it often creates an unnatural result, particularly in the younger patient who requires little additional augmentation. Even in the best surgical hands, the risk of an unnatural outcome may be significant. This treatment modality should be reserved for women who are more advanced in age and fully comprehend the limitations of this technique. Even more important, these ladies must be willing to wear lipstick as a camouflaging agent on a routine basis. If the patient does not meet these selective, exclusion factors, then the surgeon should resist the temptation to operate.

INTRAOPERATIVE CONSIDERATIONS: TECHNIQUE AND SALIENT TECHNICAL POINTS

DVD Permanent and Semipermanent Rejuvenation

Expanded Polytetrafluoroethylene Acellular Dermis (Nasolabial Fold, Labiomandibular Fold)

Besides the preparation of acellular dermis or harvesting of SMAS, the actual procedure of insertion for acellular dermis, ePTFE, or SMAS are identical and discussed herein as one procedure (Fig. 8-2). Acellular dermis, ePTFE, and SMAS tissue are henceforth referred to collectively as the implant. This procedure can be undertaken with local anesthesia alone (1% lidocaine with 1:100,000 epinephrine) or some Versed sedation depending on the patient's disposition and temperament. Clearly, SMAS insertion implies a full rhytidectomy has been performed concurrently, and the reader is directed to Chapter 5 for further details concerning SMAS harvesting and implantation during rhytidectomy. For details of acellular–dermal preparation, the reader is referred to the following section that describes acellular–dermal implantation for lip augmentation. The amount of acellular dermis that is required for labiomandibular, nasolabial, and lip augmentation is also discussed in the following section and summarized in Table 8-1. The preferred type of ePTFE is fibrillar in nature. A 1-mm size is used for a shallower groove and 2-mm for a deeper groove.

For the nasolabial fold, a stab incision is made with a Bard-Parker No. 15C or No. 11 blade parallel and within the crease of the nasolabial fold about 5 mm away from the alar–facial groove and another stab incision is made at the lowest extent of the nasolabial fold. For the labiomandibular fold, the stab incision is made at the inferior extent of the fold (Fig. 8-3B) and inside the buccal mucosa that parallels the fold (Fig. 8-4). Starting from the inferior incision, a standard passer, or introducer, device is used to tunnel in the subcutaneous plane along the fold toward the distal incision (Fig. 8-5A,B). The nondominant hand should guide and control the tunneling of the instrument. Furthermore, the tunnel should be made just large enough to accommodate the implant. For the nasolabial fold, the surgeon should create the tunnel along the nasolabial fold crease, erring slightly medially rather than laterally. Because the nasolabial fold is defined as a mound laterally and a valley medially, the surgeon should place the implant medially to raise the depression and soften the transition between the two elevations.

After the tunnel has been successfully created, one end of the implant is securely fastened to a 0-silk on a Keith-style needle about 0.5 to 1 cm from the end of the implant to avoid slippage of the suture off the implant.** The needle is then passed into the groove of the introducer (Fig. 8-6), and then the introducer is withdrawn leaving the needle in place. The wound edges of one stab incision are retracted laterally and upward with opposing tiny, double hooks. Expanded polytetrafluoroethylene, which has a higher likelihood of implant infection, does not require any preparatory soak in povidone-iodine, or equivalent solution, as the material is hydrophobic and does not benefit from immersion in a disinfectant. The implant is gently pulled through the tunnel until it fully occupies the space (Fig. 8-7). The nondominant hand again should guide the implant so that it does not kink or fold onto itself during insertion.

The length of the implant should be at least 1 cm longer than the tunneled pocket so that the ends may be tucked further distal to both incisions by 2 to 3 mm (Fig. 8-8). For the side of the implant that passes into the buccal mucosa, a more conservative amount should be visible (i.e., less than 5 mm rather than 1 cm in length) (Fig. 8-9). The portion of the implant fastened to the 0-silk suture is amputated and discarded. As mentioned, the distal aspects of the implant then are tucked distal to the incision on both ends, using a tiny double hook and Bishop forceps to facilitate ease of entry and placement. The rationale for the extension of the implant past the incision site is several-fold. First, if the implant terminates at the incision site, a tendency may arise for the wound to contract downward over a void: The implant buttresses against this possibility. Second, if the end of the implant buckles somewhat over time, it may tend to apply pressure against the wound edge and have a greater likelihood for extrusion. Third, the implant may tend to contract over time so the implant is placed as distally as possible to protect against this event. The incisions then are closed using 6-0 polypropylene in a simple, interrupted fashion with two to three sutures placed for each incision site, as determined by wound length (Fig. 8-10). These sutures are removed at 1 week.

DVD Lip Augmentation with Acellular Dermis

As mentioned, the authors believe that for semipermanent to permanent lip augmentation, acellular dermis is the preferred method because of the safety profile of the material and the ultimate natural look and feel. Although a fuller lower lip has sensuous appeal, most patients have a more attenuated upper lip and also generally derive greater satisfac-

---

**The introducer device that the authors use comes with a needle that inserts into a central groove of the introducer. However, the authors do not use the needle that comes supplied with the introducer, but instead the Keith needle (6 cm long) that is attached to the 0-silk suture is used. The introducer itself resembles a Freer elevator with the aforesaid central groove that accommodates the long needle.

Instrumentation and Equipment

Instrumentation and Equipment for Acellular Dermis and Expanded Polytetrafluoroethylene Augmentation

Prep Stand:
Nonsterile gloves
10-cc syringe (2), 27-gauge (1¼-inch long) needle (2) with lidocaine 1% and 1:100,000 epinephrine
Surgical marking pen

Instruments:
Introducer, also known as a Passer—a device that resembles a Freer but has a sharper edge as well as a central groove that accommodates a needle used to draw the implant through the pocket.
Hemostat (to grasp the free end of the implant so as to prevent pulling the implant accidentally too far into the pocket).
Tiny, double-hooks (2)
Metzenbaum or Mayo scissors

Sutures:
0-silk with a 60-mm Keith-type KS (SC2, CS-1) [SC2] <SE-1>* needle (to suture the implant)
6-0 polypropylene, P-3 (P-13, PRE-2) needle (to close the skin incision)
5-0 chromic, P-3 (PRE-2, P-13) <RE-3> needle (to close the lip incision)

Other Supplies:
No. 11 or 15c blade
Acellular–dermal graft, 3 × 7 cm graft (Table 8-1)
ePTFE, Fibrillar Form (1-mm size for a more superficial depression and 2-mm for a deeper groove)

Instrumentation/Equipment for Advancement Cheiloplasty

Prep Stand:
Nonsterile gloves
10-cc syringe (2), 27-gauge (1¼-inch long) needle (2) with lidocaine 1% and 1:100,000 epinephrine
Surgical marking pen
Castroviejo calipers

Instruments:
Tiny, double-hooks (2)
Bishop forceps

*The first needle size refers to the Ethicon code. The second parenthetical code refers to the equivalent needle size manufactured by US Surgical/Davis & Geck. Of note, the first code within the parentheses refers to US Surgical and the second number within the parentheses refers to the older Davis & Geck code. The third bracketed code refers to the equivalent needle size made by Look. For Gore-Tex sutures, all needle sizes refer only to those manufactured by W.L. Gore. The fourth code in angle braces refers to the Deknatel needle equivalent.

Sutures:
6-0 silk, P-1(P-10, PRE-1) [C1] <EDR-1> needle

Other Supplies:
No. 15 blade

Instrumentation/Equipment for Geometric Broken-Line Repair for Deep, Vertical Glabellar Rhytidosis

Prep Stand:
Nonsterile gloves
10-cc syringe (2), 27-gauge (1¼-inch long) needle (2) with lidocaine 1% and 1:100,000 epinephrine
Surgical marking pen
Castroviejo calipers

Instruments:
Wide double hooks
Tiny double hooks
Dissecting (iris or tenotomy) scissors

Sutures:
4-0 polydioxanone, PS-3 (P-11, PRE-3) [PC-34] needle
6-0 fast-absorbing suture, PC1 (PC-13, SBE-2) <BLE-1> needle

Other Supplies:
No. 11 blade
Bipolar cautery
Wire brush dermabrader (at additional session 6 weeks later if necessary for maximal scar camouflage)

Instrumentation and Equipment for Botulinum-Toxin Injection

Reconstitution (Recommended Dilution):
4.5 cc preservative-free saline
18-gauge needle
5-cc syringe

Injection:
30-gauge, 1/2″ needle
1-cc tuberculin syringe

Instrumentation and Equipment for Collagen Injection

Collagen Test Patch
Zyplast 1.5 cc. Recommended for most augmentation purposes.
Zyplast 1.0 cc. Recommended for conservative lip augmentation in the younger patient.
30-gauge needle or special injection needle (both come supplied with the Collagen kit). The specialized needle permits reducing the length of the exposed tip to control depth of the injection.

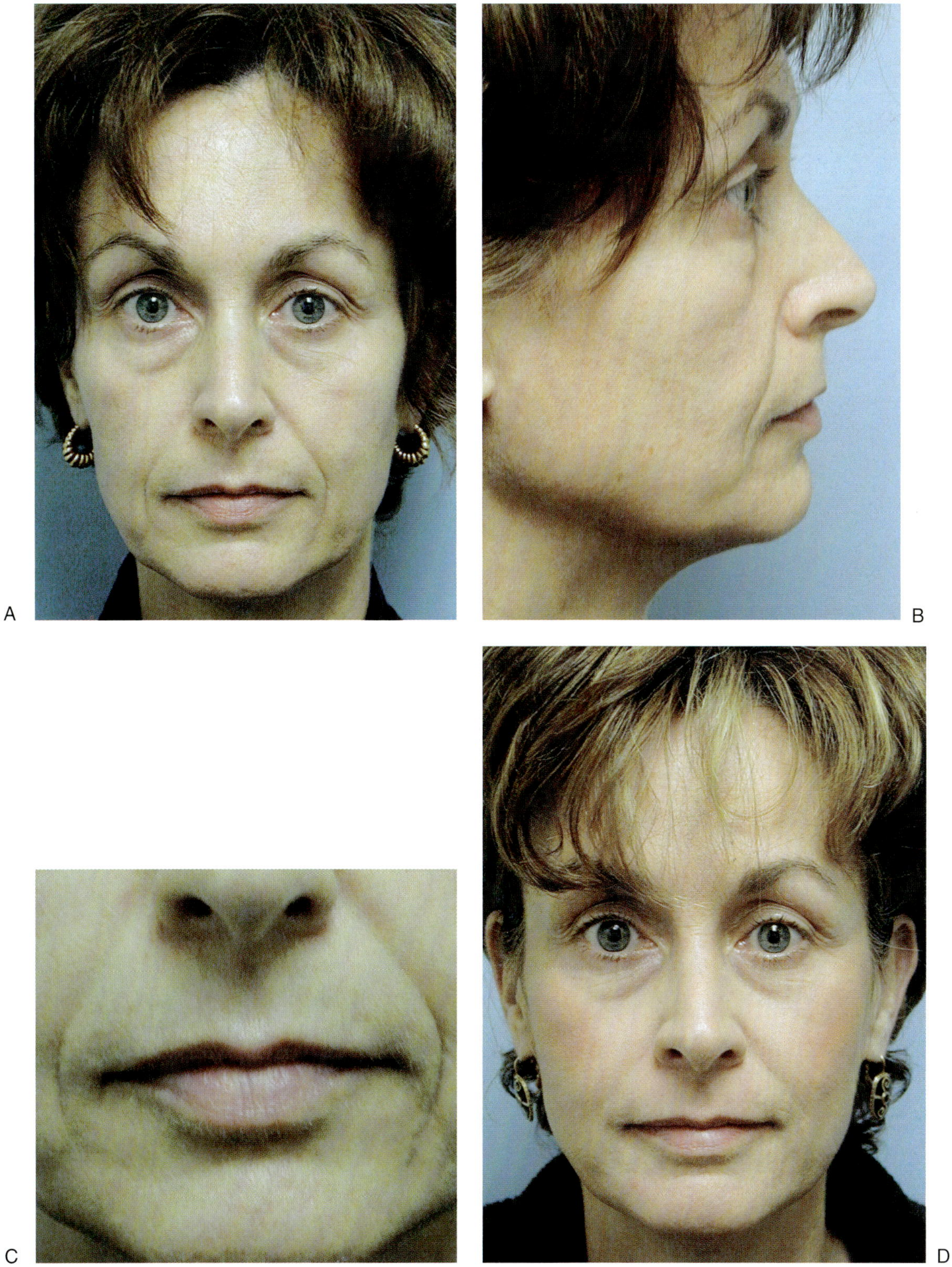

FIGURE 8-2. ePTFE Smile-Line Insertion, Step 1. A–D. This is a 44-year-old woman who was particularly concerned with her deep nasolabial folds, which she noted was present for most of her life and was a familial trait. Although she exhibited some early signs of aging in her lower eyelid, brow, and jaw line, she only desired correction of her deep nasolabial lines. She was offered temporary enhancement with collagen, semipermanent to permanent enhancement with acellular dermis (Alloderm), and permanent enhancement with expanded polytetrafluoroethylene (ePTFE; Gore-Tex). The patient did not want collagen because of its temporary nature, nor ePTFE because of the explained sequela of palpability. The patient understood that acellular dermis would be variably resorbed depending on one's physiology but could endure for many years. *(continued)*

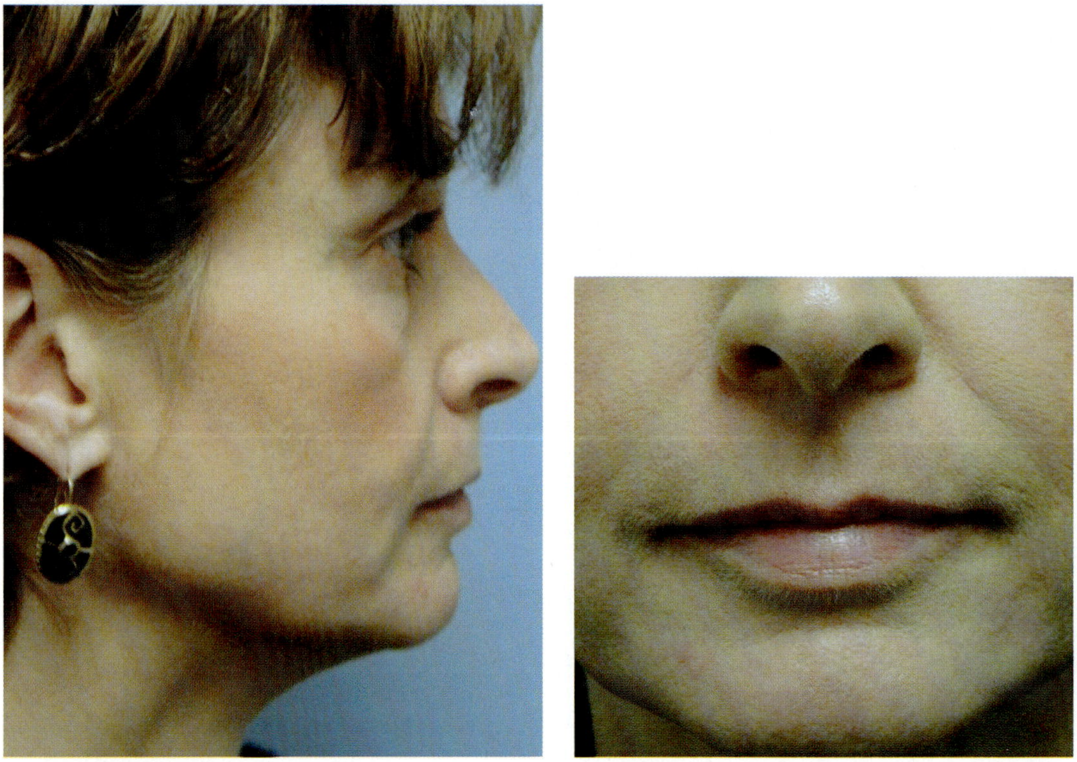

E F

FIGURE 8-2. *(Continued)* **E–F.** The patient is shown with good aesthetic improvement 6 months after augmentation.

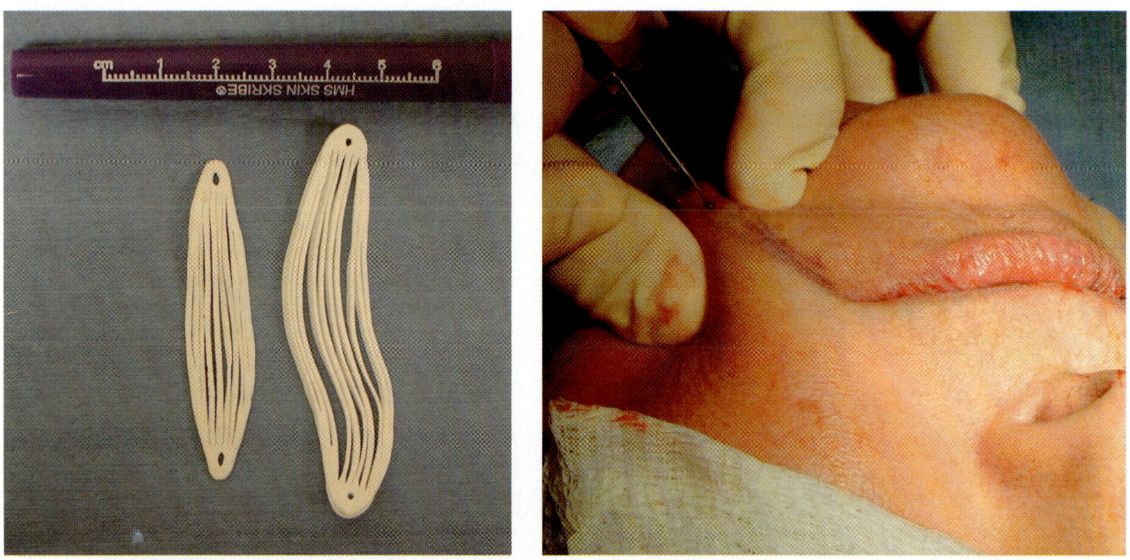

A B

FIGURE 8-3. ePTFE Smile-Line Insertion, Step 1. A: Various types of expanded polytetrafluoroethylene (ePTFE; Gore-Tex) implants can be used for nasolabial- and labiomandibular-fold augmentation. The fibrillar strands of ePTFE are preferred for their stability, tissue ingrowth, and minimal palpability. (N.B.: The following photographic sequence shows insertion of a solid ePTFE implant.) **B:** After appropriate local anesthesia (1% lidocaine with 1:100,000 epinephrine) has been infiltrated, a stab incision is made at the inferior aspect of the desired fold along the length of the fold.

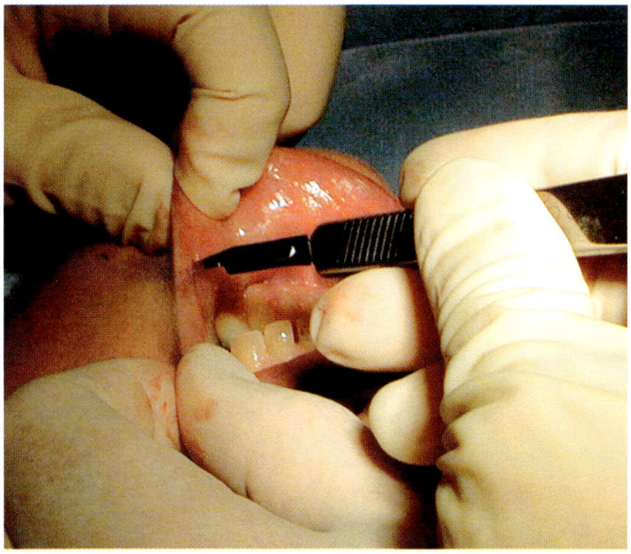

FIGURE 8-4. ePTFE Smile-Line Insertion, Step 2. For the labiomandibular fold, an incision may be made in the buccal mucosa to help camouflage the incision. (Alternatively, the superior incision may be made in the skin near the mouth rather than in the mucosa.)

A

B

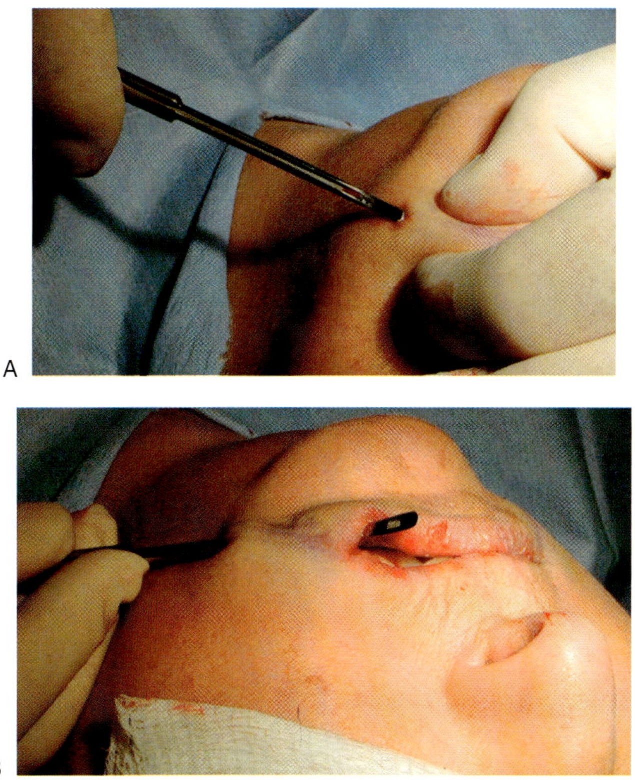

FIGURE 8-5. ePTFE Smile-Line Insertion, Step 3. A,B: Starting from the inferior incision, a standard passer, or introducer, device is used to tunnel in the subcutaneous plane along the fold toward the distal incision.

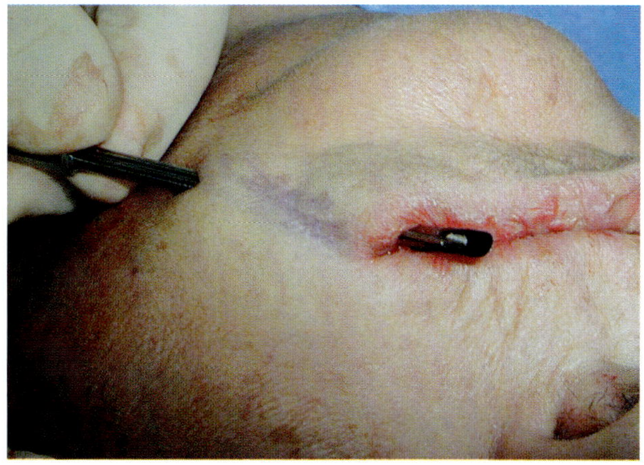

FIGURE 8-6. ePTFE Smile-Line Insertion, Step 4. The straight needle that fits into the groove of the introducer is tied to a 0 silk on one end and to the implant on the other, and then the needle is inserted into the groove of the introducer. The introducer is then withdrawn with the needle kept in place.

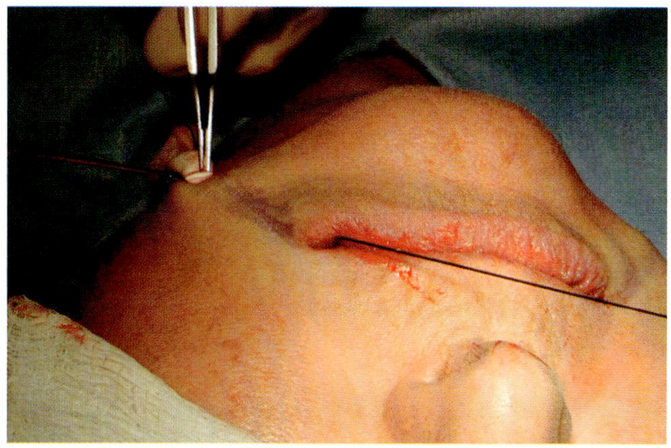

FIGURE 8-7. ePTFE Smile-Line Insertion, Step 5. The needle is then pulled through until the implant has been positioned into the pocket with a 1-cm tail of the implant left exposed.

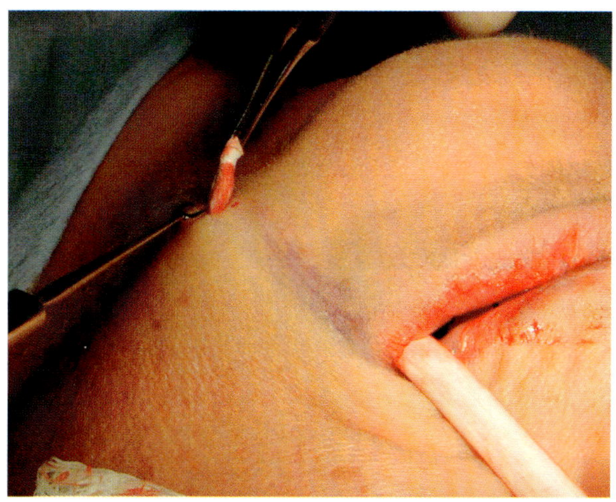

FIGURE 8-8. ePTFE Smile-Line Insertion, Step 6. The exposed 1-cm tail of the implant is then tucked further distal to the incision site using fine-toothed forceps and tiny, double-hook retractors.

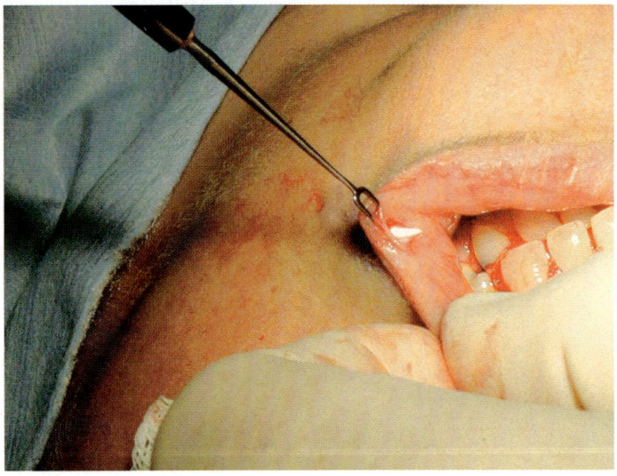

FIGURE 8-9. ePTFE Smile-Line Insertion, Step 7. For the side of the implant that passes into the buccal mucosa, a more conservative amount should be visible (i.e., less than 5 mm rather than 1 cm in length).

TABLE 8–1. ACELLULAR DERMIS SIZES FOR LIP, LABIOMANDIBULAR, AND NASOLABIAL AUGMENTATION

Location	Amount	
Upper and lower lip	3 × 7 cm:	2/3 of implant into upper lip, 1/3 of implant into lower lip (conservative, standard augmentation)
	3 × 7 cm (2):	1 entire roll in upper lip 1 entire roll in lower lip (aggressive augmentation)
Upper lip alone	3 × 7 cm:	2/3 to entire implant into upper lip
Nasolabial folds	3 × 7 cm:	1/2 of implant into each side
Labiomandibular folds	3 × 7 cm:	1/2 of implant into each side

tion with augmentation of the upper lip (Fig. 8-11). Accordingly, often patients desire only selective augmentation of the upper lip. However, simultaneous upper- and lower-lip augmentation remains a more common request.

One percent lidocaine and 1:100,000 epinephrine is infiltrated into the upper lip, and 10 minutes are allowed to transpire, during which time the acellular dermis is properly prepared (Fig. 8-12). Typically, a 3- × 7-cm acellular–dermal graft is sufficient to augment both the upper and lower lips in a conservative fashion. Two thirds of this graft is sectioned lengthwise (i.e., along the long axis of the graft), to be used for the upper lip, and the remaining one third is reserved for the lower lip. This amount of augmentation is particularly well suited for a more mature woman who desires subtle but definitive augmentation. As acellular dermis comes in different thicknesses, the thickest 3- × 7-cm sheet should be ordered to achieve maximal augmentation. Use of two 3- × 7-cm grafts for lip augmentation (i.e., one for the upper lip and one for the lower) is an aggressive augmentation that may risk extrusion and also increase the period of postoperative edema. Nevertheless, this amount of augmentation can be used for the more outspoken patient who demands significant increase in lip volume. Given the expense of acellular dermis, routine use of two sheets may not be financially justifiable except for the vocal patient who insists on considerable lip augmentation. If the patient desires only selective augmentation of the upper lip, then usually the entire 3- × 7-cm graft is placed into the upper lip so that none

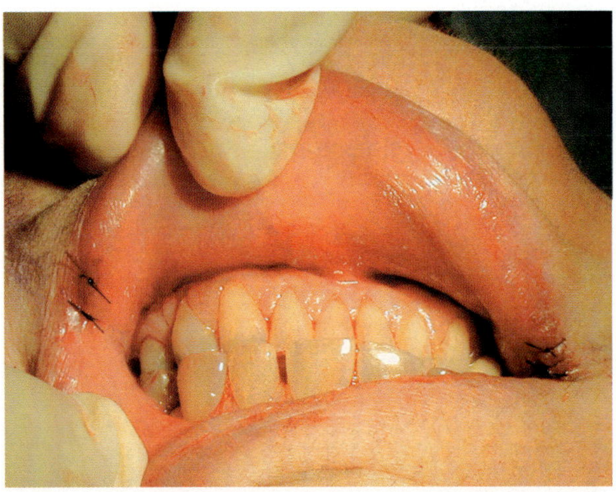

FIGURE 8-10. ePTFE Smile-Line Insertion, Step 8. The incisions are then closed with 6-0 polypropylene in a simple, interrupted fashion with two to three sutures placed for each incision site, as determined by wound length.

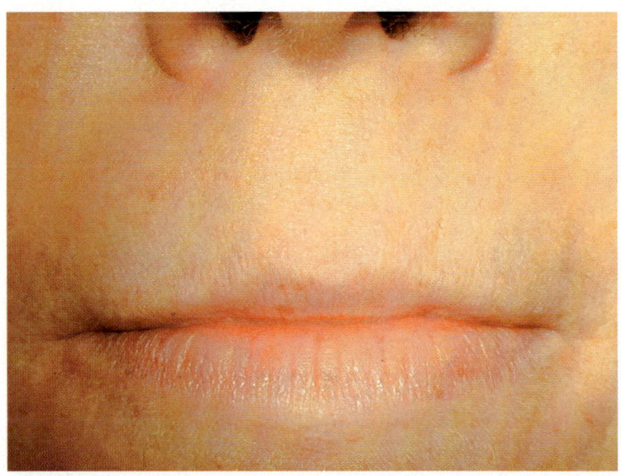

FIGURE 8-11. A typical patient who exhibits a more attenuated upper lip and desires selective augmentation of the upper lip.

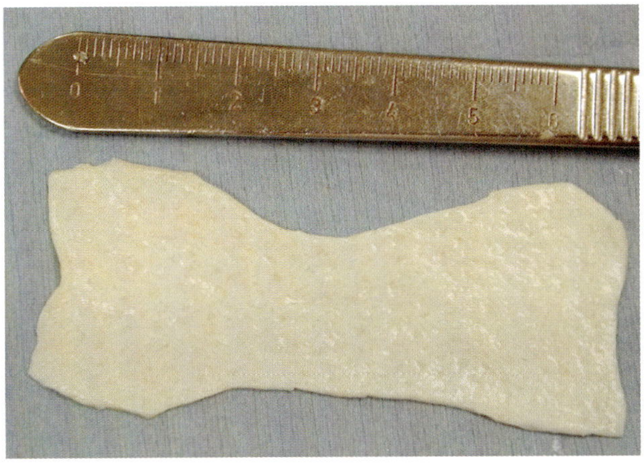

FIGURE 8-12. Acellular-Dermis Lip Augmentation, Step 1. A 3- × 7-cm sheet of acellular dermis is reconstituted with hydration according to the package instructions. The acellular dermal graft is cut lengthwise (i.e., along its long axis) into two-thirds and one-third portions, with the former designed for upper lip augmentation and the latter for the lower lip.

is wasted. However, if the lip appears too full after this degree of augmentation, a more conservative amount can be used as aesthetically demanded. For nasolabial augmentation, one half of the 3- × 7-cm graft is inserted into each smile line. Similarly, one half of the 3- × 7-cm graft is inserted into each marionette line. Table 8-1 summarizes these recommendations. The acellular dermis is rolled and sutured with a 5-0 chromic suture (Fig. 8-13) and tied at one end to the 0-silk, which in turn is affixed to the straight needle that is designed to fit into the groove of the introducer (Fig. 8-14). It is imperative that the 0-silk suture be firmly tied to the end of the implant using a square knot, because it may easily slip off the end of the implant during the forceful draw through the pocket. Stab incisions are made with a No. 15 blade approximately at the junction of the wet and dry lip on either end of the upper lip about 4 to 5 mm medial to the oral commissure (Fig. 8-15). The introducer is then passed through the upper lip using the nondominant hand to guide the device toward the other side (Fig. 8-16A–C). The proper plane of passage is below the outer mucosa but above the orbicularis-oris muscle. The instrument should be advanced slowly and deliberately in order to avoid inadvertent puncture through the outer lip with control provided by the nondominant hand. The straight needle is then passed into the groove of the introducer and pulled through as the introducer is withdrawn (Fig. 8-17A,B). Before the implant is drawn through, the free end of the implant (i.e., the end without the attached suture) should be clamped with a hemostat to prevent the implant from being pulled too far into the pocket. The straight needle is drawn through until the implant is situated properly in the pocket with only a short 1-cm tail showing on the proximal side (Fig. 8-18). When properly situated, the suture is cut free from the implant, and the hemostat clamp removed. The distal end is trimmed to the same 1-cm length tail. The acellular–dermal graft is then tucked further distal to each incision using fine-toothed forceps with tiny, double-pronged hooks for retraction (Fig. 8-19). The incisions are closed with two interrupted 4-0 chromic sutures (Fig. 8-20).

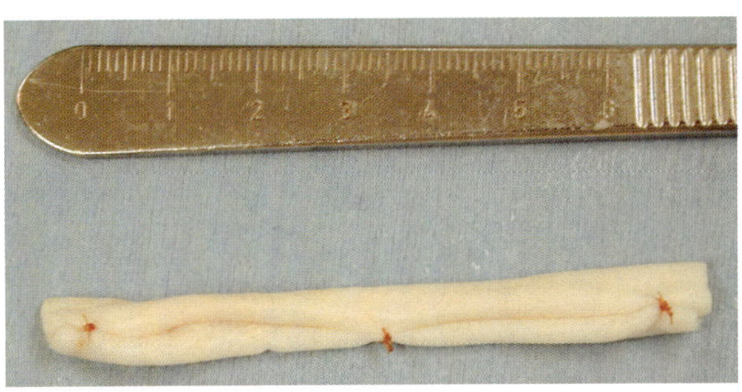

FIGURE 8-13. Acellular-Dermis Lip Augmentation, Step 2. The acellular dermis is rolled and sutured with 5-0 chromic suture before implantation.

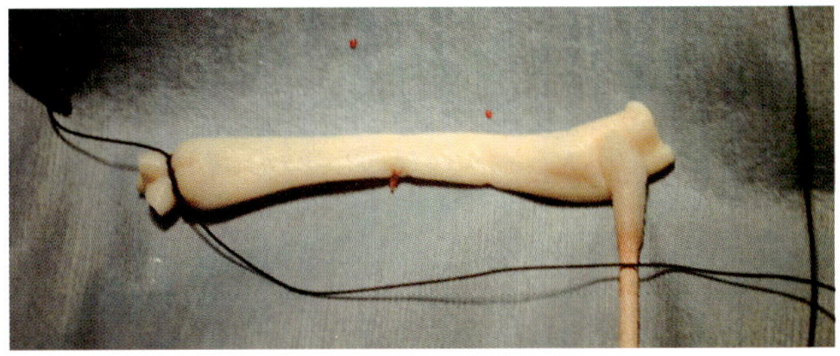

FIGURE 8-14. Acellular-Dermis Lip Augmentation, Step 3. The acellular dermis is tied at one end to a 0 silk which in turn is attached to the straight needle that is designed to fit into the groove of the introducer. The suture should be firmly tied to the implant to prevent slippage during implantation.

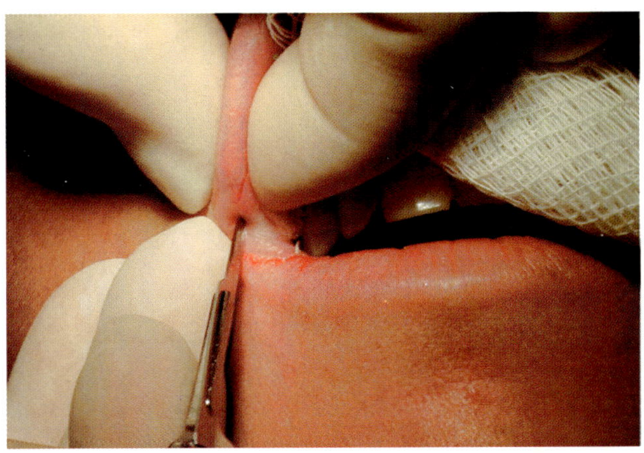

FIGURE 8-15. Acellular-Dermis Lip Augmentation, Step 4. Stab incisions are made with a No. 15 blade approximately at the junction of the wet and dry lip on either end of the upper lip about 4 to 5 mm medial to the oral commissure.

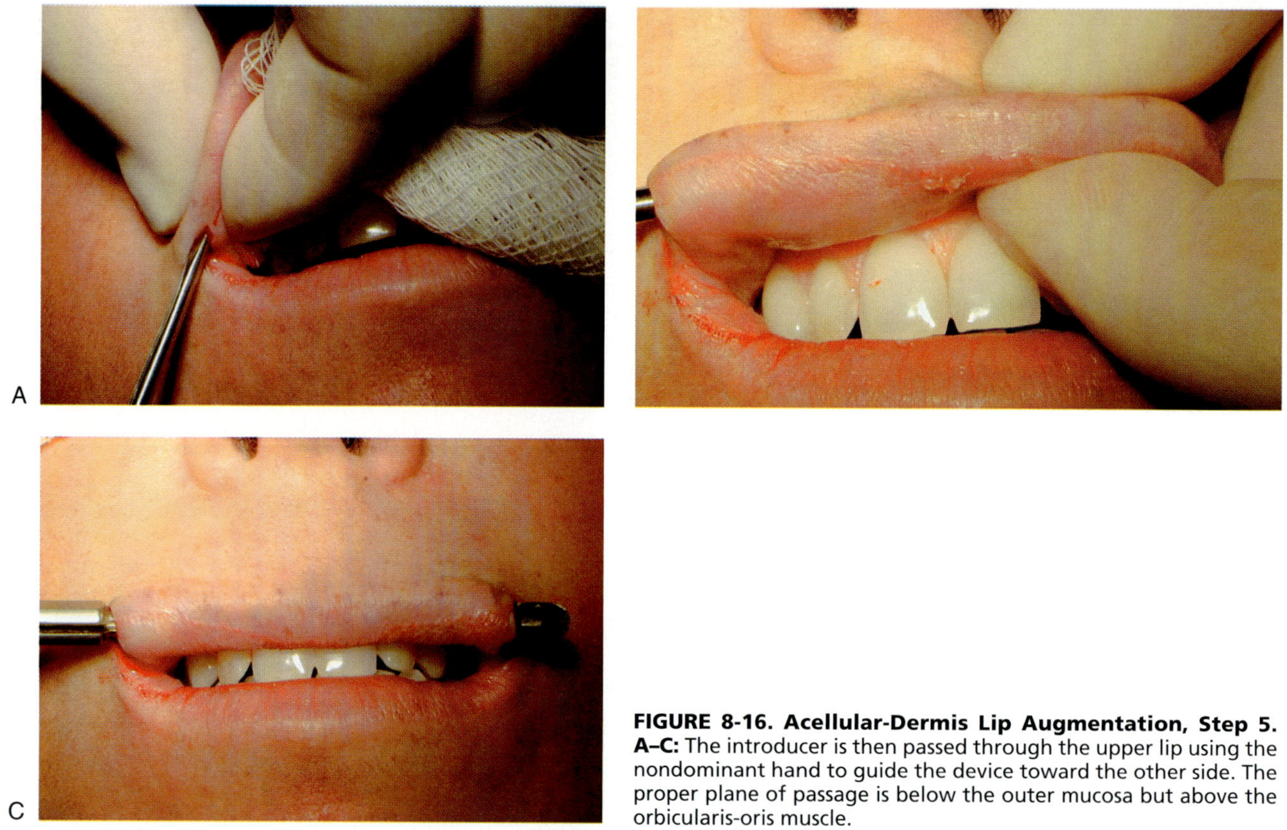

FIGURE 8-16. Acellular-Dermis Lip Augmentation, Step 5. A–C: The introducer is then passed through the upper lip using the nondominant hand to guide the device toward the other side. The proper plane of passage is below the outer mucosa but above the orbicularis-oris muscle.

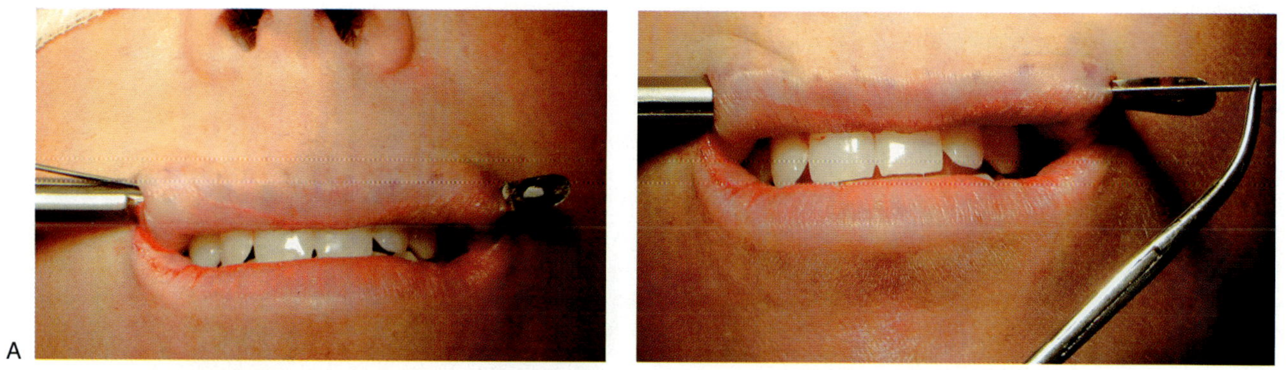

FIGURE 8-17. Acellular-Dermis Lip Augmentation, Step 6. A,B: The straight needle is then passed into the groove of the introducer and pulled through as the introducer is withdrawn. A hemostat should be affixed to the free end of the implant so as to prevent the implant from being inadvertently pulled too far through the pocket.

Of note, if Cupid's bow appears to be too full, the implant should be removed and a small wedge excised from the superior aspect of the implant along its central aspect to reduce this fullness. Some texts recommend that the implant should be placed as two separate segments, with each portion falling on either side of Cupid's bow. However, because of inevitable and unpredictable contraction of the implant, the aesthetic result may be suboptimal over time. Therefore, the authors do not advocate this technique. The exact same technique is used to augment the lower lip as explained for the upper lip, except the implant is proportionally narrower (as mentioned) in a 1-to-2 ratio but retains the same length as that of the upper-lip implant.

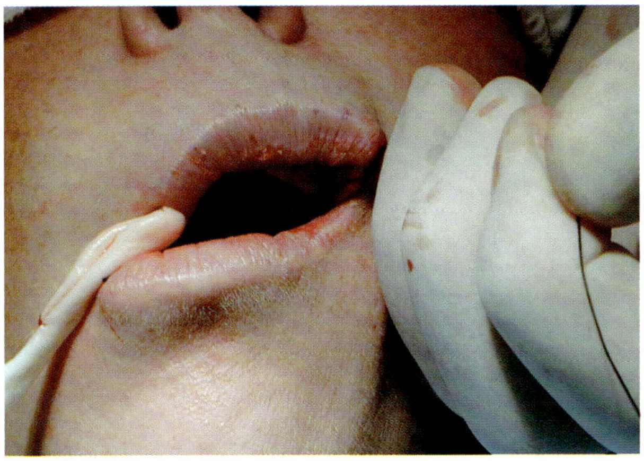

FIGURE 8-18. Acellular-Dermis Lip Augmentation, Step 7. The straight needle is drawn through until the implant is situated properly in the pocket with only a short 1-cm tail showing on the proximal side. The distal end is trimmed to the same 1-cm length tail.

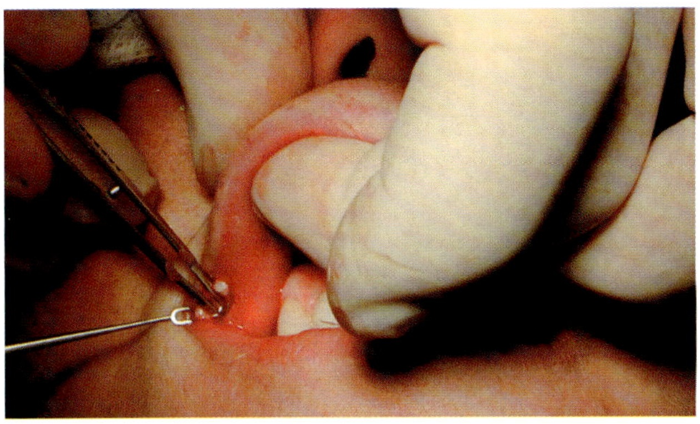

FIGURE 8-19. The acellular dermis is then tucked further distal to each incision using fine-toothed forceps and tiny double-pronged hooks.

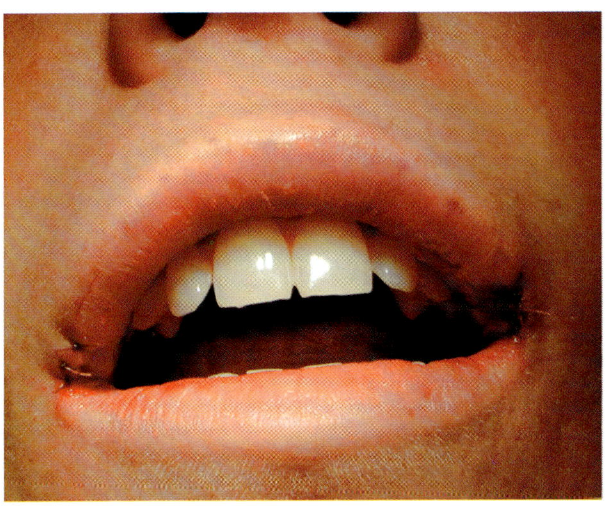

FIGURE 8-20. Acellular-Dermis Lip Augmentation, Step 8. The incisions are closed with two interrupted 4-0 chromic sutures.

Direct Excision (Glabellar)

If the patient presents with extremely advanced, canyonlike fissures in the glabellar region, the most effective modality for this type of pathology is direct excision of the rhytid and reconstruction (Case #3; Figs. 8-21 and 8-22). Of note, direct excision is only recommended for vertical rhytids and, as explained, is neither indicated nor aesthetically pleasing for horizontally oriented rhytids. It is worth repeating here that direct excision of the nasolabial fold is contraindicated in all circumstances because of the inevitable, unfavorable widening of the wound over time caused by repeated motion in this area.

Direct excision of the rhytid may take many forms, according to scar revision principles: straight-line excision, multiple z-plasties, a running w-plasty, or geometric broken line. This last technique represents the definitive technique for optimal camouflage and is reviewed here because it is the most technically intricate and ideal technique for glabellar rhytidosis.

A fusiform outline centered over the rhytid (about 1 to 2 mm on each side) is drawn with a surgical marking pen. Then the alternating geometric configurations (squares, rectangles, trapezoids, and triangles) that line either side of the wound edge are drawn in the following manner. The shapes should extend approximately 3 to 4 mm from the proposed wound edge because smaller shapes experience compromised vascularity and are difficult to handle surgically, whereas larger shapes create undue wound tension and are harder to camouflage. Smaller, 3-mm sized shapes are ideal near the medial eyebrow to avoid distortion in this region; and larger, 4-mm limbs may be used higher in the forehead area. First, a dotted line is drawn parallel to and 3 to 4 mm from the fusiform excision line, which represents the edge of the proposed geometric limbs. A pair of calipers or a ruler should be used so that the limbs are exactly the same size on each side of the wound edge along the entire length to ensure that the geometric shapes fit precisely into the corresponding, contralateral defects (Fig. 8-23). The surgeon then marks out the geometric shapes that fit within the 3- to 4-mm limb distance by drawing one shape at a time and the corresponding contralateral defect thereafter (Fig. 8-24A,B). If the surgeon elects to draw one entire side of geometric shapes before venturing to the contralateral, matching side, he or she will find it difficult to ensure that an error is not made in pairing shape with defect.

Local anesthesia (1% lidocaine with 1:100,000 epinephrine) is infiltrated into the incision and adjacent tissue, and the standard 10 minutes are allowed to transpire for maximal hemostasis and anesthetic effect. The geometric shapes are created using a Bard-Parker No. 11 blade (Becton, Dickinson, and Company, Franklin Lakes, NJ) again in an alternating fashion between sides to ensure that no error is committed. In order to maintain the integrity of the dermal sling, the skin is only perforated with the No. 11

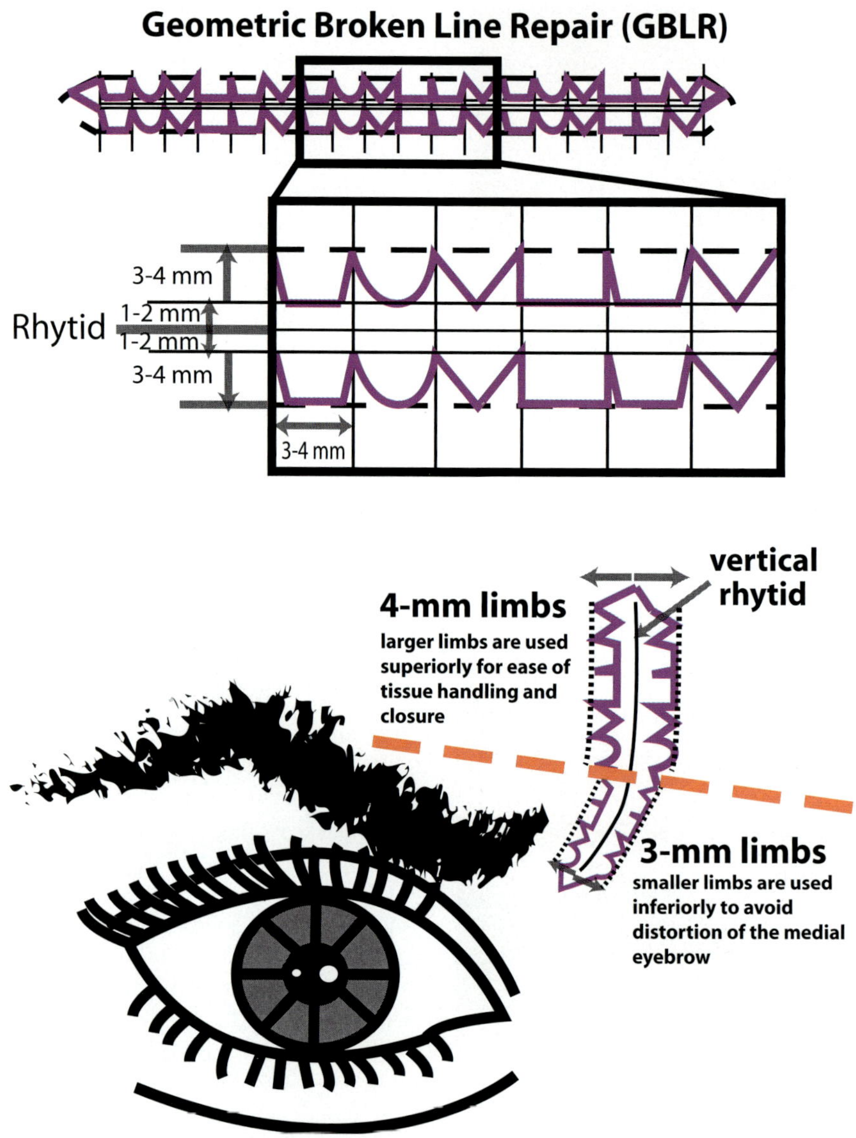

FIGURE 8-21. The illustration shows the proper technique for geometric broken-line repair to excise a vertical, glabellar rhytid. The geometric shapes should be fashioned around the rhytid, measuring approximately 3 to 4 mm in length. Three-millimeter limbs are ideal for the shapes located near the medial eyebrow to avoid distortion from excessive tissue resection, and 4-mm limbs are preferred superiorly to permit ease of tissue handling and closure. Wound closure should proceed in a bidirectional fashion with the surgeon suturing toward himself or herself going from "ship to shore" (i.e., the freely mobile shape should be sutured to the corresponding defect side). After one side has been undertaken in this fashion, the surgeon should move to the other side of the patient and suture from "ship to shore" so that the remaining shapes have been brought to the corresponding defects. *(continued)*

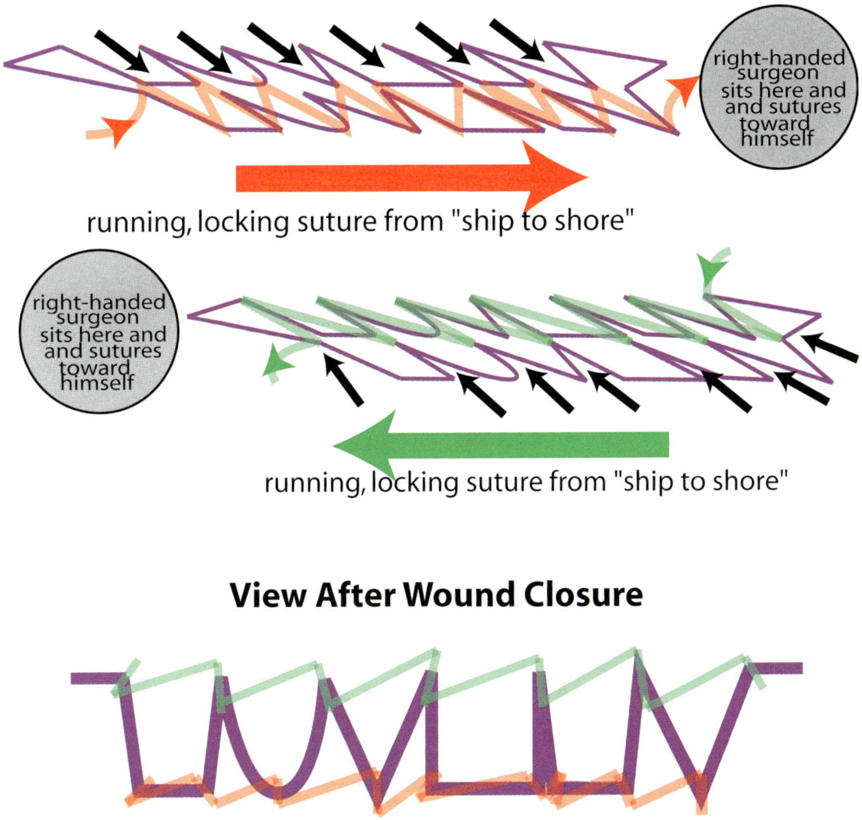

FIGURE 8-21. *(Continued).*

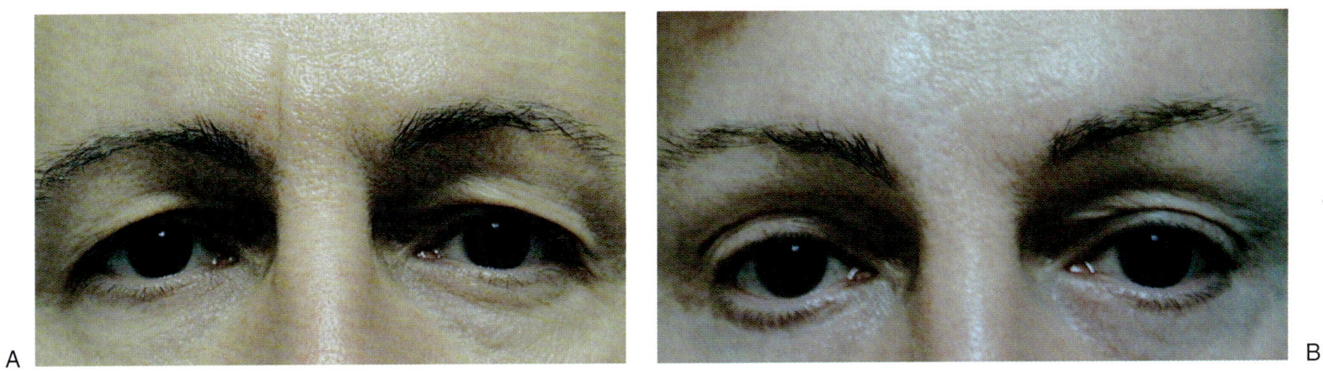

FIGURE 8-22. A,B: This is a 49-year-old entertainer who initially presented for facial rejuvenation surgery. The patient underwent brow-, midface-, and facelift surgery in conjunction with upper-eyelid blepharoplasty, a transconjunctival lower-eyelid blepharoplasty, and a 35% trichloroacetic acid chemical peel. This patient was still very bothered by the vertical glabellar furrow, which was indicated to him on his preoperative visit. Despite his satisfaction with the previous surgery, he was very motivated to have this area addressed. On examination the vertical furrow was just medial to the club of the right upper eyebrow extending deep and vertically and present during both rest and animation. He underwent successful geometric broken-line repair with subsequent dermabrasion 6 weeks later.

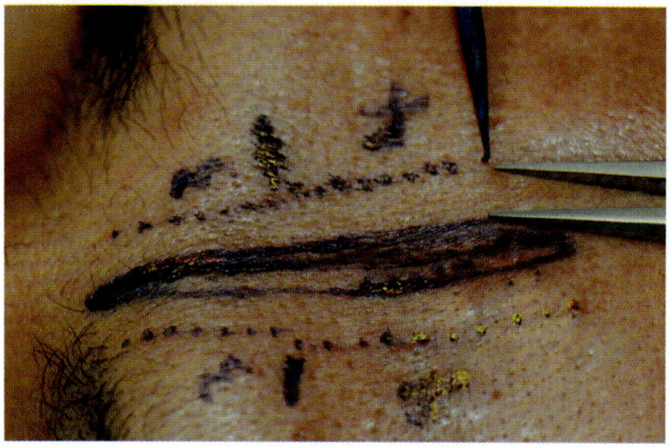

FIGURE 8-23. Geometric Broken-Line Repair, Step 1. A fusiform outline is drawn centered over the rhytid to be excised (about 1 to 2 mm on each side of the rhytid). A dotted line approximately 3 to 4 mm distance from the fusiform line is precisely measured and drawn with calipers. Three-millimeter limbs have been drawn near the medial eyebrow to avoid tissue distortion, and 4-mm limbs have been designed more superiorly to permit ease of tissue handling.

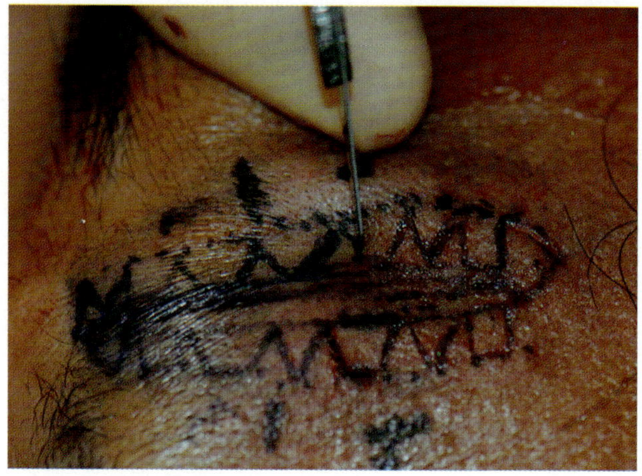

FIGURE 8-25. Geometric Broken-Line Repair, Step 3. After infiltration of local anesthesia, the shapes are incised again in an alternating fashion from one side of the incision to the other in order to ensure that the incorrect lines are not inadvertently incised. Tiny skin bridges between the incisions are kept intact until all of the principal incisions have been made to facilitate ease of dissection. A No. 11 blade is preferred for tissue transection.

blade so that tiny bridges of epidermis remain intact between perforations (Fig. 8-25). This technique permits wound tension to be maintained during the entire excisional process. The tiny skin bridges then are transected with the No. 11 blade before dissecting the skin island from the underlying muscular bed and discarded. Dissection is carried out laterally several millimeters in the subcutaneous plane to permit wound eversion and reduce wound tension.

The corrugator is then transected on either side of the wound with sharp scissors and partially avulsed (Fig. 8-26). Dissection should remain primarily in the central aspect of the wound to minimize inadvertent injury to the supratrochlear neurovascular bundle. In addition, over dissection of the corrugator complex may yield mild depression in the void created below the incision line. After hemostasis is achieved with selective cautery, the wound edges are approximated in the following prescribed fashion. First one to two deep sutures of 4-0 polydioxanone are placed as needed in an inverted orientation to reduce superficial wound tension and promote proper wound healing (Fig. 8-27). A 6-0 fast-absorbing suture is fastened at one end of the wound and run in a locking fashion toward the other end by suturing only the free corners of the created shapes on the surgeon's right side to the corresponding defects on the left side as a right-handed surgeon faces the wound. This technique follows the surgical technique of always suturing "ship to shore" (i.e., from free edge to anchored defect). Similarly, a 6-0 fast-absorbing suture is fastened on the contralateral end of the wound and run toward the other end of in a running, locking fashion. Because the surgeon is now situated on the

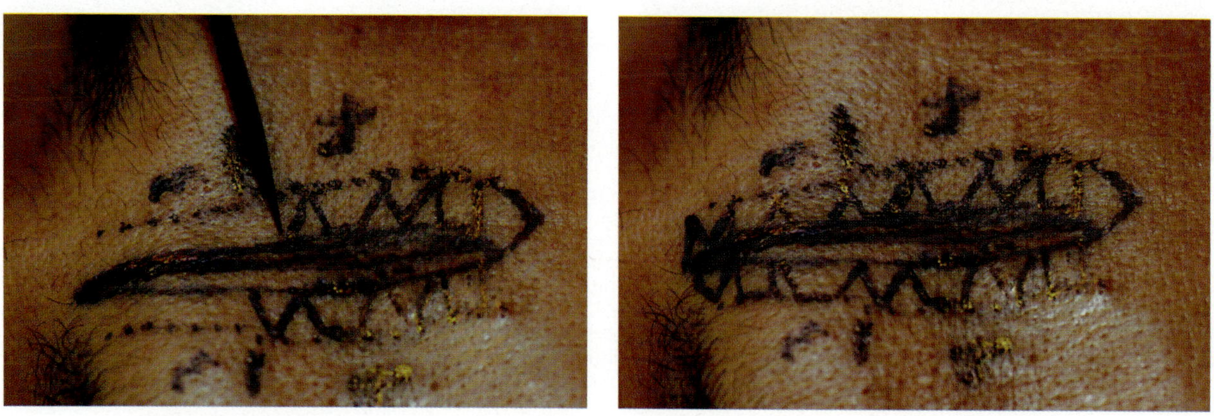

A B

FIGURE 8-24. Geometric Broken-Line Repair, Step 2. A: The geometric shapes (squares, rectangles, trapezoids, and triangles) should be drawn to fit within the 3- to 4-mm dotted line by alternating sides so that no confusion exists about matching a particular shape to its corresponding defect. **B:** The photograph shows all of the shapes drawn out.

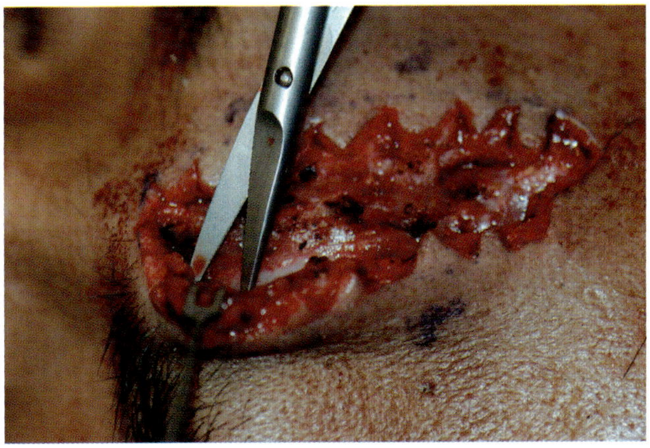

FIGURE 8-26. Geometric Broken-Line Repair, Step 4. The corrugator muscle is then transected on either side of the wound with sharp scissors and partially avulsed.

other side of the wound, the remaining unsutured shapes are again on the right and approximated to the defects on the left (Fig. 8-28A–C). Steri-Strips are applied in a transverse direction to the wound in order to minimize tension. The skin sutures may remain in place, as they are dissolvable, but may be properly trimmed at 1 week. If any irregularities exist at 6 weeks, the incision line can be dermabraded to achieve an inconspicuous scar. Botulinum toxin may be required to reduce muscle activity if corrugator resection is ineffective or returns over time.

Advancement Cheiloplasty

As mentioned, advancement cheiloplasty should be reserved only for select cases: mature women who request this procedure and are willing to wear lipstick on a routine basis to camouflage any obvious scarring. This technique is not recommended in younger women. Further, a subnasal excision of skin rather than a vermilion excision of skin is also discouraged because of a higher likelihood for an unnatural result in the authors' opinion. However, other surgeons have reported good results with this technique. Before the advent of soft-tissue augmentation options, advancement cheiloplasty was the mainstay for lip rejuvenation, but current techniques (e.g. collagen and acellular dermis) have made this technique antiquated and more of historical interest in the authors' opinion. Further, perioral rhytidosis should not be treated with an augmentation technique but deep resurfacing (CO_2 laser, phenol, or dermabrasion) instead.

If the patient consents to these limitations, then the surgeon can carry out the procedure with good conscience. The operation begins with the patient in the upright position for marking. The surgeon marks the anticipated extent of advancement, generally twice the distance that is desired, because some loss of vertical height occurs over time. Use of Castroviejo calipers can provide the most precise and accurate measurements. The surgeon should begin to mark the proposed line of excision at 5 mm medial to the oral commissure to avoid scarring from excessive lateral dissection. The surgeon should mark the line of skin excision at slightly less than a 2-to-1 ratio (proposed excision to desired vermilion height) for the majority of the lip and slightly more than a 2-to-1 ratio at the philtrum (i.e., at the peaks of Cupid's bow) (Fig. 8-29A,B). However, restraint should be exercised in making the points of Cupid's bow too exaggerated, because this peaked appearance is an identifiable stigma of a surgically operated lip. If the lip appears too high at Cupid's bow several months after the operation and the patient is dissatisfied, then the surgeon can elect to reduce the height at the philtrum via a V-to-Y advancement.

After the patient is carefully marked out and anesthetized with the standard mixture of 1% lidocaine with 1:100,000 epinephrine, the surgeon can begin to excise the intended skin. A No. 15 blade should be used to score the skin superficially along the entire perimeter of the incision just to the depth of the mid-dermis, all the while beveling away from the center of the wound. Bishop forceps or tiny, double hooks are used to retract the skin upward as the surgeon meticulously dissects the skin at the middermal level with a No. 15 blade: The white dermis should be noted above and below the knife blade as dissection continues. The remaining dermis is left intact as a platform so that after the lip is closed, it will not retract downward (Fig. 8-29C). In addition, the intact dermis provides volumetric fullness to the lip, which is a favorable aesthetic objective. The wound edges are everted and approximated with interrupted vertical-mattress sutures of 6-0 silk at the key anatomic landmarks (i.e., at the height of Cupid's bow and at the central depression point between Cupid's bow). Similarly, interrupted vertical mattress sutures of 6-0 silk are used to close the remainder of the wound in an everted fashion. (Alternatively, a simple, running 6-0 silk suture can be used to complete the remaining wound closure.) Sutures may be removed at 1 week postoperatively.

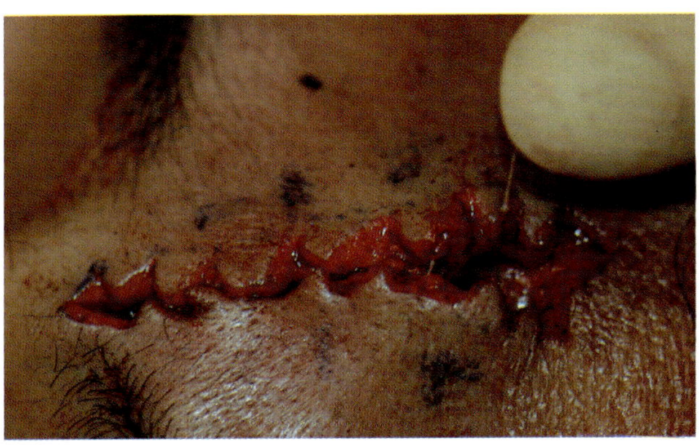

FIGURE 8-27. Geometric Broken-Line Repair, Step 5. One to two deep sutures with 4-0 polydioxanone are placed in an inverted fashion to reduce superficial wound tension.

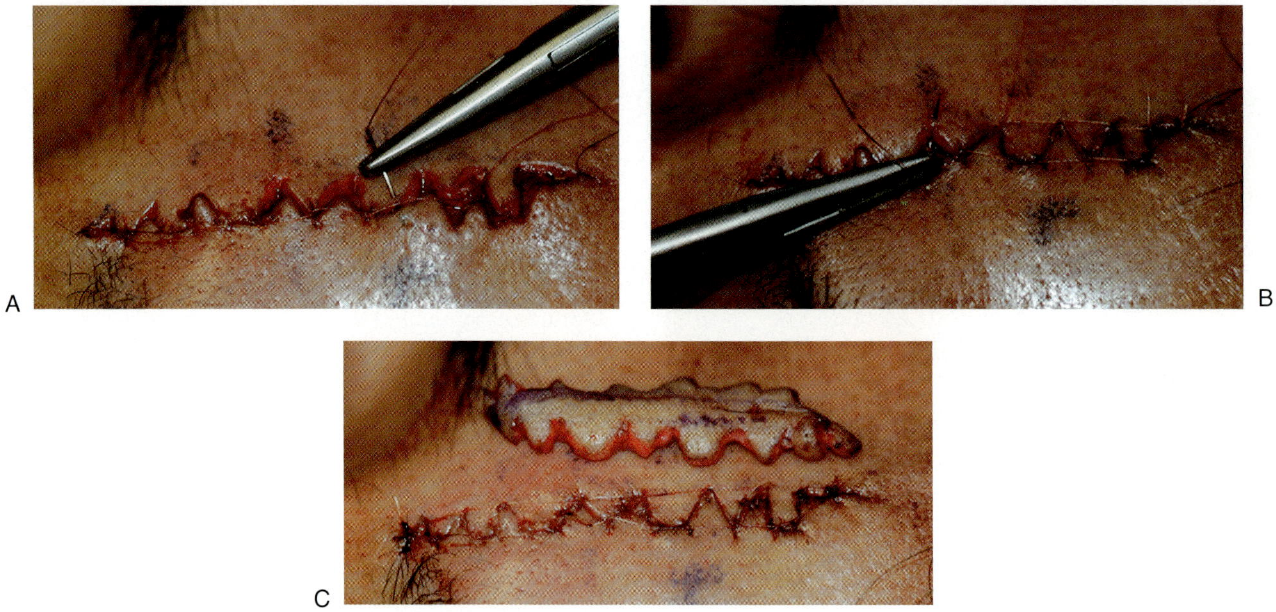

FIGURE 8-28. Geometric Broken-Line Repair, Step 6. A: A 6-0 fast-absorbing suture is fastened at one end of the wound and run in a locking fashion toward the other end by suturing only the free corners of the created shapes on the surgeon's right side to the corresponding defects on the left side as a right-handed surgeon faces the wound. This technique follows the surgical technique of always suturing "ship to shore" (i.e., from free edge to anchored defect). **B:** Similarly, a 6-0 fast-absorbing suture is fastened on the contralateral end of the wound and run toward the other end of the wound in a running, locking fashion as described in the preceding: The surgeon is now situated on the other side of the wound; therefore, the remaining unsutured shapes are again on the right and approximated to the defects on the left. **C:** The photograph shows the wound edges completely approximated with the excised rhytid lying on the adjacent skin. Six weeks later the wound should be dermabraded to ensure maximal improvement in appearance.

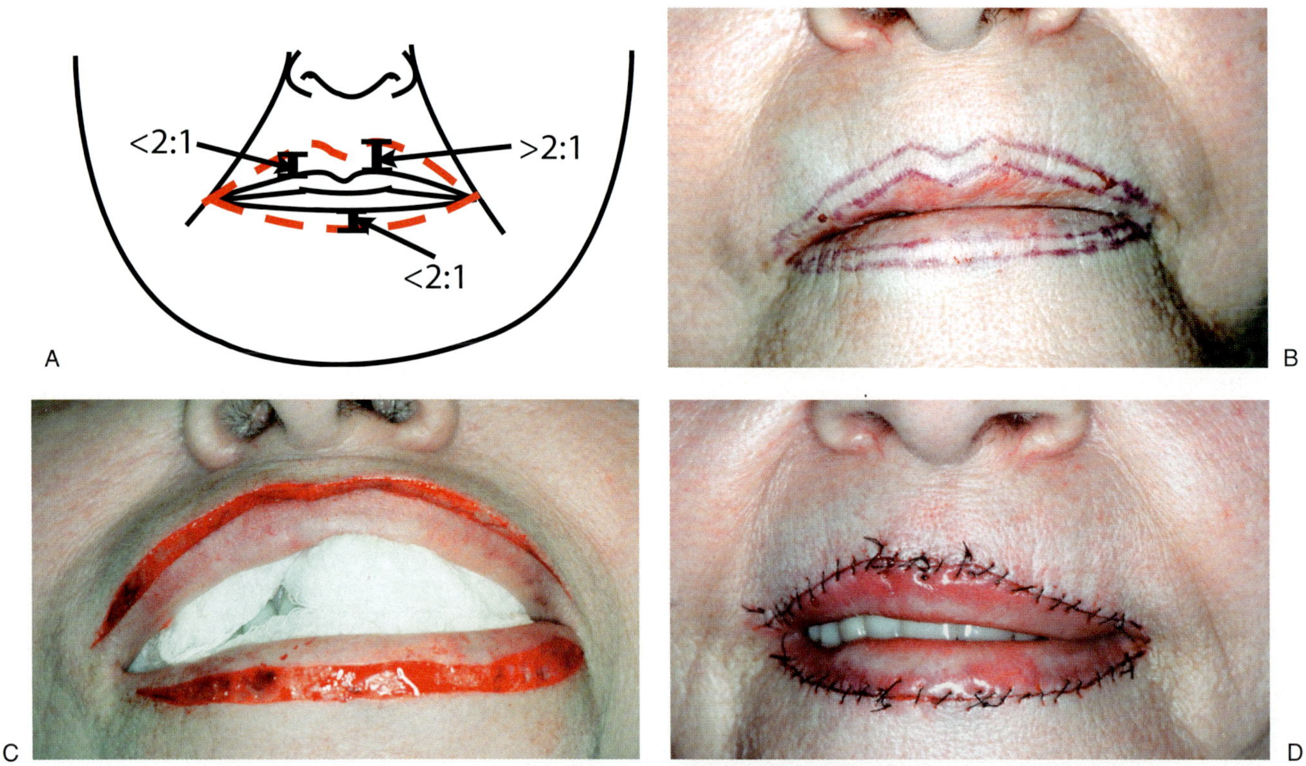

FIGURE 8-29. Advancement-Cheiloplasty Sequence. A: Illustration showing the current vermilion border, the desired vermilion border, and the proposed excision line. The proposed excision line to desired vermilion height should be slightly less than a 2-to-1 ratio for the majority of the lip and slightly above this ratio at the peak of Cupid's bow. **B:** Intraoperative photograph showing the desired marking for proposed skin excision. **C:** The photograph shows the excision of the skin through the mid-dermal plane. **D:** The incision is closed with interrupted, vertical-mattress sutures of 6-0 silk at the key anatomic landmarks (e.g., Cupid's bow and at a few, select points along the inferior-lip border) followed by a running 6-0 silk suture for the remaining lip.

Temporary Rejuvenation

Collagen (Zyplast)

As a review, the authors advocate use of collagen only below an imaginary line drawn through the nasal base, principally to soften the nasolabial and labiomandibular lines and to augment hypoplastic lips. It is not recommended to augment fine wrinkles around the lips, which should be effaced with an appropriate resurfacing modality. However, if the patient has a few deep crevices at the vermilion border that he or she would like effaced, then collagen may be a suitable temporizing agent. Further, apart from using collagen for rejuvenation of the aging face, it may be safely used throughout the entire malar region for acne scarring. (This is an exception to the horizontal-line rule illustrated in Figure 8-1.)

As a reminder to the reader, the patient must undergo an antecubital test patch with 0.1 cc of bovine collagen injected in the intradermal plane approximately 30 days before planned treatment (Fig. 8-30). During this time, the patient observes for any induration or erythema that correlates with an allergic reaction according to symptoms outlined in the package insert. Although the instructions advocate repeating the test patch at a 30-day interval, most patients do not tolerate this delay for an intervention that appeals to the "quick fix" mentality. Furthermore, a double negative test does not necessarily confirm a lack of allergy. The authors have not experienced any adverse reactions to date after a primary negative test.

Although cross-linked Zyplast is more stable and longer lasting than Zyderm, Zyplast is more prone to beading, or a lumpy-bumpy appearance, if injected too superficially or rapidly. Therefore, Zyplast should be infiltrated cautiously, requiring a learning curve to master the proper technique. The preferred plane of injection for Zyplast is deep dermis to ensure maximal longevity and minimize bead formation. The skin should either manifest delayed or no blanching after injection, and the surgeon should technically not feel the needle give way through the reticular dermis into the subcutaneous adipose tissue. Injection can be carried out either with a 30-gauge needle or the specialized needle that comes supplied with every collagen kit. The specialized needle permits reducing the length of the exposed tip to control depth of the injection. If implanted into the subcutaneous tissue, Zyplast may not endure as long a time as intradermal placement. However, the authors stress that even in the most experienced hands, some beading inevitably occurs and that the surgeon should err on the side of placing the collagen too deeply than superficially. If beading does arise, then the surgeon should gently massage the area to even out the contour and further recommend that the patient do likewise until the area returns to a smooth contour.

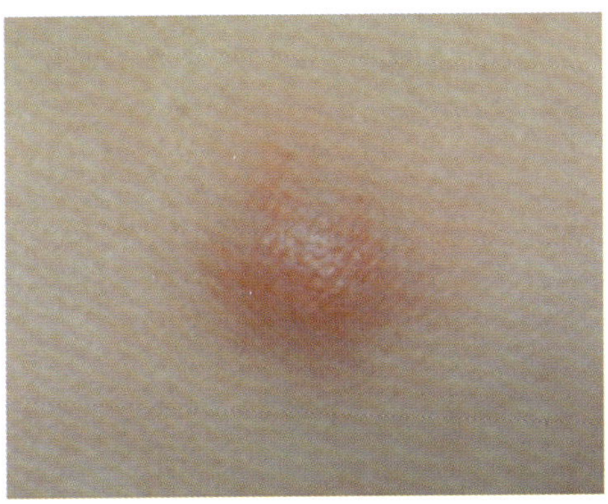

FIGURE 8-30. This patient shows a hypersensitivity response to the collagen test patch that manifested 2 days after injection and has persisted for quite some time. This photograph was taken at 1 month postinjection and exhibits ongoing erythema, induration, tenderness, and pruritus. The patient underwent needle aspiration first to rule out an abscess. With a negative result, the site was injected with 0.1 cc of triamcinolone 10 mg/mL and showed complete resolution of symptoms including induration, erythema, and pruritus over the next day except for some minor ecchymosis that lingered for another week.

Zyplast is packaged in 1-, 1.5-, 2-, and 2.5-cc syringes. Generally speaking, 1.5 cc is preferred for nasolabial fold, labiomandibular fold, and moderate lip augmentation. For all the preceding indications, 1.5 cc is more cost effective for the patient in terms of per dollar augmentation than 1.0 cc; therefore, it is more versatile. However, if a younger woman (less than 35 years old) requests some mild to moderate lip augmentation or if an individual would like only a few cutaneous depressions raised, then the 1-cc allotment may be a better choice. The authors do not use the 2- and 2.5-cc syringe sizes.

For the nasolabial fold, the surgeon should inject at the nasolabial crease or slightly medially to soften the fold (Fig. 8-31A,B). The marionette, or labiomandibular, fold is only present along the upper one third at rest. This depression near the oral commissure cannot really be easily overaugmented, as it usually requires quite a substantial amount of collagen to efface it (Fig. 8-31C). The lower two thirds of the labiomandibular fold only appears in motion and cannot be readily addressed. In addition, collagen should not be used to correct jowling. As mentioned, correction of perioral rhytids is often less desirable with collagen because Zyplast is less forgiving in these finer lines and Zyderm has less longevity. Zyplast can be used for discrete areas of deeper, crevicelike rhytids and used with discretion in finer lines if the surgeon elects not to stock both Zyplast and Zyderm (Fig. 8-32). For lip augmentation, the collagen should be injected at the vermilion–cutaneous junction aiming slightly toward the underlying vermilion. Two thirds of the collagen should be placed into the upper lip and the remaining one third should be reserved for the lower lip. Although a full lower lip may be associated with a pouty, seductive appeal, most patients desire a fuller upper lip, as it tends to be more visible to them. In addition, the flattened contour of the aged upper lip is a particularly more unpleasant feature to the patient than a more attenuated lower lip. Therefore, the

A
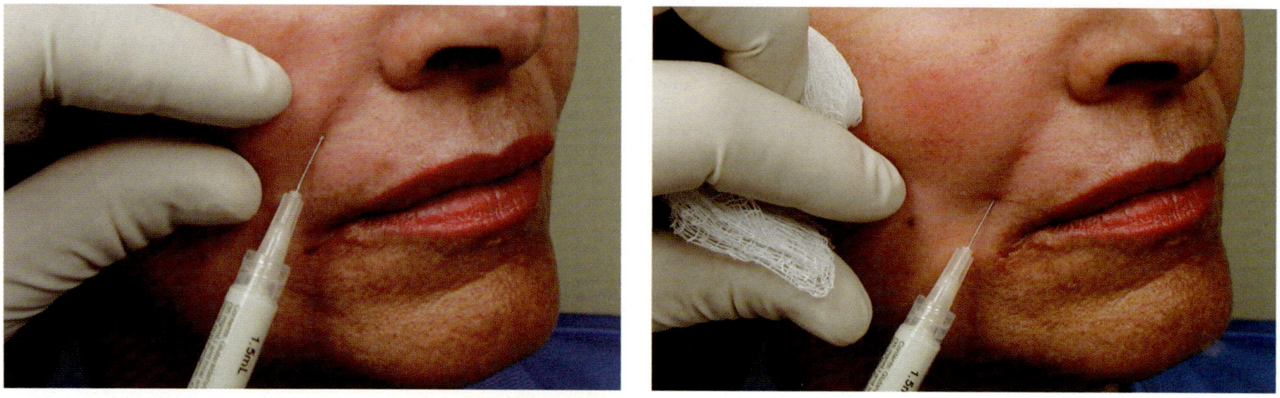
B

C
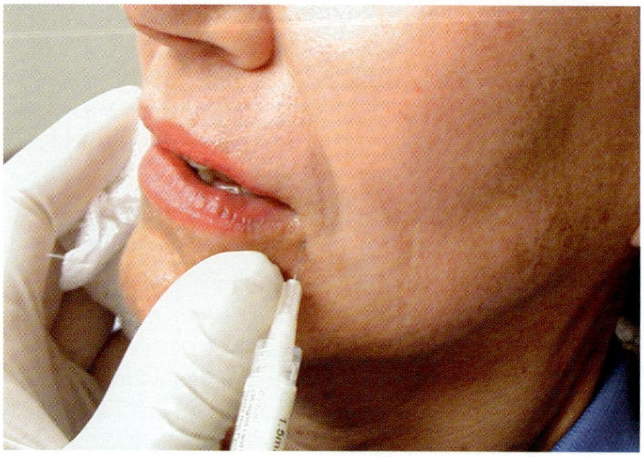

FIGURE 8-31. Collagen Injection Sequence. A,B: The nasolabial fold is shown being augmented with Zyplast. A 30-gauge needle is used here to inject the material into the deep dermis/upper subcutaneous plane. **C:** Only the upper third of the marionette line can be safely augmented with Zyplast. Generally, it requires a substantial amount to ameliorate this fold, and over-injection is unlikely (but still possible).

surgeon should not only try to augment the aged upper lip but focus on restoring a disproportionate amount in the flattened central aspect of Cupid's bow. The surgeon should infiltrate only 90% of the collagen and then have the patient assess the augmentation with a hand-held mirror to determine where the remainder of the collagen should be placed (Fig. 8-33A,B). This technique minimizes patient dissatisfaction and accords some responsibility to the patient for the ultimate outcome of the procedure.

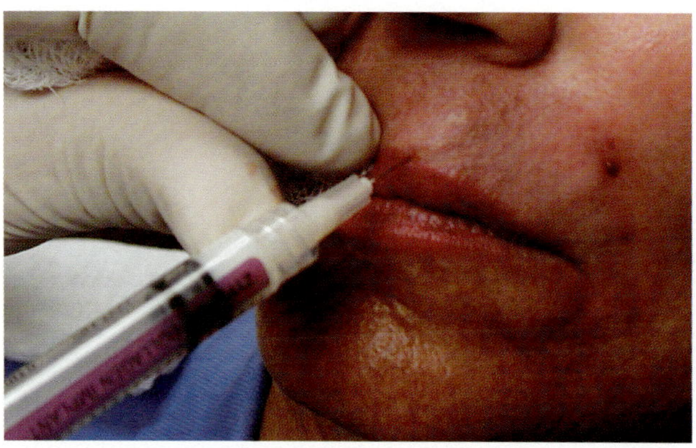

FIGURE 8-32. Collagen Injection Sequence. Zyplast can be used for deeper perioral crevices but is less forgiving in the typically finer rhytids that circumscribe the mouth.

DVD Botulinum Toxin

Botulinum toxin should be used to efface rhytids observed in motion only or incipient lines at rest and is reserved for wrinkles that occupy the upper half of the face (above the imaginary line drawn through the nasal base). In this section, the reader is presented a systematic fashion in which to inject BTX according to outlined zonal patterns of the upper face. Zone I is defined as the glabellar region; Zone II is the forehead; and Zone III refers to the lateral–canthal region, which in turn is subdivided into vertical thirds (Zones IIIA–C) (Fig. 8-34). The rationale for this zonal design will become apparent as the reader completes the study of this section.

The first step in BTX preparation is reconstitution of the refrigerated solid form. Preservative-free saline (4.5 cc) is used for reconstitution (Fig. 8-35): This amount is twice the recommended dilution: The authors have found that increased volume permits more even distribution across a wider expanse of tissue than a more concentrated mixture. However, no greater dilution than this advised amount should be undertaken, because very dilute (more than 15 cc)

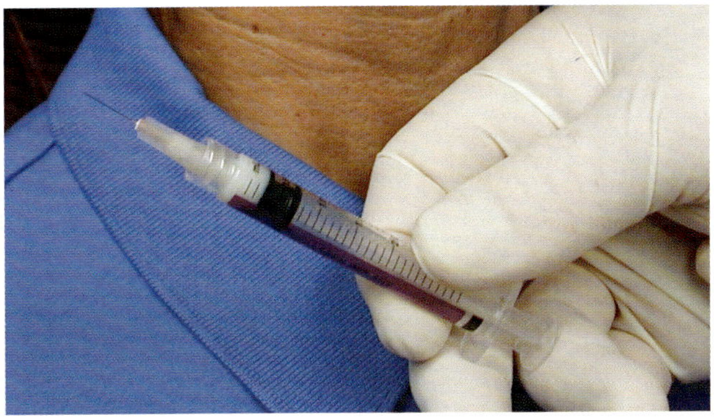

A

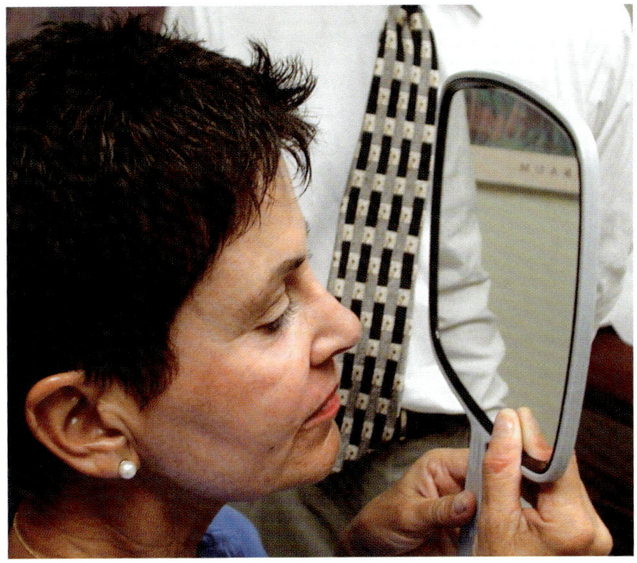

B

FIGURE 8-33. Collagen Injection Sequence. A,B: The patient should have 90% of the collagen infiltrated and given the opportunity to determine where the remaining 10% should be implanted after inspection with a hand-held mirror.

mixtures markedly decrease the potency of BTX. Further, a greater chance of toxin migration may occur at the higher volumes (more than 10 cc) that may lead to complications such as blepharoptosis or brow ptosis. A 5-cc syringe outfitted with an 18-gauge needle is used to draw up 4.5 cc of preservative-free saline, which is then in turn injected into the BTX bottle containing the unreconstituted solid. The mixture is gently swirled to ensure full dissolution of the unreconstituted BTX. It is very important not to shake the bottle vigorously because the toxin is easily denatured. The recommended dilution yields a concentration of five units per 0.2 cc of reconstituted BTX. Zone I (the glabella) typically requires 15 to 20 units (0.6 to 0.8 cc) depending on the extent of rhytidosis and the desired degree of restricted expression. Even though Zone II (the forehead) covers a greater expanse of tissue, the frontalis is less active than the medial–brow complex and requires usually 10 to 15 units (0.4 to 0.6 cc). Zone III (the lateral–canthal area) deserves between 10 to 20 units (0.4 to 0.8 cc) total, depending on the number of subdivided zones treated, requiring five to seven units (0.2 to 0.3 cc) for each subzone.

Before needle injection of BTX is carried out, the patient typically is asked to apply an ice pack to the proposed treatment areas for 5 to 10 minutes. The ice pack acts to anesthetize the area and reduce ecchymosis. Ecchymosis is diminished via two mechanisms: vasoconstriction of the muscular bed, which in turn minimizes the chance of needle laceration of a vessel, and diminution of the inflammatory cascade. Ice packs immediately after injection also can benefit the patient in a similar fashion. For the particularly sensitive patient, eutectic mixture of lidocaine and prilocaine (EMLA) cream—containing 2.5% lidocaine and 2.5% prilocaine—should be applied to the area at least 1 hour before the treatment time and held in place with transparent cling wrap (e.g., Saran Wrap). If the physician elects to use an alcohol preparatory wipe before BTX injection, he or she must wait until the alcohol has completely evaporated prior to injection because the alcohol can reduce the efficacy of the toxin.

Two principal techniques exist for BTX injection: fanning and percutaneous injection methods. Each technique has its benefits and drawbacks and is selected based on the intended Zone of treatment. The fanning method involves a single percutaneous insertion with multiple fanning strokes of the needle through the muscle belly. This method permits a more even distribution of BTX through the bulk of the muscle than the percutaneous technique. However, the 30-gauge needle attached to a 1-cc tuberculin syringe that is recommended for BTX injection is shorter (1/2″) as compared with the 27-gauge needle that has a 1¼″ length. Nevertheless, given the less traumatic caliber of the 30-gauge needle, the authors recommend use of this needle for BTX injection, whether for the fanning or percutaneous technique. The percutaneous technique involves multiple transcutaneous injections that are oriented perpendicular to the skin. Zone I (the glabella) has a particularly thick muscle (the corrugator) in a more discrete location, and the fanning method is recommended for an even and controlled treatment of this area. Conversely, Zone II (the forehead) is a larger, flatter muscle that benefits from the percutaneous technique in order to deliver adequate botulinum toxin over a greater territory. Zone III (the lateral canthus) is similar to Zone I in that the muscle surface area is more discrete and benefits from the even distribution afforded by the fanning technique.

Treatment for Zone I, the glabellar region, is addressed first. As mentioned, a total of 15 to 20 units (0.6 to 0.8 cc) is required to treat the area of rhytidosis effectively. The first time a patient is treated, the authors recommend a more conservative amount of toxin, especially if multiple areas are

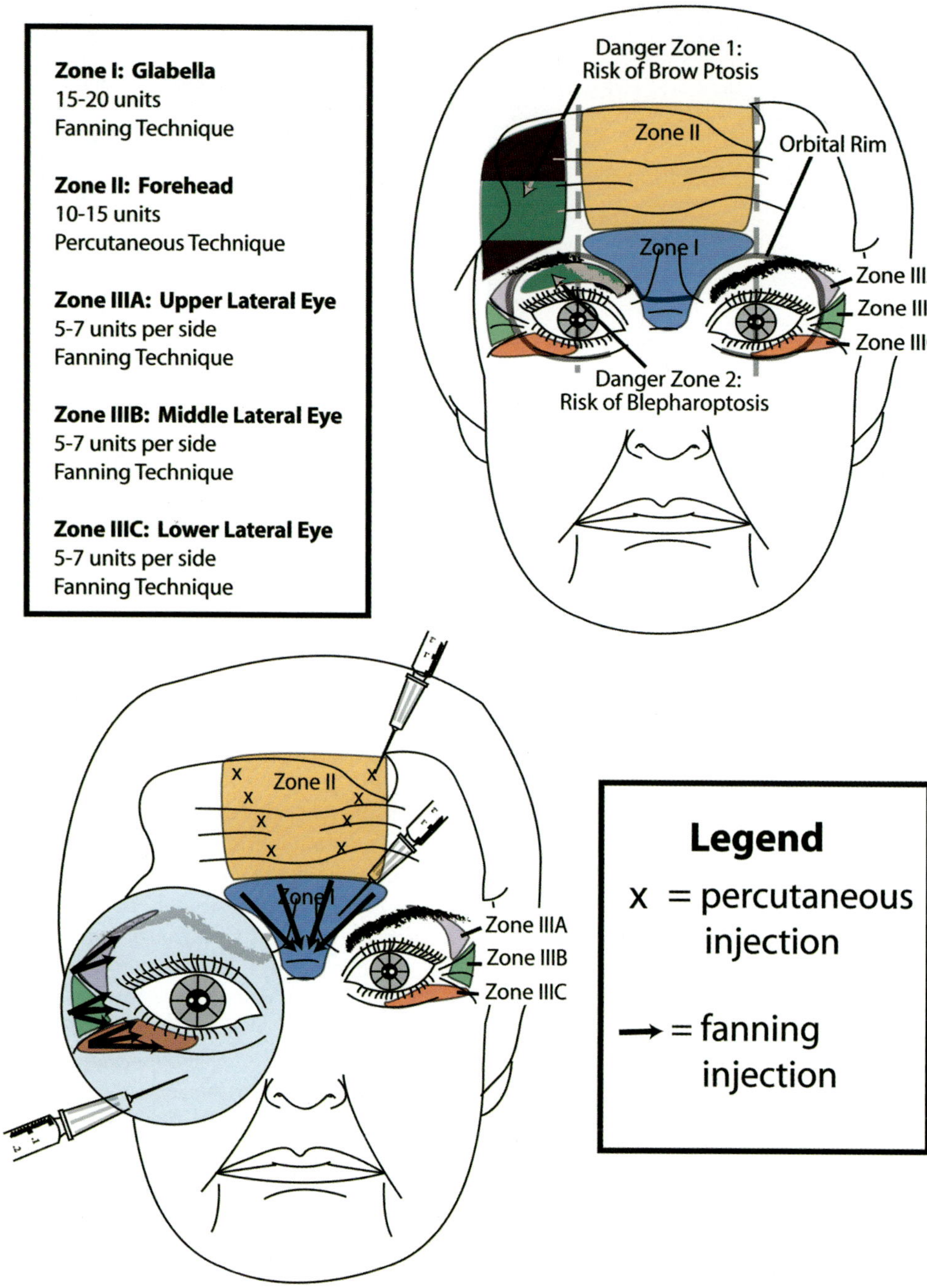

FIGURE 8-34. Illustration shows the three zones for botulinum toxin injection. Zone I is defined as the glabellar region; Zone II is the forehead; and Zone III refers to the lateral–canthal region, which in turn is subdivided into vertical thirds (Zones IIIA–C). The two danger zones to be avoided are the upper-eyelid region (which can lead to blepharoptosis) and the lateral-brow region (which can lead to brow ptosis). Preferred injection amounts and techniques are shown also.

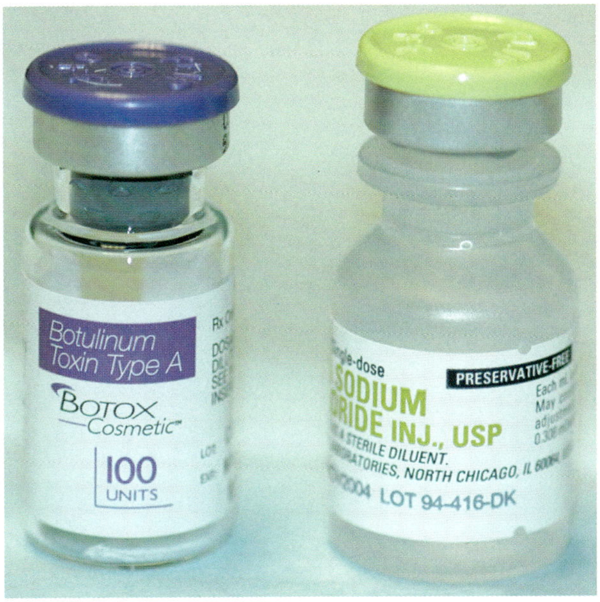

FIGURE 8-35. Botulinum toxin as manufactured by Allergan as Botox comes with 100 units of the unreconstituted form, which should be reconstituted with 4.5 cc (as the authors recommend) of preservative-free normal saline. After reconstitution, the bottle should not be vigorously shaken to avoid deactivation of the toxin. Instead, it should be gently turned upside down and right side up several times until complete dissolution of the powder.

to be treated or if the patient expresses concern about the inability of emotional display. The perimeter of Zone I that should be respected for safety and efficacy is as follows: between the medial club of the eyebrows down to the sellion (or deepest recess) of the nasal root, remaining at all times on the bony prominence of the glabella (Fig. 8-34). Superiorly, Zone I blends into Zone II above the root of the corrugator muscle. If the injection is placed down the slopes of the orbital rim toward the eye, the levator aponeurosis (the lid opening mechanism) or the central preseptal/pretarsal orbicularis-oculi muscle may be affected, impairing lid opening or closing. Injection further inferiorly past the sellion does not improve any horizontal rhytidosis, because the procerus muscle fibers become attenuated at this level. The patient should be asked to squint and frown so that the rhytidosis can be reproduced and the overactive muscles targeted. Usually the corrugators are more developed and cause the more apparent rhytidosis. During active squinting and frowning, the surgeon rolls the corrugator muscle between the index finger and thumb of the nondominant hand and injects the toxin in the described fanning technique with the other hand (Fig. 8-36A–C). The 30-gauge needle is short (1/2″), so two to three injections may be required to cover the entire muscle. The surgeon should be cognizant at all times of the amount of delivery so that an equal amount of toxin is applied to each side. The double-dilution method ensures a more even delivery and avoids the inadvertent delivery of too much toxin in an overly localized area. The remainder of BTX, if properly planned, may be used to treat the procerus according to the presence of horizontal rhytidosis.

Zone II refers to the forehead region and is defined as the area extending above Zone I from the medial club of the eyebrow upward and laterally toward the trichion (hairline) at the midpupil level (Figs. 8-34 and 8-37A–C). The recommended dose for this area is 10 to 15 units, with the upper end of the suggested dosage used particularly in men, who may have a more developed frontalis muscle. If the surgeon ventures too far laterally past the proposed perimeter of Zone II, he or she may accidentally cause brow ptosis. Therefore, a very active frontalis muscle may be reduced in activity in its central zone but not completely effaced in its lateral zone, which is a favorable outcome: Complete inactivity of the muscle looks unnatural and expressionless. Unlike the fanning technique that should be used for Zone I, the surgeon should use the multiple, percutaneous approach for the frontalis muscle in order to ensure adequate and even treatment of the central aspect of the frontalis. If Zone I and II should be concurrently treated, Zone I should be performed first, then Zone II starting from the inferior aspect in order to avoid accidental overlap of toxin injection.

Zone III defines the final area suitable for aesthetic BTX injection (i.e., the lateral–canthal region). In turn, this area is subdivided into three smaller zones. Zone IIIA refers to the upper third of the lateral orbicularis oculi that extends from the lateral canthus (medially) to the orbital rim below the eyebrow (superiorly) down to the upper crow's foot noted on squinting (inferiorly) to 1 cm lateral to the orbital rim (laterally). Zone IIIA is treated in order to effect a chemical browlift of the redundant lateral-brow tissue and to raise the hairy eyebrow to a more aesthetically pleasant configuration. However, this may be the most treacherous area to inject, because too medial an injection (over the preseptal or pretarsal orbicularis oculi) may cause blepharoptosis or interfere with the blink mechanism, and too far superiorly above the eyebrow (over the frontalis) may induce brow ptosis. Therefore, it is recommended that the surgeon stay in the lateral aspect of this area over the bony orbital rim but below the eyebrow, using five to seven units total per side or a more conservative amount initially (Fig. 8-38A–C). In rare circumstances, an overactive temporalis muscle may pull the unopposed eyebrows up dramatically, making the patient appear actually angry, which can be ameliorated with injections into the temporalis muscle. (The authors have never personally encountered this situation but have observed an anecdotal case.) In addition, excessive medial or superior injection gains little aesthetic benefit. The preferred technique of injection in this area is the described fanning technique for a more even infiltration of toxin.

Zone IIIB refers to the middle third of the lateral orbicularis oculi that spans from the upper to the lower rhytid

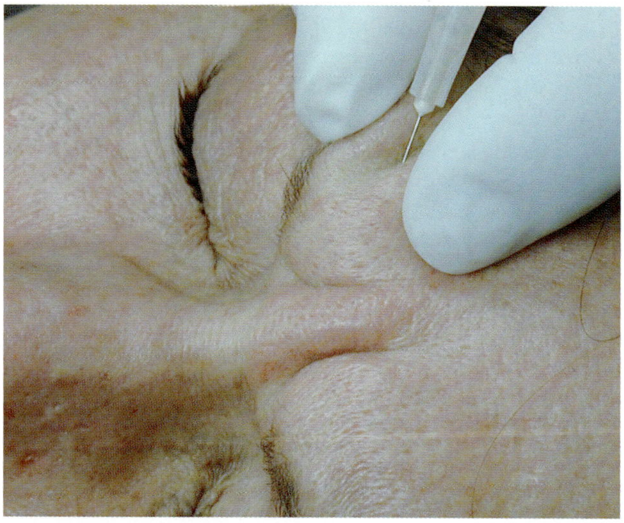
A

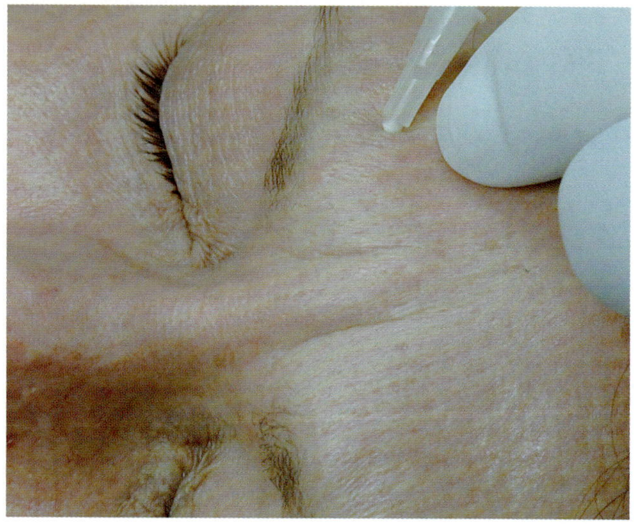
B

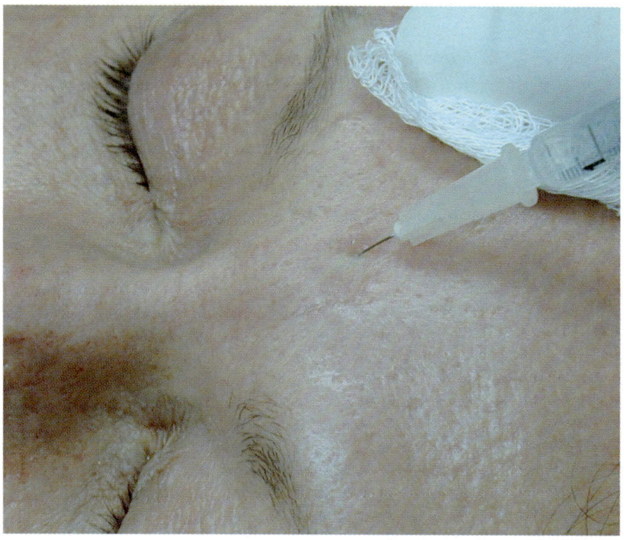
C

FIGURE 8-36. Botulinum Toxin Injection Sequence, Zone I. A–C: During active squinting and frowning, the surgeon rolls the corrugator muscle between the index finger and thumb of the nondominant hand and injects the botulinum toxin in the described fanning technique with the other hand. Because the 30-gauge needle is rather short (1/2″), two to three injections may be required to cover the entire muscle. The surgeon should be cognizant at all times of the amount of delivery so that an equal amount of toxin is applied to each side. A total of 15 to 20 units should be injected into Zone I.

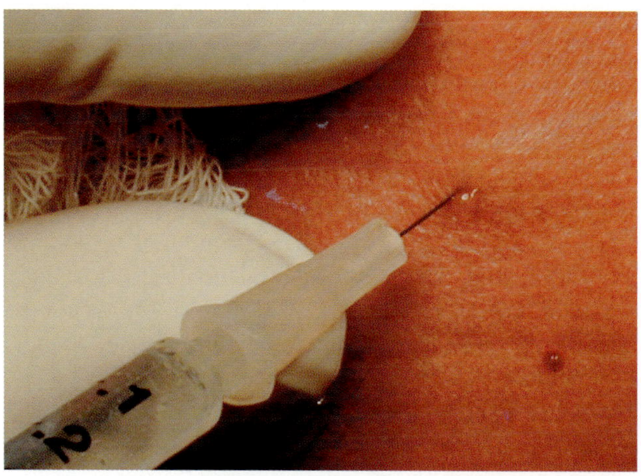
A

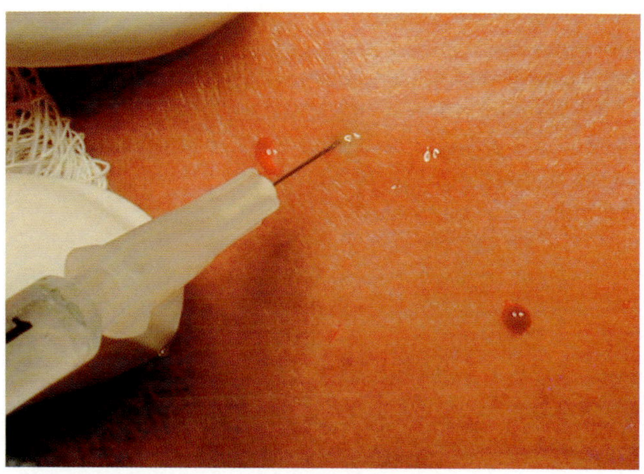
B

FIGURE 8-37. Botulinum Toxin Injection Sequence, Zone II. A–C: Zone II (the forehead) is injected using the percutaneous technique for a total of 10 to 15 units, ensuring distribution of toxin in a symmetrical fashion. The perimeter of Zone II is defined as the area that extends above Zone I upward and laterally toward the trichion at the midpupil level. More lateral placement of toxin risks inadvertent brow ptosis. *(continued)*

C
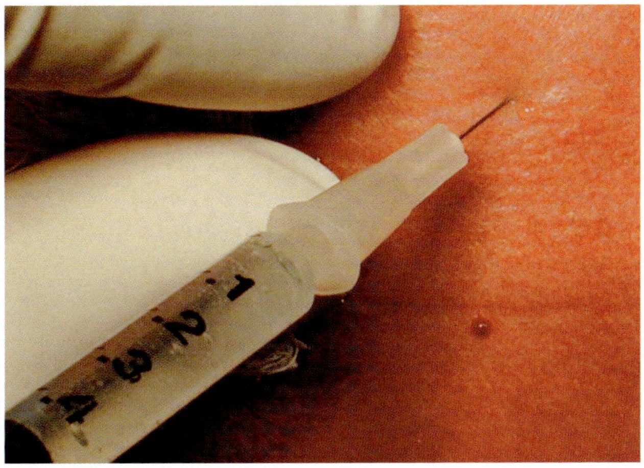

FIGURE 8-37. *(Continued).*

A B C
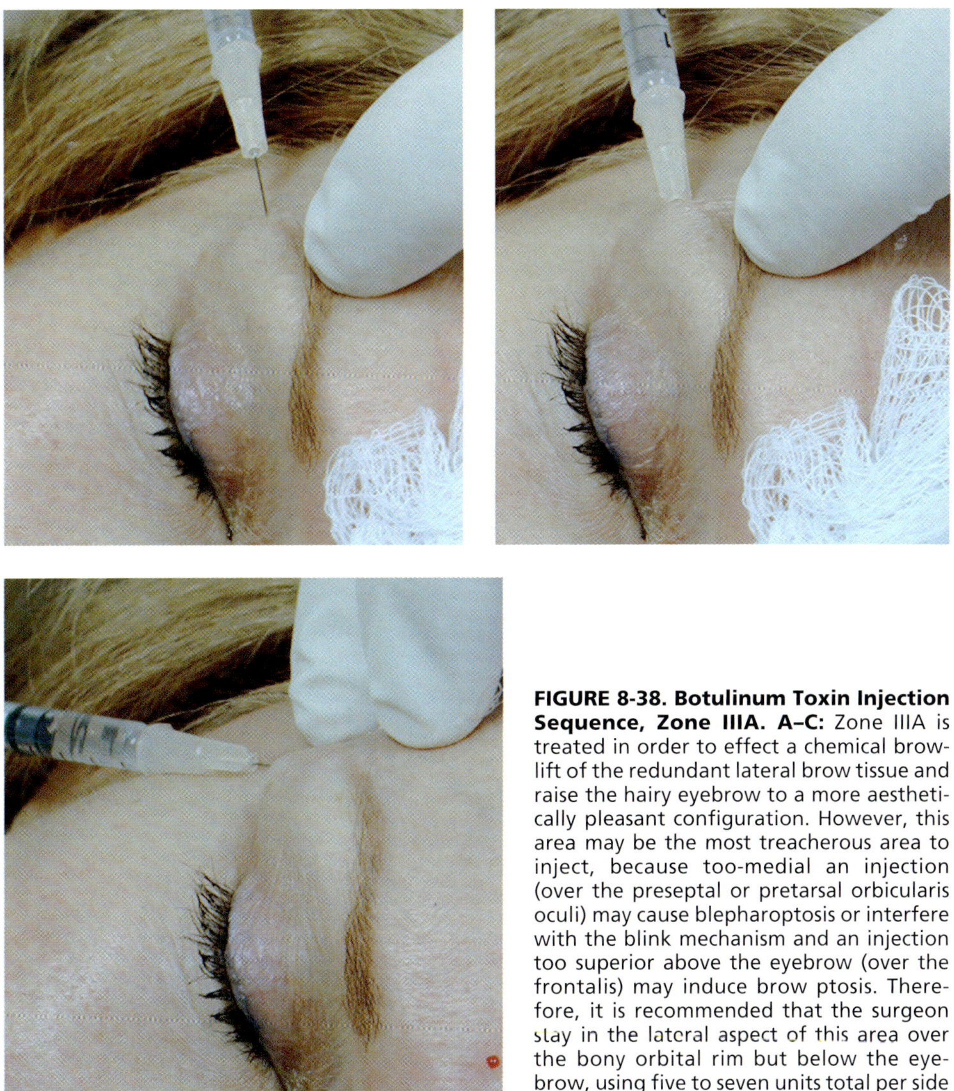

FIGURE 8-38. Botulinum Toxin Injection Sequence, Zone IIIA. A–C: Zone IIIA is treated in order to effect a chemical browlift of the redundant lateral brow tissue and raise the hairy eyebrow to a more aesthetically pleasant configuration. However, this area may be the most treacherous area to inject, because too-medial an injection (over the preseptal or pretarsal orbicularis oculi) may cause blepharoptosis or interfere with the blink mechanism and an injection too superior above the eyebrow (over the frontalis) may induce brow ptosis. Therefore, it is recommended that the surgeon stay in the lateral aspect of this area over the bony orbital rim but below the eyebrow, using five to seven units total per side or a more conservative amount initially.

Salient Technical Points

Acellular Dermis and Expanded Polytetrafluoroethylene Augmentation of the Nasolabial, Labiomandibular, and Labial Regions

1. The technique for acellular dermis, ePTFE, and SMAS insertion for augmentation is identical except for preparation of the implant. Details on SMAS insertion are included in Chapter 5 because it is inserted during a rhytidectomy. As mentioned therein, SMAS should not be used for lip augmentation. For the amount of acellular dermis required for augmentation, the reader is referred to Table 8-1. Also, before acellular dermis insertion, it should be rolled lengthwise and sutured in that configuration using 5-0 chromic suture in an interrupted fashion. From experience, acellular dermis has been safely used in lip augmentation as well as nasolabial and labiomandibular augmentation, whereas ePTFE has not been a viable material for lip augmentation (Table 8-1).
2. After appropriate infiltration of local anesthesia, stab incisions should be made for insertion of the implant:
   a. For the nasolabial fold, the incision should be made parallel and within the crease about 5 mm away from the alar–facial groove and another stab incision, at the lowest extent of the nasolabial fold.
   b. For the labiomandibular fold, the stab incision should be placed at the inferior extent of the fold and inside the buccal mucosa that parallels the fold (for a deeper groove) or just at the vermilion–cutaneous junction (for less substantial augmentation).
   c. For the lips, the stab incisions should be placed at the junction of the wet and dry lip approximately 4 to 5 mm medial to each oral commissure for both the upper and lower lips.
3. The implant is then tied very securely to a 0-silk suture that carries a 60-mm Keith needle.
4. The introducer is inserted through one stab incision and guided using the nondominant hand toward the other incision in the subcutaneous plane for the nasolabial and labiomandibular folds and in the plane between the mucosa and orbicularis oris for the lip.
5. With the introducer left in the tunnel, the 60-mm needle is guided into the introducer's groove until it is visible through the other incision. The introducer is withdrawn, keeping the needle in place.
6. A hemostat is placed on the free, untied end of the implant to prevent the implant from being overpulled through the pocket.
7. The needle is drawn through the tunnel in order to guide the implant into position. With the silk held in one hand and the hemostat in the other, the implant can be pulled back and forth until it feels to be in the proper position.
8. The silk suture is cut free from the implant. With proper retraction using tiny, double hooks at the incision site, the implant is tucked further distal to the incision site by 5 to 10 mm on both ends.
9. The incision is then closed with 6-0 polypropylene on the skin and 5-0 chromic on the lip.

Advancement Cheiloplasty

1. This technique is reserved only for the mature patient who is willing to accept a visible scar that must be camouflaged with lipstick.
2. The surgeon marks the anticipated extent of advancement, generally twice the distance that is desired, because some loss of vertical height will occur over time. Use of Castroviejo calipers can provide the most precise and accurate measurements. The surgeon should begin to mark the proposed line of excision at 5 mm medial to the oral commissure to avoid scarring from excessive lateral dissection. The surgeon should mark the line of skin excision at slightly less than a 2-to-1 ratio (proposed excision to desired vermilion height) for the majority of the lip and slightly more than a 2-to-1 ratio at the philtrum (i.e., at the peaks of Cupid's bow). Care should be taken not to exaggerate the flare of Cupid's bow too much because this is a glaring stigma of poor surgery.
3. A No. 15 blade should be used to score the skin superficially along the entire perimeter of the incision just to the depth of the mid-dermis, all the while beveling away from the center of the wound. Bishop forceps or tiny, double hooks are used to retract the skin upward as the surgeon meticulously dissects the skin at the middermal level with a No. 15 blade: The white dermis should be noted above and below the knife blade as dissection continues.
4. The wound edges are everted and approximated with interrupted, vertical mattress sutures at the key anatomic landmarks (i.e., at the height of Cupid's bow and at the central depression point between Cupid's bow). Similarly, interrupted, vertical mattress sutures of 6-0 silk are then used to close the remainder of the wound in an everted fashion.

Geometric Broken-Line Repair for Deep, Vertical Glabellar Rhytidosis

1. This technique is indicated for very deep, vertical glabellar rhytids.
2. The rhytid is outlined in a fusiform configuration.

3. Castroviejo calipers are used to measure a precise 3- to 4-mm dotted line on both sides of the fusiform border.
4. Geometric shapes (squares, rectangles, triangles, and trapezoids) should be drawn out in an alternating fashion from one side of the line to the other along the entire length of the proposed incision to fit within the 3- or 4-mm limbs. The surgeon should not undertake drawing shapes along one entire side and then the other side to limit confusion about trying to match each shape to the corresponding defect.
5. Local anesthesia of 1% lidocaine and 1;100,000 epinephrine is infiltrated into the area.
6. A No. 11 blade is used to incise each shape and its corresponding defect in the same alternating fashion as used to draw the shapes. In order to maintain the integrity of the dermal sling, the skin is only perforated with the No. 11 blade so that tiny bridges of epidermis remain intact between perforations.
7. The tiny skin bridges are joined and the rhytid excised. The wound edges are undermined laterally several millimeters in the subcutaneous plane to facilitate wound eversion and reduce wound tension.
8. The corrugator muscle is transected on either side of the wound with sharp scissors and partially avulsed. Dissection should not stray too far laterally to avoid injury to the supratrochlear neurovascular bundle.
9. One to two deep sutures of 4-0 polydioxanone are used to approximate the deep tissues and reduce wound tension.
10. A 6-0 fast-absorbing suture is fastened at one end of the wound and run in a locking fashion toward the other end by suturing only the free corners of the created shapes on the surgeon's right side to the corresponding defects on the left side as a right-handed surgeon faces the wound. Similarly, a 6-0 fast-absorbing suture is fastened on the contralateral end of the wound and run toward the other end of the wound in a running, locking fashion as described.
11. Steri-Strips are applied in a transverse direction to the wound in order to minimize tension.
12. Wire-brush dermabrasion should be used at 6 weeks to achieve an inconspicuous scar.

Botulinum Toxin

1. Botulinum toxin should be reserved for treatment of wrinkles above the imaginary, horizontal line drawn through the nasal base (Fig. 8-1).
2. For a summary of indications and techniques, the reader is referred to Tables 8-2 and 8-3.

Collagen

1. The patient must undergo a collagen test patch in the antecubital area a minimum of 30 days before administration of collagen. For equivocal results, a second test patch is recommended with another 30-day observation period.
2. For ease of stocking and for the benefit of greater longevity, the authors only use the Zyplast form of collagen.
3. The 1.5-cc syringe contains a more cost effective amount for typical augmentation required for the aging face. The 1.0-cc syringe should be reserved for younger patients who desire limited lip augmentation. For ease of inventory, the physician can elect to stock only the 1.5-cc syringes.
4. Injection can be carried out either with a 30-gauge needle or the specialized needle that comes supplied with every collagen kit. The specialized needle permits reducing the length of the exposed tip to control depth of the injection.
5. Injection of Zyplast should be carried out in the deep dermis to minimize contour irregularities and provide maximal longevity.
6. Any notable contour irregularities should be managed by rolling the area between one's fingers and encouraging the patient to do the same thereafter.
7. The physician should retain about 10% of the collagen at the end of treatment and offer the patient a hand-held mirror to determine where else the patient feels should be augmented. This technique minimizes patient complaints that more should have been injected in a particular area of concern.
8. Generally, a greater proportion of collagen is injected into the upper lip than in the lower lip, because the patient typically perceives a greater benefit in this area. For the labiomandibular fold, only the upper one third should be injected, as the lower two thirds usually cannot be effaced. Often, the upper portion of the labiomandibular fold requires significant amount of collagen to achieve the desired effacement.

TABLE 8–2. SUMMARY OF IDEAL AND ALTERNATIVE AUGMENTATION MATERIALS AND TREATMENT FOR VARIOUS FACIAL LINES

Location	Treatment
Glabella	Botulinum toxin: Motion only or early wrinkles at rest. Trichloroacotic acid (TCA) peel: Early, minimal wrinkles at rest. CO_2 laser: Moderate to deep wrinkles at rest. Geometric broken-line repair: Deep to very deep wrinkles at rest. Collagen: Contraindicated, risk of blindness. Expanded polytetrafluoroethylene (EPTFE), acellular dermis: Acceptable alternative to resurfacing for moderate to deep wrinkles. Should not be used for very shallow wrinkles and is less effective than the geometric broken-line repair for very deep wrinkles. May risk palpability and visibility and are not preferred techniques for this area.
Lateral-canthal region	Botulinum toxin: Motion only or early wrinkles at rest. TCA peel: Early, fine wrinkles at rest. CO_2 laser: Deep, coarse wrinkles at rest.
Nasolabial and labiomandibular folds	Acellular dermis: For semipermanent to permanent augmentation, may lose volume over time, may be less palpable than ePTFE. EPTFE: Permanent augmentation, may be more palpable than acellular dermis. Superficial musculoaponeurotic system (SMAS) insertion: For semipermanent to permanent augmentation, harvested during a facelift (Chapter 5). Collagen (Zyplast): For temporary augmentation. Botulinum toxin: Not recommended by the authors.
Lips	Acellular dermis: For semipermanent to permanent augmentation (see above). Collagen (Zyplast): For temporary augmentation. Advancement cheiloplasty: Reserved for patients who are more mature and are willing to wear lipstick to camouflage a potentially visible scar. EPTFE: Not recommended by the authors. SMAS: Not recommended by the authors. Botulinum toxin: Not recommended by the authors.
Peri-oral rhagades	CO_2-laser resurfacing: Ideal for numerous, fine wrinkles (Chapter 9). Dermabrasion: Good alternative to laser resurfacing but technically more demanding. TCA peel: Not very effective. Collagen: Zyderm is easier to fill these wrinkles but has less longevity than Zyplast. For ease of stocking and for greater longevity, Zyplast is preferred by the authors but should be used with discretion to avoid contour irregularities. Botulinum toxin: Not recommended by the authors.

TABLE 8–3. SUMMARY OF BOTULINUM-TOXIN TREATMENT STRATEGY

	Zone I	Zone II	Zone IIIA	Zone IIIB	Zone IIIC
Area	Glabella	Forehead	Upper lateral periocular region	Middle lateral periocular region	Lower lateral periocular region
Muscles targeted	Corrugator and procerus	Frontalis	Upper lateral orbicularis oculi	Middle lateral orbicularis oculi	Lower lateral orbicularis oculi
Objective	Eliminate medial depressor rhytidosis	Attenuate forehead rhytidosis	Effect chemical browlift	Eliminate lateral rhytids, or crow's feet	Eliminate lower-lid hypertrophic roll of orbicularis oculi and lower-lid rhytidosis
No. units	15–20 Units	10–15 Units	5–7 Units*	5–7 Units	5–7 Units
Volume	0.6–0.8 cc**	0.4–0.6 cc	0.2–0.3 cc	0.2–0.3 cc	0.2–0.3 cc
Technique	Fanning	Percutaneous	Fanning	Fanning	Fanning
Cautions	Eye opening and closing dysfunction, ptosis	Brow ptosis	Brow ptosis, eye opening and closing dysfunction, ptosis, ecchymosis†	Eye opening and closing dysfunction, ptosis, ecchymosis†	Ectropion, ecchymosis,† worsening of festooning

* Five to seven units total are used per side and per subzone (i.e., for Zone IIIA, IIIB, or IIIC).
** Volume calculated based on the double-dilutional method (0.2 cc = five units)
† Direct digital pressure should be applied for ten sustained minutes using a 4 × 4 gauze immediately after injection to minimize ecchymosis.

noted during squinting or at rest to 1 cm lateral to the orbital rim. Zone IIIB is treated in order to efface the lateral periocular rhytidosis, or crow's feet. Again, the surgeon should be wary of excessive medial infiltration over the preseptal or pretarsal orbicularis oculi, especially superiorly toward the levator. The fanning technique is recommended, starting 1 cm lateral to the orbital rim and injecting the span of the needle length (1/2″) with the recommended 30-gauge needle using five to seven units per side and per subzone (i.e., for each Zone IIIA, IIIB, and IIIC).

Zone IIIC represents the area that traverses the lower eyelid and appears as the fine rhytids and hypertrophy of the orbicularis muscle that develops either on animation or at rest. The perimeter of this zone is defined superiorly by the lowest lateral rhytid (crow's foot) down to the orbital rim inferiorly, laterally, and medially toward the midpupil below the ciliary margin by 3 mm. The surgeon may more safely inject the preseptal and even pretarsal orbicularis oculi to efface the hypertrophic roll of the orbicularis oculi or lower-lid rhytidosis without any notable adverse effect on the blink mechanism. (Eye closure is primarily derived from upper-lid closure.) However, the lower-lid tone must be carefully evaluated before injection because any lower-lid laxity may lead to postinjection rounding or ectropion. Therefore, astute attention must be paid to the patient's anatomy to determine the level of impunity that the surgeon may exercise. The same technique and recommended dosage as for Zones IIIA and IIIB are advocated for Zone IIIC as well. An important contraindication should be mentioned for treatment of Zone IIIC: Malar bags or orbicularis festooning may be exacerbated by BTX as the muscle then becomes more lax, causing further outpouching of the muscle.

In general, Zone III reveals the greatest extent of ecchymosis postoperatively that should be addressed with immediate and sustained digital pressure with a 4 × 4 gauze for a period of 10 minutes. The assistant should resist the urge to remove the gauze temporarily for inspection, because this will compromise the effect of pressure application. Further, ice is not used in combination with pressure because the ice interferes with the ability for maximal and even pressure on this area. At the conclusion, patients are handed postoperative-care instructions that inform them not to massage the treated area because this behavior disperses the toxin to unintended regions.

POSTOPERATIVE CONSIDERATIONS: CARE, FOLLOW-UP, AND COMPLICATIONS

Postoperative Care and Follow-Up

Postoperative care for the adjunctive procedures is relatively straightforward for the surgical, incision-based procedures (e.g., routine antibiotic ointment applied to incision sites and suture removal at 1 week postoperatively). However, a few salient points should be mentioned regarding proper postoperative care for collagen and BTX patients.

For BTX patients, a postoperative care sheet should be given to remind them of one essential preventative measure, not to massage the treated areas. (Refer to the end of Chapter 3 for a copy of this form.) The risk of massaging the toxin into adjacent muscles such as the levator complex that would lead to blepharoptosis is a real concern. Some caveats that often have been suggested by other physicians—such as to reduce physical activity for a day and maintain an upright posture for several hours—have not been found to be necessary in the authors' clinical experience. The other purpose of the care sheet is to inform the patient of the 2- to 3-day (and at times up to 1-week) latency of toxin activity and to encourage them to call if any problems or inquiries arise.

Collagen and Botulinum Toxin

As patients who have undergone collagen or BTX injection do not require any formal postoperative care visits (e.g., suture, drain, or dressing removal), the surgeon is advised to contact the patient by telephone if a scheduled visit has not been made. This personal communication is much appreciated by the patient and permits the surgeon to establish whether the intended aesthetic objective has been properly met. Generally, a postoperative call to the patient regardless of procedure facilitates good rapport and is always recommended. If the surgeon does not have time to contact all of his or her patients who have undergone minor office procedures, then his nurse or office assistant should place the call instead. The phone call should be made about 3 to 5 days postoperatively, and the surgeon should inquire as to patient satisfaction and as to whether any adverse outcomes were encountered (e.g., allergic reaction, bruising, asymmetry, etc.). If the patient expresses any concern about the aesthetic result, he or she should be promptly scheduled for a postoperative visit. At the postoperative visit, the surgeon will be able to assess whether the patient's complaints are justified or whether they reflect ignorance on the part of the patient regarding a projected outcome. Education using a hand-held mirror often alleviates the frustration or misperception about the intended result. Furthermore, preoperative photographs may further enhance patient education and can be used if necessary. If the surgeon and patient agree that no discernible result is evident, then the patient should be offered retreatment without payment. Although this policy may seem costly to the surgeon's practice, the long-term dividends reaped by patient retention and satisfaction are incalculable.

Complications and Management

Botulinum Toxin

Fortunately, complications arising from BTX injections remain relatively rare in properly trained hands. The principal complication that may arise after BTX injection is asymmetry. However, asymmetry was often present preoperatively but went unnoticed by the patient until subjected to the obsessive scrutiny that is characteristic of the postoperative period. If asymmetry results from improper technique, then the surgeon should attempt to ameliorate the condition with additional BTX as deemed achievable. For instance, if a unilateral brow ptosis arises from laterally placed injection in the frontalis muscle, then the surgeon may opt to restore symmetry by carefully placing additional toxin in Zone IIIA on the affected side to weaken the depressor effect of the orbicularis and thereby elevate the brow. However, care should be taken not to venture too far medially and disturb the levator mechanism, compounding the problem. If blepharoptosis arises after a BTX injection, then injury to the levator, albeit temporary, most likely has transpired. The surgeon should then assess whether any visual field deficit has occurred and attempt to correct this condition with appropriate topical eye drops (e.g., phenylephrine 2.5%, Neo-Synephrine). Phenylephrine has an onset of action within 30 to 60 minutes with a duration that lasts 3 to 5 hours. However, narrow-angle glaucoma is an important contraindication to remember. Furthermore, because pupillary dilation also results, near vision and accommodation may be compromised during usage. If lagophthalmos arises, then the surgeon's primary goal is ocular protection from exposure keratitis. Vigorous and attentive ocular lubrication is mandatory if the patient cannot protect the globe. The surgeon also should advise the patient to engage in squinting exercises in order to strengthen any of the still-viable muscle fibers that have not been paralyzed.

Collagen

As alluded to earlier, the most technically difficult aspect of Zyplast injection is placement in the proper plane (i.e., deep dermis). Irregular contour that may arise should be addressed with careful massage until the irregularity resolves. If the collagen is placed too superficially into the dermis, more evident contour irregularity will be apparent and massage may be less successful in immediate improvement of this problem. The surgeon always should be observing how the collagen appears during injection and ensures that only minute discrete injections are placed in any single locus to avoid this problem.

The most serious consequence of improper or unfortunate collagen injection is blindness and skin slough. However, if the surgeon remains below the proposed imaginary line drawn through the nasal base, this complication should never arise. Furthermore, the thin, periocular skin is particularly difficult to achieve uniformity in contour with the less forgiving Zyplast. If the reader elects to proceed with periocular collagen injection, then Zyderm I or II should be used. As mentioned, the glabella should be avoided at all costs because this particular area has been noted to have the highest incidence of complications.

Acellular Dermis and Expanded Polytetrafluoroethylene

The complications that may arise with acellular dermis and ePTFE are applicable to any alloplast (e.g., visibility, palpability, malposition, mobility, extrusion, and infection). Palpability is less often a problem with acellular dermis, but it is a known postoperative result rather than a complication of ePTFE implantation, and the patient should be advised accordingly in the preoperative period. Visibility may arise owing to technical error in that the implant was improperly placed too superficially or in the wrong site (e.g., laterally over the prominence of the nasolabial fold) (Figs. 8-39A,B). Limited mobility may be tolerated unless the patient complains of this problem, in which case removal and delayed

A

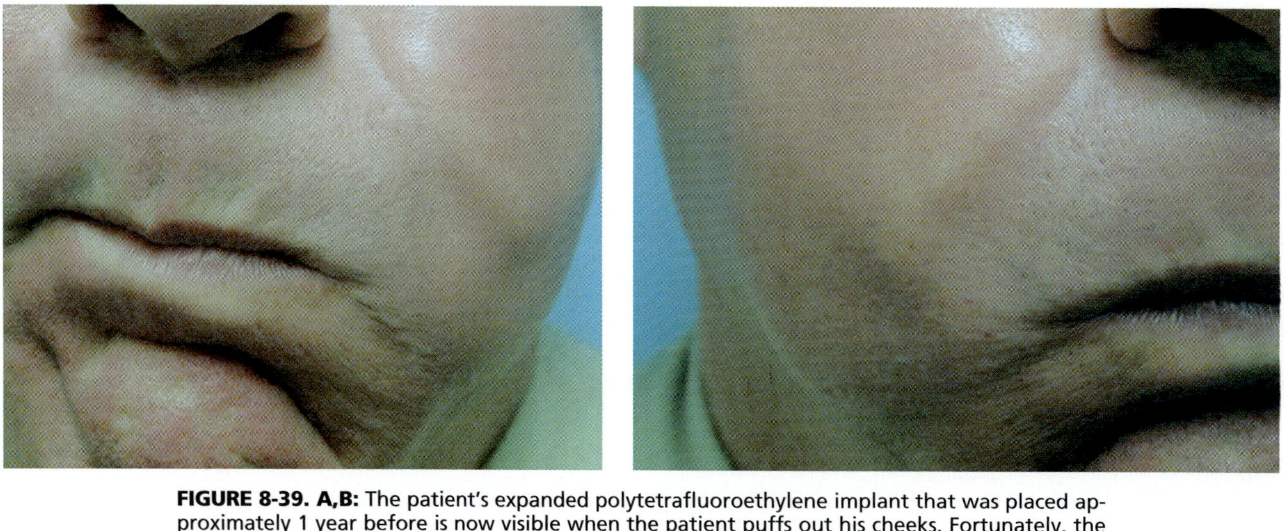

B

FIGURE 8-39. A,B: The patient's expanded polytetrafluoroethylene implant that was placed approximately 1 year before is now visible when the patient puffs out his cheeks. Fortunately, the implants remain camouflaged in the resting or less animated state.

reimplantation may correct this situation. Malposition should be taken care of by careful repositioning of the implant if possible or trimming the malpositioned portion with or without reinsertion of it. Extrusion may be handled in a similar fashion (i.e., repositioning, trimming, and reinsertion of the implant). An infection should be promptly treated with a single dose of intravenous antibiotics that cover gram-positive flora and an equivalent oral antibiotic for a full 10 days. If purulence is noted, then culture should be obtained, and the same antibiotic regimen prescribed. However, frank abscess usually invariably mandates implant removal and reinsertion at a later date after the infection has cleared (Fig. 8-40).

Direct Excision and Geometric Broken-Line Repair of Glabellar Rhytids

This section does not review basic management strategies for complications that arise after incision-based surgery (e.g., hematoma, infection, and wound dehiscence) but aim to describe the peculiar problems that may be associated with this adjunctive procedure. If overresection of the corrugator muscle is undertaken, a postoperative depression may result. This complication is particularly difficult to treat, but patience may prove to be a most valuable asset. An alloplast (e.g., ePTFE) may serve to fill in this defect should it arise but is less than optimal. Alternatively, the wound can be revised by further undermining and rotating some adjacent muscle under the incision line. Aggressive corrugator dissection also can lead to injury of the supratrochlear bundle, which usually returns over time. Unfortunately, no real treatment exists for this complication except patient reassurance. Any visible scar irregularity should be addressed with dermabrasion staged 6 weeks after the initial surgery. Patients should be advised of this likelihood before the primary surgery. Finally, any return of muscle function can be addressed with adjuvant BTX therapy if needed.

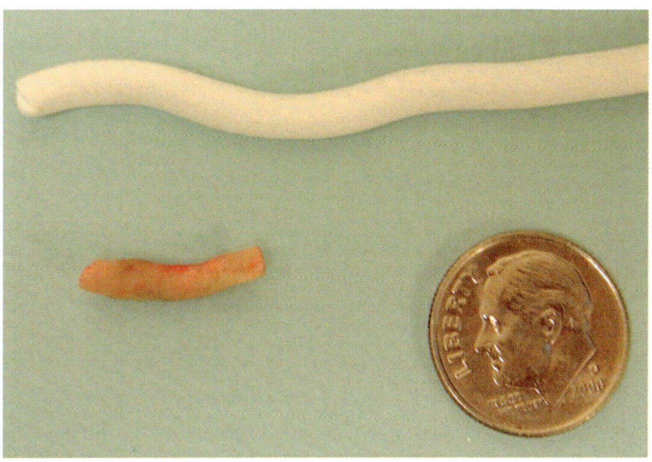

FIGURE 8-40. This expanded polytetrafluoroethylene (ePTFE) implant *(below)* was placed into a patient's lips and after repeated bouts of infection required removal. The implant was noted to be indurated and contracted, which may or may not have been related to the episodes of infection. The original ePTFE implant *(above)* is shown for contrast. Because of the high incidence of palpability, visibility, extrusion, and infection in the lip region, the authors have turned away from ePTFE for lip augmentation in favor of acellular dermis. Expanded polytetrafluoroethylene has been noted to be a safe alternative for areas of less animation such as the nasolabial and labiomandibular folds.

CLINICAL PRESENTATIONS: A SYNTHESIS OF APPROACH

Case #1 (Fig. 8-41A–D)

This is a 58-year-old patient who was referred by her dermatologist for BTX therapy. On questioning the patient, her only real concern was the deep vertical furrow that emanated medial to her right eyebrow. On examination, this patient exhibited an entrenched furrow that was present even in a resting state. On animation, the furrow became only slightly more obvious. Based on this patient's examination and her desires, it was felt that she would not receive considerable improvement from BTX therapy alone. Because the only area that troubled her was the very pronounced, vertical, glabellar rhytids rather than any neighboring rhytidosis in her forehead or lateral periocular regions, she was counseled that a surgical option (e.g., a geometric broken-line repair) would probably offer her the best solution to her particular concern. She was also informed that subsequent dermabrasion with or without CO_2-laser resurfacing would most likely be required 6 weeks after initial treatment to ensure optimal scar camouflage. Further, she was carefully advised that the procedure also would target the underlying corrugator muscle that engendered this problem, but that attenuation of this muscle would not be complete nor would it be likely permanent owing to reattachment and hypertrophy of the existing muscle fibers. Accordingly, based on postoperative evaluation and the patient's own inspection, BTX therapy at that point would be indicated to maintain the surgical result if the patient so desired.

Procedures

Excision of the vertical furrow, lysis of corrugator and procerus muscles, and a geometric broken-line repair followed by a combined technique using dermabrasion and CO_2-laser resurfacing 6 weeks later.

Discussion

Botulinum toxin therapy can prevent wrinkles from arising with consistent and ongoing treatment and can even soften early or incipient wrinkles but fails to address deep wrinkles that are present at rest. Browlift surgery also fails to eliminate glabellar rhytidosis and, according to the authors' opin-

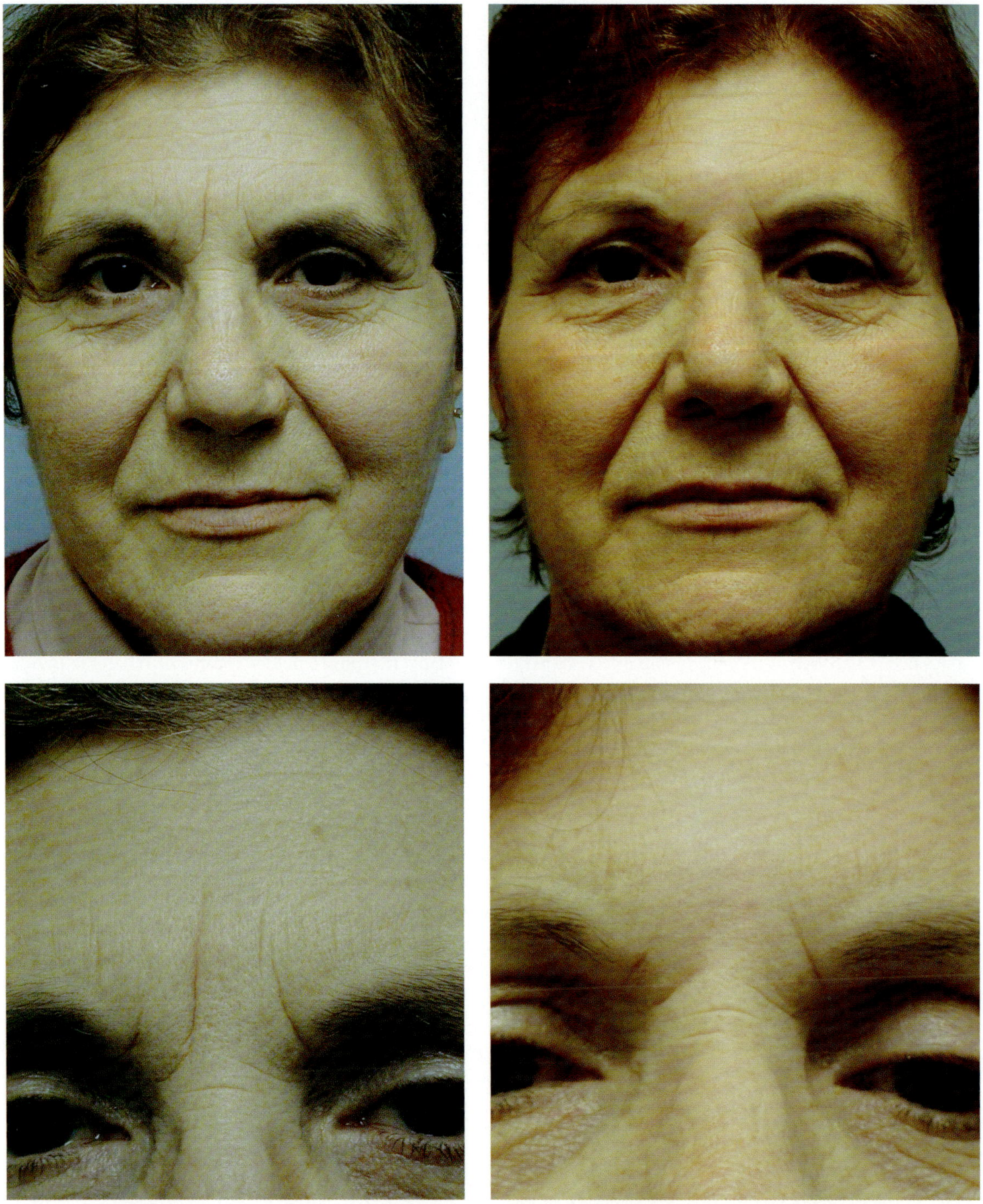

A C B D

FIGURE 8-41. A–D: This is a 58-year-old woman who was referred by her dermatologist for botulinum toxin (BTX) treatment of her deep, vertical glabellar lines. The patient was informed that BTX therapy would be ineffective for her deeply inscribed lines but that a scar-revision technique would be more suitable if she was only interested in treatment of this select area. She underwent direct excision of the scar and attenuation of the underlying corrugator muscle followed by geometric broken-line repair. She then had the area of scar revision refined with staged dermabrasion and CO_2-laser resurfacing 6 weeks later. She is shown 2 years later.

ion, is not a reliable method to prevent wrinkles by dissection of the underlying musculature, because muscle function inevitably returns. Nevertheless, attenuation of the muscle bed during direct excisional surgery is undertaken because of the immediate access to this site and the little additional labor or morbidity involved in removal of some underlying muscle. As mentioned, the patient should be counseled that not all muscle activity is eliminated and return of muscle strength can reach the preoperative level over time. In particular, care is taken not to resect muscle that lies very far past the wound edges because of the risk of permanent sensory impairment of the supratrochlear nerve that courses through the corrugator muscle.

If the patient requires a browlift as well, then browlift surgery should be undertaken before direct excisional surgery. If the browlift is performed after a direct excision, the tension on the wound during release of the arcus marginalis along the periorbital rim may disrupt the delicate suture line for several months after the procedure. Concurrent browlift and direct excision are also not recommended, because the increased edema that arises with a browlift can adversely affect wound healing in the area of scar revision and also impair judgment as to how to approximate the wound edges precisely. If the patient is unwilling to accept a staged repair of this area, then concurrent resurfacing with a CO_2 laser may help improve (but not necessarily entirely eliminate) a very deep rhytid (see the following). The reader is reminded that resurfacing over the brow region can be carried out safely concurrently with a minimally invasive browlift so long as the plane of dissection is maintained at the subperiosteal level.

A resurfacing modality may be a reasonable option to address the problem of an intermediate-depth rhytid. Certainly, resurfacing is a much less labor-intensive modality than scar revision using the geometric broken-line technique. Unfortunately, Jessner's and 35% TCA are not particularly effective for medium to deep rhytidosis in this area. CO_2-laser resurfacing is a better option and can be combined with a full-face TCA peel to achieve a more uniform appearance to the resurfaced skin if the patient is willing to tolerate the recovery. CO_2 laser alone can be used in a targeted approach to the glabellar rhytid. Although resurfacing may address moderate rhytidosis, direct excision still provides the optimal aesthetic result.

Other techniques for scar revision that are less technically demanding and labor intensive can be substituted for the geometric broken-line repair. For example, a running w-plasty closure can be undertaken to achieve the same goal but may fall short of the aesthetic outcome that is achievable with the more sophisticated geometric broken-line technique. Besides scar revision techniques, the underlying soft tissue may be augmented with solid fillers such as ePTFE or acellular dermis, but the authors feel that these alloplasts provide suboptimal improvement. These materials may soften the fold but not entirely eliminate the well-demarcated cutaneous crease that has formed over time. Further, these materials are often not well tolerated in terms of palpability and visibility in the glabellar region. The reader is reminded that injectable fillers (e.g., collagen) have been reported (albeit rarely) to risk blindness and are not considered a safe or viable alternative. Proper preoperative consultation ensures selection of the most suitable technique to accommodate the patient's specific aesthetic deficit and level of motivation.

Case #2 (Fig. 8-42A,B)

This is a 53-year-old registered nurse who had undergone prior facelift surgery and was satisfied with the aesthetic out-

A 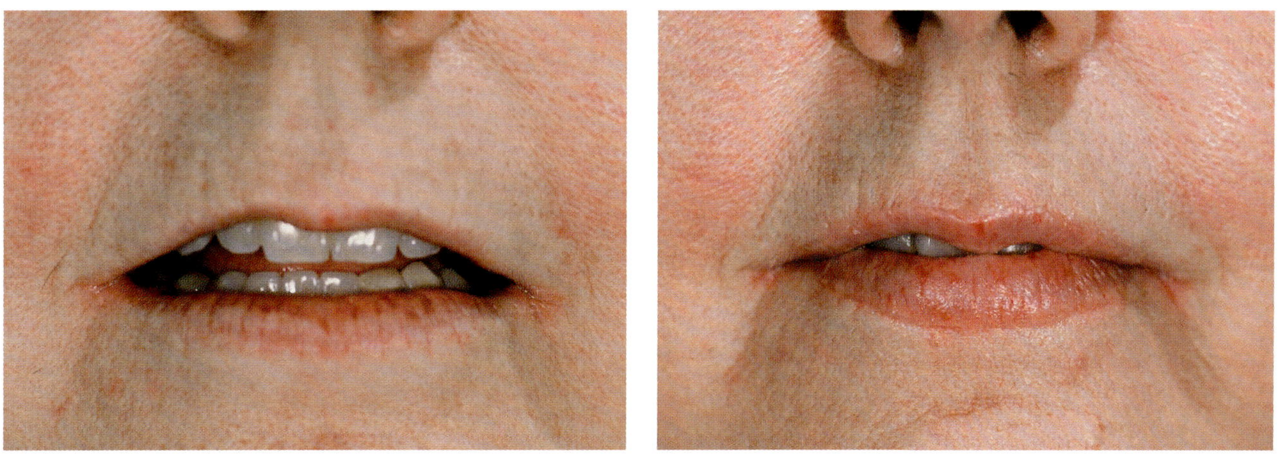 B

FIGURE 8-42. A,B: This is a 53-year-old woman who had undergone prior facelift surgery who desired to have augmentation of her lips but disavowed any use of implants. She stated that her lips always appeared very hypoplastic even since a very young age. Because of her mature age and willingness to wear lipstick on a routine basis, she was an eligible candidate for advancement cheiloplasty. She underwent 4-mm advancement of her upper and lower lips with a resulting 2-mm vermilion show at 1 year postoperatively.

come. Nevertheless, she stated that her lips have always been very attenuated and hypoplastic in appearance even during her youth. The patient disavowed alloplastic techniques in favor of advancement cheiloplasty, which she had heard about from a friend but had not directly witnessed the results of herself. The patient was asked how often she wore lipstick and stated that she did so all the time but that application was difficult owing to the limited expanse of exposed red-vermilion lip. After the patient understood that a visible scar would be present along the vermilion-cutaneous junction and that lipstick would have to be worn on a routine basis to camouflage the line of incision, she acknowledged her consent to these potential limitations but elected to proceed with advancement cheiloplasty. Given the patient's mature age and stated compliance with postoperative lipstick camouflage, surgery was scheduled.

Procedure

The procedure was advancement cheiloplasty with 4 mm of upper- and lower-lip excision, each to achieve the goal of a 2-mm advancement for each lip.

Discussion

As stated in the preceding text, the patient who is a suitable candidate for this type of surgery is one who is more advanced in age and is willing to accept a visible line at the vermilion–cutaneous junction that must be camouflaged with lipstick. If these limitations are not clearly articulated, the patient may be quite dissatisfied with the surgical outcome. At the time of this patient's presentation, few options were available for lip augmentation, and the senior author had been practicing advancement cheiloplasty more frequently. With experience, advancement cheiloplasty is now only rarely offered to the patient who must meet the selective criteria outlined in the preceding. During the preoperative consultation, the surgeon and patient should also agree to the precise amount of augmentation or advancement that is desired but understand that variable scar contracture may make the ultimate amount of advancement less predictable. This patient desired about 2 mm of advancement for both the upper and lower lips, which is a relatively conservative goal. In order to achieve this target, the surgeon generally should outline a distance that is approximately twice the desired amount of vermilion show but also parallel the patient's natural lip lines (see text under intraoperative considerations for details). Some salient technical points about the procedure are worth reiterating.

1. The plane of dissection should remain at the mid-dermal level throughout the procedure in order to provide a platform for advancement and minimize loss of lip volume during advancement.
2. No tissue undermining should be performed.
3. Incision lines should start approximately 5 mm from the oral commissure for both the upper and lower lip to prevent scar contracture around the commissure.
4. Interrupted vertical-mattress sutures are placed using 6-0 silk that facilitates proper wound eversion and accurate wound alignment.

The patient is shown 1 year after surgery with a reasonably good result for a conservative advancement. The patient was ecstatic about her aesthetic improvement.

For the patient with perioral rhytids and attenuated lips, a combined approach can be used to address each of these distinct pathologies. A resurfacing modality should be used (e.g., CO_2-laser therapy or dermabrasion) in order to eliminate perioral rhagades. Dermabrasion is more technically challenging than use of the CO_2 laser but can be just as effective. Then, advancement cheiloplasty or soft-tissue augmentation (e.g., collagen or acellular dermis) can be done to improve the attenuated nature of the lips. It is imperative that any kind of resurfacing be carried out before advancement cheiloplasty, because the incision line is easily disrupted by the laser or the dermabrader. Collagen therapy also should follow resurfacing but for a different reason: The rhytids should be clearly visible so that proper effacement can be undertaken in a directed fashion. With acellular dermis, both reasons hold true, and resurfacing should precede alloplastic insertion. With advancement cheiloplasty, resurfacing may not be necessary if the amount of skin tissue excised extends over the entire expanse of the perioral rhytids.

Case #3 (Fig. 8-43A–F)

This is a 36-year-old receptionist who noticed that she has been looking more tired and angry over the past several years. When she came to the office for consultation, she had heard about BTX and inquired whether this modality would be suitable for her. She pointed to the glabellar (Zone I) and the lateral-periocular regions (Zone IIIB,C) as areas of particular concern. She stressed that she really did not want to be subjected to any protracted downtime and also was somewhat fearful about undergoing any kind of surgical procedure. With a hand-held mirror, she was asked to squint, frown, and elevate her forehead. The periocular and glabellar rhytids were early in their development and only truly visible with animation. In addition to these wrinkles, she was shown how BTX could effect a chemical browlift by placing it judiciously in Zone IIIA and had this effect demonstrated to her by gently lifting the ptotic, lateral brow tissue. She said that she had never heard of this benefit because all of her friends have only remarked on the toxin's potential to efface wrinkles but expressed interest in this use of BTX. Although the patient was hesitant about having any more involved surgery, she was counseled that BTX eventually would exceed the cost of a surgical browlift and that she should consider this treatment given her younger age and the related cost that would accrue over time. However, she

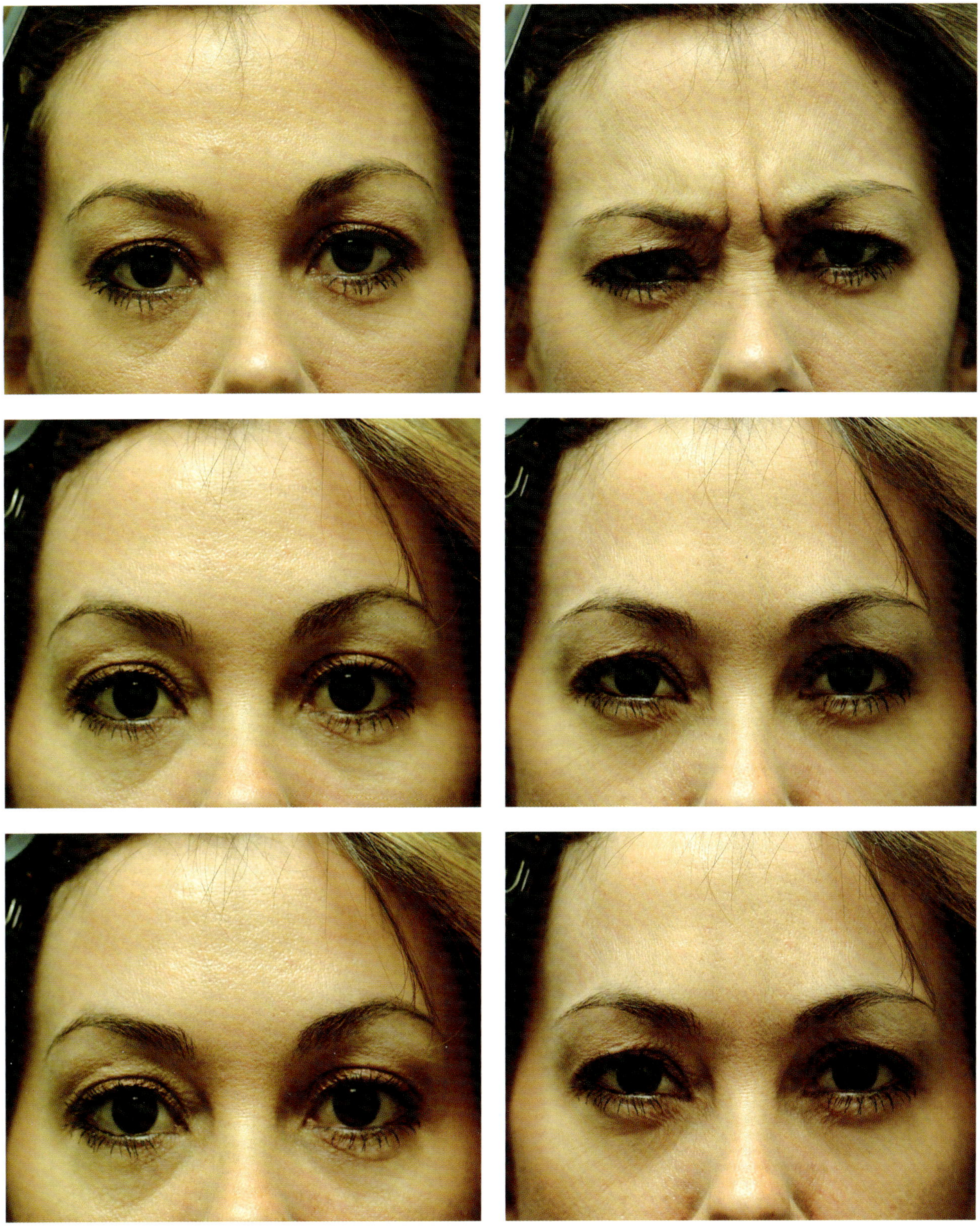

A B C D E F

FIGURE 8-43. A–F: This is a 36-year-old woman who desired rejuvenation of her eye region but did not want any surgical intervention. Her friend had told her about botulinum toxin (BTX), and she was interested in knowing if that modality would improve her look. The patient underwent treatment with BTX in all zones (Zone I, II, IIIA–C) with notable improvement in all areas. She is shown 3 days after injection in both relaxed and frowning views **(C,D)** and at 2 weeks with the same poses **(E,F).**

was told that BTX was a reasonable first step to "try on" a browlift to see if that particular look was desirable for her.

When strategizing which area would be most beneficial for the patient, she was offered the opinion that the following order would be applicable to her situation: Zone IIIA, I, IIIB/IIIC, and II in decreasing order of priority. Zone IIIA would offer her a browlift; Zone I would preclude her from excessive frowning; Zone IIIB/IIIC would minimize the periocular wrinkling; and Zone II would decrease the horizontal furrows along the forehead. More precisely, she was told that Zones IIIA and I would be the least expensive option to achieve a very good result, but she desired treatment of all zones.

The patient was informed about the exact nature of botulinum toxin and the temporary effects of the treatment that could last as short as 3 months but as long as 6 months depending on her body's metabolic elimination. The potential side effects also were elaborated, including but not limited to potential brow and blepharoptosis, asymmetry, bruising, swelling, temporary headache, ineffectiveness, and eventual but unlikely resistance to the toxin. She was informed that although the toxin is absolutely temporary in its effect, some patients have remarked on how they have actually forgotten or unlearned bad habits of expression and did not require more treatment after a few sessions. Nevertheless, these reports were only anecdotal in nature and definitely did not apply to the effect of a chemical browlift in Zone IIIA. As with any surgical procedure, the patient signed an informed consent and had all of her questions answered. In addition, photographic documentation was obtained with close-up views in both animated (frowning/squinting and elevating brow) and resting states to improve patient dialog, particularly in the postinjection setting when the patient may complain of the toxin having no effect.

Procedure

Botulinum toxin was infiltrated in the following amount, distribution, and order: Zone I (20 units), II (10 units), IIIA (seven units per side), IIIB (five units per side), IIIC (five units per side) for 64 units. Zone III was undertaken last so that firm, digital pressure could be applied with a 4 × 4 gauze for a period of 10 minutes to minimize bruising in this highly vascular area. Of note, the patient also underwent 5 minutes of preicing. As each Zone was injected, the ice packs were moved to the next area of injection to anesthetize that area and limit bruising before injection.

Discussion

The most noticeable improvement that the patient observed (and is corroborated in the accompanying photographs) is the remarkable brow elevation that BTX wrought. The typical patient who is desirous of BTX therapy usually is interested in a quick fix and, as with any cosmetic patient, wants to see a material benefit immediately. Unfortunately, some of the benefits of BTX are more preventative in nature rather than immediately apparent in that wrinkles that could develop over time owing to repeated motion are prevented from arising because of ongoing and consistent treatment sessions. However, if the wrinkles that appear on animation are troublesome to the patient, then a material benefit is noted during expressive motion of the upper face. As a chemical browlift (placed in Zone IIIA), BTX can afford a notable improvement to the patient's look even in the resting state. Therefore, treatment of this Zone often results in the most satisfied patient who then raves about the effect to all of his or her friends. Further, the patient who is a good candidate for BTX therapy usually starts in his or her mid to late thirties when some initial brow ptosis and incipient rhytidosis may be the only signs of premature aging. Therefore, BTX offers a potent adjunct to stave off the signs of aging in a targeted approach without the accompanying stigma or downtime of surgery for a young, industrious individual who would otherwise shun this latter option. Nevertheless, if the patient exhibits significant brow ptosis, then a surgical browlift may be the most cost-effective solution for that patient over time. In educating the patient about this type of surgery, it is important that the patient fully understands that the wrinkles during frowning in Zone I, the horizontal rhytids in Zone II, and the periocular rhytids in Zones IIIB,C are not affected by browlift surgery and that continued BTX therapy is required to treat these areas of concern. A surgical browlift only targets Zone IIIA, and this limitation should be well articulated.

The patient was given her comparative preinjection and postinjection photographs for her personal use. The authors have found that doing so improves patient rapport and provides tangible evidence to others who may be interested in seeing the benefit that BTX can offer and thereby become potential future patients. The reader is reminded about the importance of placing a telephone call 3 to 5 days after injection to confirm the benefit that the treatment session provided and having the patient return immediately if he or she thinks that no real benefit was evident. Often, an experienced clinical eye helps assuage the patient's concern, and comparative clinical photographs can offer the most convincing proof that BTX worked. However, if no benefit is manifest even after 7 days, then the patient should be offered additional treatment at no extra cost, because the authors suggest maintaining favorable patient rapport.

Case #4 (Fig. 8-44A,B)

This is a 31-year-old woman who was seen in consultation concerned about very thin lips. She stated that she always had thin lips but was becoming increasingly self-conscious about this feature. On frontal inspection, the patient was noted to have inadequate vertical height of both her upper

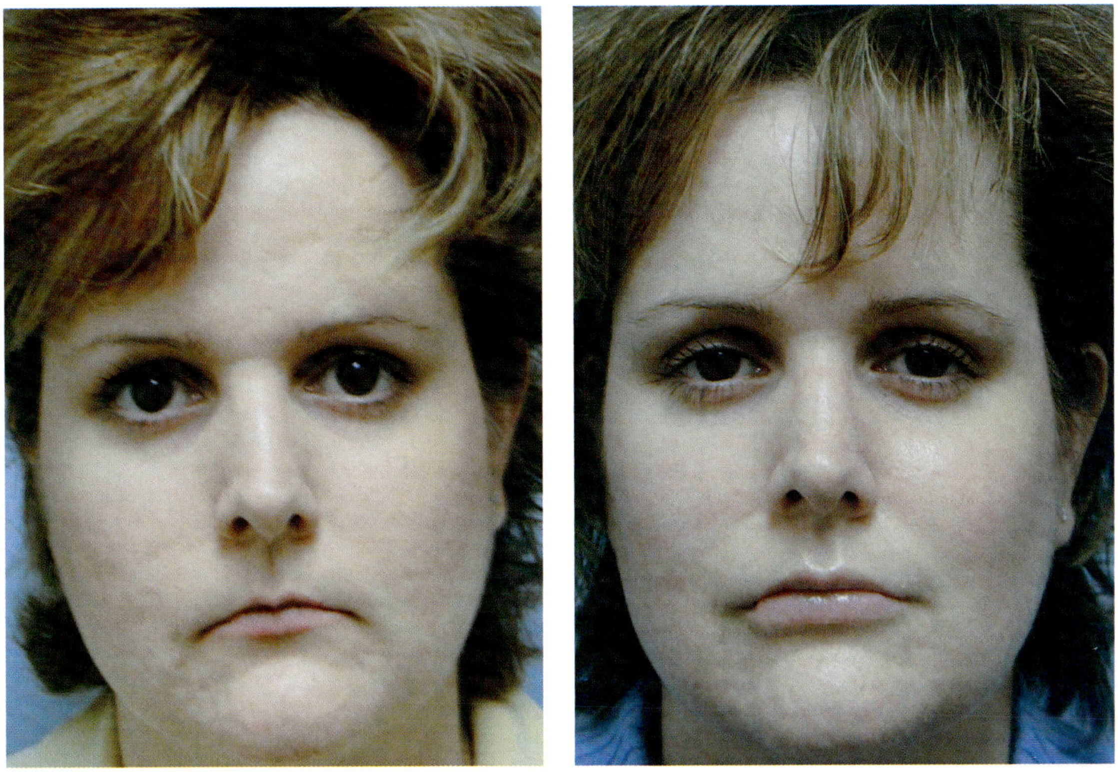

A B

FIGURE 8-44. A,B: This is a 31-year-old woman who desired lip augmentation, stating that she has always had very hypoplastic, attenuated lips. She was quite motivated to seek a permanent solution to her problem and was counseled on the benefit of acellular–dermal augmentation. She underwent successful augmentation using a 3- × 7-cm graft with two thirds of the graft inserted into the upper lip and the remaining one third into the lower lip. She is shown 6 months after surgery.

and lower lips, and on profile view, a proportionately limited amount of lip projection also was evident. Given the patient's relatively young age and the need for lifetime treatment to maintain the result, collagen injection was not the best long-term solution. Nevertheless, the patient should be encouraged to try collagen if she expresses uncertainty about whether lip augmentation is a suitable aesthetic endeavor. She understood the financial obligation that would be entailed with ongoing treatment sessions with collagen and was motivated enough to seek a more permanent solution to her deficiency. She was informed of the precise nature of acellular dermis, namely, that it was derived from harvesting irradiated cadaveric skin and for which infectious transmission had been appropriately screened but could never be entirely ruled out. Further, acellular dermis exhibits a variable degree of resorption based on a patient's particular physiological response to the foreign matter but that results have been seen to endure for several years if not more indefinitely. Other implant materials (e.g., ePTFE forms) were not recommended owing to the authors' limited success with these types of implants in the lips given their observed predilection toward palpability, induration, contracture, infection, and extrusion.

Procedure

The procedure was a lip augmentation with a 3 × 7 cm acellular–dermal graft in which two thirds of the graft was placed into the upper lip with the remainder allocated for the lower lip.

Discussion

When counseling a patient about lip augmentation, several key factors should be elaborated. For the younger patient who has a less mature body image or exhibits only a minor deficiency, it is often advisable to encourage the patient to have lip augmentation with collagen first to determine if the patient's expectations are realistic. This is less of an issue in the younger patient with obvious hypoplastic lips or in the middle-aged woman with lip hypoplasia related to the progression of the aging process.

Although many materials have been advocated for lip augmentation, the authors contend that the solid form of acellular dermis provides the most natural feel, optimal safety, and aesthetic appearance for long-term enhancement. In the senior author's practice, patients have been so far observed to retain their acellular–dermal graft for over 7 years without any clinical evidence of resorption. However, if the patient is predisposed toward rapid resorption, the implant may disappear after as little as 3 months. To reiterate, lip augmentation can be the most anxiety-provoking surgical procedure for the surgeon and patient alike when other solid materials are used due to the omnipresent risk of infection, extrusion, palpability, and mobility. Because the lip is a highly mobile structure and proximal to the contaminated oral flora, complications can arise despite the best technical efforts. It is worth reiterating an important philosophical point: No implant that cannot be removed (e.g., certain permanent liquid injectables) should ever be placed, especially in the lip, which may require mutilating surgery to remove and only partially at best. Although no ideal implant material has been found at this time, acellular dermis has remained a steadfast augmentation material for the lips in the armamentarium of the authors' practices.

REFERENCES

1. Requena C, Izquierdo MJ, Navarro M, et al: Adverse reactions to injectable aesthetic microimplants. Am J Dermatopathol 2001; 23:197–202.
2. Hoffmann C, Schuller-Petrovic S, Soyer HP, et al: Adverse reactions after cosmetic lip augmentation with permanent biologically inert implant materials. J Am Acad Dermatol 1999;40: 100–102.
3. Rudolph CM, Soyer HP, Schuller-Petrovic S, et al: Foreign body granulomas due to injectable aesthetic microimplants. Am J Surg Pathol 1999;23:113–117.
4. Castillo GD: Management of blindness in the practice of cosmetic surgery. Otolaryngol Head Neck Surg 1989;100: 559–562.
5. Friedman PM, Mafong EA, Kauvar AN, et al: Safety data of injectable nonanimal stabilized hyaluronic acid gel for soft tissue augmentation. Dermatol Surg 2002;28:491–494.
6. Lowe NJ, Maxwell CA, Lowe P, et al: Hyaluronic acid skin fillers: adverse reactions and skin testing. J Am Acad Dermatol 2001; 45:930–933.
7. Micheels P: Human anti-hyaluronic acid antibodies: is it possible? Dermatol Surg 2001;27:185–191.

9

CUTANEOUS REJUVENATION

SAMUEL M. LAM
EDWIN F. WILLIAMS III

Although the principal focus of this book is surgical, incision-based, intervention for the aging face, a thorough understanding of cutaneous resurfacing modalities also must be sought to offer the patient the most complete rejuvenative regimen. Patients who only exhibit actinic damage, such as superficial dyschromias and textural skin changes, without actual ptosis of tissues are more suitable candidates for resurfacing than traditional lifting procedures. In addition, resurfacing may be effectively combined with lifting procedures for patients who exhibit both tissue ptosis and photodamage if flap integrity may be ensured (e.g., with subperiosteal elevation of the brow the skin may be safely resurfaced concurrently) or deferred for several months until flap vascularity is restored.

The facial aesthetic surgeon must not only master the technical aspects of some of the myriad resurfacing modalities that abound but know when to select a particular technique and further when to combine techniques to achieve maximal benefit for the patient. The authors stress the importance of careful selection of a few, reliable techniques that have proven efficacy rather than the quixotic quest to implement all of the techniques available today.

As important as technical mastery is the commensurate understanding of the complicated and often confusing postoperative management of the resurfaced patient, which involves an intensive, almost daily encounter to guide the patient successfully through the process. To date, no text has lucidly revealed this aspect of patient care in a pragmatic, detailed, and systematic fashion. Complications such as dermatitis and (rarely) scarring during the postoperative period may arise and must be swiftly identified and treated to minimize adverse outcomes.

This chapter concludes with a primer on basic skin care and rejuvenative topical agents, such as tretinoin-based products, for those patients who are not yet ready for any surgical therapy or those who would like to maintain the longevity of their surgical result. Physicians often relegate this type of care to the aesthetician and disavow the necessity to learn more about skin care. However, the physician should be partly responsible for this knowledge at minimum, because he or she must decide when it is safe for the resurfaced patient to use camouflaging products and effectively answer simple queries regarding which products may be appropriate for the newly resurfaced skin.

PREOPERATIVE CONSIDERATIONS: PATIENT SELECTION AND RELEVANT ANATOMY

Before considering what technique would be appropriate for a particular patient, the surgeon must have a well-structured understanding of the types of resurfacing modalities available. Basically, cutaneous resurfacing may be divided into two principal categories: nonablative and ablative therapy. The former represents a recent advance in resurfacing that promotes dermal remodeling via collagen synthesis without any epidermal effacement. Accordingly, the epidermis is entirely untouched during nonablative therapy; therefore, no benefit is obtained for the photodamaged outer skin. Instead, limited fine-to-moderate rhytidosis may be addressed with multiple treatment sessions over a period of several months to permit sufficient time for collagen–dermal remodeling to occur. Similarly, because the epidermal layer is maintained intact, the patient experiences no downtime and is subjected only to a brief, painless treatment session that leaves no residual edema, ecchymosis, or erythema. Again, it should be emphasized that this new technique must be selectively employed in the suitable patient with the individual fully cognizant of the inherent limitations for facial rejuvenation.

The authors have investigated the potential benefit of this newer technique in a blinded, prospective, histologic analysis using a porcine model.[1] The results of this study were quite revelatory: The histologic specimens harvested from the nonablative, pulsed-dye laser-treated skin demonstrated statistically significant collagen remodeling in both a quantitative (collagen band width, nuclei per high-powered field) and qualitative (overall dermal thickness) fashion as compared with untreated skin. The dermal depth could not be quantitatively measured because the thickness exceeded the punch-biopsy instrument in all the laser-treated (both ablative and nonablative) skin. Further, the degree of collagen remodeling favorably compared with that of ablative, carbon dioxide laser-treated areas. However, this preliminary data must be cautiously assessed, as these results were obtained in an animal model; human clinical trials are warranted to establish the precise role that nonablative therapy should play in facial rejuvenation.

The early clinical trials have been somewhat equivocal. Fitzpatrick's study showed a statistically significant aesthetic improvement in patients' hemifaces that were treated with a nonablative, pulsed-dye laser as compared with a placebo-controlled (cryogen spray alone) side.[2] All photographic analyses were conducted in a blinded, prospective method. These findings were further corroborated with histologic samples taken from each side that revealed significant collagen synthesis on the treated side compared with the controlled, untreated side. Despite histologic improvement, one study showed limited clinical patient satisfaction.[3] However, other studies have corroborated the benefit of nonablative techniques for mild to moderate skin pathologies.[4–8]

The authors have found that the best results obtained with this technology may be obtained in patients with mild to moderate fine rhytidosis, particularly in the periocular region (e.g., crow's feet at the lateral canthus and crepelike wrinkles that traverse below the eye). The ideal candidate for this treatment strategy is the younger individual (in his or her thirties) who exhibits minimal photodamage (dyschromias and other epidermal damage) with fine, periocular rhytidosis. These patients are also very well suited to botulinum toxin (BTX) injections, which may be used in combination or independently of nonablative laser therapy. Patients who exhibit more marked rhytidosis, actinic damage, or ptotic tissues do not significantly benefit from this technique and should be dissuaded from undertaking nonablative therapy.

Cutaneous, ablative resurfacing represents the more traditional method of facial skin rejuvenation in which the entire outer layer of the epidermis is removed along with a partial thickness of the underlying dermis to effect a favorable aesthetic result. Ablative resurfacing may be undertaken via three principal methods: mechanical abrasion, chemical exfoliation, and laser therapy. Each modality has its own unique characteristic benefits and drawbacks, and at times combination of these techniques may offer the patient the most favorable means of obtaining the desired objective. Mechanical abrasion may range from the least invasive microdermabrasion (which effectively acts as a nonablative method of facial rejuvenation) to the more aggressive technique of dermasanding to fully ablative dermabrasion. The latter offers precise control of uneven cutaneous contour and texture and is particularly well suited in the acne-scarred skin. Although acne scarring does not strictly fall within the confines of the topic of the aging face, a discussion of this clinical scenario is conducted, because treatment of this pathology clearly illustrates the role of effective combined resurfacing. Similar to the varied mechanical methods of resurfacing, chemical peeling agents differ in their potency from the light glycolic and Jessner's solutions to the more invasive higher-strength trichloroacetic acid (TCA) and phenol mixtures. Thirty-five percent TCA and phenol prove their incontestable benefit to reverse significant photoaged skin with moderate rhytidosis. Laser therapy for facial rejuvenation may be entirely nonablative (as discussed in the preceding) via laser and light therapies intended for this purpose, such as the intense pulsed-light devices or the pulsed-dye laser adjusted to lower fluences. Alternatively, traditional ablative lasers such as the CO_2 laser efface the epidermis to effect the desired rejuvenation and may be more appropriate for severely photodamaged skin. The other ablative laser that has been widely advocated, the Erbium:YAG (Er:YAG) laser, has theoretical advantages over the CO_2 laser, including less thermal injury and more specific collagen photothermolysis, but has fallen short in practical usage because of poor hemostasis and limited effect. Therefore, the authors do not advocate use of this particular type of laser whether as an adjunct to the CO_2 laser or alone, as there is no real perceived advantage that the Er:YAG offers over comparable chemical peeling.

However, any ablative resurfacing modality carries with it considerable morbidity, which includes risk of hyperpigmentation and hypopigmentation, dermatitis, perioperative edema, protracted erythema, milia and acne outbreaks, physical discomfort, an involved cleaning and occlusive regimen, need for solar protection, and the most dreaded outcome, potential scarring. Despite these limitations, ablative resurfacing achieves remarkable success in rejuvenating severely photodamaged skin and is still a mainstay of therapy for those patients who require intensive rejuvenation and who are willing to accept the expected recovery period. All patients are thoroughly counseled that the postoperative period will be complex and should fully comprehend that their appearance will be analogous to that of a burn victim. Patients are informed of their expected postoperative appearance at the outset so that they may be psychologically well equipped to handle the temporary disfigurement. Proper preoperative counseling is an essential element to successful postoperative care.

The various resurfacing techniques that are available today offer the aesthetic facial surgeon an unprecedented ability to achieve a desired cosmetic outcome. However, every resurfacing technique should not be viewed as flawless or universal in its clinical benefit. The reader is advised to avoid a "compartmentalized" perspective in which every cutaneous problem is solved by a single technique. As addressed in the following, each modality has inherent drawbacks as well as distinct advantages, which offer the patient the optimal result if appropriately combined with other resurfacing techniques.

An important consideration is that resurfacing cannot address all cutaneous problems, namely, skin redundancy or volume excess. If the patient presents with dermatochalasis, or excessive upper-eyelid skin, the surgeon should remove the redundant skin to restore a youthful countenance. Similarly, brow ptosis or cheek jowling should be corrected with a brow lift or rhytidectomy, respectively. Steatoblepharon, or pseudoherniation of fat of the eyelids, is amenable to fat removal or repositioning. Deep or fine rhytids, which are the product of continuous facial motion, may be better served with a paralytic agent (e.g., botulinum toxin). However, the authors admit that ablative (and even nonablative) resurfacing has been observed to yield a more tightened facial appearance by virtue of the collagen stimulation.

When deciding which resurfacing technique to employ, one should reflect on three key guidelines: (a) the subunits of the face; (b) the depth of the facial pathology; and (c) the Fitzpatrick skin grade of the patient.[9] The face may be divided into so-called subunits (perioral, periocular, nasal, brow, and cheek), which tolerate different resurfacing modalities to varying degrees. For example, the lower eyelid tends to withstand the pigmentary ablation of the CO_2 laser better than the jaw line. It has been noted that the line of demarcation between hypopigmented face and pigmented neck may become more pronounced over the years as the facial skin continues to undergo some progressive depigmentation. Therefore, full-face laser resurfacing should be undertaken with caution, especially considering the protracted erythema that the patient must bear. The depth of the facial lesion (scar, rhytid, etc.) should be considered when deciding what resurfacing modality may be best suited. For example, deep acne scarring may be more effectively addressed with dermabrasion than TCA peel. Finally, the patient's Fitzpatrick score has significant impact on the short- and long-term tendency toward hyperpigmentation and hypopigmentation. Accordingly, laser resurfacing should be used with greater restraint in darker-skinned individuals, especially when considering the greater disparity in color (lighter face and darker neck) that may arise along the jaw line.

Generally speaking, any kind of resurfacing should not be carried out concurrently with a surgical procedure in which the resurfaced area is undermined. However, the authors have achieved favorable results with minimal morbidity in select patients (nonsmokers, nondiabetics) in which a shorter, cutaneous flap is dissected and a lighter end point of the chemical peel (less frosting) is achieved or only a single CO_2 pass is undertaken. In addition, the peel and laser are feathered gently toward the distal aspect of the flap to limit risk of flap compromise. However, caution always must be exercised if combined surgery and resurfacing are performed and may not be advisable, especially to the neophyte surgeon. As a rule, patients who have undergone a surgical undermining procedure should wait at least a period of 9 months before being resurfaced. Similarly, a patient who recently underwent aggressive resurfacing procedure should expect to wait 9 months before a surgical undermining procedure.

Besides an assiduous assessment of the patient's aesthetic deficits, the surgeon must review a pertinent clinical history that may adversely contribute to the patient's outcome. Clearly, conditions that inhibit proper wound healing should be assessed, which include prior history of keloid or hypertrophic scarring, tobacco use (of any kind), diabetes mellitus, and active and ongoing acne. Of note, the authors have not witnessed any adverse scarring even in patients who have a history of hypertrophic or keloid scarring if resurfacing is confined to the face, because the unique healing properties of the face limit the potential for these exuberant forms of scarring. Also, if the patient continues to engage in daily and protracted sun exposure, this activity, especially in the postoperative period, should be highly discouraged for risk of poor healing, scarring, dermatitis, and marked hyperpigmentation. Patients who have considerable bodily actinic damage should be advised that their rejuvenated face might not appropriately match the advanced nature of the sun-damaged skin of their body; and this disparity might prove troublesome to them if proper preoperative advice is not delivered. As is well known, the most significant medicine that is an absolute contraindication to ablative resurfacing is use of isotretinoin (Accutane) for any duration over the prior year. The reduction of the pilosebaceous glands that this medication engenders predisposes the patient to the very real risk of uncontrolled scar formation. Also, patients who have undergone prior undermining of their skin (e.g., a rhytidectomy or brow lift) are at a slightly increased risk of scarring owing to injury to the regenerative pilosebaceous glands. The very rare cases of scarring that the authors have witnessed have all occurred in patients who have undergone a prior facial surgical procedure in which cutaneous undermining was undertaken. Nevertheless, the physician should not unduly frighten the patient regarding this limited risk but should remain vigilant in the postoperative period for this potential outcome.

As part of the preoperative regimen, an oral antiviral medication is commenced 2 days prior to the actual procedure if resurfacing is planned in the perioral region. If the patient manifests a herpetic outbreak despite prophylaxis (which is rare), he or she remains on the antiviral medication at twice the dosage for an additional week from the onset of the outbreak. Usually, herpetic lesions may be distinguished from acne or milia in the timing of onset (typically 6 to 7 days postoperative), characteristic clustering and vesicular nature of the lesions, and intense burning sensation in the affected areas. If the patient manifests these symptoms, the authors instruct the patient to contact the office immediately so that proper intervention may be initiated. Perioperative antibiotics that target the skin flora, such as cephalexin, are also routinely implemented in patients for a 1-week duration postoperatively although their proven efficacy may be debated. In the past, hydroquinone and retinoic acid were dispensed to the patient a few weeks prior to the planned procedure for daily topical application, but

Ideal Candidates for Resurfacing

Nonablative
- Younger patient (thirties)
- Fine periocular rhytidosis
- Limited photodamage
- Limited tissue ptosis (also consider adjuvant Botox)

Ablative
- Chemical peel (Jessner's/35% TCA)
  - Any age with epidermal photodamage
  - Mild to moderate rhytidosis
  - Limited perioral rhytidosis
  - Limited tissue ptosis
- Laser resurfacing
  - Generally older patient with deeper rhytidosis not amenable to chemical peel (e.g., perioral or glabellar rhytidosis)
  - Consider limiting laser resurfacing to discrete subunits (best-tolerated areas are the periocular, perioral, and glabellar regions) because of risk of hypopigmentation, especially demarcated at the jaw line, and morbidity of laser resurfacing
  - Combined resurfacing for acne and rhinophyma
  - Patients understand the longer recovery time (several months of erythema)

Mechanical dermabrasion
- Depressed surface irregularities (e.g., acne scarring)
- Rhinophyma
- In conjunction with scar revision (6 weeks after)
- Deeper wrinkles (perioral) in lieu of laser resurfacing

Instrumentation and Equipment for Chemical Peel (Fig. 9-1)

Jessner's Solution*
(Resorcinol 14 g, salicylic acid 14 g, lactic acid 14 cc, QS ethanol 100 cc)
35% TCA solution

*A local pharmacist can make the preceding solutions and may need to know the ingredients of Jessner's solution, as listed, when formulating the mixture and should know that the formulation of TCA is based on a percentage by weight.

100% Acetone (may be purchased at a local hardware store)
Cotton-tipped applicators
Cotton balls
4 × 4 gauzes
Nonsterile gloves
Cooling fan
Balanced saline solution (for eye flush if chemical peel inadvertently enters the eye)
Intravenous Versed sedation (optional but recommended)

this regimen has since been abandoned. Alster's study of 100 prospectively evaluated and controlled patients showed no benefit of either agent in the reduction of postinflammatory hyperpigmentation—which corroborates the authors' empirical observations. Her rationale for this lack of efficacy was attributed to the removal by the peel or laser of all superficial melanocytes that were treated by the preceding topical agents.[10]

INTRAOPERATIVE CONSIDERATIONS: TECHNIQUE AND SALIENT TECHNICAL POINTS

Nonablative Laser Therapy (Pulsed-Dye Laser)

As mentioned, various devices that emit broadband light or, alternatively, true lasers, have been used as a nonablative instrument. The authors have had extensive experience with the pulsed-dye laser and have found that this type of laser has an unparalleled safety profile and is well tolerated by the patient (Fig. 9-2A,B). In addition, the pulsed-dye laser also may be used to eradicate superficial vascular ectasias, such as cherry angiomas or spider veins (Fig. 9-3). Because the epidermis should be protected during treatment, a cooling spray should be employed (20 ms duration, 20 ms prior to laser emission), which is equipped with Candela pulsed-dye laser models. In the cited animal study, the authors noted that the only variable that did not negatively affect collagen remodeling was the use of the cryogen spray, which did serve to limit the risk of epidermal hyperpigmentation. Therefore, cryogen spray is advocated in nonablative therapy. Increasing fluence, spot size, and pulse duration statistically affected the amount of collagen remodeling. Nevertheless, practically speaking, a safe parameter for nonablative laser resurfacing that virtually ensures limited to no ecchymosis, edema, or discomfort but still achieves a favorable clinical improvement is a 10-mm spot size, set at 4 J/cm^2 with use of the cryogen spray.

Proper laser precautions should be observed (e.g., posted laser signs, eye protection, and trained staff). Both physician and staff should don appropriate laser goggles tailored to the 585- to 595-nm wavelength. Because the laser needs to pass in close proximity to the patients' eyes to address the peri-

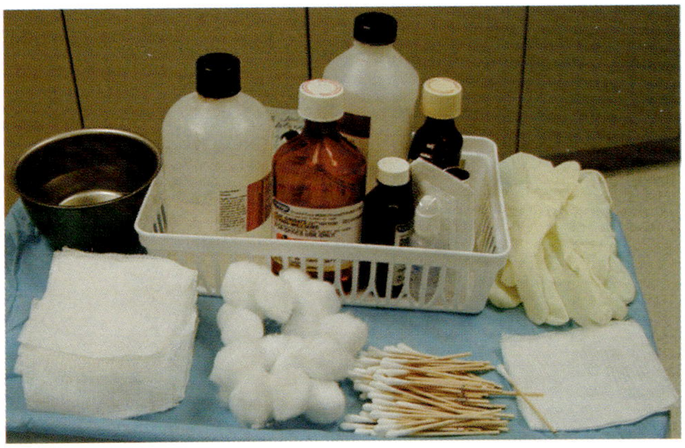

FIGURE 9-1. The physician should have all of the necessary equipment for the chemical-peel session readily available on a nearby table. The physician will require 100% acetone, Jessner's solution, and TCA of varying concentrations. 4 × 4 Gauze is needed to abrade the skin with the acetone and to apply the cold water onto the face at the end of treatment to dilute the chemical reaction. Cotton-tipped applicators are used to apply the chemical solutions in the lower-eyelid region and cotton balls or pads are used for the remainder of the face. Balanced saline solution or water in a spray bottle always should be ready for use in case the patient complains of any ocular irritation from inadvertent entry of peel solution. A cooling fan is also needed to blow upward onto the face to cool it during a session. All chemical peels must be applied with gloves (nonsterile are acceptable) so as to avoid injury to the physician's hands. A trash can should be accessible so that every used cotton-tipped applicator, gauze, or cotton ball can be immediately discarded to limit the risk of recycling it.

ocular rhytids, it is advisable to have the physician hold the patients' eyes firmly shut with the nondominant hand rather than use protective eyewear for the patient. The patient should be forewarned that the laser light is quite bright, especially when passed near the eye, even when the eye is completely closed. In addition, the patient may be gently startled by the cooling spray that immediately precedes laser delivery and should be informed of the initial laser pulse. Of note, one to two passes of the laser are sufficient for each treatment session. Full-face laser treatment also may be performed if the patient exhibits fine rhytidosis elsewhere that is amenable to nonablative therapy. Generally, three to four treatment sessions administered at 1-month intervals are advocated to achieve maximal benefit for the patient. As emphasized, proper patient selection and education are prerequisites to patient satisfaction.

Chemical Exfoliation (Jessner's/35% Trichloroacetic Acid)

For patients with epidermal actinic damage, even those who are still quite young (i.e., in their thirties), who have mild to moderate rhytidosis, chemical exfoliation with combined Jessner's/35% TCA proves to be a reliable and effective treatment modality. This section discusses the technical aspects involved in achieving a uniform, safe, reproducible result.

Unquestionably, vigorous and thorough cleansing of the skin with 100% acetone is a critical first step to ensure that an even peel is attained. The acetone solution should be applied with a 4 × 4 gauze, which more effectively abrades the skin than a cotton ball or a cotton-tipped applicator can. The purpose of the acetone is twofold: to remove the outer layer of oil and function as a keratolytic of the stratum corneum, both of which may serve as physical barriers to attain a deep and uniform peel. The patient should be informed that the application of acetone might be somewhat unpleasant because of the noxious odors and vigorous application.

A

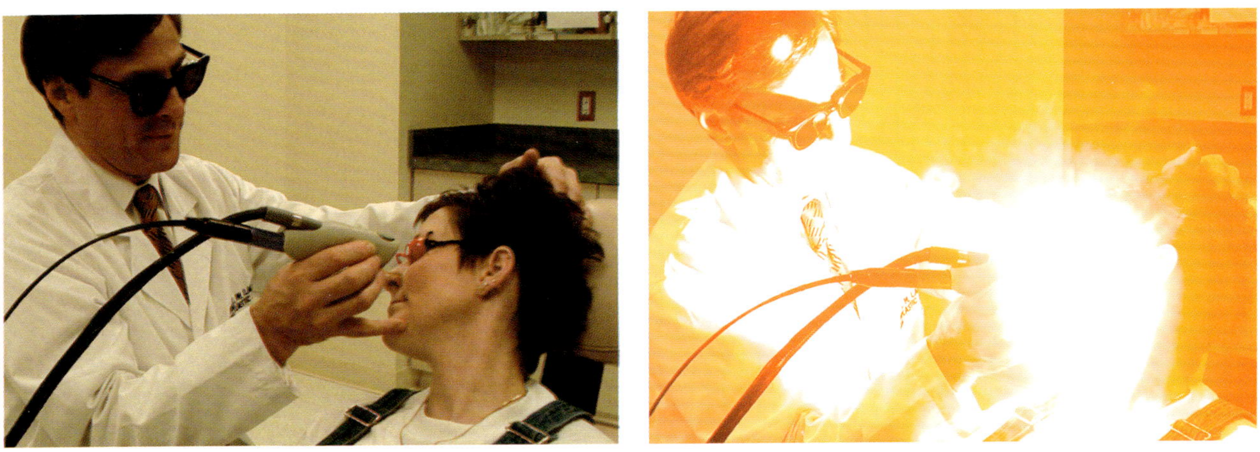

B

FIGURE 9-2. A,B: The authors have extensive experience with the pulsed-dye laser for nonablative resurfacing. This treatment modality is designed for fine, periocular rhytids principally in the younger patient. Proper eyeglasses designed to block the 585- to 595-nm wavelength should be donned to avoid any ocular injury for the patient and physician. The recommended treatment parameter is 10-mm spot size, 4 J/cm^2 with use of the cryogen spray that permits rejuvenation without noticeable bruising or swelling. One to two passes are generally sufficient per session with a total of three to four treatment sessions administered at 1-month intervals.

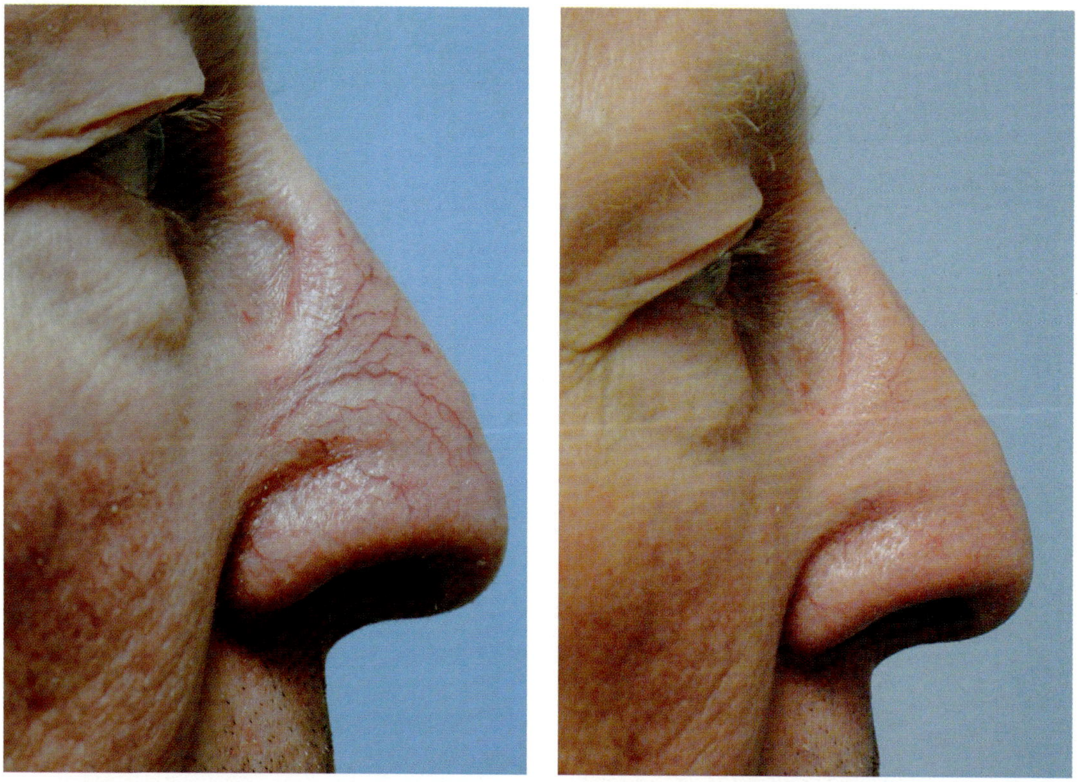

A B

FIGURE 9-3. A,B: This is a 64-year-old man who has experienced progressive vascularity of his nose consisting of superficial, axial type vessels with a pattern of distribution limited only to his nose. He has never sought treatment before but would like targeted intervention for this problem. He underwent treatment with a pulsed-dye laser (595 nm) using a 2 × 7 mm hand piece set at a fluence of 15 J/cm^2 and is shown 8 weeks after treatment with notable improvement. The pulsed-dye laser is an ideal treatment modality to efface superficial, red-hued vessels and is slightly less effective for deeper, blue-colored vessels. Selective cautery of these vessels is often a less than an ideal alternative because of the bleeding that ensues, the risk of scarring, and the likelihood of a shorter interval for return of this pathology. As with all dermatologic procedures, the patient must understand that the underlying disease process, which remains, may engender further outcropping of these vascular lesions and that repeat treatment often is required at a later date.

The Jessner's solution, which is comprised principally of alpha hydroxy acids (see preceding text box), acts to complete the keratolytic process. Jessner's solution may be applied with relative impunity as the liberal application usually only penetrates into the outer epidermal layer. Often, a light frost may be evident but only indicates a reversible salt deposition rather than the irreversible blanching that ensues owing to protein coagulation when the actual TCA peel is applied. Unlike the TCA peel, no visual change of the skin color is targeted, because the superficial nature of the Jessner's solution usually does not impart any color change. The patient does not require any sedation for this part of the procedure, because the Jessner's solution usually only engenders a mild tingling sensation and only rarely frank discomfort.

Like application of TCA, the subunit principle is followed with application of Jessner's solution. First, attention is paid to the lower eyelid/periocular region in the same fashion as described for the TCA peel. The patient is placed in an upright position, inclined approximately 60 degrees from the horizontal. This semiinclined orientation minimizes inadvertent entry of solution into the eyes during application over the lower-eyelid region while maintaining patient comfort. The assistant gently holds cotton-tipped applicators at both the lateral and medial canthi in order to prevent tears from unevenly diluting the peeled area and, more important, to minimize peel solution from entering the eye via capillary conduction. A bottle of balanced-saline solution (BSS) should always be on the table side should the patient report any ocular irritation or burning. (If the patient does complain of ocular discomfort, the surgeon should recline the patient to a supine position and gently flush the eyes with BSS with the stream targeted at the medial canthus. This method minimizes reflex closure of the eye that would impair proper ocular irrigation.) The Jessner's solution is applied with a cotton-tipped applicator in the lower eyelid region and with a cotton ball for the remainder of the face. It is important that the cotton ball be squeezed semidry before applying the solution to avoid unintentional trickle of solution onto the neck. Furthermore, the used cotton-tipped swabs and cotton balls should be promptly discarded into the waste bin so that confusion does not arise as to which cotton ball was used for which peel solution.

After each lower-eyelid/periocular region has been treated, the surgeon should advance in a systematic fashion by subunit from forehead/temple region, right-cheek region, left-cheek region, the upper-lip/lower-lip/chin region, and then nasal region. The order is not important, but it is recommended that the surgeon proceed in the same order every time to ensure that no area is repeeled or missed. The nasal and upper-lid areas are relatively recalcitrant to significant rejuvenation with a peeling agent but are treated nonetheless to achieve a complete and uniform peel. However, the upper-lid area is treated very superficially given the attenuated skin in this area and the attendant risk of scarring. Also, the cheek and chin subunits should be gently feathered for about a centimeter onto the neck to curtail an abrupt transition. If a lifting procedure is entertained concurrently or independently, the transposition of ptotic tissues upward may result in the unpeeled area of the neck also moving upward into the facial region.

After the Jessner's has been completed, the TCA may be applied immediately. First, the patient is marked out along subunits with a surgical marking pen, as the application of TCA must rigorously conform to the subunit principle to avoid overtreatment, undertreatment, or retreatment of areas (Fig. 9-4). If the patient is marked out before the Jessner's solution, the marked areas are lost or markedly diminished by the Jessner's peel. Before the patient is sedated, the lower-eyelid area is again treated first with the same technique and patient positioning described in the preceding for the Jessner's application (Fig. 9-5A–C). Although the patient will experience noteworthy burning discomfort, the lower-eyelid application must be undertaken with the patient fully awake or only minimally sedated so that he or she may report any ocular burning due to entry of peeling solution into the eyes. In order to offset the burning sensation, a cooling fan is held by the second assistant at the level of the patient's waist and aimed tangentially upward toward the face: A more direct gust may cause undesirable tearing and reflexive blinking.

Unlike with Jessner's application, the blanched appearance of the skin is a critical factor in determining when the desired end is achieved. The skin first assumes a mild erythema as the papillary dermis is entered, then a light frost, to finally a more complete, opaque white (Figs. 9-6A–D and 9-7A–C). After a few minutes, the skin may begin to regress back to a light erythema, fooling the physician into thinking that the area is undertreated. The return to erythema is a major reason that the subunit principle should be adhered to in order to avoid retreatment of areas known to be treated already. Generally, the end should be a completely uniform frost but not excessively opaque, which may risk scarring. Experience dictates proper depth of the peel, and review of the enclosed DVD further enhances education. As mentioned, the upper eyelids should be only lightly treated (light frost), because this particular area exhibits much thinner skin. The nose and forehead tend to withstand a deeper peel, but a deeper peel generally is not effective for the nasal area in any case. If the peeled area appears to have been overtreated, immediate application of gauze impregnated with water should be undertaken to dilute the peel solution and retard the action of the peel.

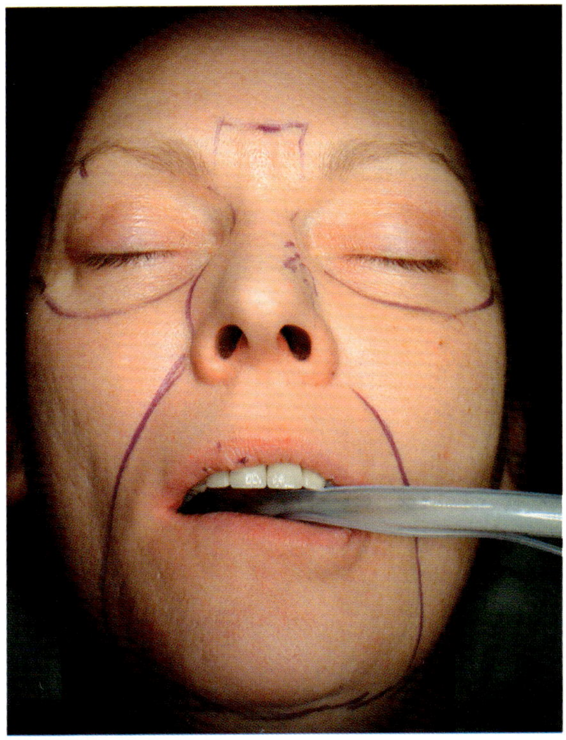

FIGURE 9-4. TCA Peel, Step 1. After the patient has undergone acetone and Jessner's preparation according to the prescribed method, he or she is marked out along facial subunits to guide treatment in a systematic manner. The physician should progress in an orderly fashion to avoid retreating or missing a subunit. If the physician advances in a haphazard technique, areas will be only partly treated or the physician will re-treat areas that have now faded from the initial frost, thinking that these areas were missed, and thereby overtreat that area. (Note: The patient is photographed under general anesthesia because she will be undergoing a brow and midface lift after completion of the peel.)

The authors advocate application of the TCA peel to discrete areas of deep rhytidosis first, if such areas are present, before evenly applying the solution to the entire subunit because the edema and frost that follow a coat of TCA effectively camouflage the linear areas of rhytidosis. Immediately after the subunit is treated, the area is covered with a gauze soaked in iced water in order to minimize patient discom-

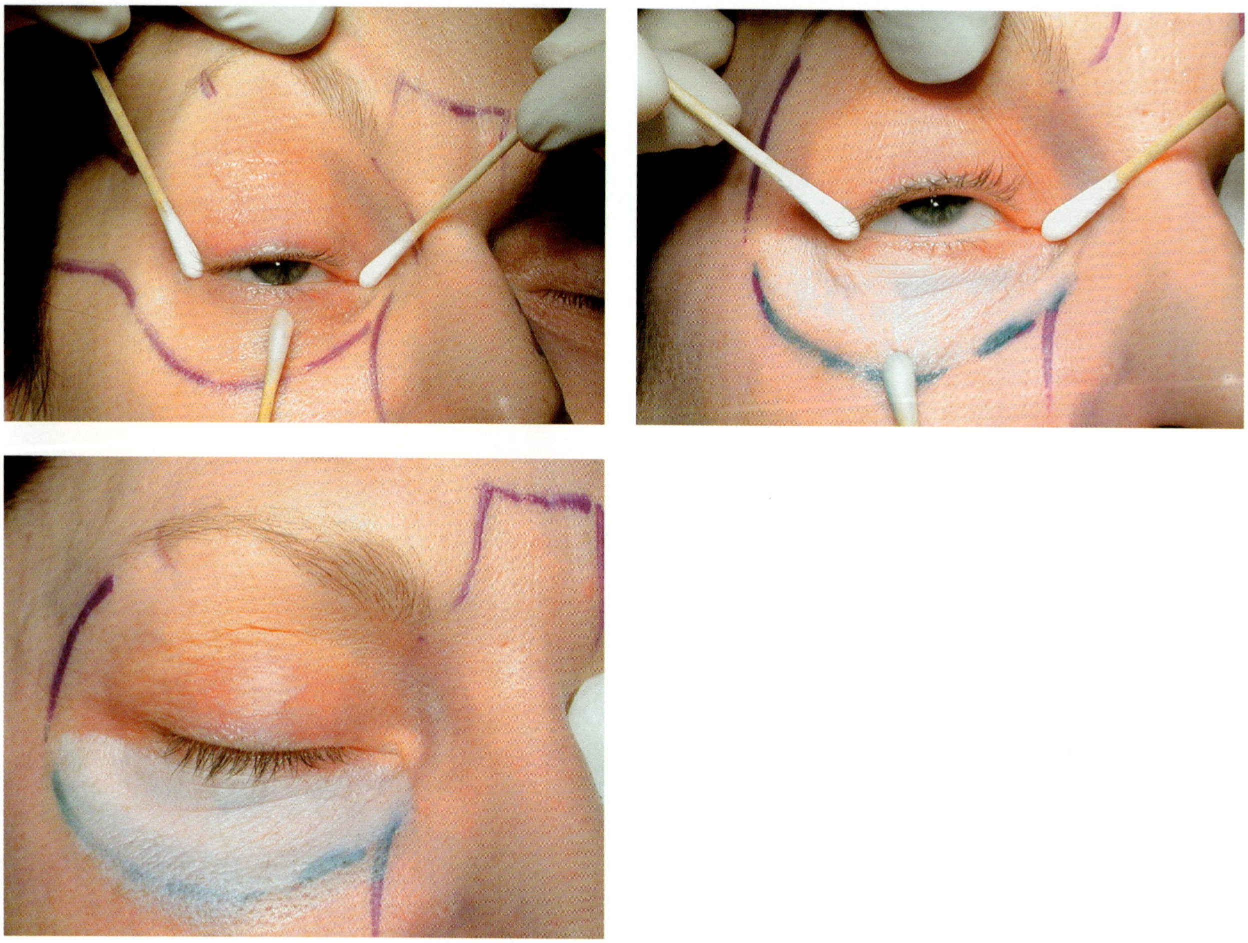

A B C

FIGURE 9-5. TCA Peel, Step 2. A: The lower-eyelid region is always treated first with the patient ideally under no sedation and in a 60-degree incline. The patient should focus upward toward a fixed point to ensure that the lower-eyelid skin remains taut during treatment. However, if general anesthesia is undertaken, then the upper eyelid should be held upward and the eye carefully examined for any evidence of peel entry. In addition, because the patient cannot report any symptoms of burning or irritation that accompany contact of peel onto the globe, the eye should be routinely irrigated at the conclusion of lower-eyelid treatment and at the end of the entire peeling session. The assistant should stand behind the patient and gently hold cotton-tipped applicators at both the medial and lateral canthi to avoid entry of peel onto the globe and limit tearing that will run down and dilute the peel unevenly. The assistant should only hold gentle pressure and not force the applicators downward with vigor, which will trigger increase in reflexive tearing. If the patient is awake or only lightly sedated, a fan should be blowing upward across the patient's abdomen up toward the face and eye region to cool the treated area without forcibly blowing into the eye and again causing undue tearing and irritation. Unlike the remainder of the face, a cotton-tipped applicator should be used to apply the chemical agent. **B,C:** Close-up views of the treated area show the desirable level of semitranslucent to fully opaque white that should manifest toward the end of treatment of a particular area. The reader is reminded that the color will fade in a few minutes and the area should not be mistakenly treated again. Immediately after treatment, a 4 × 4 gauze or eye pad soaked in iced saline or water should be placed onto the treated area to dilute the chemical reaction and provide relief (if the patient is awake) of the burning sensation that accompanies the peel.

fort and terminate the chemical process. Iced pads may be reapplied as necessary to maintain patient comfort.

The neck and décolletage area may be treated with a lighter TCA peel (e.g., 15% to 25%). However, the reader is cautioned that aggressive and repeated application of a lighter-strength TCA eventually equals that of a higher concentration. The desired color change should be a light and semitranslucent white and not assume a completely opaque appearance.

After the peeling is complete, Aquaphor ointment (Beiersdorf, Wilton, CT) is generously applied over all peeled areas of the face with a tongue depressor. As the epidermis remains intact for several days, no occlusive dressing is required.

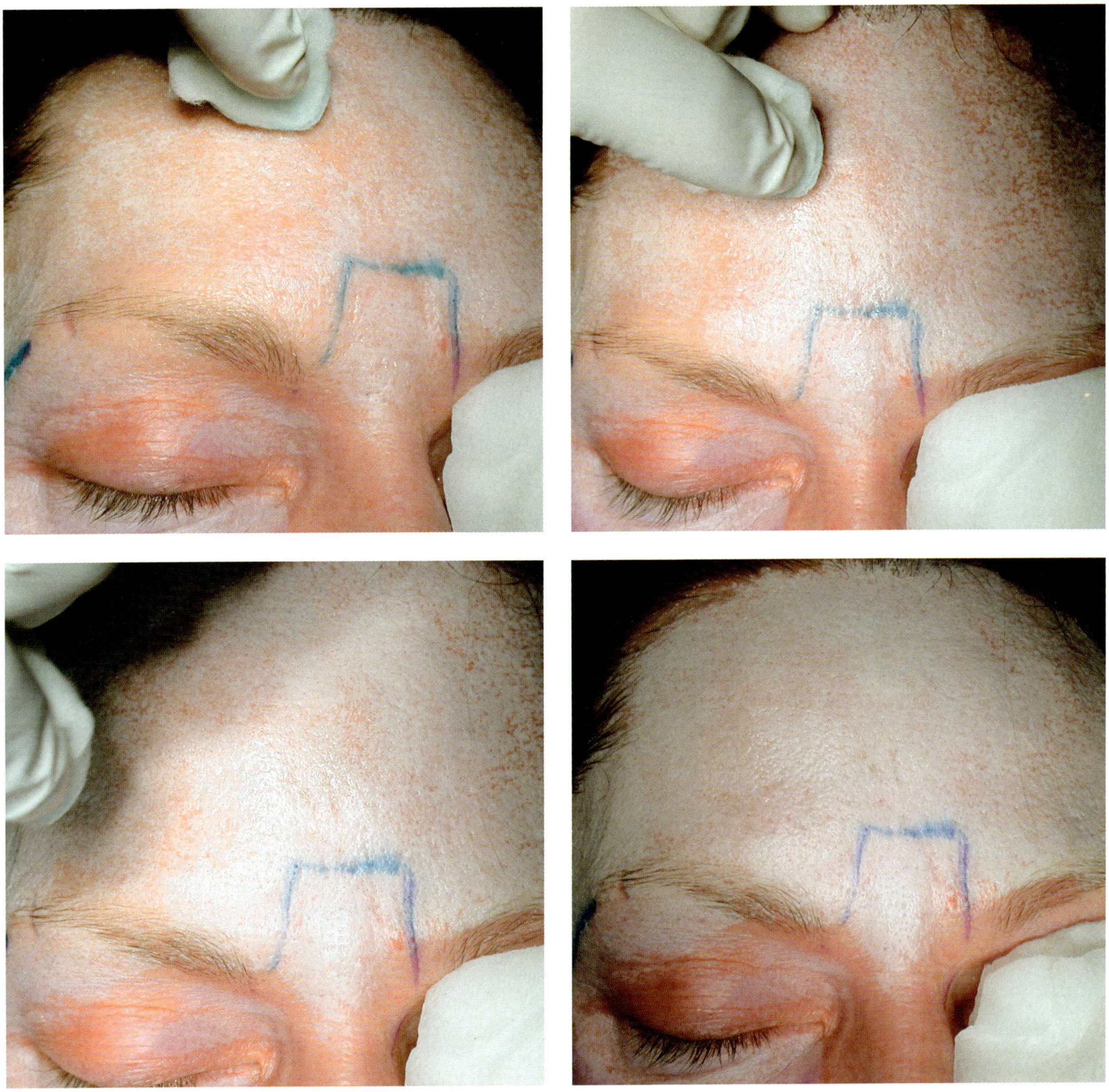

A B C D

FIGURE 9-6. TCA Peel, Step 3. A–D: The forehead is addressed after both lower-eyelid regions have been treated. Application of the chemical peel is undertaken with a cotton ball or cotton pad. The photographs show after several passes of application, the color of the skin begins to change from a semitranslucent to a uniform opaque white. Beyond this point, the color may become a heavily opaque white or even slight gray, which may be the first signs of overtreatment. After treatment (or to abort further reaction), a 4 × 4 gauze soaked in iced water should be placed onto the treated subunit before continuing to the next subunit.

CO_2 Laser Resurfacing

As discussed in the preoperative section of this chapter, CO_2 laser resurfacing should be reserved for deeper rhytidosis, particularly the perioral rhagades, and for patients who are willing to contend with the longer recovery period (Fig. 9-8). Deeper rhytids of the glabella and perioral areas are only minimally addressed with a Jessner's/TCA peel, and patients should recognize that limitation. An alternative to the laser is the phenol peel, but the authors have more limited experience with this peeling technique, which is not discussed herein. The reader is advised to be facile with various resurfacing techniques that have different advantages but not to feel obligated to master the Byzantine number of techniques available today.

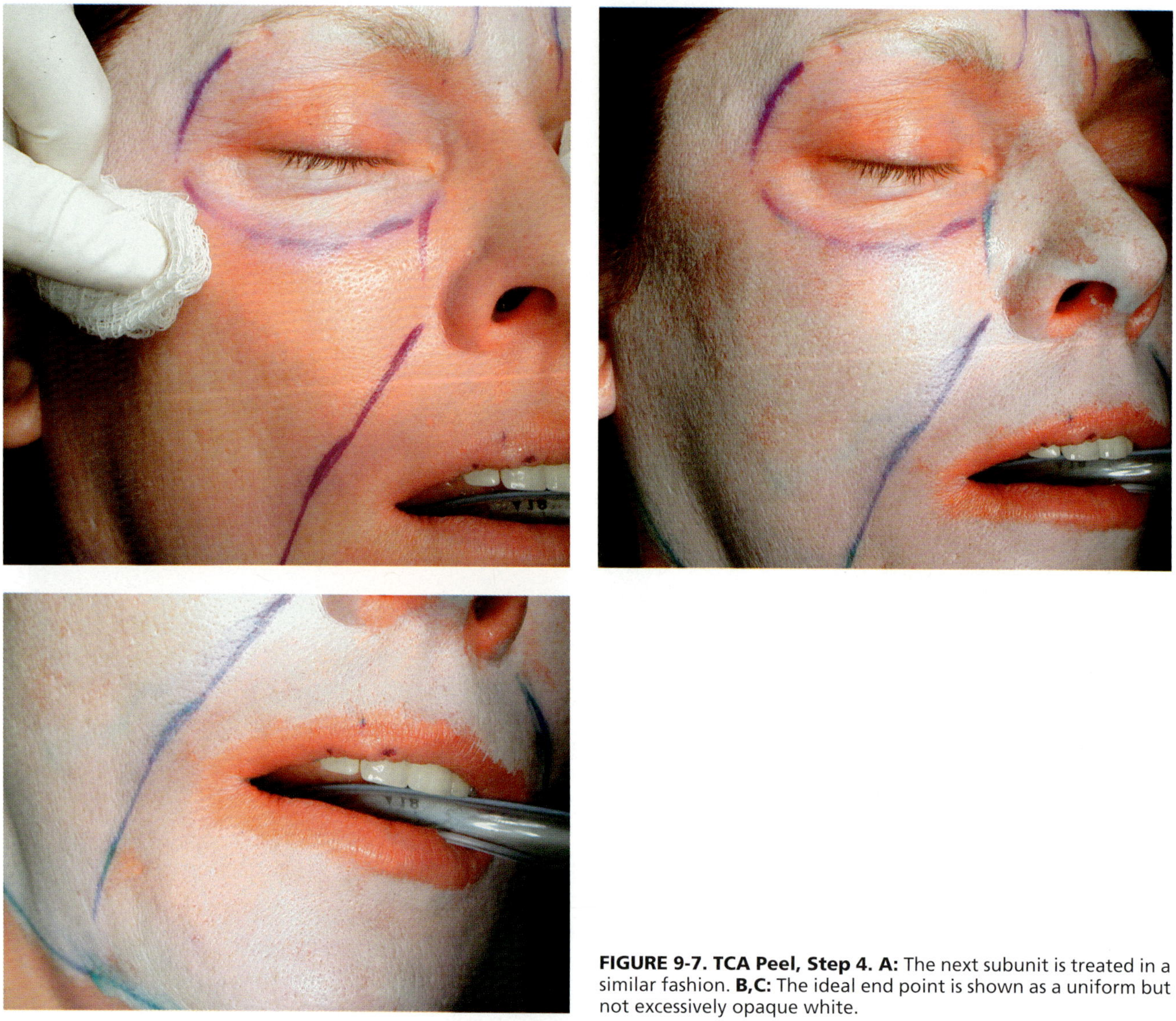

A B C

FIGURE 9-7. TCA Peel, Step 4. A: The next subunit is treated in a similar fashion. **B,C:** The ideal end point is shown as a uniform but not excessively opaque white.

As of the last few years, the authors have been reluctant to subject patients to a full-face laser except in the rarer instances when deeper, panfacial rhytidosis mandates use of this modality. The facial areas that tend to be best suited for laser resurfacing are the glabellar, lower eyelid, and perioral regions. If the laser is applied only to discrete areas of the face, then a chemical peel should be considered in the adjacent areas to blend in the areas of resurfacing. Obviously, all areas should be peeled first before laser is applied to adjacent areas to avoid uncontrolled depth of the peel in areas that have been laser resurfaced. Like the TCA peel, the laser is generally applied by subunit so that adjacent TCA-peeled areas may blend effectively with the laser-treated areas. The laser is set at the recommended start-safe parameters that correspond with a power density for tissue ablation (10 J/cm^2). The laser is held perpendicularly to the skin but aimed tangentially at the perimeter of the resurfaced area to camouflage the transition with the peeled areas. The second pass of the CO_2 laser is undertaken to effect greater collagen remodeling and dermal ablation and is applied almost exclusively in a tangential fashion to minimize excessive thermal injury and depth of resurfacing. Beyond these enumerated technical considerations, laser resurfacing is technically much less demanding than chemical exfoliation and does not require further elaboration in this section. Unlike the TCA peel, the resurfaced areas are fully denuded of epidermis and require both Aquaphor ointment and an occlusive dressing to facilitate reepithelialization and principally to lessen discomfort.

Dermabrasion

The most established resurfacing technique is mechanical dermabrasion. The authors favor a wire-brush over the dia-

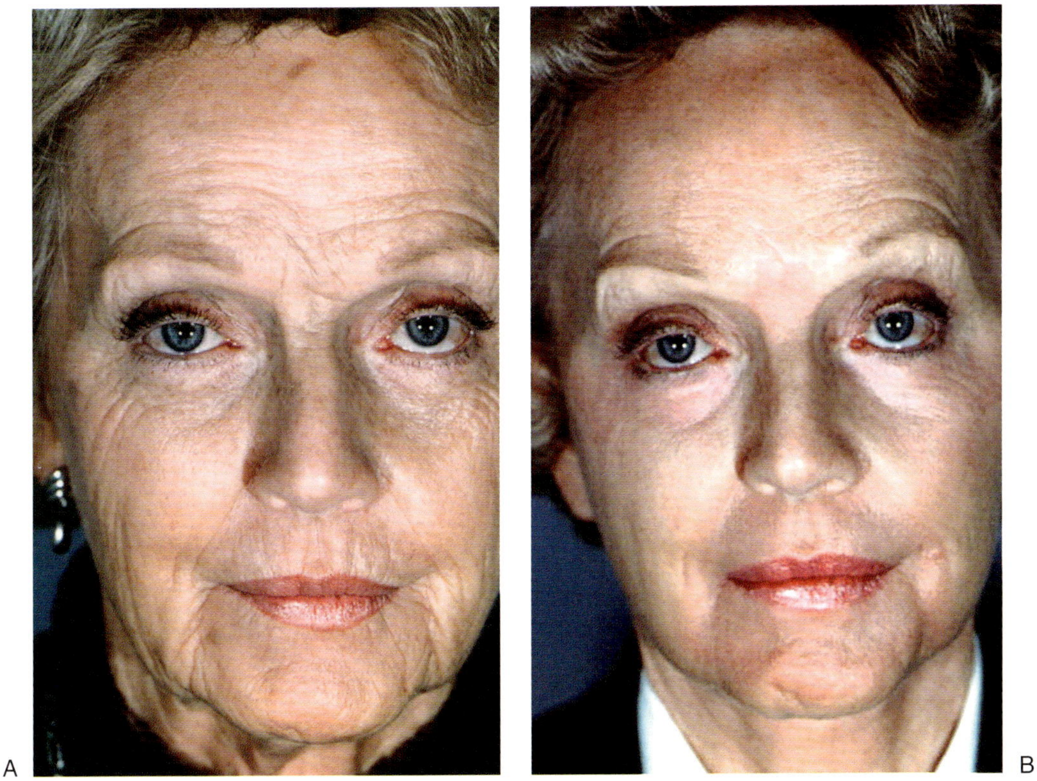

FIGURE 9-8. A,B: This is a 69-year-old woman who was interested in facial rejuvenation prior to renewing her wedding vows. She showed significant photodamage of her skin. She underwent CO_2 laser in the forehead, glabellar, lower-eyelid, and perioral regions and is shown 9 months after resurfacing with notable improvement. This procedure was performed many years ago, and this case highlights the evolution in treatment strategies. The patient would have benefited from a Jessner's/35% trichloroacetic acid peel in the remaining areas for more even and global rejuvenation. The deep and coarse rhytids are more suitable to the CO_2 laser, especially in the perioral region, if the patient is willing to undergo the more protracted recovery period.

mond fraise for its speed and more effective abrasion. Diamond fraises tend to be more forgiving for the novice operator and hold less risk of injury and scarring. The authors have observed no scarring in the patients after dermabrasion or after the use of combined resurfacing techniques. Dermabrasion is the most technically demanding resurfacing tool and should be used with proper training and with a gentle touch. It is more time consuming to achieve a uniform abrasion and appropriate feathering than other modalities. It is obviously restricted from use near the eye in the surrounding periocular region. Another disadvantage is the relative aerosolization and splatter of blood-borne particles that may transmit viruses and other infectious agents to the operator and personnel. (The surgeon and all assistants in the immediate proximity of the dermabrader should be adequately covered with surgical gowns and face-masks outfitted with clear visor shields to avoid contamination with aerosolized splatter of blood and skin particles.) Hypopigmentation also may develop after dermabrasion, especially in the higher Fitzpatrick patients; and the authors caution against deep dermabrasion in darker skin-toned individuals in favor of sequential lighter dermabrasion. However, the authors feel that laser still promotes greater hypopigmentation than dermabrasion for the same depth-of-wound injury because of the thermal effects of the laser.

Dermabrasion offers the undisputed advantage for addressing deeper scars, such as cystic acne scarring, and deeper rhytids, as found periorally. However, in patients with very deep "ice-pick" acne scarring, direct excision of the pitted area with a No. 11 blade followed by wound closure with 6-0 polypropylene should be undertaken as an initial step before subsequent dermabrasion is carried out 6 weeks later. Unlike CO_2 laser intervention, dermabrasion avoids thermal injury, allowing for faster healing time and less protracted erythema than with the laser. However, the laser may be better than dermabrasion for the perioral region as one study suggests,[11] but this matter is controversial. Further, dermabrasion has been successfully used to treat deep, perioral rhagades. Many have touted the beneficial collagen remodeling seen with the CO_2 laser, but one study that compared the histologic changes in dermabrasion and CO_2 laser found no difference in a porcine model.[12] Dermabrasion proves to be a superior instrument when treating the recalcitrant and deeply embedded scars of severe

Salient Technical Points

Chemical Exfoliation (Jessner's/35% Trichloroacetic Acid)

1. Vigorous application of acetone with a 4 × 4 gauze is required to ensure adequate oil removal and a consequently uniform peel.
2. Jessner's may be liberally applied, and no skin color end is targeted.
3. The patient should be then marked out with a surgical marking pen to define the subunits, which the surgeon should rigorously follow.
4. Always begin application of the TCA to the periocular region first, because the patient should be minimally sedated to report any discomfort and in an upright position so that the chemical solution has less of a chance to enter the eye.
5. Always have BSS on standby to irrigate the eye if any irritation is reported.
6. Apply TCA first to discrete rhytids before applying a more even coat over the particular subunit. Edema erases any evidence of rhytidosis after one pass of the TCA.
7. Always squeeze out the TCA-impregnated cotton ball before application to minimize accidental excess trailing down the neck.
8. Discard every used cotton ball into the waste bin to minimize potential confusion over what solution remains on the cotton ball.
9. Use discretion when peeling the upper-lid region, which benefits little from peeling and has a risk of scarring because of the thinness of the skin.
10. Abort any peel reaction that appears to have passed too deeply with moistened gauze because water dilutes the peel concentration.

CO_2 Laser Resurfacing

1. Ensure that the patient understands the protracted recovery period.
2. Treat only discrete areas of deep rhytidosis (lower eyelid, glabellar, and perioral regions) rather than the entire face if possible because of the longer recovery time and the risk of progressive jaw line depigmentation.
3. Ensure that all laser-treated areas are symmetrical, because patients may express undue concern over areas that are not perceived to be perfectly symmetrical.
4. The second pass of the laser should be aimed only tangentially over a broader area to effect collagen tightening.
5. If a concurrent chemical peel is planned in adjacent areas to achieve a more even resurfacing, the peel always should be completed first.

Dermabrasion

1. Dermabrasion is an excellent modality for acne scarring, second-stage scar revision, and rhinophyma refinement.
2. It is the technically most challenging resurfacing modality.
3. The diamond fraise may be more forgiving (but less efficient) than the wire brush and may be particularly well suited for the novice surgeon.
4. The surgeon and proximal operating staff should be gowned and protected with visored facemasks because of the aerosolization of blood and skin particles.
5. The weight of the dermabrader should never fully rest on the skin surface but should be gently controlled to permit superficial abrasion.
6. After the first dermabrasion pass, the second should be directed perpendicular to the first in order to effect even cutaneous abrasion and maximal microlaceration of the dermis.
7. The periocular region should not be resurfaced with a dermabrader for risk of lacerating the delicate eyelid skin.
8. When working near the lips, the dermabrader should be directed toward the lip to avoid accidental and disastrous ensnarement of the lip. Similarly, 4 × 4 sponges should remain some distance from the rotating dermabrader head.
9. The depth of dermabrasion should not greatly exceed the initial bleeding encountered at the level of the papillary dermis to avoid potential scarring.

acne. Although dermabrasion may be viewed as a "low-tech" modality, its unique advantages should recommend this treatment option in many different clinical scenarios. Therefore, the facial plastic surgeon should keep this invaluable tool in his or her armamentarium.

Mechanical dermabrasion may be best carried out under general anesthesia when a significant area must be resurfaced for several reasons. First, use of local anesthesia may be limited to minimize tissue distortion that may interfere with correct identification of tissue depth. Second, patient movement is reduced, which is critical to safe and successful dermabrasion. Third, a curious phenomenon of unconscious, reflexive patient quivering, which is witnessed when dermabrasion is carried out under sedation, is avoided.

However, limited dermabrasion should be conducted under the minimum anesthesia that would aid patient comfort and secure patient compliance.

When dermabrasion is carried out near the lip, the surgeon should ensure that the rotation of the dermabrader head is toward the lip edge to lessen the chance of the lip being caught in the dermabrader. Similarly, 4 × 4 gauzes used to wipe the blood from the resurfaced area should remain away from the dermabrader head to minimize ensnarement. Dermabrasion is carried out with a firm hand and gentle touch. The full weight of the instrument should not rest on the skin surface but only the lightest contact established. The surgeon observes the microlaceration of the skin and the bleeding that ensues as the papillary dermis is violated. After the initial pass of the dermabrader has been completed, the surgeon then should rotate the direction of the dermabrader head perpendicular to the first pass to achieve uniform resurfacing and laceration of the dermis. The depth of dermabrasion is dependent on the depth of the pathology but generally should not greatly exceed the level of initial bleeding observed at the level of the papillary dermis. At the end of the procedure, all dermabraded areas are dressed with Aquaphor ointment and an occlusive dressing similar to laser-treated areas.

DVD Combined Resurfacing Techniques

The following clinical scenarios should help the reader better appreciate how these disparate resurfacing modalities may be effectively combined to achieve a desired effect.

Acne Scarring

Acne scarring offers a prime example of how various resurfacing modalities may be combined to achieve an improved cosmetic result (Fig. 9-9A–C). First and foremost, the patient must fully appreciate the limitations of aesthetic improvement possible. The deep scars that descend into and interdigitate with the underlying subcutaneous tissue are refractory to complete elimination but may be realistically improved 30% to 50%, as patients are counseled. However, the literature quotes best improvements of 70% to 80%.[13] Further, the patient must have all active acne lesions resolved for at least 9 months prior to considering any treat-

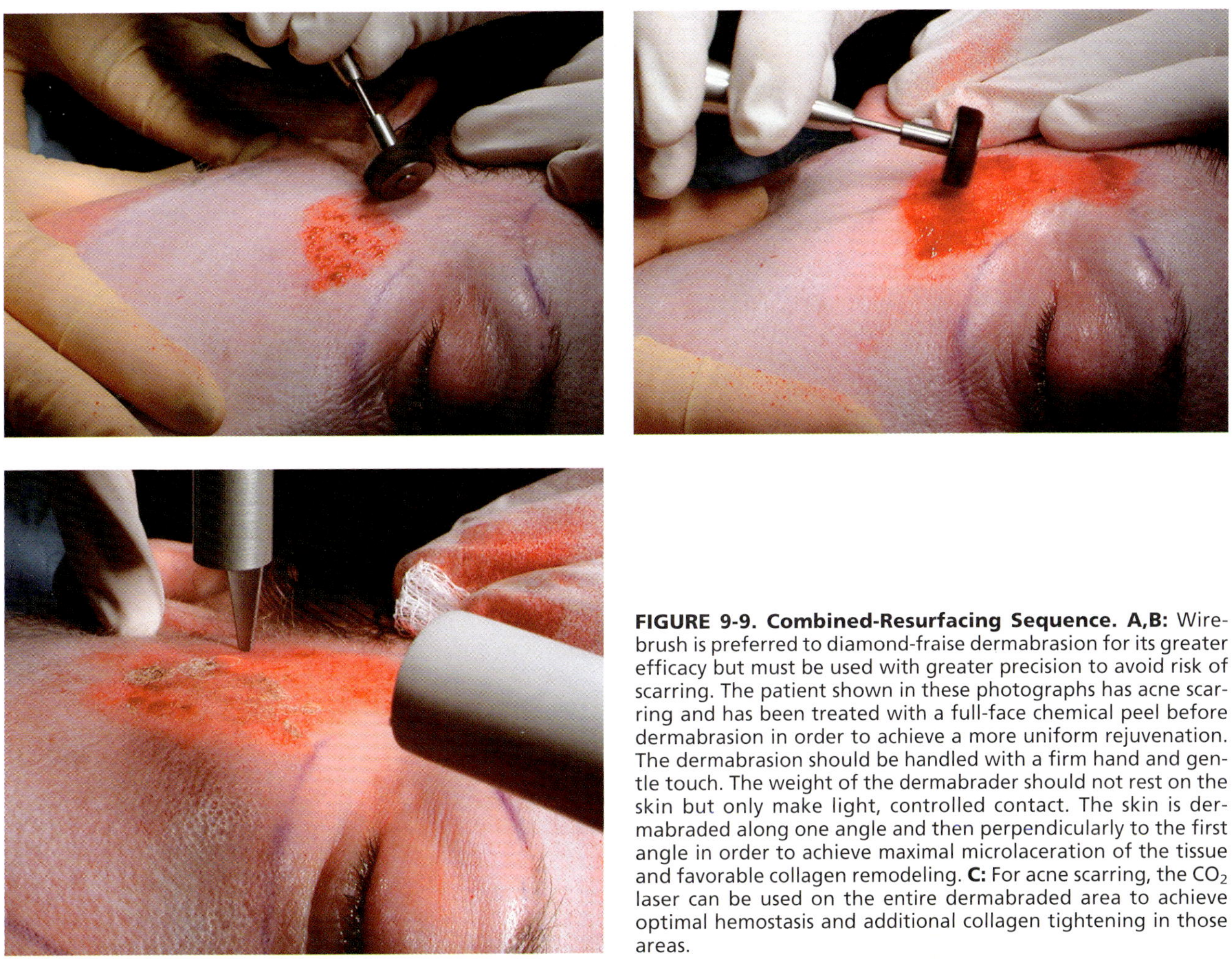

A B C

FIGURE 9-9. Combined-Resurfacing Sequence. A,B: Wire-brush is preferred to diamond-fraise dermabrasion for its greater efficacy but must be used with greater precision to avoid risk of scarring. The patient shown in these photographs has acne scarring and has been treated with a full-face chemical peel before dermabrasion in order to achieve a more uniform rejuvenation. The dermabrasion should be handled with a firm hand and gentle touch. The weight of the dermabrader should not rest on the skin but only make light, controlled contact. The skin is dermabraded along one angle and then perpendicularly to the first angle in order to achieve maximal microlaceration of the tissue and favorable collagen remodeling. **C:** For acne scarring, the CO_2 laser can be used on the entire dermabraded area to achieve optimal hemostasis and additional collagen tightening in those areas.

ment. The collagenases that predominate during active eruptions can lead to significant scar formation if resurfaced. Additionally, as mentioned, the patient must have terminated any isotretinoin (Accutane) use for a minimum of 6 months or, better yet, 1 year.

Acne scarring tends to be worse in the malar region but also may affect the chin, temple, and forehead areas. Often, a TCA peel may be employed to address concomitant photodamage in less scarred areas as well as to feather the deeper resurfaced skin with the surrounding areas. In higher Fitzpatrick patients (III or IV), TCA peels are applied more widely with spot-focused dermabrasion in only the deeper scars to minimize inflammatory hyperpigmentation. Further, as stated, the authors only dermabrade to the superficial papillary dermis in these darker-skinned patients with the intention of further dermabrasion sessions to minimize possible hypopigmentation that may otherwise occur with deeper dermabrasion. If a chemical peel is performed, it should be done first for two reasons: (a) the eyelid region (if resurfaced) should be done first when the patient is more awake to avoid inadvertent entry of peel solution into the eye; and (2) *the peel should be performed on intact epidermis and dermis prior to any dermabrasion or CO_2 laser to avoid an uncontrolled full-thickness injury in denuded areas.*

Dermabrasion is then carried out on areas of deep, acne scarring in the previously described transverse fashion. (The skin is abraded in one direction and then redirected perpendicular to the original path.) Patients also should be cautioned that pore size may increase (and rarely decrease in size) with dermabrasion, especially over the central areas of the face. It is imperative to observe the change in pore size during dermabrasion and to abort any further passes of the dermabrader if the pore size appears to be enlarging.

The laser is then passed over the dermabraded areas once or twice in order to tighten the collagen further and provide some limited hemostasis. The CO_2 laser is selectively delivered to only the areas of severe acne scarring and feathered into the surrounding areas. At the conclusion of the procedure, the exposed, treated areas are coated with Aquaphor ointment, and the laser-treated areas have an additional N-terface (Winfield Laboratories, Inc., Richardson, TX) dressing applied to minimize air exposure and resulting discomfort.

Rhinophyma

Rhinophyma serves as another excellent model for combined facial resurfacing. The disfiguring, bulbous quality of the rhinophymatous nasal tip has such excessive volume that laser resurfacing alone[14] or cautery may take an unnecessarily long time to debulk the tissue. The thermal damage of either of these modalities alone also has led to unfavorable scar contracture and at times nasal valvular collapse and obstruction. Cold-knife excision alone is imprecise and tends to cause significant hemorrhagic loss. What the authors have found to work well is a combination of hot and cold techniques that allow rapid debulking, fine-tuning, and hemostasis. Review of the disease process and details of the surgical technique may be found in Chapter 7.

Facial Rhytidosis

For thicker, discrete lesions such as actinic keratoses and seborrheic keratoses, the lesion should be first removed by a No. 10 (or No. 15) blade in a shave resection followed by CO_2 laser to vaporize the remaining tissue and restore a more even contour. Conversely, dyschromias and fine to moderate rhytids respond more favorably to a TCA peel. As noted, the TCA peel offers a faster recovery period and diminished risk of hypopigmentation or depigmentation than the CO_2 laser. Deeper rhytids, such as perioral rhagades, may be better treated with the CO_2 laser, if patients accept the sequela of protracted erythema and risk of hypopigmentation. An acceptable alternative to the CO_2 laser for thick keratoses and deep rhytids is dermabrasion. Dermasanding with silicon–carbide sandpaper may be used for relatively small lesions of actinic keratosis.

POSTOPERATIVE CONSIDERATIONS: CARE, FOLLOW-UP, AND COMPLICATIONS

DVD Postoperative Care and Follow-Up

Postoperative care may be overwhelming for many patients, and a strict, daily postoperative visit schedule (at least for the first five consecutive days) is followed to reassure patients about the expected sequelae and instruct them on the daily care regimen.[15] Prior to establishing a daily follow-up routine, the office staff received numerous phone calls into the evening hours from fearful and concerned patients. Now, practically no telephone communication transpires except for the routine policy of contacting patients the night of surgery to answer questions and promote a positive physician–patient rapport. Also, the intensive teaching that trained staff members disseminate to patients in the postoperative period is most suited to be undertaken at that time and not in the preoperative phase for fear that the worried patient would unduly elect not to undergo the procedure. Further, postoperative instructions given before the procedure most likely will be forgotten if relayed verbally or confuse the patient if presented in a detailed written format.

The First 5 Days

The initial few days after resurfacing must involve good physician (or staff)–patient communication to mitigate patient fears and provide the requisite instruction as to the proper cleaning regimen to which the patient should adhere.

TABLE 9–1. POSTOPERATIVE CARE FOR THE CHEMICALLY RESURFACED PATIENT*

Postoperative Days	Ointment Regimen	Cleaning Regimen	Makeup Regimen
1–5 Days	Aquaphor	Vinegar and water** b.i.d. for the first postoperative day, then q.i.d. thereafter	None
5–10 Days	Aquaphor (until epithelialization is complete)	Cetaphil cleanser (without sunscreen)	None
10–30 Days	Ceptaphil lotion	Cetaphil cleanser (without sunscreen)	Natural, powder-based makeup with titanium dioxide or zinc oxide sunblock (when epithelialization is complete)

*The laser-treated patient follows the same regimen except he or she has an occlusive dressing for the first 2 postoperative days. Accordingly, the patient cannot clean the skin during this period when the occlusive dressing is applied.
**1/2 tablespoon of vinegar mixed with 1 cup of distilled water, then rinsed off with distilled water, and dried with a cotton-tipped applicator. Patients may begin showering on postoperative day 3 as tolerated.

An important principle to which the authors subscribe is the early application of iced cold packs to the treated areas. A marked reduction in postoperative edema has been witnessed with the liberal use of cold packs in patients who have undergone any type of resurfacing as well for those patients who have undergone surgical procedures, such as rhytidoplasty, browlift, or blepharoplasty. Ice packs should be initiated immediately after the resurfacing procedure is complete. (In fact, iced gauze is applied immediately to each subunit after that area has undergone chemical peeling.) Patients are asked to apply cold packs routinely, as tolerated, for the next 24 hours. They also are advised preoperatively to acquire a pack of frozen peas that they can use as an effective cold pack when they arrive home. Clearly, vigilant icing should never be a substitute for a gentle surgical hand and good operative technique.

The patient who has undergone a chemical peel** has a markedly different experience than that of his or her postlaser counterpart. Accordingly, treatment protocols differ somewhat to reflect this divergence in experience (Table 9-1). Postlaser patients have an exposed dermis, which causes significant discomfort, especially when the dermal layer lies in direct contact with the ambient air (Fig. 9-10). Therefore, laser-treated skin is covered with a thick coating of Aquaphor and an occlusive dressing (N-terface), followed by additional Aquaphor ointment, and then trimmed 4 × 4 gauze. This multilayer protection serves to reduce patient discomfort from a perceived 6 to 8 (of 10) on a pain scale to 1 to 2 (as gleaned from the authors' survey of their patients). A recent study has confirmed the reduction of pain in individuals with closed dressing versus open wounds in laser-resurfaced

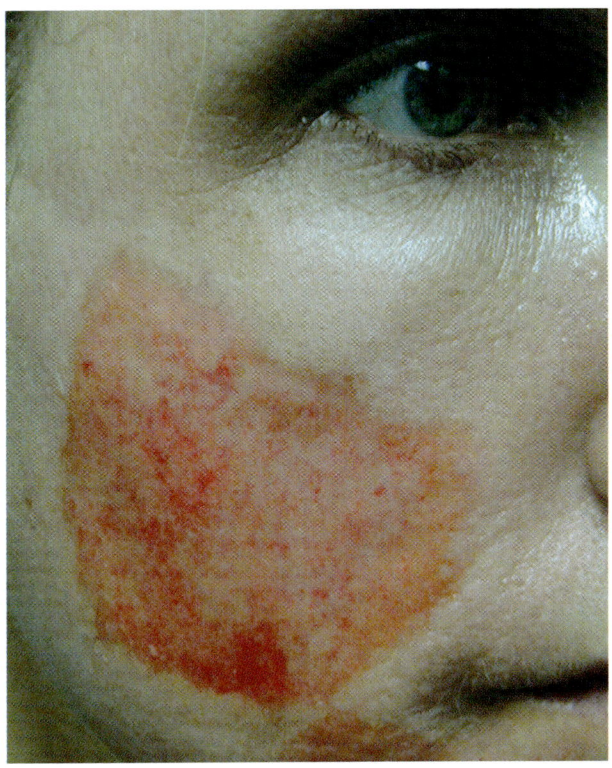

FIGURE 9-10. This is a close-up, right-lateral view of a patient who is postoperative day 1 from a full-face trichloroacetic acid (TCA) peel as well as bilateral cheek dermabrasion and CO_2 laser treatment for acne scarring, for which she had already undergone laser and dermabrasion treatment to the cheeks in the remote past. The photograph demonstrates the old epithelial covering still present on the TCA-peeled areas compared with the exposed dermis in the dermabraded and laser-treated areas.

**The authors prefer Jessner's solution followed by 35% TCA for the majority of patients.

patients, as well as the absence of any increase in bacterial infections or contact dermatitis.[16] If the occlusive dressing should become displaced, patients are asked to apply additional Aquaphor ointment over the exposed area rather than trying to readjust the dressing, for patients typically adjust only the overlying gauze and not the N-terface dressing, which exacerbates rather than alleviates any dryness.

The following day after resurfacing, the patient is examined to ensure that a sufficient coating of Aquaphor is in place (usually 1 to 2 mm in thickness) and that the multilayered dressing is correctly situated. The occlusive dressing is maintained for a period of 2 days, after which the patient follows the same regimen as the chemically exfoliated patient. If the dressing has fallen away, then a fresh N-terface/gauze dressing is applied and trimmed accordingly to reduce bulkiness and fit the contours of the face. Additionally, the N-terface/gauze dressing is removed from the perioral region and reapplied postoperative day 1 in order to clean the area that is typically prone to exudative buildup.

Unlike the laser-treated patient, the chemically resurfaced patient still maintains an epidermal layer after the procedure for several days (Fig. 9-11A–D). The discomfort that the chemically resurfaced individual experiences usually lasts about 4 hours after the procedure, then dissipates to some extent. No occlusive dressing is applied, but a thick coating of Aquaphor ointment is evenly distributed over the treated areas. The patient should be instructed to begin

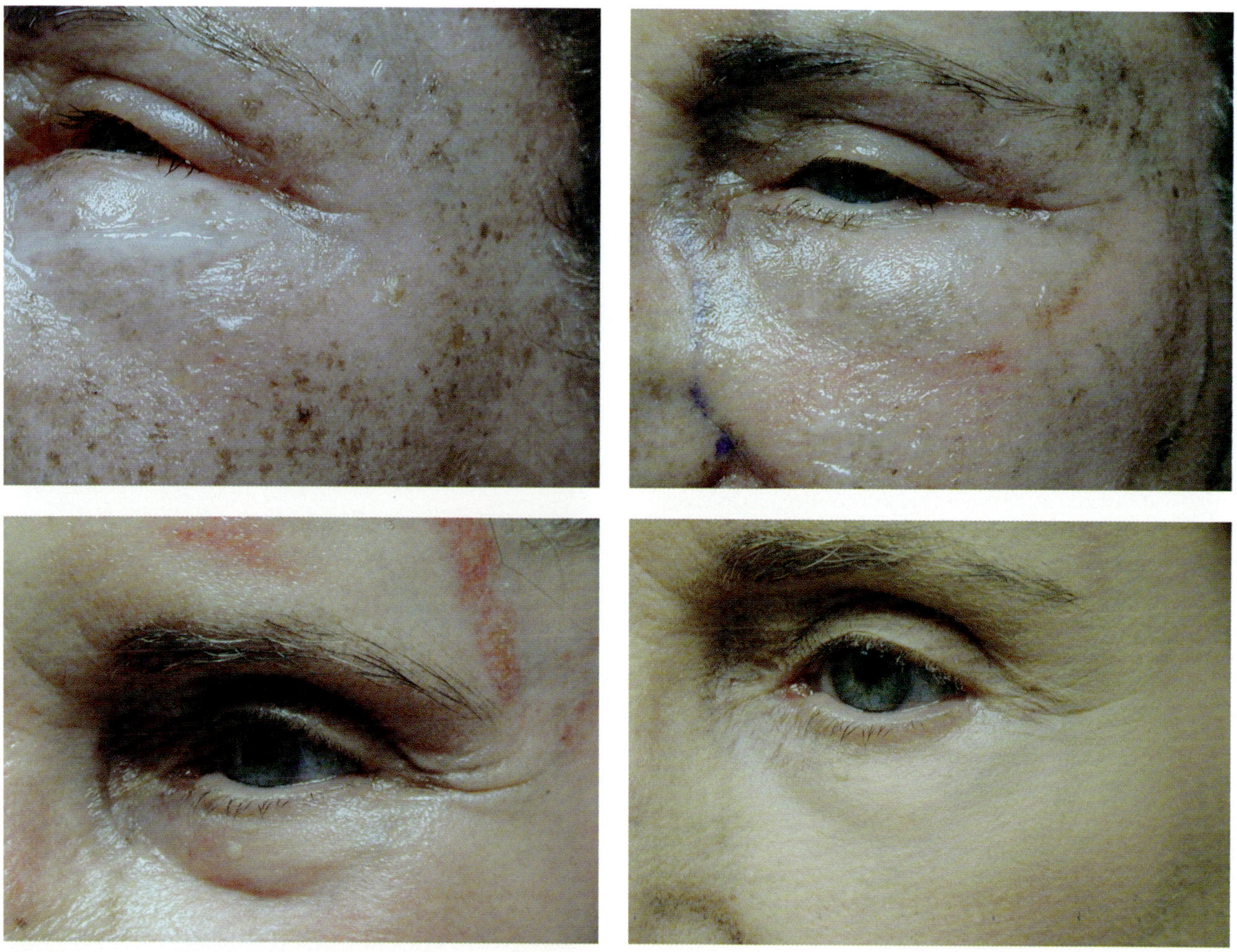

A B C D

FIGURE 9-11. A: The patient is shown the second day after a peel with marked edema that is typically the worst on the second day and dissipates slowly thereafter. The darkened spots signify the old epidermis that has yet to shed, and the lighter pink area in the lateral-canthal region indicates a denuded area that has lost the old epidermal covering already. **B:** The same patient is shown on the third day with more shedding of the old epidermis and a marked reduction in edema. **C:** The patient is shown on the tenth day after peeling with almost entirely new epidermal covering except for two areas that have yet to heal in the forehead region. These exposed areas were selectively treated with Aquaphor until complete epithelialization. **D:** The patient is shown on the fourteenth day after undergoing makeup treatment with a mineral powder-based makeup that is suitable for the newly resurfaced skin.

cleaning the affected areas on the first postoperative day. However, the patient should be advised to remove all the Aquaphor ointment with a cotton ball moistened with distilled water before attempting to clean the resurfaced areas. The cleaning regimen involves 1/2 tablespoon of white vinegar mixed with 1 cup of distilled water. This mixture is gently applied with a cotton ball to the affected areas twice a day for the first postoperative day and four times daily thereafter. The vinegar and water should be rinsed off with distilled water. The resurfaced area may be dried by rolling a cotton-tipped applicator over the cleaned areas. The authors have found that conventional faucet water may cause more irritation than distilled water but recognize that water purity is a regionally dependent variable. Further, cleaning the skin more frequently or less so has led to either discomfort and protracted healing or build-up of exudate, respectively. Although the epithelial layer is maintained for several days, the patient still may report some discomfort whenever the skin is cleaned.

During the first few postoperative days, the photodamaged skin of the chemically resurfaced patient will begin to turn ashen and fall away in a piecemeal fashion. The patient may be alarmed at the abrupt darkening of the skin and the subsequent erythematous base that arises underneath the old epithelial remnants but should be appropriately assuaged that all of this is expected. Both the laser and chemically treated patients should continue the described cleaning regimen during the initial 5 days. In addition, after the first 3 days, patients should be able to tolerate showering with tepidly warm water cascading down their forehead, which not only effectively soothes the treated areas but also soaks the skin, encouraging sloughing of dead epithelial cells. Before this period, premature showering will cause undue discomfort and should be avoided. The laser-treated patient usually needs to wait 4 to 5 days before warm water may be tolerated against the face. Shampooing may be permitted if the shampoo is mild and kept away from the affected areas during the period of reepithelialization.

Many topical ointments have been tried on the resurfacing patient with varying success. Plain petroleum products tend to evaporate much more quickly than Aquaphor and thereby prove to be less desirable. More sophisticated products, such as copper-peptide solutions (Neova, Procyte Corp., Redmond, WA), result in an undesirably high incidence of dermatitis in the authors' experience. After trying many high-end specialty skin care lines, the authors have returned to simple, less expensive products that tend to have fewer ingredients and that the authors contend contribute to the lower incidence of adverse skin reactions that have been witnessed. The single most important factor that contributes to the onset of dermatitis—which can lead in turn to pruritus, erythema, delayed healing, and even scarring—is application of products too early (prior to completed epithelialization) and that are chemically irritating to the skin.

Of note, patients are instructed to sleep in a semiinclined posture to alleviate some of the expected edema. Further, maintaining a supine position also prevents unintended removal of ointment, which can both soil the sheets and expose the healing skin to excessive dryness. However, patients who have failed to follow this prescribed policy have healed equally well and are not compelled to subscribe to this regimen if they cannot tolerate it.

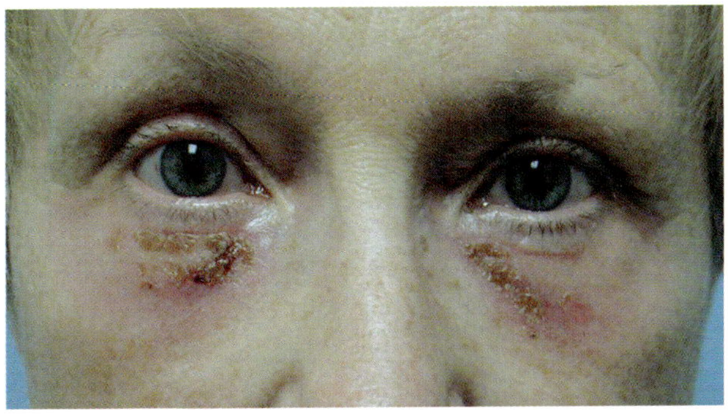

FIGURE 9-12. Close-up, frontal view of a patient who is 10 days postoperative from a lower-lid transconjunctival blepharoplasty with pinch excision for dermatochalasis as well as a lower-lid trichloroacetic acid peel. The photograph demonstrates the exudative buildup that resulted from inadequate cleaning and insufficient application of ointment. She was advised not to pick at the exudate or scabs but to soak the areas with vinegar and water and attempt gentle removal with a cotton-tipped applicator afterward. She also was admonished to apply a thicker coating of Aquaphor ointment until she was completely epithelialized and free of exudates.

From 5 to 10 Days

Treatment protocols do not differ significantly between the first and the following 5 days. Attention to moisture with a thick coating of Aquaphor is still the most important aspect to successful and rapid healing. As is well documented in the literature, uneven and delayed healing may be attributed to desiccation and exudative covering of a wound. Gentle, yet vigilant, cleaning and soaking remove the unwanted exudate that can transform into an encrusted scab if left without moisture (Fig. 9-12). Likewise, a wet, fibrinous exudate retards effective epithelialization and should be appropriately removed. Furthermore, a moistened exudate may foster the colonization and possible infection in the treated areas, leading to slower epithelialization and irritative dermatitis. However, patients are strongly cautioned about refraining from picking at their scabs or crusts to avoid potential scarring.

Epithelialization rate is quite variable (Figs. 9-13A and 9-14) but is usually complete by 10 days. Aquaphor ointment must be continued until full epithelialization is realized. Epithelial breaks may be observed under crusting or, conversely, in areas aggressively cleaned. The cleaning regimen should be followed carefully to avoid unnecessary delay in epithelial growth. Even if the occlusive ointment results

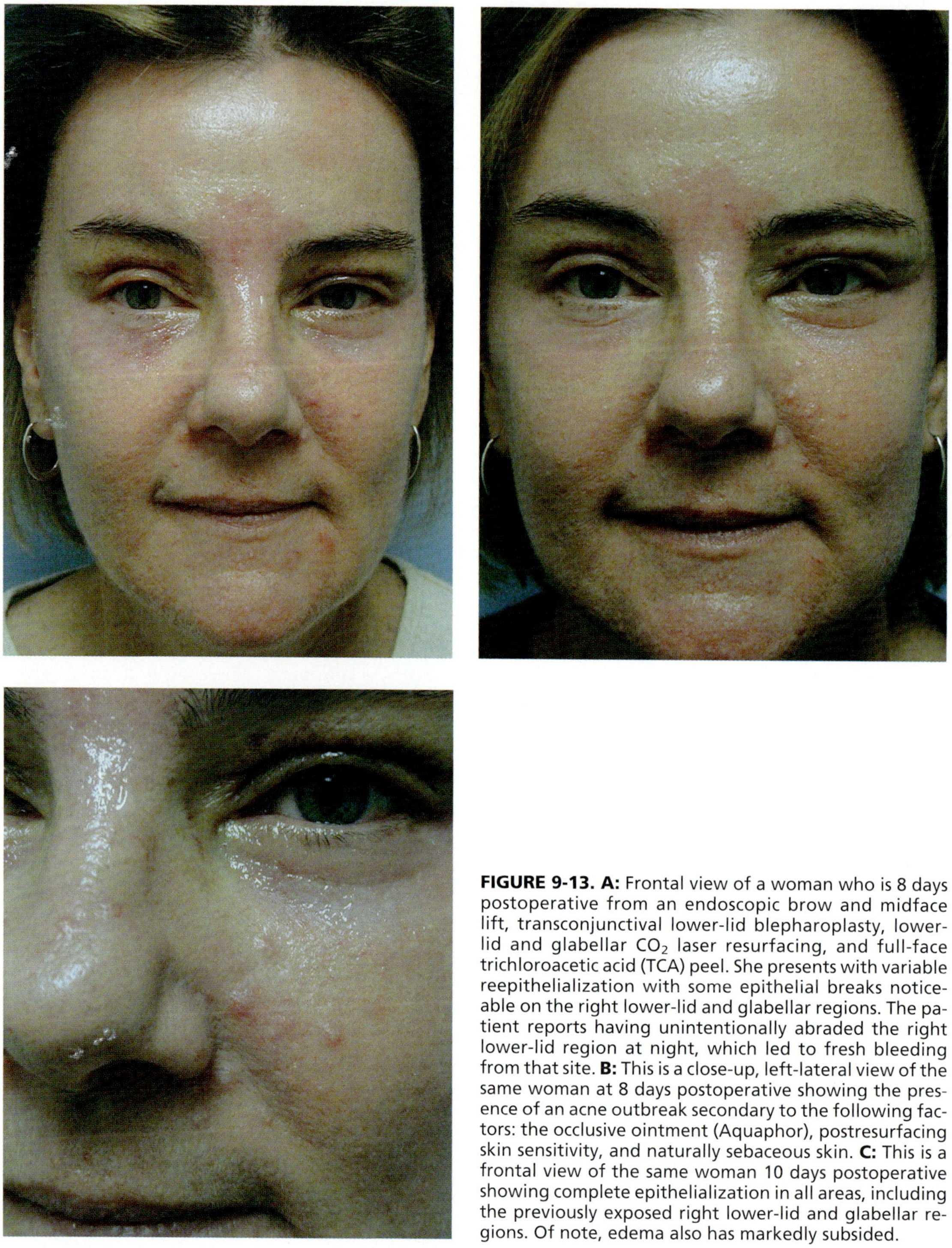

FIGURE 9-13. A: Frontal view of a woman who is 8 days postoperative from an endoscopic brow and midface lift, transconjunctival lower-lid blepharoplasty, lower-lid and glabellar CO_2 laser resurfacing, and full-face trichloroacetic acid (TCA) peel. She presents with variable reepithelialization with some epithelial breaks noticeable on the right lower-lid and glabellar regions. The patient reports having unintentionally abraded the right lower-lid region at night, which led to fresh bleeding from that site. **B:** This is a close-up, left-lateral view of the same woman at 8 days postoperative showing the presence of an acne outbreak secondary to the following factors: the occlusive ointment (Aquaphor), postresurfacing skin sensitivity, and naturally sebaceous skin. **C:** This is a frontal view of the same woman 10 days postoperative showing complete epithelialization in all areas, including the previously exposed right lower-lid and glabellar regions. Of note, edema also has markedly subsided.

in milia or acne formation, it must be continued until all the epithelialization is complete. To simplify matters, all patients are kept on Aquaphor ointment for at least 10 days (or longer if epithelialization has not been concluded) unless full epithelialization is completed earlier and considerable milia have plagued the patient.

Unlike the cleaning regimen outlined during the first 5 days in which vinegar and water are preferred, Cetaphil (Galderma, Alliance, TX) cleanser has proven to be a safe and reliable agent that works more vigorously than vinegar and water solution and may be tolerated by the patient after 5 days of healing have transpired. As with all treatment protocols, careful attention must be paid to tailor a plan on an individual basis. If the patient finds that Cetaphil proves to be too harsh an agent at that stage, then a vinegar and water preparation should be maintained instead.

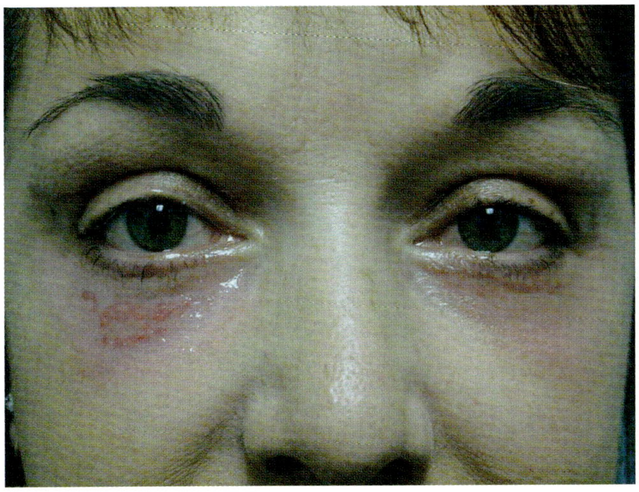

FIGURE 9-14. Close-up, frontal view of a patient who is 14-days status post–TCA peel to the lower lids and transconjunctival lower-lid blepharoplasty with pinch excision of redundant skin. She demonstrates complete epithelialization of the left eye with some residual exposed dermis under the right eye, for which she is being maintained on Aquaphor ointment. This photograph demonstrates the variability in healing that may be partially attributed in this case to an aggressive cleaning regimen. We advised her to decrease her cleaning to only twice a day.

After 10 Days

The most critical period in healing involves the first 8 to 10 days, during which the denuded skin undergoes reepithelialization. As mentioned, if reepithelialization has not fully occurred by 10 days, then Aquaphor ointment should be continued until that time arrives (Fig. 9-14). Once epithelialization is completed, a gentle moisturizer may be used, such as Cetaphil lotion (Galderma). The patient should be cautioned to avoid Cetaphil lotion that has any sunscreen contents because this chemical element may contribute to irritative (immediate) or contact (delayed) dermatitis. After epithelialization is concluded, Cetaphil lotion is better tolerated than Aquaphor because the thickness of the coating is less, which minimizes the chance of milia formation and is more cosmetically acceptable. However, if the patient begins to experience significant dryness, then he or she should alternate Aquaphor ointment at night followed by Cetaphil lotion during the day until the dryness subsides.

After epithelialization is completed, the patient may begin to don cosmetic camouflage as desired. However, if the patient does not desire entry into the public eye, usage of cosmetic products is discouraged for as long as possible to expedite healing and minimize dermatitis. Consultation with a trained aesthetician may be required to determine the best products that hold minimal potential for dermatitis. Liquid-based products tend to have more preservatives and should be avoided for the first 30 days. Conversely, mineral-based, all natural, powder foundations may be better tolerated by the newly resurfaced skin. After trying many product lines, the authors have experienced almost no dermatitis with the Jane Iredale (Iredale Mineral Cosmetics, Ltd., Denver, CO) concealing makeup that contains a titanium-dioxide sun block. Also, chemical sunscreens that contain octyl methoxycinnamate tend to be more irritative than physical blocking agents such as titanium dioxide or zinc oxide and should be avoided for at least 30 days.[17]

Men can begin shaving 15 days after a chemical peel if all epithelialization has occurred by that time. Typically, men heal faster than women because they have greater vascularity and a higher density of pilosebaceous units. An electric razor should be used for the next 30 days after shaving is begun in order to avoid injury to the newly epithelialized skin.

After the initial 3 to 4 weeks, the patient should be enrolled on a regimen of topical retinoic acid to maintain the benefits of the chemical peel or laser-treated skin. The regimen should be started on an every-other-day or every-third-day basis to ensure that no sensitivity develops and should be advanced to a daily dosage if the patient's new skin tolerates it. In order to minimize sensitivity, the skin should be cleansed and completely dry (approximately 10 to 30 minutes after cleaning) before any retinoic acid is applied. In addition, only a pea-sized amount should ever be used, and the immediate lower-lid area (between the lid margin and the orbital rim) should be carefully avoided so that no inadvertent entry of solution into the eye occurs. *If the patient still has erythema, then retinoic acid should be deferred until all erythema subsides.* As a reminder, erythema typically resolves by 2 to 3 weeks after a TCA peel and often only after 2 to 3 months for CO_2 laser-treated areas.

Complications, Sequelae, and Management

Milia and Acne Outbreaks

Usually milia develop after the first 8 to 10 days and are unusual before this period. If some lesions occur early on, they most likely represent acne uncovered by the recent resurfacing (Fig. 9-13B). However, all these lesions should be delineated carefully from herpetic outbreaks, which exhibit clustering of lesions, vesicular appearance, and intense burning. Milia formation may be exacerbated by prolonged use of an occlusive petroleum-based ointment, such as Aquaphor. Most milia should be left undisturbed because the majority spontaneously resolve. However, if they persist for several weeks or prove to be troublesome to the patient, they may be unroofed with an 18-gauge needle (or No. 11 Bard-Parker blade), and the contents expressed with two opposing cotton-tipped applicators applied with pressure to the milial site. Numerous milia that present or persist after 3 to 4 weeks may be effectively treated with topical retinoic acid applied daily until resolution. Acne, on the other hand (which at times may be indistinguishable from milia) may be treated with a course of tetracycline. Antibiotic administration may be required even several weeks to months after resurfacing as the body adapts to the newly formed skin.

Postinflammatory Hyperpigmentation

As mentioned, a preoperative course of hydroquinone fails to address the deeper melanocytes that persist after a resurfacing procedure. Instead, hyperpigmentation commonly develops after 3 to 5 weeks postprocedure and should be treated with hydroquinone, or an alternative, lightening agent. Prophylactic usage of hydroquinone prior to 3 weeks should be discouraged because this agent tends to be irritative to the new skin. Prophylactic 4% hydroquinone has been used at 3 weeks postoperatively, starting every other day at bedtime for 1 to 2 weeks followed by daily application in those patients exhibiting a Fitzpatrick III or higher skin grade. Glyquin (ICN Photonics, Ltd., Orangeburg, NY), which contains 4% hydroquinone, has been found to be less irritative than other hydroquinone formulations. This product also contains a sun protection factor (SPF) 15 among its ingredients. Fortunately, hyperpigmentation is readily treatable.

Hypopigmentation

Unlike postinflammatory hyperpigmentation, which is reversible, hypopigmentation proves to be a more recalcitrant entity. Hyperpigmentation usually results from injury of the melanocytes superficially that leads to melanin stimulation, whereas hypopigmentation is a product of a deeper level of dermal injury in which the melanocytes are ablated. Hyperpigmentation typically occurs several weeks after resurfacing, whereas hypopigmentation arises after several months to even years postprocedure. Hypopigmentation rarely occurs after a medium-depth chemical peel, such as with the authors' choice of Jessner's solution followed by 35% TCA. However, phenol peels may be more prone to develop hypopigmentation (the so-called "porcelain-mask" appearance), particularly if the croton-oil component is increased.[18–21] Ablative laser resurfacing may also lead to hypopigmentary changes that become more evident as time advances. This is particularly noticeable at the jaw line and may be progressive in nature. Because of this fact, laser resurfacing has been limited to discrete areas of the face that, in the authors' experience, tend to tolerate laser resurfacing better such as the lower-lid, glabellar, and perioral regions.

Hypopigmentation must be carefully delineated from frank depigmentation. Hypopigmentation may resolve, but true depigmentation is not easily managed. If complete depigmentation occurs, all the underlying melanocytes have been destroyed and therefore may not repopulate. Hypopigmentation, on the other hand, involves a reduction in melanocyte number and consequent melanin production. To regain pigmentation, the hypopigmented patient must be subjected to the arduous undertaking of repeated application of psoralen agents exposed to ultraviolet light, which has been successfully used to treat vitiligo for over 50 years.[22] The authors confess lack of experience with this corrective formula and refer interested (and motivated) patients to their dermatologic colleagues for further evaluation and management.

Erythema

Erythema is a known sequela of resurfacing and may persist for several months in the laser-treated patient but usually resolves within 1 to 2 weeks for the chemically treated patient. The thermal injury imparted by the laser may contribute to this longer recovery period. Although erythema may last for a protracted period, long-standing erythema may predispose toward dermatitis or scarring. *The continuum of erythema, dermatitis, and scarring must be carefully understood by the physician so that aggressive management may be employed to abort this chain of events (vide infra).* The erythematous skin is still sensitive to sun exposure, irritative topical agents, and other noxious stimuli. Therefore, it should be managed to minimize exposure to substances that may stimulate dermatitis. If erythema persists for longer than the typical period delineated in the preceding, then active treatment should be initiated as if dermatitis were present. Topical or oral steroids should be considered to treat the erythema to abort the development of dermatitis, which can in turn transform into scarring. Any signs that the erythema has changed in nature, usually turning a more inflamed red, may be suggestive of an incipient dermatitis.

Dermatitis

Dermatitis usually occurs between 10 to 30 days postresurfacing and is manifest by a constellation of signs and symptoms, including significantly increased erythema, raised or irregular contour to the affected skin, and associated pruritus (Figs. 9-15 and 9-16). In the authors' experience, dermatitis has been more prevalent in laser- than chemically treated skin, which may be a product of the prolonged erythema associated with laser-resurfaced skin. As mentioned, this erythema predisposes the patient to dermatitis and must be carefully followed. Dermatitis has been noted to occur principally in the lower-eyelid and perioral region. The authors have chosen to confine laser treatment to these specific areas to avoid the morbidity of full-face laser resurfacing (e.g., prolonged erythema, hypopigmentation at the jaw line, etc.). In the past, when the authors treated patients with full-face laser resurfacing, patients exhibited broader areas of dermatitis. Therefore, in the authors' experience, physicians should be more attentive to laser-treated areas for signs and symptoms of developing dermatitis.

The main objective in treating dermatitis is early identi-

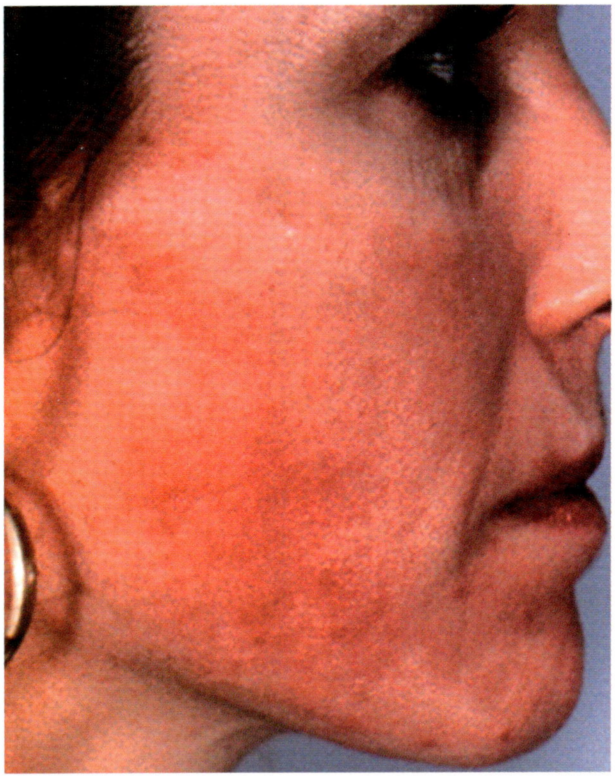

FIGURE 9-15. Close-up, right-lateral view of a patient who is 8 weeks postoperative from a full-face CO_2 laser resurfacing, who demonstrates a contact dermatitis secondary to introduction of a fragrance product. She was advised to stop all topical products, including makeup. In addition, she was started on topical steroid treatment (desonide cream) and followed very closely. She demonstrated complete resolution within 2 weeks.

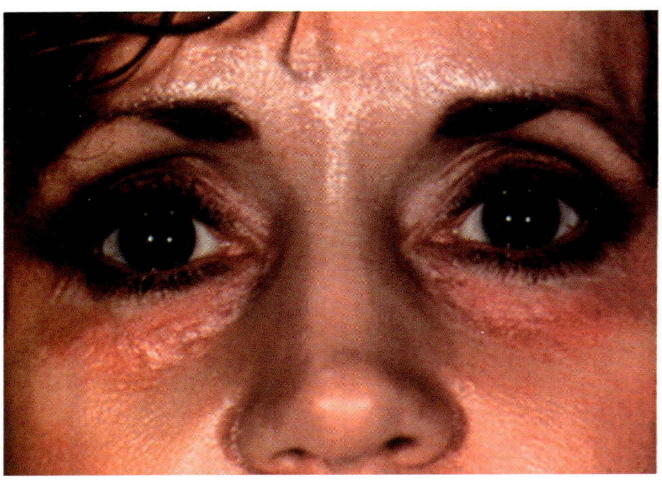

FIGURE 9-16. Close-up, frontal view of a patient who is 6 weeks status post–CO_2 laser resurfacing of her lower eyelids and who demonstrates focal areas of increased erythema and induration consistent with dermatitis. No specific etiologic agent could be elicited from a detailed history. However, the patient was treated with intralesional steroids and closely followed up on a weekly basis with complete resolution of her symptoms within 2 weeks.

fication and removal of the offending agent that is causing the dermatitis. One should interview the patient to determine what agent may have been introduced to engender the dermatitis flare-up. *The importance of early recognition and treatment cannot be overemphasized.* Dermatitis that smolders for a protracted period of time may be increasingly difficult to break: This vicious cycle becomes more tenacious as time progresses. Pathophysiologically, dermatitis stimulates fibroblast activity and collagen synthesis, which directly serves as constituent elements for scar formation. Over time, the temporary dermatitis may transform into more permanent scarring if not addressed early.

Treatment should begin with flurandrenolide tape (Cordran tape, Oclassen Pharmaceuticals, Corona, CA), which contains a potent corticosteroid and has been observed to be impressive in reversing dermatitis. Cordran tape should be applied only to intact, dry skin and works well in discrete areas of dermatitis. It should be applied at night and left in place until the following morning when it can be gently removed by allowing shower water to loosen its adhesive qualities. For more generalized areas, desonide cream (DesOwen, Galderma)—which contains topical corticosteroid to combat dermatitis—is favored. As mentioned, if dermatitis is allowed to persist, the chance of scarring also rises. Therefore, if the preceding methods fail to rid the dermatitis, then intralesional or systemic steroids should be entertained. Intralesional steroid injection may be administered in discrete areas afflicted with dermatitis: triamcinolone acetonide (Kenalog) 10 mg/mL strength dosed at 1 mg/kg is preferred. Alternatively or concurrently, a Medrol dose pack or oral-prednisone equivalent regimen may be started. In addition, pulsed-dye laser therapy has proved very effective as an adjunctive measure in the authors' experience.[23]

Scarring

Fortunately, scarring remains a rare complication of cutaneous resurfacing. However, if erythema or dermatitis persists, some scarring may develop from the chronic irritation to the skin. If such an outcome arises, then treatment should be directed at minimizing the scarring through aggressive and diligent attention to the situation. Similar to management of dermatitis, corticosteroid application (topical, intralesional, systemic) may be administered in a stepwise fashion until a favorable response is evident. Further, early and frequent pulsed-dye laser treatment (about every 3 to 4 weeks) also may control and hopefully eliminate scar formation. Patients who develop scars should be followed weekly until resolution of their complication.

BASIC SKIN CARE

Many physicians who provide aesthetic services relegate knowledge of basic skin care to their aestheticians.

Although, aestheticians have often received extensive training in skin care and cosmetic camouflage, the aesthetic surgeon should not rest on his or her laurels about proper understanding of basic skin care. The surgeon should fully comprehend if the patient's skin care regimen may adversely affect the healing of the resurfaced skin, detect topical agents that may be contributing to dermatitis, and recommend basic products that would promote healing without irritation. Further, the physician should advise the patient on products that will maintain the longevity of the peel or educate the patient on alternative, noninvasive, topical therapy other than ablative resurfacing.

This section does not endeavor to undertake an exhaustive review of all products that are currently on the market, which would otherwise be confusing, unnecessary, and outdated by press time. After reading this section, the physician should understand basic concepts in daily skin care and answer straightforward questions that patients may pose. Perhaps the simplest method of understanding proper skin care is through the requisite products that the patient should use to ensure healthy and vital skin (i.e., daily skin care products: cleansers, toners, moisturizers, sunscreens/blocks, and night creams; and rejuvenative agents: tretinoin and alpha hydroxy acids).

Daily Skin Care Products

Cleansers

Cleansers are the first step toward healthy skin. Unfortunately, most individuals are accustomed to harsh, drying soaps that are counterproductive to good skin care, especially for the postresurfaced skin. Traditional soaps are alkaline by nature and strip essential oils and protective lipids from the skin, leaving it dry and raw. The "antibacterial" soaps may be safely used on the body but are too astringent and alkaline on the more sensitive facial skin and furthermore unnecessary for proper cleaning. Abrasive components, such as pumice, only serve to irritate the skin and may exacerbate conditions such as acne or otherwise sensitive skin. Unlike conventional soaps (pH 8 to 9), cleansers are pH balanced to the skin (pH 5.5) and maintain the acid mantle, which is particularly critical for oilier skin types. Alkaline soaps excessively remove oil and stimulate increased oil production, leaving the skin even oilier.

Cleansers may be divided into two principal types: creamy and foaming. The former type is particularly suited for dry skin, as it maintains greater moisture than the foaming type. Creamy cleansers work well with the postresurfaced skin or in older patients who tend to have more desiccated skin. In addition, creamy cleansers are better at removal of cosmetics than foaming cleansers. However, foaming cleansers offer the patient the visual appeal of lather like traditional soap products and may more effectively clean oilier skin than cream-based cleansers are capable.

Cleansers only should be used once daily, preferably at night, especially if used to remove cosmetics. Twice daily is unnecessary and potentially drying and irritating to the skin. After the face is rinsed, a washcloth may be used to pat dry the skin. If the skin should require additional cleansing during the day, water alone will suffice unless an unusual amount of dirt or debris is accumulated.

Toners

Toners are designed to balance the pH (if an alkaline cleanser is used) and remove any residual debris (e.g., lingering makeup) after use of a cleanser. Toners that contain salicylic acid may benefit the acne-prone skin but may at times promote acne flare-up. However, quality, pH-balanced cleansers have effectively made toners in most cases superfluous. If a toner is used, one should avoid a product that contains alcohol or acetone, both of which are detrimental to the skin owing to the caustic nature of these agents.

Moisturizers

After any kind of cleansing (or toning) of the skin, no matter how gentle, the skin is left somewhat dehydrated and requires effective moisturization. Even oily skin that appears to need no moisturization benefits from a good moisturizer. In fact, a moisturizer will assist in keeping the oil production in check, especially after a cleanser has stripped some of the native oils away.

In general, moisturizers may be either water- or oil-based. The former is better for acne-prone or oily skin, whereas the latter is better designed for drier skin types. Combination skin (oily skin distributed along the central T-zone of the face) should be treated with a water-based product. However, during the winter months when the air may be quite dry, then a water-based product may be used in combination with an oil-based product for areas that remain dry despite water-based moisturization.

A moisturizer should be used once in the morning and once at night. The morning moisturizer may contain a sun protection factor (SPF), which is a critical element to healthy skin. The lip also should be protected with a moisturizing balm that contains an effective SPF. Prolonged, direct sun exposure, particularly between 10 a.m. and 4 p.m. during the height of direct rays, should be avoided as much as possible. Sun protection may consist of a physical blocking agent (e.g., titanium dioxide or zinc oxide) or a chemical block (e.g., octyl methoxycinnamate). A combination of a physical and chemical block works together synergistically to achieve the best protection, while minimizing the chemical load that is imparted by a pure chemical blocking agent. Generally speaking, an SPF 15 is all that is required for indirect, daily sun exposure with only a nominal gain with higher SPF strengths. However, if one should elect to be outdoors for more than 1 hour, then an SPF 30 should be used, with a higher percentage of a physical block again to minimize chemical irritation. Conversely, the body can tolerate much higher chemical and physical blocks than can the face. All patients that have undergone ablative resurfacing should avoid any product with a chemical block for the first 30 days to reduce the likelihood of irritation and dermatitis.

A different moisturizer should be used at night that contains no SPF but instead has a higher lipid content, which acts to nourish and replenish the skin. The skin undergoes its maximal replenishment during the nighttime hours of rest; therefore, nightly moisturization with proper lipid-based ingredients is critical to ensure healthy skin. As part of any moisturizing program, the patient should drink plenty of water during the day. Water spray mists to the face add little benefit but may instead dry the skin further when evaporated.

Rejuvenative Agents

In addition to a strict daily regimen of skin care, certain topical agents may serve a medicinal purpose to rejuvenate aging skin. The two types that are discussed are alpha hydroxy acids and vitamin A derivatives.

Alpha Hydroxy Acids

Alpha hydroxy acids (AHA) are antioxidants that also act to reduce the signs of aging by gently peeling the outer part of the epidermis. Glycolic acid is a type of AHA derived from sugar cane, whereas lactic acid represents another AHA, which is a constituent of milk. Alpha hydroxy acids may come packaged in high-end moisturizers or antiaging creams, or alternatively as a separate product. Usually, 8% to 12% AHA may act as an effective exfoliant and may be used up to twice daily after cleansing and before application of a moisturizer. Higher strengths of AHAs exist (70%) that act as a physician-strength chemical peel, which violates the full expanse of the epidermis. However, TCA peels may offer the physician more control and efficacy than these higher-potency AHA solutions. Alpha hydroxy acids are particularly useful for the younger face that exhibits early signs of aging, or may be used as an alternative to the more irritating vitamin A derivatives (e.g., tretinoin; Retin-A, Renova). Alternatively, AHAs may be used for a couple of months as a transition before engaging in a full program of tretinoin in order to prime the skin and minimize unwanted irritation.

Vitamin A Derivatives

Tretinoin, a vitamin A derivative, comes in different forms (e.g., Retin-A, Retin-A Micro, and Renova). The effect that these agents have on ridding the face of the stigmata of aging is much more pronounced than that of AHAs. However, tretinoin products are quite harsh and drying on most types of skin. Actually, some erythematous irritation is desired as an end point, which signals that the skin is responding appropriately to the product. Retin-A comes in different strengths (0.025%, 0.05%, and 0.1%) with the latter two concentrations more suited to facial rejuvenation as well as different formulations (cream and gel) with the former better for facial rejuvenation and the latter appropriate for oily, acne-prone skin. Retin-A Micro reportedly offers a more sustained release of the active ingredient over a 24-hour period and may be used instead. Renova has had great success as an alternative to Retin-A and has been considered less irritating to the skin, because the creamier base relieves the drying effect engendered by the medicine.

The method of application is as critical to success as compliance and may considerably influence the level of compliance if done properly. The authors usually recommend that patients start slowly on tretinoin-based products, perhaps every third day and advancing to every other day and finally to every day as the skin tolerates it. Retin-A or Renova is applied only at night after the face is gently cleansed. At least 10, and preferably 30 minutes are allowed to transpire before application of the medicine because moist skin may accelerate the absorption leading to undesired sensitivity. Only a pea size of the cream is placed on the index finger and equally distributed at four points on the face: the central forehead, each cheek, and the chin. Then this modest aliquot is spread evenly over those four quadrants. A night moisturizer then may be immediately applied. It is very important that the patient remain out of direct sunlight during use of the product because it causes photosensitivity. Therefore, a good sun block should always be used in conjunction with Retin-A or Renova. The patient will only observe the benefit of the medicine after several weeks to months of consistent usage. Unfortunately, the beneficial effects may be erased if the product is discontinued. Patients are recommended to begin Retin-A or Renova after all the erythema has subsided after a peel or other resurfacing in order to maintain longevity of the procedure.

CONCLUSIONS

The nondermatologically oriented surgeon may refuse to hassle with the time- and labor-intensive process involved during the postresurfacing period. However, traditional lifting procedures are often not indicated or fall short of the intended effect. As part of the armamentarium, resurfacing offers the facial aesthetic surgeon the most comprehensive capacity to rejuvenate the aging face.

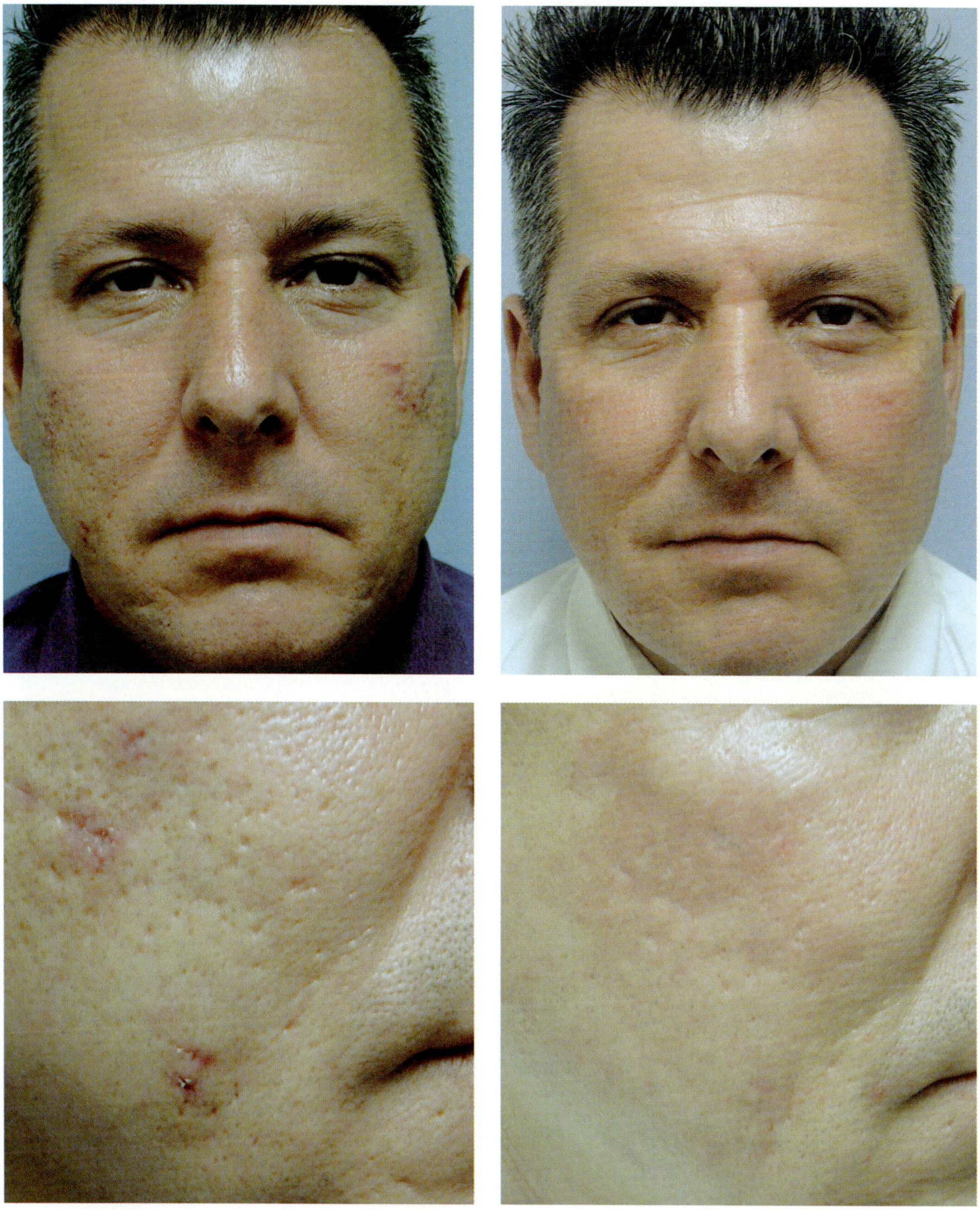

A C B D

FIGURE 9-17. A–D: These photographs show a 40-year-old patient who suffers from acne scarring along both malar regions. He exhibits both ice-pick scarring and cystic-acne scarring. He underwent direct excision and closure of his ice-pick scars, followed 6 weeks later by combined resurfacing, which involved a full-face Jessner's/35% trichloroacetic acid chemical peel, bilateral wire-brush dermabrasion to his malar region, and CO_2 laser resurfacing over the dermabraded areas.

CLINICAL PRESENTATIONS: A SYNTHESIS OF APPROACH

Case #1 (Fig. 9-17A–D)

This is a 40-year-old state officer who presented for improvement of his skin texture and complexion. He stated that he has had acne his entire life but no serious episodes since his twenties. In the wake of his prior severe cystic form of acne, he has been left with an extremely disfigured malar region. In particular, he exhibited multiple, deep "ice-pick" scars in the setting of an irregular and uneven cutaneous topography. He was noted to have very thick skin and moderate to marked sebaceous activity. The patient possessed brown eyes and a Fitzpatrick-III skin classification. To achieve the optimal aesthetic result, the patient was advised that a staged treatment protocol would be warranted. First, the deep ice-pick scars would be excised and closed followed later by a combined resurfacing approach that involved CO_2 laser resurfacing, chemical peeling, and wire-brush dermabrasion. He was informed that only 50% improvement would most likely occur despite the most aggressive treatment strategy because of the recalcitrant nature of acne scarring. Also, the patient was told that subsequent sessions might be required for further refinement if desired.

Procedure

The procedure consisted of surgical excision of multiple "ice-pick" scars (a total of nine) and wound approximation followed by a combined resurfacing technique with Jessner's/35% TCA peel to the entire face, wire-brush dermabrasion to the cheek regions, and CO_2 laser over the dermabraded areas 6 weeks later.

The patient initially underwent excision of nine separate, large ice-pick type scars, which was carried out with a No. 11 blade in the orientation of relaxed skin tension lines and repaired with good apposition of the wound edges and closure using 6-0 polypropylene. After a period of 6 weeks, a combined-resurfacing technique using laser, peel, and dermabrasion was undertaken to achieve an improved contour to the remaining malar skin. First, the patient underwent full-face Jessner's/35% TCA chemical peel until a uniformly opaque frost was observed. A chemical peel was enlisted first to improve his overall skin texture, eradicate moderate photodamage, and ensure an imperceptible transition between treated and untreated dermabraded areas. Once the chemical peel was completed, wire-brush dermabrasion was undertaken to address the principal cutaneous pathology (i.e., the uneven texture). A CO_2 laser was then used to achieve hemostasis in the dermabraded-treated areas and effect further collagen tightening in these areas. Aquaphor ointment was applied, and he subscribed to the intensive postoperative regimen for a resurfaced patient.

Discussion

This patient demonstrates the two principal types of acne scarring that are possible: "ice-pick" scarring and cystic-acne scarring. As evident, the treatment strategy is divergent in that discrete ice-pick depressions must be excised and closed, whereas cystic acne must be resurfaced using combined techniques. A staged procedure provides the best solution to the problem, in which the ice-pick scars are addressed first. Combining three resurfacing techniques permits the advantage that each modality provides: The chemical peel facilitates even transitions between treated and untreated dermabraded areas; the dermabrader provides maximal improvement to the areas of acne scarring; and the CO_2 laser adds the benefit of hemostasis and further tissue contraction in dermabraded-treated areas. The reader is reminded that a chemical peel always must be completed first in intact skin before either laser or dermabrasion is attempted. For darker complexioned patients, the depth of dermabrasion should be more conservative and the chemical peel used more extensively to achieve a uniform result. Additional treatment sessions may be required for patients with higher Fitzpatrick scores owing to the conservatism advocated for each session. Prophylactic treatment with 4% hydroquinone 2 to 3 weeks after resurfacing may preclude the onset of unfavorable postinflammatory hyperpigmentation in these patients. Above all else, the patient should be fully cognizant of the limited benefit (no greater than 70%) that resurfacing achieves for acne scarring.

Case #2 (Fig. 9-18A–D)

This is a 55-year-old business owner who presented for facial rejuvenation. She acknowledged that her lifelong sun exposure had contributed significantly to her present aged appearance. Different resurfacing modalities were discussed with the patient, including full-face Jessner's/35% TCA peel alone, full-face CO_2-laser resurfacing, or a combination of both modalities. Given her extensive photodamage—namely, deep rhytids and coarse, leathery skin—it was felt that full-face CO_2-laser resurfacing would be justifiable in this patient's particular case to achieve the maximal aesthetic benefit. The protracted recovery period and potential for postresurfacing pigmentary problems concomitant with this treatment modality were carefully elaborated to the patient so that she could render a reasonable decision about which resurfacing method she would be more willing to endure. Given the risks, benefits, and alternatives, the patient elected to proceed with full-face CO_2-laser resurfacing.

Procedure

The procedure consisted of full-face CO_2 laser resurfacing. The patient underwent resurfacing with Sharplan's CO_2 laser

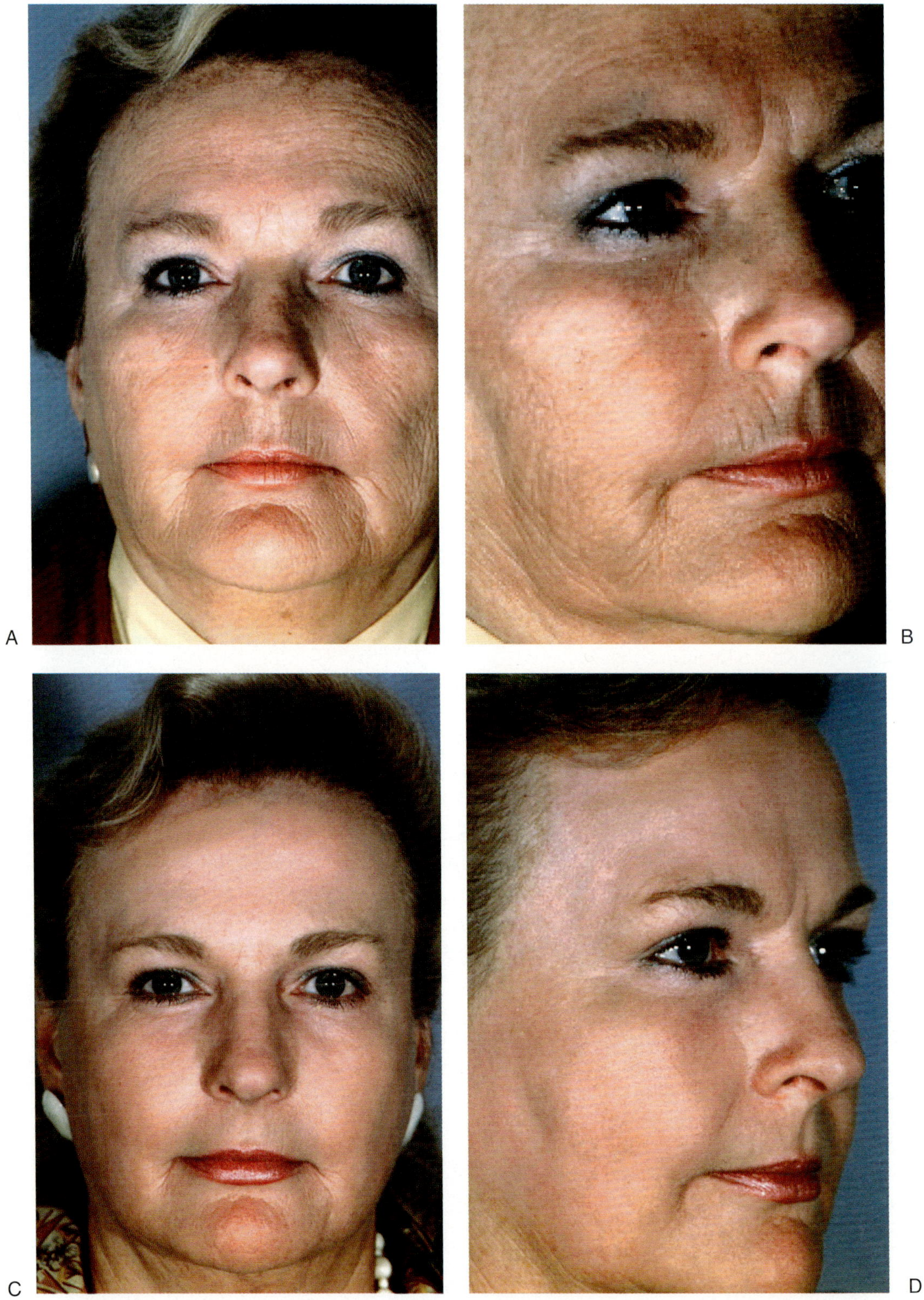

FIGURE 9-18. A–D: These photographs show a 55-year-old patient who exhibits significant photodamage with deeply etched rhytids and coarse, leathery skin. She underwent full-face CO_2 laser resurfacing with a total of three passes except only one pass along the jaw line for better feathering and transition to the untreated cervical skin and two passes along the thinner periorbital region excluding the sensitive pretarsal skin altogether. She is shown approximately 1 year after laser resurfacing with notable cutaneous improvement.

outfitted with the silk-touch hand piece using the manufacturer's recommended start-safe parameters. Under general anesthesia, the patient was subjected to three full passes of the CO_2 laser in a systematic fashion progressing from facial subunit to subunit. Only one pass was executed along the jaw line to provide a gentle transition to the untreated neck. The thinner periorbital area was resurfaced, including the upper eyelids but excluding the pretarsal skin using only two passes of the laser. At the conclusion of the procedure, the patient was dressed with Aquaphor ointment and N-terface occlusive dressing for the first 48 hours. The patient subscribed to the intensive postpeel regimen and was followed in the office on a daily basis. The patient's erythema persisted for 11 weeks and resolved without sequelae. The postoperative photograph is taken 1 year after resurfacing. The patient underwent a facelift and browlift 4 years after the initial resurfacing.

Discussion

Although the Jessner's/35% TCA chemical-peel combination has become the workhorse of facial rejuvenation in the authors' practices for cutaneous rejuvenation of the White face, the CO_2 laser has proved its value in select facial areas that are more recalcitrant to treatment by the Jessner's/35% TCA peel, namely, the perioral and glabellar regions. In the past, the senior author used the CO_2 laser more widely, but has retreated from this staunch position because of the extended recovery period and risk of progressive hypopigmentation that becomes particularly notable along the jaw line. Nevertheless, certain circumstances justify this more aggressive modality for the entire face. Although this patient was managed during the era of liberal CO_2 resurfacing, the patient would have been treated likewise today given her entrenched, cutaneous pathology. For very coarse, leathery skin and deeply etched, widespread rhytidosis, CO_2 laser remains the mainstay of therapy. Clearly, phenol chemical exfoliation is a suitable alternative but has not represented a significant part of the authors' practices and therefore cannot be authoritatively discussed.

Case #3 (Fig. 9-19A,B)

This is a 74-year-old patient referred by her dermatologist to evaluate her candidacy for cosmetic rejuvenation of her skin.

A

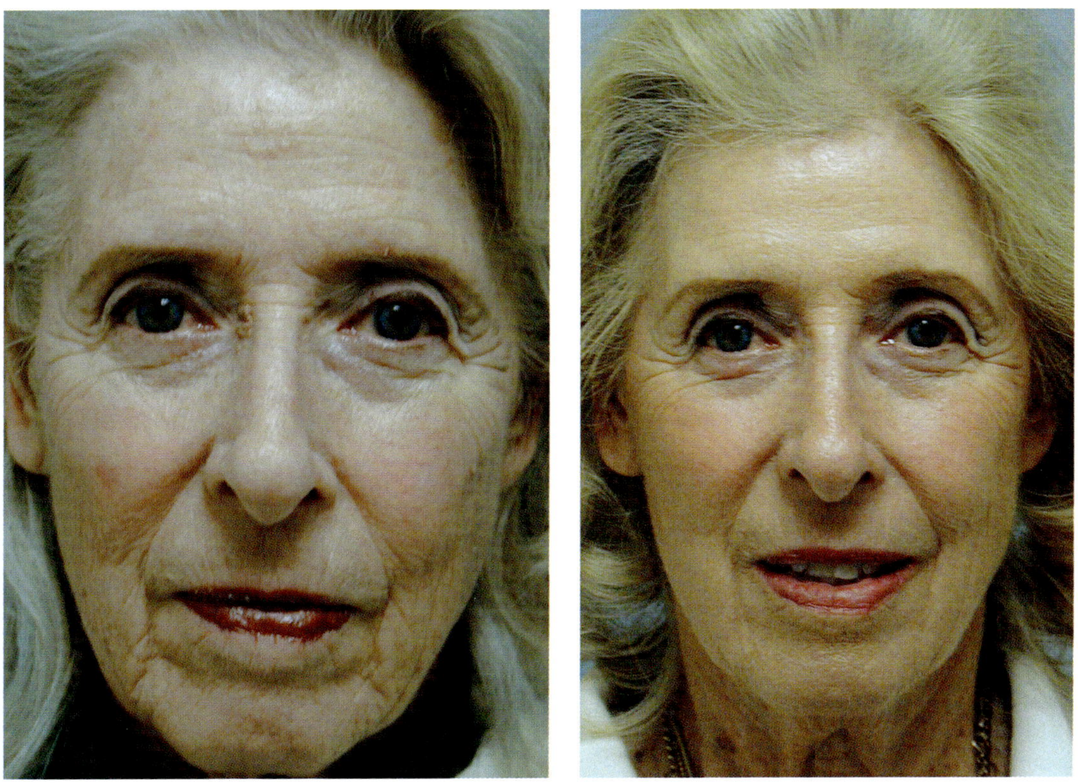

B

FIGURE 9-19. A,B: These photographs show a 74-year-old woman who was referred by her dermatologist for cutaneous rejuvenation of her skin. She had been treated with fluorouracil-based topical therapies without notable improvement to her multiple hyperkeratotic lesions. The patient was desirous of cosmetic improvement of her overall photodamaged skin rather than continued medical management of discrete keratotic lesions. Although CO_2 laser therapy would have been beneficial at least to provide maximal rejuvenation in the periocular and perioral regions, the patient's advanced age and hesitant disposition precluded use of this modality. Instead, full-face chemical peel with Jessner's and 35% trichloroacetic acid was used after shave excision of her numerous hyperkeratotic lesions. She is shown 1 year after a one-time chemical peel that brought about significant improvement in her photodamaged skin.

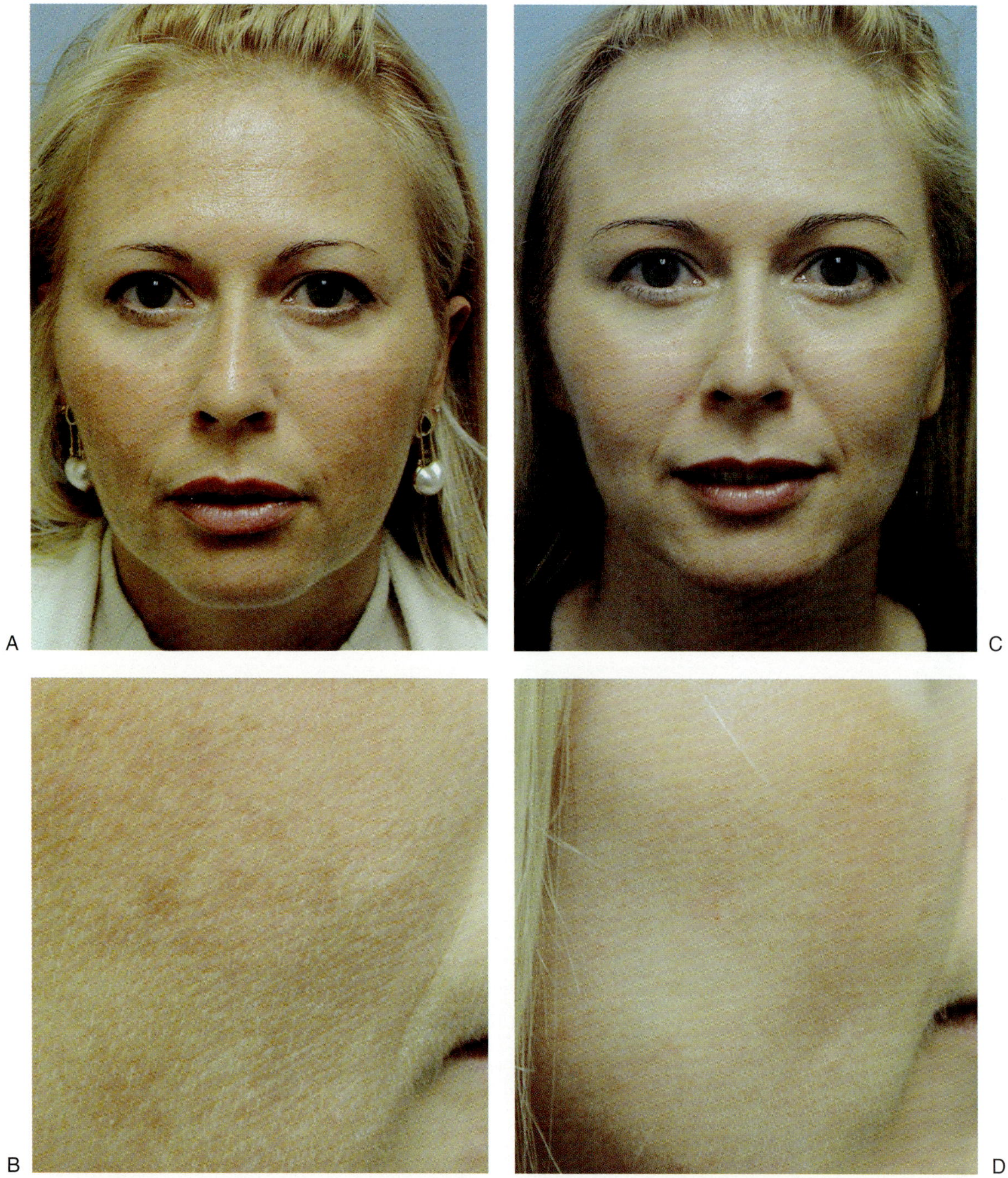

FIGURE 9-20. A–D: These photographs show a 39-year-old woman who suffers from a significant bronzed appearance to her skin because of prior oral contraceptive use and chronic sun exposure. She also has some mild horizontal rhytidosis across her forehead with finer wrinkles in the remaining facial skin. The patient underwent a Jessner's preparation followed by a 35% trichloroacetic acid peel to her entire face and is shown 15 months after resurfacing. After the peel, she exhibits a more even complexion free of sun-induced dyschromias and a tighter appearance to her overall skin.

The patient admitted to chronic sun exposure but denied any history of prior skin cancer in herself or her immediate family. The referring dermatologist had been treating her for numerous precancerous lesions using fluorouracil-based topical therapies but with limited success. The patient was motivated to seek treatment because she desired global rejuvenation that could restore her skin to a more youthful state. On examination, she was noted to have fair skin and blue eyes. In addition, she had numerous hyperkeratotic lesions consistent with actinic keratoses but without any frank evidence of malignancy. Overall, the skin appeared to be desiccated, uneven, and leathery in texture consistent with significant photodamage, particularly in the perioral and periocular regions. The patient was counseled on the benefits and limitations of CO_2 laser resurfacing versus TCA peel or combined treatment modality using both laser and peel. Although the patient would have been an excellent beneficiary of full-face or partial-face CO_2 laser therapy from an aesthetic perspective, she was a less than ideal candidate given her advanced age and hesitant disposition. Instead, full-face TCA peel was elected for optimal rejuvenation given the enumerated constraints.

Procedure

The procedure consisted of a full-face 35% TCA peel after pretreatment with Jessner's solution. The patient underwent shave excision of her hyperkeratotic and actinic-keratotic lesions using a No. 10 blade before the application of the peel solution. Care was taken to maintain a full layer of epidermis below the level of each shave excision.

Discussion

Given the patient's significant photodamage, CO_2 laser therapy would have been an ideal choice for at least partial ablation of the more severely affected areas, such as the perioral and periocular regions. Nevertheless, the patient expressed some trepidation over the proposed recovery period that might last several weeks to months. In addition, the senior author's experience has revealed that mature patients poorly tolerate a protracted postoperative course that accompanies laser resurfacing. Even in younger patients, the CO_2 laser often can be an overwhelming experience and has now been mostly relegated to select facial zones that tend to require its higher ablative efficacy (e.g., the glabellar, periocular, and perioral regions). Except for these more recalcitrant areas, the TCA peel provides exceptional rejuvenation without the concomitant downtime of laser rejuvenation and has become the mainstay of cutaneous resurfacing in the authors' practices.

Case #4 (Fig. 9-20A–D)

This is a 39-year-old consultant who presented to the office to discuss various options for facial rejuvenation. The patient stated that she was not interested in any kind of surgical intervention but was primarily bothered by the uneven pigmentation of her skin. She commented that she had been on oral contraceptives periodically over the past several years. She also admitted to a moderate amount of sun exposure and felt that her complexion made her face "look dirty." Clinical examination revealed some mild to moderate horizontal rhytidosis of the forehead but only minimal wrinkling in the remaining facial skin. She is classified as a Fitzpatrick-II skin type.

Procedure

The procedure was a full-face 35% TCA chemical peel following pretreatment with Jessner's solution.

Discussion

The 35% TCA chemical peel has become the workhorse of the authors' practices for the patient with fair skin, minimal rhytidosis, and extensive facial dyschromia. At times it is warranted to reduce the concentration of the TCA to 20% to 25% in a patient with primarily uneven pigmentation and only minimal rhytids. Similarly, a lighter peel can be used for areas that require less rejuvenation, and the full 35%, reserved for facial subunits that manifest greater photoaging. However, the reader is reminded that any concentration of TCA can be used aggressively (i.e., repeated application and prolonged contact time of the peeling agent before water dilution) in order to achieve the intended result. Therefore, all peels should be used judiciously and systematically to avoid an unintended result. The technical details of chemical-peel application that are elaborated in the principal text are not reiterated herein. However, it is worth emphasizing that consistent, reproducible, and safe results are dependent on correct patient selection and compliance with proper technique.

Patients with darker complexions may be better served with a lighter peel (e.g., Jessner's/20% TCA peel) rather than the more potent 35% concentration. Aggressive peeling of discrete facial zones in Fitzpatrick IV to V patients may result in visible lines of demarcation between peeled and unpeeled areas. Fitzpatrick VI patients generally are unsafe to resurface, whereas Fitzpatrick V patients must be approached very cautiously. Serial peel application using Jessner's alone at 2-week intervals for four treatment sessions also may be a suitable alternative treatment strategy for darker skin types. Diligent application of topical 4% hydroquinone after complete epithelialization in these types of patients can also abort the rise of postresurfacing hyperpigmentation. However, use of this noxious product should be used only after a minimum of 2 weeks postresurfacing and be carefully followed for the risk of dermatitis owing to its irritating effects. As the preceding text has suggested, not only is the cutaneous pathology (mild to moderate rhytids and related photodamage) a critical aspect to selection of treatment modality, but also the patient's overall Fitzpatrick scale to determine how that individual will tolerate the effects of the peel and how vigorous a peel can be attempted.

REFERENCES

1. Dahiya R, Lam SM, Williams EF: A systematic histologic analysis of nonablative laser therapy in a porcine model using the pulsed-dye laser. Arch Facial Plast Surg 2003;5:218–223.
2. Roston E, Bowes LE, Iyer S, et al: A double-blind, side-by-side comparison study of low fluence long pulse dye laser to coolant treatment for wrinkling of the cheeks. J Cosmet Laser Ther 2001; 3:129–136.
3. Trelles MA, Allones I, Luna R: Facial rejuvenation with a nonablative 1320 nm Nd: YAG laser: a preliminary clinical and histologic evaluation. Dermatol Surg 2001;27:781–782.
4. Bernstein EF, Ferreira M, Anderson D: A pilot investigation to subjectively measure treatment effect and side-effect profile of nonablative skin remodeling using a 532 nm, 2 ms pulse-duration laser. J Cosmet Laser Ther 2001;3:137–141.
5. Goldberg DJ, Rogachefsky AS, Silapunt S: Nonablative laser treatment of facial rhytides: a comparison of 1450-nm diode laser treatment with dynamic cooling as opposed to treatment with dynamic cooling alone. Lasers Surg Med 2002;30:79–81.
6. Bjerring P, Clement M, Keickendorff L, et al: Selective nonablative wrinkle reduction by laser. J Cutan Laser Ther 2000;2:9–15.
7. Goldberg DJ. Nonablative subsurface remodeling: clinical and histologic evaluation of a 1320-nm Nd: YAG laser. J Cutan Laser Ther 1999;1:153–157.
8. Goldberg DJ: New collagen formation after dermal remodeling with an intense pulsed light source. J Cutan Laser Ther 2000;2: 59–61.
9. Williams EF, Lam SM: Combined resurfacing techniques: a systematic approach. Int J Cosm Surg Aesthetic Dermatol 2002;4: 88–91.
10. West TB, Alster TS: Effect of pretreatment on the incidence of hyperpigmentation following cutaneous CO_2 laser resurfacing. Dermatol Surg 1999;25:15–17.
11. Kitzmiller WJ, Visscher M, Page DA, et al: A controlled evaluation of dermabrasion versus CO2 laser resurfacing for the treatment of perioral wrinkles. Plast Reconstr Surg 2000;106: 1366–1372.
12. Campbell JP, Terhune MH, Shotts SD, et al: An ultrastructural comparison of mechanical dermabrasion and carbon dioxide laser resurfacing in the minipig model. Arch Otolaryngol Head Neck Surg 1998;124:758–760.
13. Fulton FE, Jr: Dermabrasion, chemabrasion, and laserbrasion. Historical perspectives, modern dermabrasion techniques, and future trends. Dermatol Surg 1996;22:619–628.
14. Karim AM, Streitmann MJ: Excision of rhinophyma with carbon dioxide laser: a ten-year experience. Ann Otol Rhinol Laryngol 1997;106:952–955.
15. Lam SM, Sullivan SE, Williams EF: Management of the postpeel and laser resurfaced patient: a ten-year experience. Int J Cosm Surg Aesthetic Dermatol 2002;4:189–199. (Portions of this article have been reprinted herein with the original publisher's expressed permission.)
16. Newman JP, Fitzgerald P, Koch RJ: Review of closed dressings after laser resurfacing. Dermatol Surg 2000;26:562–571.
17. Weiss JS, Ellis CN, Headington JT, et al: Topical tretinoin improves photoaged skin. A double-blind vehicle-controlled study. JAMA 1988;259:527–532.
18. Hetter GP: An examination of the phenol-croton oil peel: Part I. Dissecting the formula. Plast Reconstr Surg 2000;105: 227–239; discussion 249–251.
19. Hetter GP: An examination of the phenol-croton oil peel: Part II. The lay peelers and their croton oil formulas. Plast Reconstr Surg 2000;105:240–248; discussion 249–251.
20. Hetter GP: An examination of the phenol-croton oil peel: Part III. The plastic surgeon's role. Plast Reconstr Surg 2000;105: 752–763.
21. Hetter GP: An examination of the phenol-croton oil peel: Part IV. Face peel results with different concentrations of phenol and croton oil. Plast Reconstr Surg 2000;105:1061–1083; discussion 1084–1087.
22. Grimes PE, Bhawan J, Kim J, et al: Laser resurfacing-induced hypopigmentation: Histologic alterations and repigmentation with topical photochemotherapy. Dermatol Surg 2001;27:515–520.
23. Alster TS: Laser treatment of hypertrophic scars, keloids, and striae. Dermatol Clin 1997;15:419–429.

SUBJECT INDEX

Page references followed by *n, f,* or *t* indicate footnotes, figures, or tables, respectively.

M